AN ATLAS OF ANATOMY

AN ATLAS OF

By Regions: Upper Limb, Abdomen, Perineu
Pelvis, Lower Limb, Vertebrae, Vertebral Column,
Thorax, Head and Neck,
Cranial Nerves and Dermatom

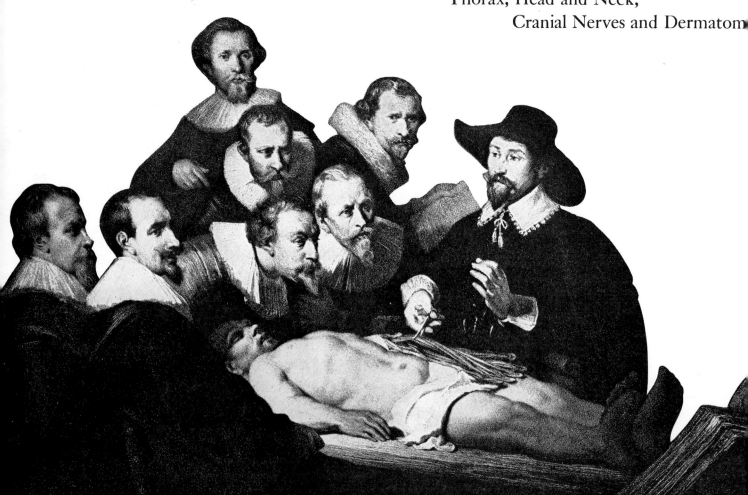

Anatomy

J. C. BOILEAU GRANT

M.C., M.B., Ch.B., Hon. D. Sc. (Man)., F.R.C.S. (Edin.)

*Professor Emeritus of Anatomy in the University of Toronto
and Curator of the Anatomy Museum; for many years and until recently
Visiting Professor of Anatomy in the University of California, Los Angeles;
formerly Professor of Anatomy in the University of Manitoba*

SIXTH EDITION

 THE WILLIAMS & WILKINS CO.

Baltimore • 1972

Library of Congress
Catalog Card Number
71-160140
SBN 683-03729-3

First Edition, 1943
Reprinted, 1944, 1945

Second Edition, 1947
Reprinted, 1948, 1949

Third Edition, 1951
Reprinted, 1953, 1954

Fourth Edition, 1956
Reprinted, 1958, 1960, 1961

Fifth Edition, 1962
Reprinted 1963, 1964, 1966
1967, 1968, 1969,
1970

Sixth Edition, 1972

Portuguese Edition, 1946

COMPOSED AND PRINTED
AT THE WAVERLY PRESS, INC.
MT. ROYAL & GUILFORD AVES.
BALTIMORE, MD. U.S.A. 21202

428 E. Preston St.
21202

Title page illustration:
THE ANATOMY LESSON OF DR. NICOLAES TULP
by Rembrandt van Rijn
FROM A MEZZOTINT IN THE BETTMAN ARCHIVE

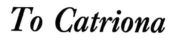

To Catriona

Preface to the Sixth Edition

This collection of illustrations depicts the structures of the human body, region by region, in much the same order as the student displays them by dissection.

In the execution of these illustrations the following preliminary steps were taken: each specimen was posed and photographed; from the negative film so obtained an enlarged positive film was made, usually one third larger than it would appear when reproduced; with the aid of a viewing box the outlines of the structures on the enlarged film were traced on tracing paper; and these outlines were scrutinized against the original specimen, in order to ensure that the shapes, positions and relative proportions of the various structures were correct. The outline tracing was then presented to the artist who transferred it to suitable paper and, having the original dissection beside her, proceeded to work up a plastic drawing in which the important features were brought out. Thus, little, if any, liberty has been taken with the anatomy; that is to say, the illustrations profess a considerable accuracy of detail.

In order that the student may be able to turn the pages and study figure after figure without requiring to re-orient himself, all illustrations of bilaterally symmetrical structures are from the right half of the body, unless it is stated otherwise.

Most of the specimens here depicted are in the Anatomy Museum of the University of Toronto.

The observations and comments that accompany the illustrations are designed to attract attention to salient points and to points of significance that might otherwise escape notice. Their purpose is to interpret the illustrations. They are not, nor are they intended to be, exhaustive descriptions.

The often recurring noun, musculus or muscle, is omitted from the names of the muscles, but by way of compensation the initial letters of the qualifying adjectives are printed in capitals, e.g., musculus trapezius and musculus rectus abdominis are printed thus: Trapezius and Rectus Abdominis.

As to terminology, the international nomenclature, Nomina Anatomica (1955) is employed in place of the Birmingham Revision (B.R., 1933) of the Basle Nomina Anatomica (B.N.A., 1895) which was originally in use. Where, however, the adopted terms differ substantially from the revised B.N.A. terms—and this is in a small minority of instances—both terms are given, the discarded terms being set within parentheses ( ). Square brackets [ ] indicate a synonym approved at the International Congresses of Anatomists held periodically.

The Publishers, finding that better pictures could be produced than formerly if newer technical methods were applied to the original art-work, decided to have every picture re-engraved. This has been done, and at the same time some have been enlarged, many have been improved and some have been replaced.

A number of half-tone illustrations and photographs have been added to this edition. These include; a median section of a child at birth (frontispiece), and cross-sections of the perineum and pelvis (191.6); considerable additions—to the eye (523.1), to the pterygopalatine fossa including the ganglion, maxillary nerve, and maxillary artery, 3rd part (560.1), and to the middle and inner ears (641.1, 650.1)

Also, olecranon bursa and nerve to Anconeus (56.1), arterial arches of hand (71.1), liver on section (160), uterus (232.1), junction of femoral and popliteal arteries (264.1), Articularis Genus (298.1), medial relations of ankle (321.1), sesamoid bones of metatarso-phalangeal joint of hallux (329.1 & 329.2), reflexions of pleura (413.2), hyperostosis frontalis interna (486), arteries of neck and base of brain (505), parasympathetic (secreto-motor) ganglia (513.1, 513.2, & 547.1), and carotid bodies (659.1).

Further, at the suggestion of students and in keeping with the times, the use of diagrams and line drawings has been extended considerably. Many of these figures first appeared in the author's *A Method of Anatomy* (now, Grant and Basmajian); others have been designed for the Atlas. They mostly appear in the lower corners of a page as secondary or supporting figures. It is hoped that these intrusions may help to anticipate a question, to solve a difficulty, to offer an explanation, or otherwise speed comprehension and attract attention to a useful point of reference.

Color has been used more freely, particularly: — pink for mucous membranes and yellow for peritoneum, excepting that of the omental bursa, where orange is used.

A guide to the plan of the book is to be found in the abbreviated list of illustrations on pages xi to xiii. As, however, most structures appear in two or more illustrations, this list is not a substitute for the index.

Source references immediately precede the index.

During the preparation of the various editions of this work I have received generous assistance from several colleagues, notably: Dr. C. G. Smith, who verified the bony attachments of the muscles of the limbs for the first edition, and who devised the schemes of the cranial nerves for the second; Dr. Allene I. Scott, who spent long hours making many of the most difficult dissections for the third edition; and Dr. J. E. Anderson, who has lavished care on some of the more intricate preparations and tracings for the fourth and fifth editions. To these I renew my thanks.

To Professor J. S. Thompson, my successor in the Chair in the University of Toronto, I express my deep thanks for the facilities of the Department so freely placed at my disposal.

I have been most fortunate in the expert assistance rendered me by a number of medical artists. I owe a particular debt to Mrs. Dorothy I. Chubb, a pupil of Max Brodel, who worked with me from the beginning, and also to Miss Nancy Joy, now Director of Art as Applied to Medicine, in the University of Toronto, who soon joined her, for without their expert skill, patience in a laborious task, and the desire to achieve accuracy and effect, this book could hardly have been made. Mrs. Chubb was mainly responsible for the art-work of the first two editions and almost solely responsible for that of this, the 6th edition. Miss Joy for those in between. To them I record again my grateful appreciation of their work so cheerfully and carefully done.

I gladly acknowledge the assistance of Miss Elizabeth Blackstock, of the Department of Art as applied to Medicine of this University, whose talent is apparent in the cross-sections of the upper limb, the paranasal sinuses, and the arteries of the stomach, pancreas, and bile passages. Mrs. E. Hopper Ross and Miss Marguerite Drummond, have provided me with occasional and excellent illustrations, for which I am very grateful.

To Mr. James B. Francis and Mr. Douglas Baker, for their early and valued assistance with the bones and muscles of the lower limb, I express my thanks.

To Mr. Charles E. Storton, who has throughout given me general expert assistance, including the preliminary photographic work, which has been of very high order, and to Mr. H. Whittaker, who at times has undertaken the photographic work, my thanks are due for their willing and very skillful help.

In this current edition I am much indebted to a number of students for their helpful suggestions and criticisms, and to them I offer my thanks. Especially would I thank Mr. Roger W. Wilson for the unusual trouble he has taken and for the value of his remarks.

Finally, to the Publishers, Messrs. Williams and Wilkins, who, through Mr. Earle V. Hart and Mr. Norman Och, have with unfailing courtesy and consideration given me loose rein and have endeavoured to meet all my requests, I express my gratitude and thanks.

J. C. B. GRANT.

Illustrations

UPPER LIMB

Figures

General: bones, arteries, superficial veins, cutaneous nerves, and motor nerves.   *1–10*

Pectoral Region and Axilla: attachment of muscles, mamma, serial dissections, brachial plexus, veins of axilla, cross-section, and Serratus Anterior.   *11–23*

Back: cutaneous nerves, superficial muscles, suprascapular & supraspinous regions, and variations.   *24–28*

Brachium and Subdeltoid Region: attachment of muscles, medial (20), lateral & posterior views, cross-section, and subacromial bursa.   *29–35*

Shoulder and Acromioclavicular Joints: coracoacromial arch, synovial capsule, ligaments, and variations.   *36–43*

Elbow Region: front view, cubital fossa, variations, elbow & proximal radio-ulnar joints, ligaments, bones, synovial capsule, cross-section, nerve to Anconeus, olecranon bursa, and posterior views.   *44–57*

Front of Forearm and Wrist: attachment of muscles, serial dissections, bones of hand, cross-sections (forearm, wrist, & hand) and front of wrist.   *58–66*

Palm of Hand: serial dissections, cross-section (finger), and radial side of wrist.   *67–76*

Back of Forearm and Dorsum of Hand: attachment of muscles, serial dissections, ulnar side of wrist, cutaneous nerves, bones of hand, synovial sheaths, extensor retinaculum, extensor tendons, and extensor expansions.   *77–89*

Joints: distal radio-ulnar, radiocarpal, intercarpal, and digital.   *90–96*

Variations, Epiphyses, and Cross-Sections of Bones.   *97–104.1*

ABDOMEN

Figures

Preview of Abdomen: skeleton of abdomen, 3 paired gland composite, gastro-intest-tract & 3 unpaired glands, and transpyloric plane.   *104.2*

Anterior Abdominal Wall: serial dissections, cutaneous nerves; inguinal canal & region; testis & spermatic cord; and female inguinal canal—all in series.   *105–123*

Digestive System: diagram, and abdominal contents in situ.   *124–125*

Stomach: in situ; parts, interior & musculature; omenta & omental bursa; peritoneal ligaments of spleen & liver; peritoneal recesses; arteries of stomach, celiac trunk, vagus nerves in abdomen, posterior wall of omental bursa, and tributaries of portal vein.   *126–135*

Liver: visceral surface, corrosion preparations, veins of liver, porta hepatis, cystic artery, variations, vessels of gall bladder & ducts (also **160**), and exposure of bile duct in series.   *136–148*

Spleen: in situ, viseral surface, reflected from kidney, and accessory spleen.   *149–152*

Duodenum and Pancreas: in situ, posterior aspect, bile passages & pancreatic ducts, blood supply, section of liver, porta-caval anastomoses, and variations.   *153–161*

Intestines: mesenteric arteries, duodenal recesses, large intestines, structure of small intestine, ileocecal region, and variations.   *162–172*

Posterior Abdominal Wall: from behind, exposing kidney.   *173–175*

Kidneys, Ureters, Suprarenal Glands, Celiac Ganglion and Plexus: in situ, relations, cross-section of abdomen, structure of kidney, segmental arteries, and variations.   *176–187*

Figures

Great Arteries & Veins and their Branches and Tributaries: blood supply of ureter, & aorta entire.   *188–189*

Posterior Abdominal Wall and Diaphragm: muscles, lumbar plexus, hiatuses in diaphragm & nerve supply. Lumbar lymph nodes & vessels, sympathetic trunk and splanchnic nerves.   *190–191.3*

PERINEUM AND PELVIS

Perineum and Pelvis: cross-sections.   *191.6*

Male Perineum: muscles, vessels & nerves; Sphincter Ani, Levator Ani & anal canal (structure & blood supply), ischio-rectal fossa & retropubic space, exposure of prostate, urinary tract, penis, interior of spongy urethra, and perineal membrane.   *192–201*

Male Pelvis: from above, median section, Levator & Sphincter Ani, bladder, seminal vesicles, prostate & bulbo-urethral glands, interior of bladder & prostatic urethra, and Levator Ani from above.   *202–209*

Side Wall of Pelvis: deferent duct & ureter; 3 paired gland composite; iliac vessels, sacral plexus & other nerves, muscles, and ligaments.   *210–217*

Bony Pelvis: male & female, and sacro-iliac joint. orientation of pelvis.   *218–223*

Female Perineum: serial dissections.   *224–230.1*

Female Pelvis: Levator Ani from above; ovaries, tubes, uterus & broad ligaments; viscera from above, in series; median section; side wall in series, and suspensory mechanism.   *231–241*

LOWER LIMB

General: bones, arteries, superficial veins, cutaneous nerves, and motor nerves.   *242–250*

Inguinal Region: superficial inguinal lymph nodes, veins & arteries; saphenous opening, femoral sheath, and valves in veins.   *251–255*

Femoral Triangle: femoral sheath; femoral vein & tributaries; boundaries, contents, and floor of triangle.   *256–259*

Front of Thigh and Adductor Region: muscles, vessels & nerves, adductor hiatus, cross-section of thigh, and attachment of muscles.   *260–266*

Gluteal Region and Back of Thigh: muscles, vessels & nerves, and short rotator muscles.   *267–273*

Figures

Hip Joint: ligaments, bony parts, blood supply, sections (cross & coronal), acetabular fossa and its vessels.   *274–284*

Popliteal Fossa: serial dissections, attachments of muscles, and anastomoses around knee.   *285–291*

Knee Joint: ligaments and their attachments, and synovial capsule.   *292–302*

Lateral and Anterior Crural Regions and Dorsum of Foot: attachments of muscles, muscles, vessels & nerves; retinacula, synovial sheaths, and cross-section of leg.   *303–310*

Bones of Foot: attachment of muscles (lateral, medial, dorsal & plantar views).   *311–314*

Posterior Crural Region: bones, attachment of muscles, serial dissections, medial side of ankle, and variations.   *315–324*

Sole of Foot: serial dissections, and sesamoid bones.   *325–331*

Ankle Joint and Joints of Foot.   *332–342*

Bones of Foot. Epiphyses. Anomalous Tarsal Bones.   *343–356*

VERTEBRAE AND VERTEBRAL COLUMN

Vertebra: functions, parts, and ossification.   *357–362*

Vertebral Column: subdivisions, homologous parts, distinguishing features, and movements. Cervical, thoracic, lumbar, sacral & coccygeal segments. Anomalies.   *363–383*

Articulations: intervertebral disc, ligaments, and vertebral venous plexus.   *384–390*

THORAX

Bones: bony thorax, sternum (features, in youth, anomalies), ribs (features, anomalies), lateral costal artery, and sternocostal joints.   *391–404*

Thoracic Wall: diagram of intercostal space, anterior wall, intercostal spaces (front & back), and costovertebral joints.   *405–411*

Diagrams of Respiratory and Cardiovascular Systems: subdivisions of mediastinum and of pleura, and pleural reflexions.   *412–413*

Lungs: in situ, costal & mediastinal surfaces, bronchial tree, pulmonary arteries & veins, and bronchopulmonary segments.   *414–427*

Mediastinum: right & left sides, pleural cupola, and diaphragm (from above).   *428–431*

Figures

Pericardium and Heart: in situ, excised, cardiac vessels, pericardial sac (interior of & posterior relations), chambers of heart, explanatory diagrams, and anomalies of aortic arch.   *432–447.2*

Superior Mediastinum: serial dissections—thymus; great vessels, phrenic & vagus nerves; pulmonary arteries; and esophagus & thoracic duct, trachea & left recurrent nerve.   *448–451*

Posterior Mediastinum: bronchi & lymph nodes, esophagus & aorta; thoracic duct; blood supply of esophagus; azygos system of veins & venous anomalies; aorta intact, and branches of thoracic aorta.   *452–457.1*

HEAD AND NECK

Head and Neck: on median section. **Skull:** front & side views, buttresses of face and of nose.   *458–464*

Face: muscles, vessels, parotid gland & facial nerve; cartilages of nose & ear; sensory nerves of face; and diagrams (eyelid, orbital contents, superficial veins, and carotid & subclavian arteries).   *456–471.4*

Posterior Triangle of Neck: serial dissections, and brachial plexus.   *472–476*

Back: serial dissections & cross-section, spinal cord & membranes, and lower end of dural sac.   *477–484.1*

Nuchal Region: skull from behind & anomalies, serial dissections & cross-section, cranial nerves in posterior cranial fossa, and posterior fossa.   *485–497*

Head from Above: diagrams of scalp & its vessels & nerves, surface anatomy, diploic veins, cranial dura mater, folds of dura, and dural venous sinuses.   *498–504*

Contents of Cranium: arterial circle, cervico-cranial arteries, cross-section of midbrain, origin of cranial nerves, interior of base of skull, nerves in middle cranial fossa, secreto-motor fibers of pterygo-palatine and otic ganglia, and coronal sections (cavernous sinus & orbital cavity).   *505–517*

Eye: orbital cavity, dissections from front & from above serially, ocular muscles, eyeball on section, dissection of eye of ox, irido-corneal region, and ciliary ganglion, ophthalmic artery, and motor nerves of orbit.   *518–525*

Front and Root of Neck: platysma, front of neck in series, root of neck in series, cross-section, cervico-thoracic ganglion, cervical nerve in situ, and thyroid gland & its variations.   *526–539*

Anterior Triangle of Neck: diagrams of the triangles, bony landmarks & digastric muscle; carotid & submandibular triangles; and diagrams of veins, arteries & branches of vagus nerve.   *540–543.3*

Suprahyoid Region: in series—Mylohyoid; Geniohyoid; medial wall of submandibular triangle; salivary glands; Hyoglossus & its relations; and lingual artery & its branches.   *544–549*

Parotid Region: Parotid gland & facial nerve; parotid bed, vessels & nerves of auricle; and structures deep to bed.   *550–552*

Mandible and Temporomandibular Joint: sections (coronal & sagittal).   *553–555*

Infratemporal Fossa: maxillary artery; bony walls; and contents, maxillary nerve, pterygo-palatine ganglion, and maxillary artery (3rd part).   *556–560*

Prevertebral Region: muscles, cervical plexus, and sympathetic ganglia.   *561*

Atlanto-Occipital and Atlanto-Axial Joints: carnial nerves piercing dura, and variations.   *562–568*

Exterior of Base of Skull and 3 Keys to that Base.   *569–571.2*

Exterior of Pharynx: from behind, & side view with relations, otic ganglion, and auditory tube (lateral views).   *572–577*

Interior of Pharynx: from behind, and cross-section through nasal cavities.   *578–579*

Palate: in series; and cross-section through mouth, tonsil & parotid gland.   *580–584*

Interior of Pharynx: side view, in series—tonsil, its blood supply & bed, and pharyngeal muscles.   *585–590*

Mouth and Tongue: coronal sections of head; tongue, hyoid bone, side of mouth, otic ganglion (medial view), Mylohyoid & Geniohyoid from above, and cross-section through larynx.   *591–600*

Teeth: their sockets, permanent teeth; skulls at birth, primary teeth, and teeth erupting.   *601–604*

Nasal Cavities: septum, nerve supply, arterial supply, and lateral wall.   *605–610*

Paranasal Sinuses and their Variations: sphenoid bone of child & adult.   *611–620.1*

Larynx: serial dissections; nerve supply, arterial supply, and interior.   *621–632*

Ear: schemes: coronal section; tympanic membrane; medial wall of cavity & facial & semi-circular canals; ossicles; auditory tube & tympanic cavity, mastoid antrum & cells, temporal bones of child, geniculate ganglion, and inner ear.   *633–650*

Distribution of Cranial Nerves.   *651–662*

Dermatomes.   *663–665*

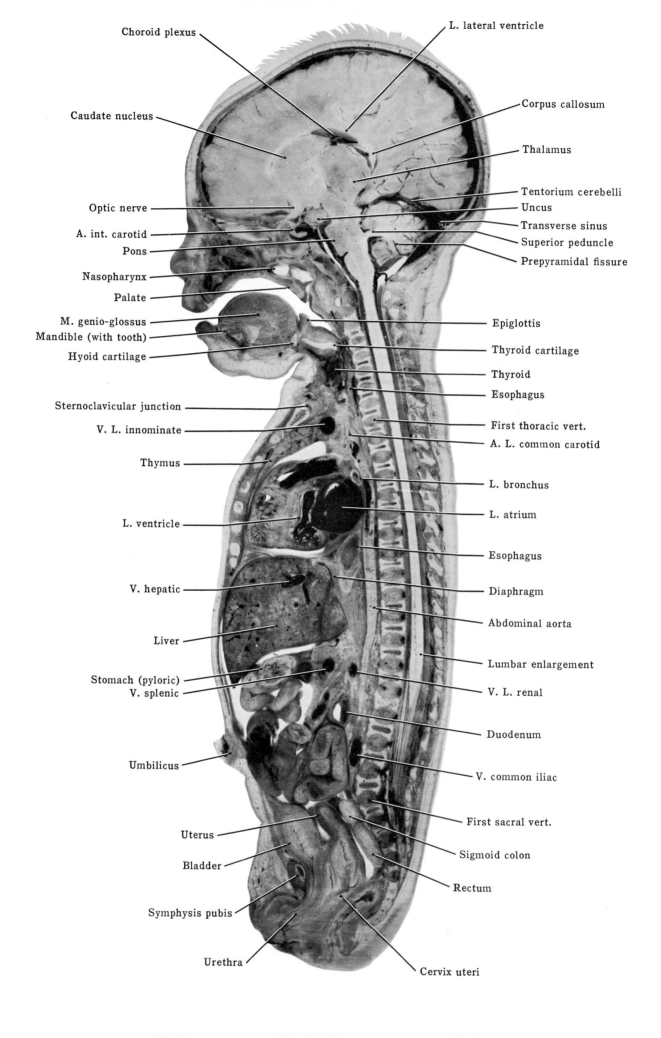

Choroid plexus

Caudate nucleus

Optic nerve

A. int. carotid

Pons

Nasopharynx

Palate

M. genio-glossus

Mandible (with tooth)

Hyoid cartilage

Sternoclavicular junction

V. L. innominate

Thymus

L. ventricle

V. hepatic

Liver

Stomach (pyloric)

V. splenic

Umbilicus

Uterus

Bladder

Symphysis pubis

Urethra

L. lateral ventricle

Corpus callosum

Thalamus

Tentorium cerebelli

Uncus

Transverse sinus

Superior peduncle

Prepyramidal fissure

Epiglottis

Thyroid cartilage

Thyroid

Esophagus

First thoracic vert.

A. L. common carotid

L. bronchus

L. atrium

Esophagus

Diaphragm

Abdominal aorta

Lumbar enlargement

V. L. renal

Duodenum

V. common iliac

First sacral vert.

Sigmoid colon

Rectum

Cervix uteri

The Upper Limb

Median Section of a Child, female, one or two days old. From a specimen in the Department of Anatomy in the University of California at Los Angeles. (Courtesy of Professor C. H. Sawyer.)

Note:
The crown-rump length is 14⅛ inches, and the maximum anteroposterior length of the head 4-11/16 inches. The remnant of the umbilical cord can be seen. Dorsally, the spinal cord is split throughout its length, and ventrally the urethra is likewise split. The sizes and positions of the various organs and parts at birth may be compared with those of the adult, as seen in the figures in the Atlas.
For example, the cranium or brain-case is enormous, but the face, there being no erupted teeth and no air sinuses, is small. The thorax and the pelvis are also small. In the central nervous system, note the cervical and lumbar enlargements of the cord, and the low vertebral level of its caudal end. In the cardio-vascular system the veins are conspicuous. In the respiratory system, the neck being short, the thyroid cartilage approaches the horizontal. In the digestive system the liver is large and low lying. In the genito-urinary system, the bladder is abdominal, and the urethra is almost adult in length. The median arcuate ligament of the diaphragm is almost in the adult position. The label on the abdominal aorta is too high. The coccyx is long. And so it goes.

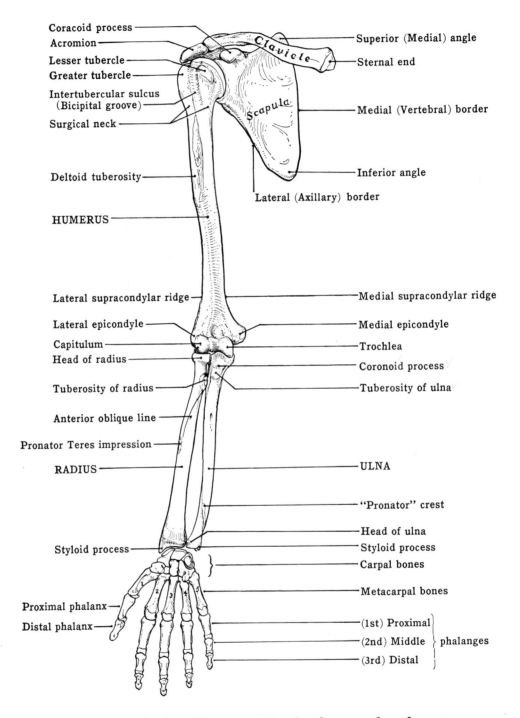

Coracoid process
Acromion
Lesser tubercle
Greater tubercle
Intertubercular sulcus
(Bicipital groove)
Surgical neck

Clavicle
Scapula

Superior (Medial) angle
Sternal end

Medial (Vertebral) border

Deltoid tuberosity

HUMERUS

Inferior angle
Lateral (Axillary) border

Lateral supracondylar ridge
Lateral epicondyle
Capitulum
Head of radius
Tuberosity of radius

Anterior oblique line

Pronator Teres impression

RADIUS

Medial supracondylar ridge
Medial epicondyle
Trochlea
Coronoid process
Tuberosity of ulna

ULNA

"Pronator" crest
Head of ulna
Styloid process
Carpal bones

Styloid process

Metacarpal bones

Proximal phalanx
Distal phalanx

(1st) Proximal
(2nd) Middle
(3rd) Distal

phalanges

1   Bones of the Upper Limb, from the front

(For bones of hand, see figs. 62 & 95; for attachments of muscles, see figs. 11, 29 & 58.)

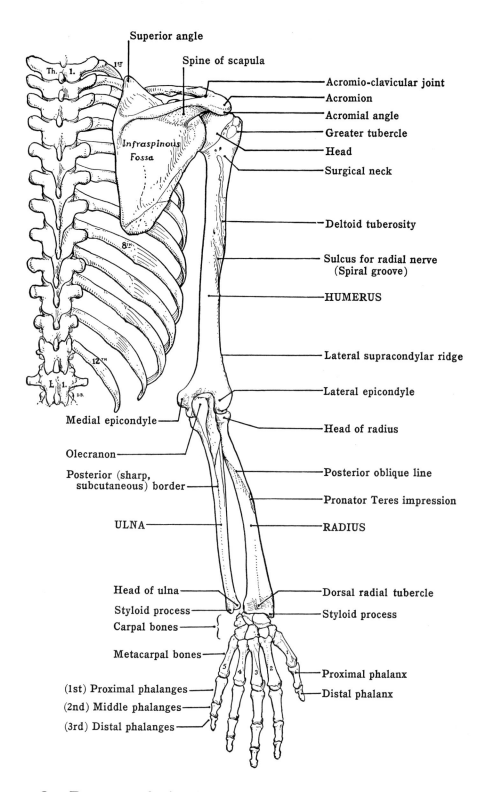

Superior angle

Spine of scapula

Acromio-clavicular joint

Acromion

Acromial angle

Greater tubercle

Head

Surgical neck

Th. 1.

1ST

Infraspinous Fossa

8TH

Deltoid tuberosity

Sulcus for radial nerve (Spiral groove)

HUMERUS

12TH

Lateral supracondylar ridge

L. 1.

D.B.

Lateral epicondyle

Medial epicondyle

Head of radius

Olecranon

Posterior oblique line

Posterior (sharp, subcutaneous) border

Pronator Teres impression

ULNA

RADIUS

Head of ulna

Dorsal radial tubercle

Styloid process

Styloid process

Carpal bones

Metacarpal bones

5 4 3 2

Proximal phalanx

(1st) Proximal phalanges

Distal phalanx

(2nd) Middle phalanges

(3rd) Distal phalanges

2 Bones of the Upper Limb, from behind

(For bones of hand, see fig. 86; for attachments of muscles, see figs. 30 & 77.)

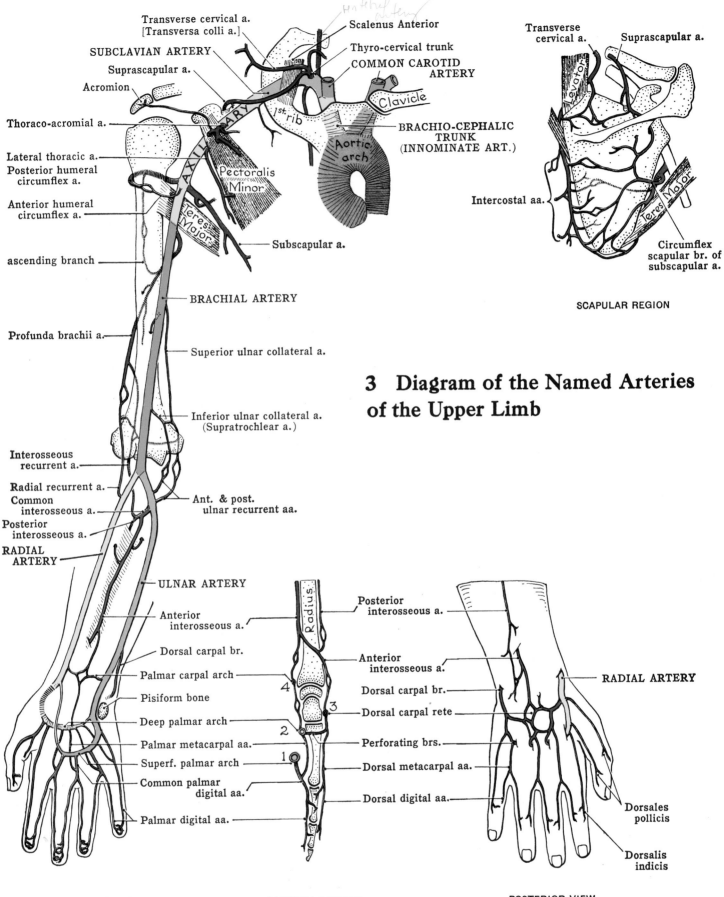

Transverse cervical a.
[Transversa colli a.]

SUBCLAVIAN ARTERY

Suprascapular a.

Acromion

Thoraco-acromial a.

Lateral thoracic a.
Posterior humeral
circumflex a.

Anterior humeral
circumflex a.

ascending branch

Profunda brachii a.

Interosseous
recurrent a.

Radial recurrent a.
Common
interosseous a.
Posterior
interosseous a.
RADIAL
ARTERY

Scalenus Anterior

Thyro-cervical trunk
COMMON CAROTID
ARTERY

Clavicle

BRACHIO-CEPHALIC
TRUNK
(INNOMINATE ART.)

1st rib

Aortic
arch

AXILLARY

Pectoralis
Minor

Teres
Major

Subscapular a.

BRACHIAL ARTERY

Superior ulnar collateral a.

Inferior ulnar collateral a.
(Supratrochlear a.)

Ant. & post.
ulnar recurrent aa.

Transverse
cervical a.

Suprascapular a.

Levator

Intercostal aa.

Teres Major

Circumflex
scapular br. of
subscapular a.

SCAPULAR REGION

3 Diagram of the Named Arteries of the Upper Limb

ULNAR ARTERY

Anterior
interosseous a.

Dorsal carpal br.

Palmar carpal arch

Pisiform bone

Deep palmar arch

Palmar metacarpal aa.

Superf. palmar arch

Common palmar
digital aa.

Palmar digital aa.

Radius

4

3

2

1

Posterior
interosseous a.

Anterior
interosseous a.

Dorsal carpal br.

Dorsal carpal rete

Perforating brs.

Dorsal metacarpal aa.

Dorsal digital aa.

RADIAL ARTERY

Dorsales
pollicis

Dorsalis
indicis

ANTERIOR VIEW

SAGITTAL SECTION

POSTERIOR VIEW

List of Named Arteries of the Upper Limb.

SUBCLAVIAN ARTERY
  Thyro-cervical Trunk
    Transverse cervical (colli) a.
      Superficial branch
      Deep branch
    Suprascapular a.
      Acromial br.
AXILLARY ARTERY
  Thoracica suprema
    (Superior thoracic a.)
  Thoraco-acromial a.
    (Acromio-thoracic a.)
    Pectoral branch
    Deltoid branch
    Acromial branch
  Lateral thoracic a.
    Lateral mammary branches
  Subscapular a.
    Circumflex scapular a.
    Thoraco-dorsal a.
  Posterior humeral circumflex a.
    Acromial branch
    Descending branch
  Anterior humeral circumflex a.
BRACHIAL ARTERY
  Profunda brachii a.
    Ascending branch
    Nutrient branch to humerus
    "Terminal descending branches"
      Middle collateral a.
      Radial collateral a.
  Superior ulnar collateral a.
  Nutrient branch to humerus
  Inferior ulnar collateral a.
ULNAR ARTERY
  Anterior ulnar recurrent a.
  Posterior ulnar recurrent a.
  Common interosseous a.
    Anterior interosseous a.
      Median a.
      Nutrient branch to radius
      Nutrient branch to ulna
    Posterior interosseous a.
      Interosseous recurrent a.
  Palmar carpal branch
  Dorsal carpal branch and rete
  Deep palmar branch
  Superficial palmar arch
    Common palmar digital aa.
    Proper palmar digital aa.
RADIAL ARTERY
  Radial recurrent a.
  Palmar carpal branch
  Superficial palmar branch
  Dorsal carpal branch
    Dorsal metacarpal aa.
    Dorsal digital aa.
  Princeps pollicis a.
  Radialis indicis a.
  Deep palmar arch
    Palmar metacarpal aa.
    Perforating branches

3   Arteries of the Upper Limb

The stem artery of the upper limb is the subclavian artery. Now, the right subclavian artery springs from the brachio-cephalic trunk (innominate artery) behind the right sterno-clavicular joint, whereas the left subclavian artery springs directly from the aortic arch and ascends behind the left sterno-clavicular joint. From this point onward the arteries of the two sides are symmetrical.

The subclavian artery arches over the apex of the lung and pleura, rising about an inch above the clavicle, and it leaves the root of the neck at the lateral border of the 1st rib to enter the axilla, as the axillary artery. The axillary artery leaves the axilla at the lower border of the Teres Major to enter the arm or brachium as the brachial artery. About 1″ below the crease of the elbow the brachial artery bifurcates into the radial and ulnar arteries, which traverse the forearm or antebrachium and enter the palm where each ends as an arterial arch. The ulnar artery forms the superficial palmar arch, which descends to the level of the web of the thumb where it is completed by a slender branch of the radial artery—commonly its superficial palmar branch. The radial artery, after crossing the floor of the "snuff box" (i.e., the hollow at the root of the thumb), to reach the dorsum of the hand, passes through the 1st intermetacarpal space and so enters the palm. It there forms the deep palmar arch, which lies half an inch proximal to the superficial palmar arch. The deep palmar arch is completed by a slender artery, the deep palmar branch of the ulnar artery.

Subdivisions: The subclavian artery is divided into 3 unequal parts by the Scalenus Anterior, and the axillary artery is similarly divided by the Pectoralis Minor.

Relationship to bone: The axillary artery passes within a finger's breadth of the tip of the coracoid process. The brachial artery lies medial to the humerus proximally and anterior to it distally. At the wrist the ulnar artery (and nerve) is sheltered from injury by the pisiform bone; its deep palmar branch curves round the lower border of the hamate bone. The radial artery is identified at the wrist by its pulse, which beats against the lower end of the radius.

Branches: The limbs are organs of locomotion and prehension, and the muscles are the motors that move them. Hence, most of the blood delivered to the limbs is for the supply of the muscles and little for the skin, fasciae, bones, and joints. The branches of the arteries are numerous, and they are for the most part muscular and nameless. Most of the named branches in the limbs are muscular too, but their claim to recognition depends mainly on the anastomoses they effect, for these are important surgically, and on their size.

Anastomoses: (a) It should be safe to tie either the subclavian or the axillary artery between the thyro-cervical trunk and the subscapular artery because of the anastomoses around the scapula; (b) it should be safe to tie the brachial artery distal to the inferior ulnar collateral artery because of the anastomoses around the elbow; (c) and it should be safe to tie either the radial or the ulnar artery in the forearm because these arteries are united by 2 palmar arches and by 2 carpal arches.

Arches: The superficial palmar arch lies deep only to skin and palmar aponeurosis—it is well-named. The three other arches lie on the skeletal plane, that is to say, on bones, joints, ligaments or interosseous membranes. Their order of magnitude (1, 2, 3, 4) is indicated. The deep palmar arch not only unites the radial and ulnar arteries, but it anastomoses with the interosseous arteries of the forearm, of the dorsum of the hand, and of the digits.

Calibers: The caliber of the axillary artery diminishes considerably just beyond the origin of the subscapular and posterior circumflex arteries, which are large arteries. The caliber of the ulnar artery is reduced to that of the radial artery beyond the origin of the common interosseous artery.

The anterior interior interosseous artery does duty for the posterior interosseous artery in the distal half of the back of the forearm.

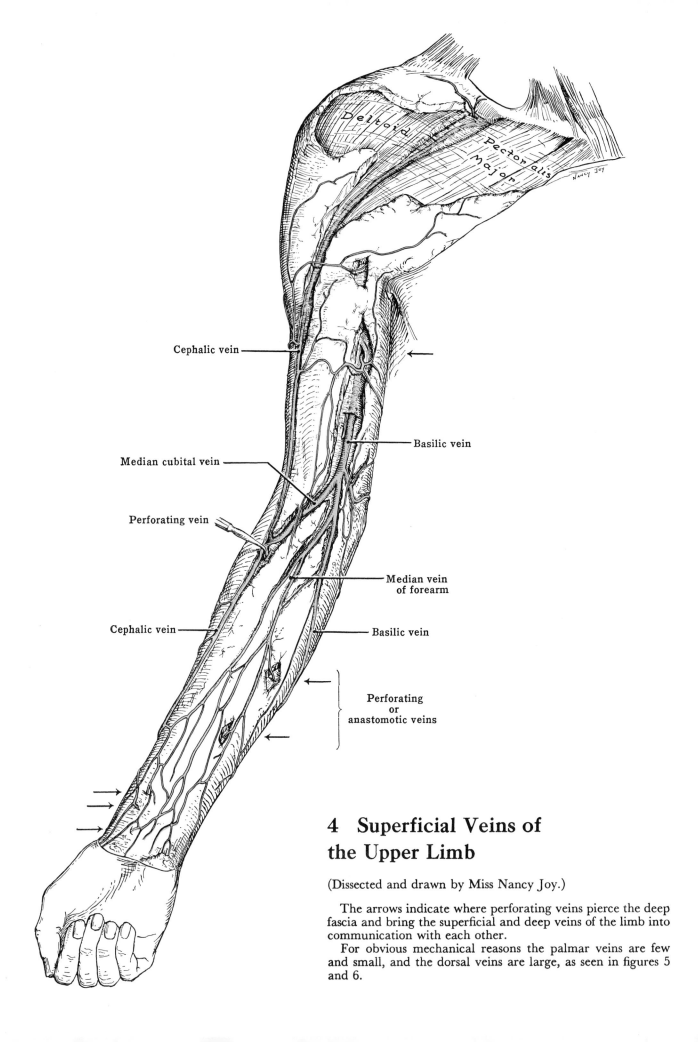

Cephalic vein

Median cubital vein

Perforating vein

Cephalic vein

Deltoid

Pectoralis Major

Nancy Joy

Basilic vein

Median vein of forearm

Basilic vein

Perforating or anastomotic veins

4 Superficial Veins of the Upper Limb

(Dissected and drawn by Miss Nancy Joy.)

The arrows indicate where perforating veins pierce the deep fascia and bring the superficial and deep veins of the limb into communication with each other.

For obvious mechanical reasons the palmar veins are few and small, and the dorsal veins are large, as seen in figures 5 and 6.

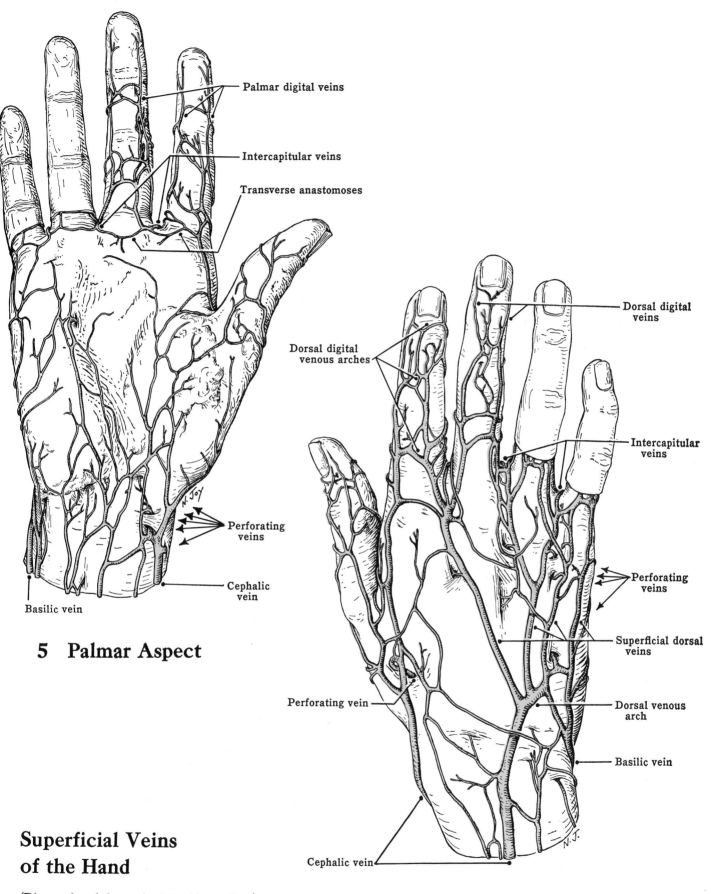

Palmar digital veins

Intercapitular veins

Transverse anastomoses

Dorsal digital
venous arches

Dorsal digital
veins

Intercapitular
veins

Perforating
veins

Perforating
veins

Cephalic
vein

Superficial dorsal
veins

Basilic vein

Perforating vein

Dorsal venous
arch

Basilic vein

5 Palmar Aspect

Cephalic vein

Superficial Veins
of the Hand

(Dissected and drawn by Miss Nancy Joy.)
See legend attached to figure 4.

6 Dorsal Aspect

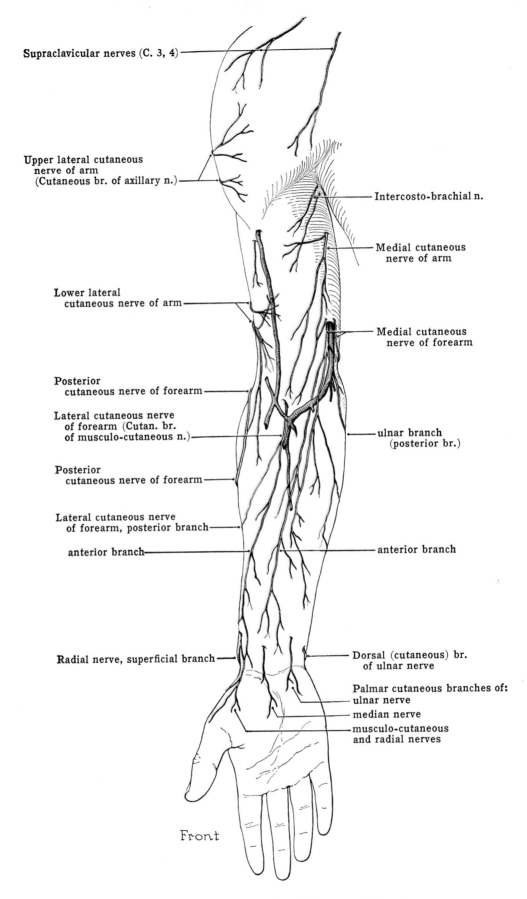

Supraclavicular nerves (C. 3, 4)

Upper lateral cutaneous
nerve of arm
(Cutaneous br. of axillary n.)

Intercosto-brachial n.

Medial cutaneous
nerve of arm

Lower lateral
cutaneous nerve of arm

Medial cutaneous
nerve of forearm

Posterior
cutaneous nerve of forearm

Lateral cutaneous nerve
of forearm (Cutan. br.
of musculo-cutaneous n.)

ulnar branch
(posterior br.)

Posterior
cutaneous nerve of forearm

Lateral cutaneous nerve
of forearm, posterior branch

anterior branch

anterior branch

Radial nerve, superficial branch

Dorsal (cutaneous) br.
of ulnar nerve

Palmar cutaneous branches of:
ulnar nerve
median nerve
musculo-cutaneous
and radial nerves

Front

7 Cutaneous Nerves of the Upper Limb

Of the 5 terminal branches of the brachial plexus (fig. 19) viz. musculo-cutaneous, median, ulnar, radial, and axillary nerves, the first 4 contribute cutaneous branches to the hand.

The posterior cord of the plexus is represented by 5 cutaneous nerves. Of these (a) one, the upper lateral cutaneous n. of the arm, is a branch of the axillary n.;

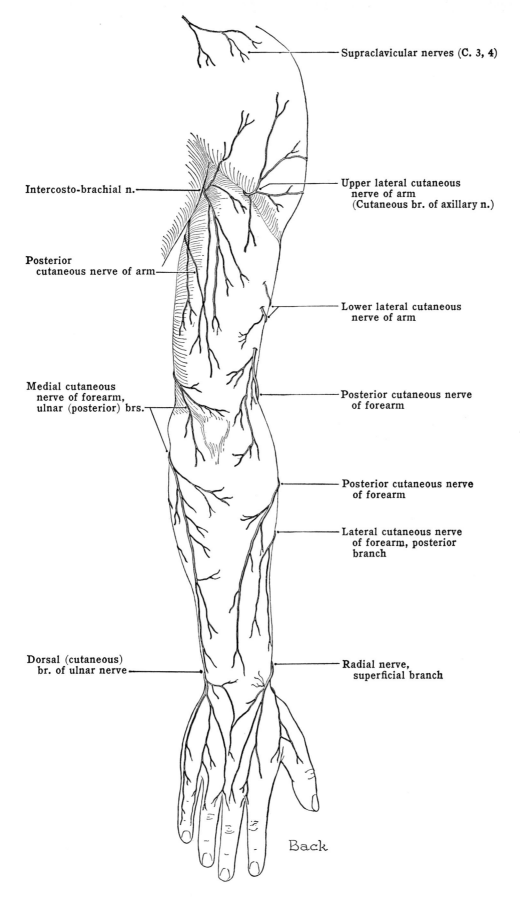

Supraclavicular nerves (C. 3, 4)

Intercosto-brachial n.

Upper lateral cutaneous
nerve of arm
(Cutaneous br. of axillary n.)

Posterior
cutaneous nerve of arm

Lower lateral cutaneous
nerve of arm

Medial cutaneous
nerve of forearm,
ulnar (posterior) brs.

Posterior cutaneous nerve
of forearm

Posterior cutaneous nerve
of forearm

Lateral cutaneous nerve
of forearm, posterior
branch

Dorsal (cutaneous)
br. of ulnar nerve

Radial nerve,
superficial branch

Back

8   Cutaneous Nerves of the Upper Limb

(b) whereas 4 are branches of the radial n. They are: the posterior cutaneous n. of
the arm, the lower lateral cutaneous n. of the arm, the posterior cutaneous n. of the
forearm, and the superficial branch of the radial nerve.

See figures 13 (pectoral region), 24 (back), 44 (elbow), 83 (hand).

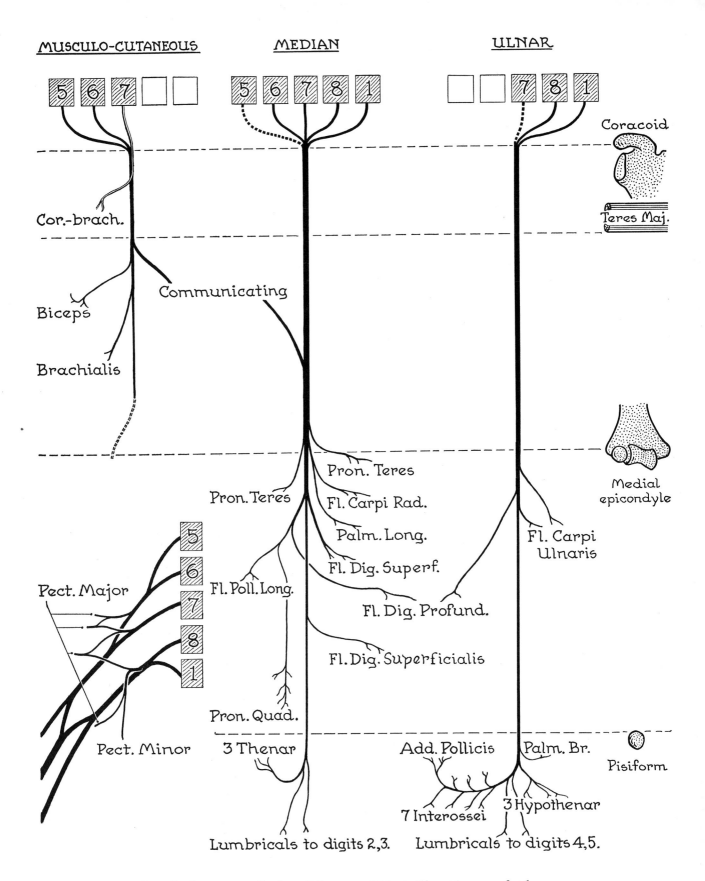

9 Scheme of the Motor Distribution of the Ventral Nerves of the Upper Limb

The average levels at which the motor branches leave the stems of the main nerves are shown with reference to the lower border of the axilla (Teres Major), elbow joint (medial epicondyle), and wrist (pisiform bone).

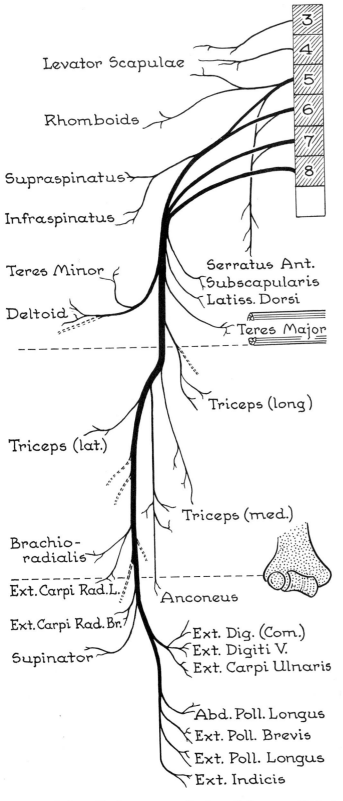

Levator Scapulae

Rhomboids

Supraspinatus

Infraspinatus

Teres Minor

Deltoid

Serratus Ant.
Subscapularis
Latiss. Dorsi
Teres Major

Triceps (long)

Triceps (lat.)

Triceps (med.)

Brachio-radialis

Ext. Carpi Rad. L.

Anconeus

Ext. Carpi Rad. Br.

Supinator

Ext. Dig. (Com.)
Ext. Digiti V.
Ext. Carpi Ulnaris

Abd. Poll. Longus
Ext. Poll. Brevis
Ext. Poll. Longus
Ext. Indicis

Trapezius
Latissimus Dorsi
Levator Scapulae
Rhomboideus Major
Rhomboideus Minor
Pectoralis Major
   clavicular part
   sternocostal part
   abdominal part
Pectoralis Minor
Subclavius
Serratus Anterior
Deltoideus
Supraspinatus
Infraspinatus
Teres Minor
Teres Major
Subscapularis
Biceps Brachii
   long head
   short head
   bicipital aponeurosis
Coraco-brachialis
Brachialis
Triceps
   long head
   lateral head
   medial head
   tricipital aponeurosis
Anconeus
Pronator Teres
Flexor Carpi Radialis
Palmaris Longus
Flexor Carpi Ulnaris
   humeral head
   ulnar head
Flexor Digitorum Superficialis
   humero-ulnar head
   radial head
Flexor Digitorum Profundus
Flexor Pollicis Longus
Pronator Quadratus
Brachio-radialis
Extensor Carpi Radialis Longus
Extensor Carpi Radialis Brevis
Extensor Digitorum Communis
Extensor Digiti Minimi (V)
Extensor Carpi Ulnaris
Supinator
Abductor Pollicis Longus
Extensor Pollicis Brevis
Extensor Pollicis Longus
Extensor Indicis
Palmaris Brevis
Abductor Pollicis Brevis
Flexor Pollicis Brevis
Opponens Pollicis
Adductor Pollicis
Abductor Digiti Minimi (V)
Flexor Digiti Minimi (V)
Opponens Digiti Minimi (V)
Lumbricales
Interossei
   Palmar
   Dorsal

A List of the Muscles of Upper Limb.

10 Scheme of the Motor Distribution of the Dorsal Nerves of the Upper Limb

The average levels of origin of the motor branches are shown as in figure 9.
There being no fleshy fibers on the dorsum of the hand, there are no motor nerves.

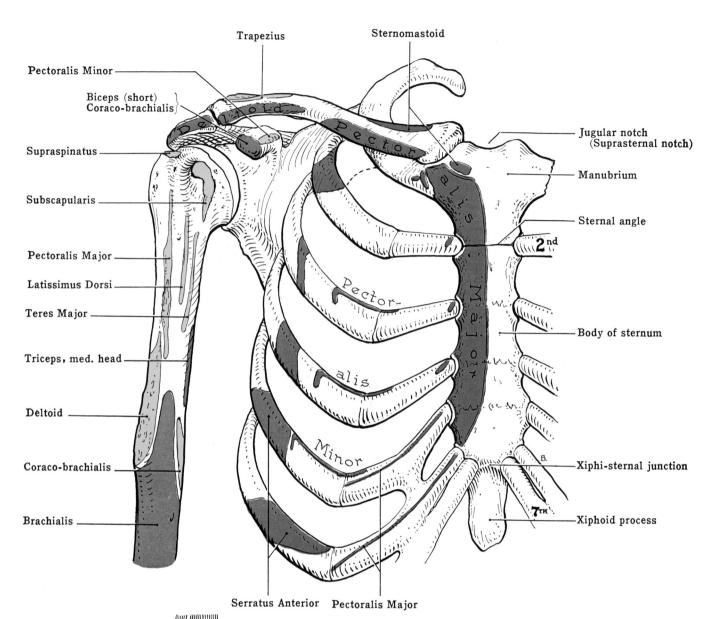

Trapezius

Sternomastoid

Pectoralis Minor

Biceps (short)
Coraco-brachialis

Supraspinatus

Subscapularis

Pectoralis Major

Latissimus Dorsi

Teres Major

Triceps, med. head

Deltoid

Coraco-brachialis

Brachialis

Jugular notch
(Suprasternal notch)

Manubrium

Sternal angle

2nd

Body of sternum

Xiphi-sternal junction

7TH

Xiphoid process

Serratus Anterior   Pectoralis Major

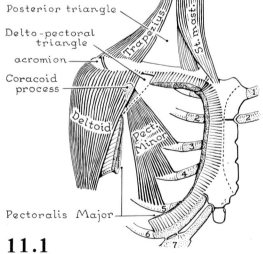

Posterior triangle

Delto-pectoral triangle

acromion

Coracoid process

Pectoralis Major

11.1

Diagram:
Some muscles of the region.

11   Bones of the Pectoral Region and Axilla showing Attachments of Muscles.
Origins (red), insertions (blue)

Observe:

1. The following muscles attached in line with each other:
    Horizontally, on the clavicle—(a) Trapezius and Sternomastoid; (b) Deltoid and clavicular head of Pectoralis Major
    Longitudinally, on the humerus—(c) Supraspinatus, Pectoralis Major and anterior part of Deltoid; and (d) Subscapularis and Latissimus Dorsi and Teres Major.

2. Pectoralis Major having a crescentic origin from the clavicle, sternum and 5th and (or) 6th costal cartilages.

3. Pectoralis Minor here arising from the 3rd, 4th and 5th ribs. It commonly arises also from either the 2nd or the 6th rib.

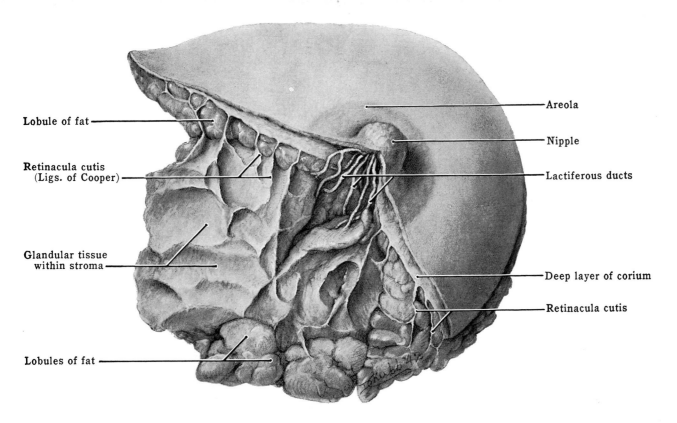

Lobule of fat

Retinacula cutis
(Ligs. of Cooper)

Glandular tissue
within stroma

Lobules of fat

Areola

Nipple

Lactiferous ducts

Deep layer of corium

Retinacula cutis

12 Mammary Gland of the Female

(*Dissection by Dr. Ross G. MacKenzie*)

With the rounded handle of the scalpel collections of superficial fat were scooped out of their compartments on the surface of the glandular tissue. The glandular tissue was incised in order to allow the ducts to be traced. A fringe of the deeper layer of the skin projects.

Observe:

1. The nipple rising from the centre of the pigmented areola.
2. The 7 of the 15 to 20 lactiferous ducts that are displayed. Traced in retrograde direction, they run at first dorsally in the long axis of the nipple, enveloped in an areolar cuff, and then spread radially and branch to the glandular tissue.
3. The glandular tissue within a dense (fibro-) areolar stroma from which septa, retinacula cutis, which imprison lobules of superficial fat, extend to the deeper layers of the skin.

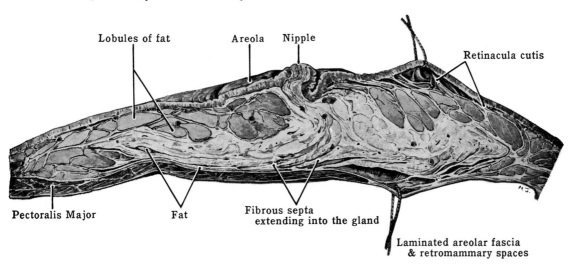

Lobules of fat

Areola

Nipple

Retinacula cutis

Pectoralis Major

Fat

Fibrous septa
extending into the gland

Laminated areolar fascia
& retromammary spaces

12.1 Mammary Gland of the Female, on antero-posterior section

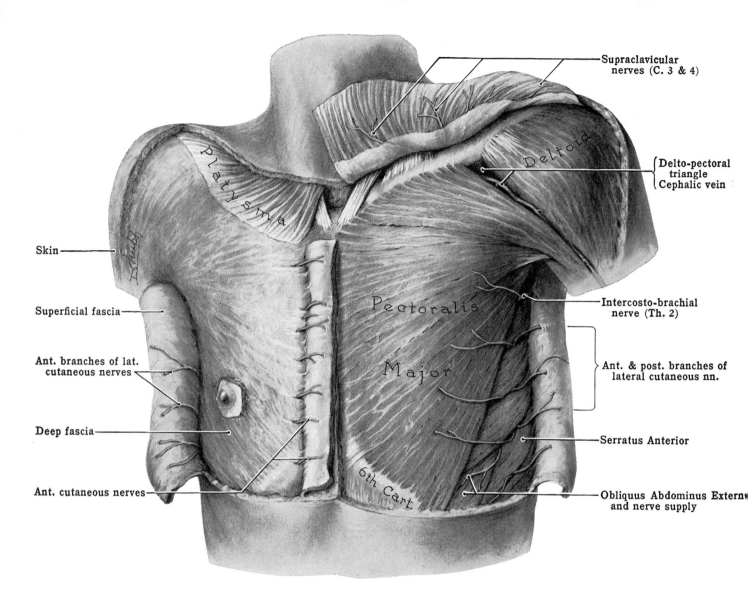

Supraclavicular
nerves (C. 3 & 4)

Delto-pectoral
triangle
Cephalic vein

Skin

Superficial fascia

Ant. branches of lat.
cutaneous nerves

Deep fascia

Ant. cutaneous nerves

Platysma

Deltoid

Pectoralis

Major

6th Cart.

Intercosto-brachial
nerve (Th. 2)

Ant. & post. branches of
lateral cutaneous nn.

Serratus Anterior

Obliquus Abdominus Extern
and nerve supply

13   Superficial Dissection of the Pectoral Region

Platysma, which descends to the 2nd or 3rd rib, is cut short on the left side of the
picture; it, together with the supraclavicular nerves, is thrown up on the right side

Observe:

1. The deep fascia covering Pectoralis Major is filmy.
2. The intermuscular bony strip running along the clavicle is both subcutaneous and
   subplatysmal. (Platysma, entire in fig. 526.)
3. The two heads of Pectoralis Major meeting at the sterno-clavicular joint.
4. The cephalic vein passing through the delto-pectoral triangle.
   Note:—The brachial plexus (C. 5, 6, 7, 8 and Th. 1) does not supply cutaneou
   branches to the pectoral region, hence the break in the numerical sequence, i.e
   branches of supraclavicular nerves C. 3 & 4 meet those of Th. 2.

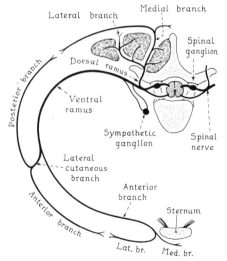

Medial branch

Lateral branch

Spinal
ganglion

Dorsal ramus

Posterior branch

Ventral
ramus

Sympathetic
ganglion

Spinal
nerve

Lateral
cutaneous
branch

Anterior
branch

Anterior branch

Sternum

Lat. br.

Med. br.

13.1

Diagram: A typical segmental nerve,
showing the source of anterior and
lateral cutaneous nerves.

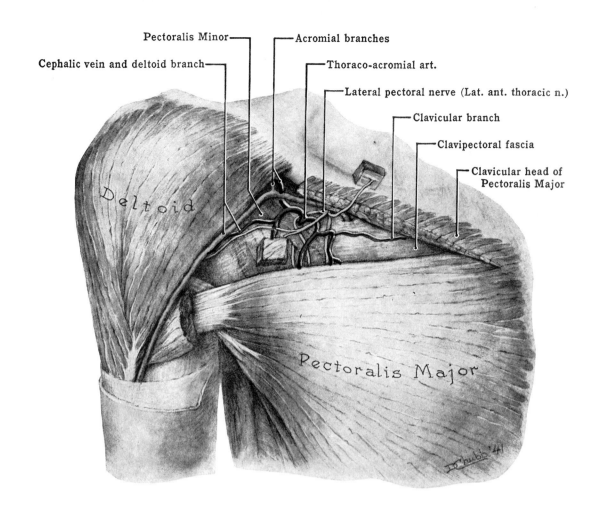

Pectoralis Minor

Cephalic vein and deltoid branch

Acromial branches

Thoraco-acromial art.

Lateral pectoral nerve (Lat. ant. thoracic n.)

Clavicular branch

Clavipectoral fascia

Clavicular head of Pectoralis Major

Deltoid

Pectoralis Major

14   Clavipectoral Fascia (Coraco-clavicular Fascia)

Clavicular head of Pectoralis Major is excised, except for 2 cubes of that muscle which remain to identify its nerves. The thoraco-acromial veins, which join the cephalic vein, are removed.

Observe:

. The part of the clavipectoral fascia above Pectoralis Minor—the costocoracoid membrane (fig. 14.1)—pierced by the lateral pectoral nerve and its companion vessels.

. The part of the fascia enclosing Pectoralis Minor. Here muscle and fascia are pierced by medial pectoral nerve (see fig. 16), thoraco-acromial art. and cephalic vein.

. The trilaminar insertion of Pectoralis Major.

. The course of the cephalic vein through delto-pectoral triangle and costo-coracoid membrane.

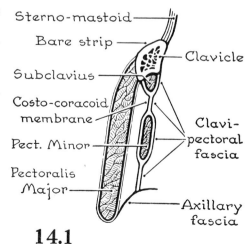

Sterno-mastoid

Bare strip

Clavicle

Subclavius

Costo-coracoid membrane

Pect. Minor

Clavi-pectoral fascia

Pectoralis Major

Axillary fascia

14.1

Diagram of anterior wall of axilla, on sagittal section.

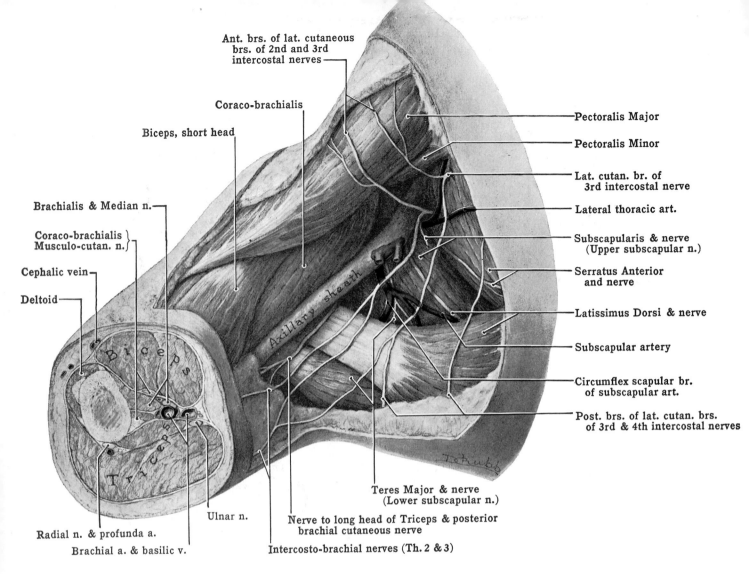

Ant. brs. of lat. cutaneous
brs. of 2nd and 3rd
intercostal nerves

Coraco-brachialis

Biceps, short head

Brachialis & Median n.

Coraco-brachialis }
Musculo-cutan. n. }

Cephalic vein

Deltoid

Pectoralis Major

Pectoralis Minor

Lat. cutan. br. of
3rd intercostal nerve

Lateral thoracic art.

Subscapularis & nerve
(Upper subscapular n.)

Serratus Anterior
and nerve

Latissimus Dorsi & nerve

Subscapular artery

Circumflex scapular br.
of subscapular art.

Post. brs. of lat. cutan. brs.
of 3rd & 4th intercostal nerves

Radial n. & profunda a.

Brachial a. & basilic v.

Ulnar n.

Nerve to long head of Triceps & posterior
brachial cutaneous nerve

Intercosto-brachial nerves (Th. 2 & 3)

Teres Major & nerve
(Lower subscapular n.)

15 Axilla, from below. Cross Section of the Arm

Observe:

1. The three muscular walls of the axilla:
   (a) Anterior wall—Pectoralis Major, Pectoralis Minor and Subclavius, but only the
   lower borders of Pectorales are in view.
   (b) Posterior wall—Subscapularis, Latissimus Dorsi and Teres Major.
   (c) Medial wall—Serratus Anterior.
   The lateral or bony wall—intertubercular sulcus (bicipital groove of the humerus)—is
   concealed by Biceps and Coraco-brachialis.

2. The axillary sheath and the cutaneous nerves crossing Latissimus Dorsi. The most lateral of
   these nerves is also the sole nerve supply of long head of Triceps (fig. 18).

3. The axillary sheath transmits the great nerves and vessels of the limb. It is a neuro-vascular
   bundle (displayed in fig. 16).

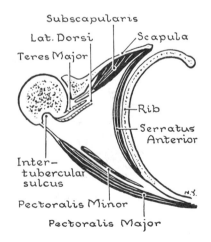

Subscapularis

Lat. Dorsi

Teres Major

Scapula

Rib

Serratus Anterior

Inter-
tubercular
sulcus

Pectoralis Minor

Pectoralis Major

15.1

Diagram of the walls of the axilla,
on cross section.

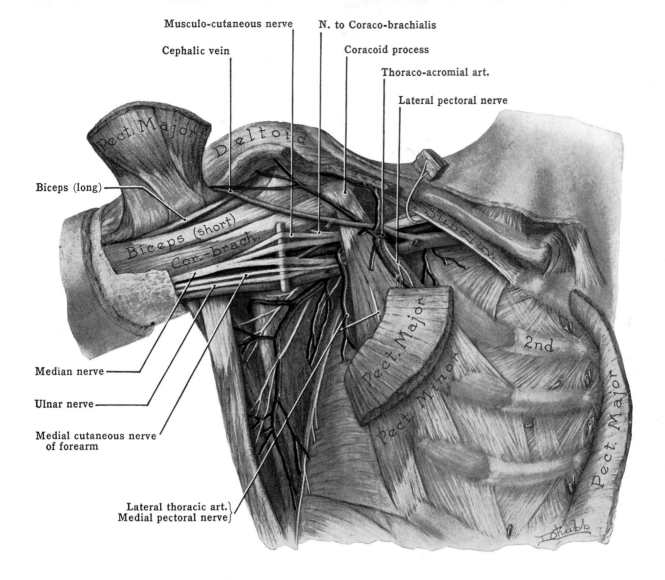

Musculo-cutaneous nerve
N. to Coraco-brachialis
Cephalic vein
Coracoid process
Thoraco-acromial art.
Lateral pectoral nerve

Pect. Major
Deltoid
Biceps (long)
Biceps (short)
Cor. brach.
Subclav.
Pect. Major
2nd
Pect. Minor
Pect. Major

Median nerve
Ulnar nerve
Medial cutaneous nerve
of forearm

Lateral thoracic art.
Medial pectoral nerve

16   Anterior Structures of the Axilla

Pectoralis Major is reflected and the clavi-pectoral fascia removed.

Observe:

1. Subclavius and Pectoralis Minor, which are the two deep muscles of the anterior wall.
2. The axillary artery passing behind Pectoralis Minor, a finger's breadth from the tip of the coracoid process, and having the lateral cord lateral to it and the medial cord medial.
3. The axillary vein lying medial to the axillary artery.
4. The median nerve, followed proximally, leading by its lateral root to the lateral cord and the musculo-cutaneous nerve, and by its medial root to the medial cord and the ulnar nerve. [These 4 nerves and the medial cutaneous nerve of the forearm are raised on a stick.]
5. The nerve to Coraco-brachialis arising within the axilla.
6. The cube of muscle above the clavicle is cut from the clavicular head of Pectoralis Major.

Note:—The lateral root of the median nerve may be in several strands.

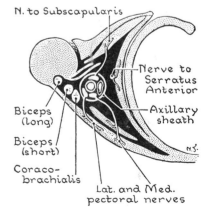

N. to Subscapularis
Nerve to Serratus Anterior
Axillary sheath
Biceps (long)
Biceps (short)
Coraco-brachialis
Lat. and Med. pectoral nerves

16.1

Diagram of the contents of the axilla, on cross section.

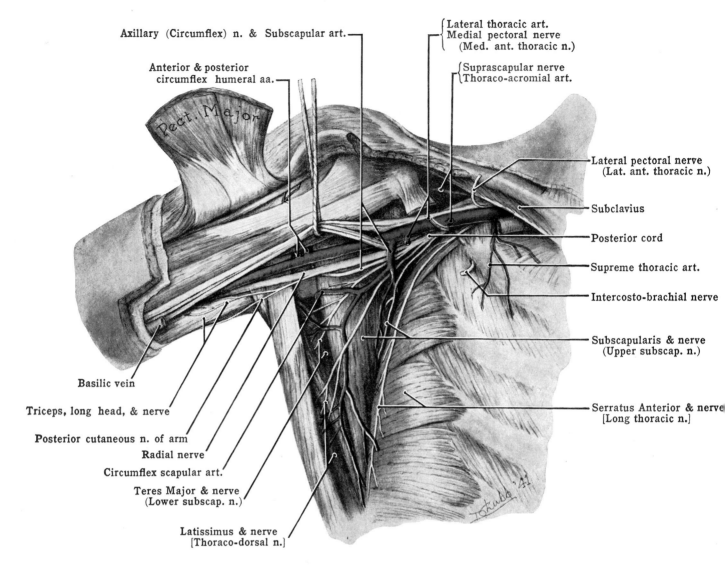

Axillary (Circumflex) n. & Subscapular art.

Anterior & posterior circumflex humeral aa.

Pect. Major

Lateral thoracic art.
Medial pectoral nerve
(Med. ant. thoracic n.)

Suprascapular nerve
Thoraco-acromial art.

Lateral pectoral nerve
(Lat. ant. thoracic n.)

Subclavius

Posterior cord

Supreme thoracic art.

Intercosto-brachial nerve

Subscapularis & nerve
(Upper subscap. n.)

Serratus Anterior & nerve
[Long thoracic n.]

Basilic vein

Triceps, long head, & nerve

Posterior cutaneous n. of arm

Radial nerve

Circumflex scapular art.

Teres Major & nerve
(Lower subscap. n.)

Latissimus & nerve
[Thoraco-dorsal n.]

17 Posterior and Medial Walls of the Axilla

Pectoralis Minor is excised; the lateral and medial cords are retracted; the axillary vein is removed.

Observe:

1. The posterior cord and its 2 terminal branches (viz. radial and axillary nerves), lying behind the axillary artery.

2. The nerves to the 3 posterior muscles. Of these:
    (a) Nerve to Latissimus Dorsi enters the deep surface of its muscle $\frac{1}{2}''$ from its free border at a point mid-way between the chest and the abducted arm.
    (b) Upper nerve to Subscapularis lies parallel to (a) but above it (fig. 18).
    (c) Lower nerve to Subscapularis and to Teres Major lies parallel to (a) but below it.

3. Nerve to Serratus Anterior clinging to its muscle throughout—high up some fat may intervene.

4. Suprascapular nerve passing towards the root of the coracoid process.

5. Subscapular artery, the largest branch of the axillary artery. Here arising high; usually it arises at the lower border of Subscapularis.

6. Posterior circumflex humeral artery accompanying the axillary nerve through the quadrangular space (fig. 18).

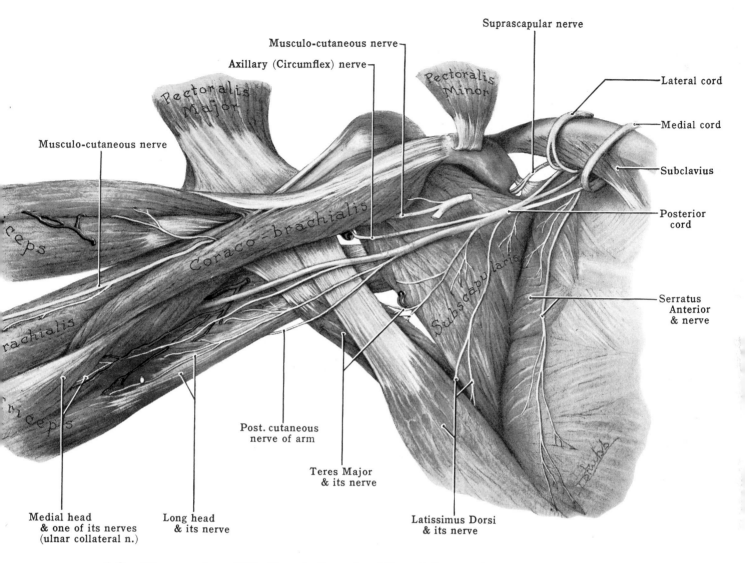

Suprascapular nerve

Musculo-cutaneous nerve

Axillary (Circumflex) nerve

Pectoralis Major

Pectoralis Minor

Lateral cord

Medial cord

Subclavius

Musculo-cutaneous nerve

Coraco-brachialis

Posterior cord

Subscapularis

Serratus Anterior & nerve

brachialis

ceps

riceps

Post. cutaneous nerve of arm

Teres Major & its nerve

Medial head & one of its nerves (ulnar collateral n.)

Long head & its nerve

Latissimus Dorsi & its nerve

18 Posterior Wall of the Axilla. Musculo-cutaneous Nerve. Posterior Cord of the Brachial Plexus

Pectorales Major et Minor are thrown laterally; the lateral and medial cords are thrown upwards; the arteries, veins, and median and ulnar nerves are removed.

Observe:

1. Coraco-brachialis arising with the short head of Biceps from the tip of the coracoid process and inserted half way down the humerus (fig. 29).

2. The musculo-cutaneous nerve piercing Coraco-brachialis, and supplying it, Biceps and Brachialis before becoming cutaneous.

3. The posterior cord of the plexus formed by the union of the 3 posterior divisions, supplying the 3 muscles of the posterior wall of the axilla, and soon ending as the radial and axillary nerves.

4. The radial nerve giving off, in the axilla, the nerve to the long head of Triceps and a cutaneous branch, and, in this specimen, the ulnar collateral branch to the medial head of Triceps. It then enters the spiral groove of the humerus with the profunda brachii artery.

5. The axillary nerve traversing the quadrangular space with the posterior circumflex humeral artery. The circumflex scapular artery traversing the triangular space.

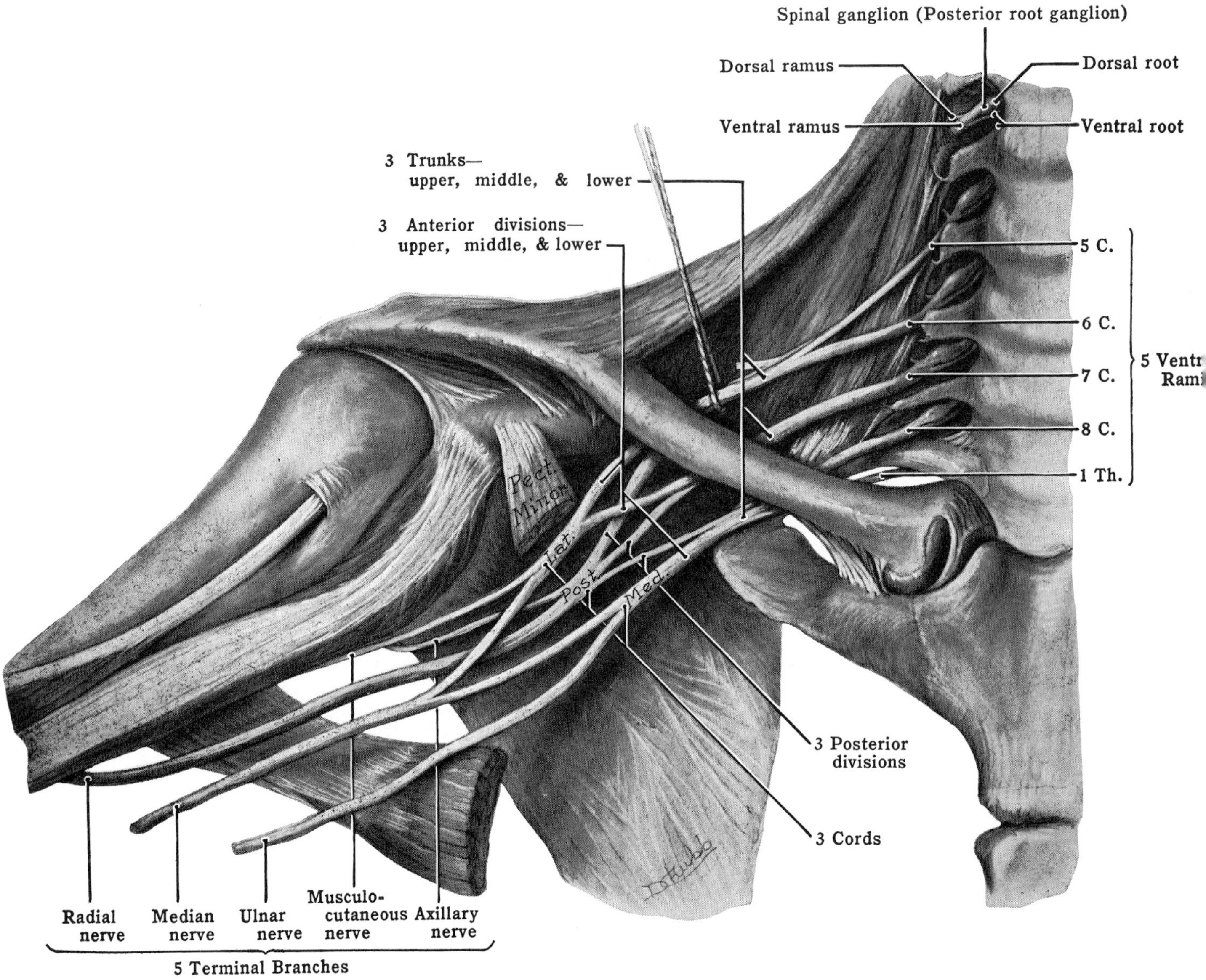

Spinal ganglion (Posterior root ganglion)

Dorsal ramus

Ventral ramus

Dorsal root

Ventral root

3 Trunks—
upper, middle, & lower

3 Anterior divisions—
upper, middle, & lower

5 C.

6 C.

7 C.

8 C.

1 Th.

5 Ventr
Rami

Pect.
Minor

Lat.

Post.

Med.

3 Posterior
divisions

3 Cords

Radial
nerve

Median
nerve

Ulnar
nerve

Musculo-
cutaneous
nerve

Axillary
nerve

5 Terminal Branches

19   Brachial Plexus: Ligaments of the Clavicle

Observe:

1. A dorsal (sensory) root of a spinal nerve larger than a ventral (motor) root.
2. The 2 roots uniting beyond the ganglion to form a very short mixed spinal nerve.
3. The mixed nerve at once dividing into a small dorsal ramus and a large ventral ramus.
4. The 5 ventral rami forming the brachial plexus. (Of these the middle ramus C.7, is the largest.)
5. These 5 rami uniting to form the 3 trunks of the plexus.
6. Each trunk dividing into 2 divisions, an anterior and a posterior.
7. These 6 divisions becoming 3 cords—a lateral, a medial, and a posterior.
8. The 3 cords lying behind Pectoralis Minor.

Note: The ligaments of the clavicle and the structures of the sterno-clavicular joint are depicted but not labelled (fig. 36).

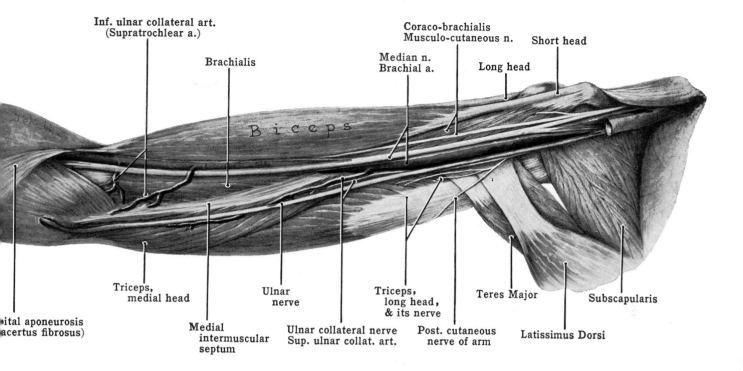

Inf. ulnar collateral art.
(Supratrochlear a.)

Brachialis

Coraco-brachialis
Musculo-cutaneous n.

Short head

Median n.
Brachial a.

Long head

Biceps

Triceps,
medial head

Ulnar
nerve

Triceps,
long head,
& its nerve

Teres Major

Subscapularis

ital aponeurosis
acertus fibrosus)

Medial
intermuscular
septum

Ulnar collateral nerve
Sup. ulnar collat. art.

Post. cutaneous
nerve of arm

Latissimus Dorsi

20 Brachium or Arm, medial view

Observe:

1. Three muscles: Biceps Brachii, Coraco-brachialis and Brachialis occupying the front of the brachium or arm; Triceps Brachii occupying the back.

2. Medial intermuscular septum separating these two muscle groups in the distal $\frac{2}{3}$ of the arm.

3. The great artery of the limb passing a finger's breadth medial to the tip of the coracoid process, and applied to the medial side of Coraco-brachialis above (proximally), and to the front of Brachialis below (distally).

4. In the axilla, the lateral and medial cords of the brachial plexus and their end branches making an M-shaped display about the front of the artery.

5. The median nerve applied to the artery throughout; crossing it from lateral to medial side.—usually crossing superficially (fig. 28D).

6. The ulnar nerve applied to the medial side of the artery as far as the middle of the arm, then passing behind the medial septum, and descending subfascially, on the medial head of Triceps, to the back of the medial epicondyle, where it is palpable (fig. 56).

7. The superior ulnar collateral art. and the ulnar collateral branch of the radial nerve (to medial head of Triceps) accompanying the ulnar nerve.

8. The musculo-cutaneous nerve supplying Coraco-brachialis, following the lateral side of the brachial the artery, and disappearing between Biceps and Brachialis accompanied by an arterial branch to these two muscles. More commonly it pierces Coraco-brachialis as in figure 18.

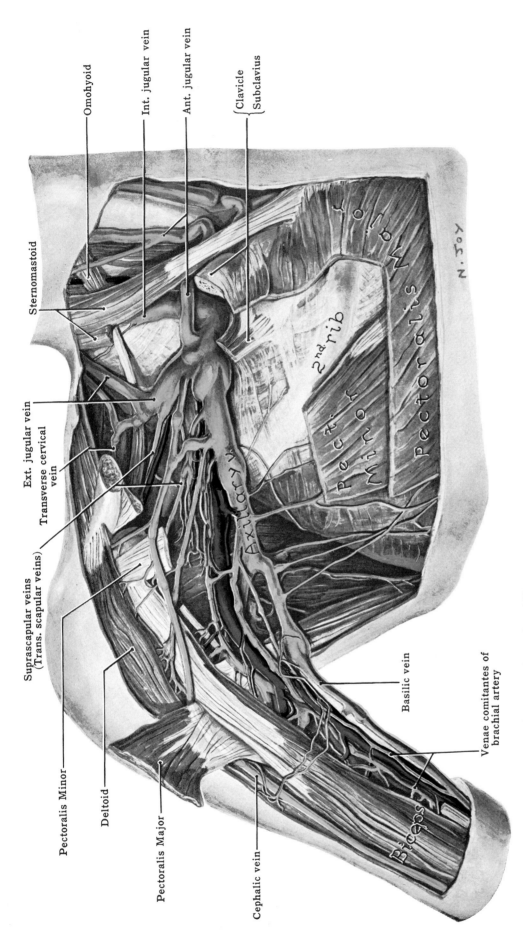

Omohyoid

Int. jugular vein

Ant. jugular vein

{ Clavicle
{ Subclavius

Sternomastoid

Ext. jugular vein

Transverse cervical vein

Suprascapular veins
(Trans. scapular veins)

Pectoralis Minor

Deltoid

Pectoralis Major

Cephalic vein

Basilic vein

Venae comitantes of brachial artery

2nd rib

Pect. Major

Pect. Minor

Pectoralis

Axillary V.

Biceps

R.N. 507

21 Veins of the Axilla

Observe:

1. The basilic vein becoming the axillary vein at the lower border of Teres Major; the axillary vein becoming the subclavian vein at the 1st rib; and the subclavian joining the internal jugular to become the brachiocephalic vein (innominate v.) behind the sternal end of the clavicle. Over 40 venous valves are shown. Note 1 in the basilic vein, 3 in the axillary, and 1 in the subclavian where it rests upon the 1st rib—the last valve on the road to the heart.

2. Venae comitantes of the brachial artery uniting and joining the axillary vein near the middle of the axilla.

4. The profunda brachii, posterior humeral circumflex, and circumflex scapular venae comitantes united and, as one large vein, joining the axillary vein.

5. Several subscapular veins, tenuous because the latex injection failed to force their valves.

6. Three suprascapular veins—1 from below the suprascapular ligament to the axillary vein, and 2 from above the ligament to the external jugular vein.

Note:—anastomotic veins are in view; obviously those on the dorsum of the scapula joining circumflex scapular and

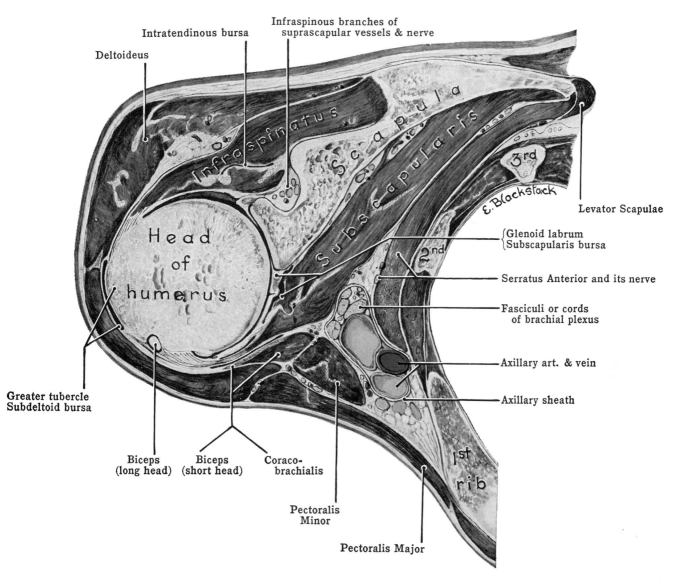

Deltoideus

Intratendinous bursa

Infraspinous branches of
suprascapular vessels & nerve

Infraspinatus

Scapula

Subscapularis

3rd

E. Blackstock

Levator Scapulae

Head
of
humerus

2nd

Glenoid labrum
Subscapularis bursa

Serratus Anterior and its nerve

Fasciculi or cords
of brachial plexus

Axillary art. & vein

Axillary sheath

Greater tubercle
Subdeltoid bursa

Biceps
(long head)

Biceps
(short head)

Coraco-
brachialis

Pectoralis
Minor

1st
rib

Pectoralis Major

22 Cross-section through the Shoulder Joint
and the Axilla, near its apex

Observe:

1. The long head (tendon) of Biceps, in its synovial sheath, facing straight forwards. The short head of Biceps and the
Coracobrachialis and Pectoralis Minor evidently sectioned
close below their attachment to the coracoid process.

2. The cartilage of the head of the humerus, extensive and very
thin peripherally.

3. The glenoid cavity of the scapula, small and with glenoid
labrum attached loosely in front but firmly behind where it
is part-origin of the long head of Biceps (Fig. 38).

4. Delicate synovial folds projecting from the labra between
head and glenoid cavity.

5. The fibrous capsulse, thin posteriorly and partly fused with
the tendon of Infraspinatus; thicker anteriorly (gleno-
humeral ligaments).

6. Bursae: (a) Subdeltoid bursa, between Deltoid and greater
tubercle (continuous above with subacromial bursa, fig. 35);
(b) Subscapular bursa, between Subscapularis tendon and
the scapula (fig. 36) (communicating with the joint cavity);
(c) Coraco-brachialis bursa, between Coraco-brachialis
and Subscapularis; (d) an Intra-Infraspinatus bursa (present).

7. Walls of axilla near apex, formed by Subscapularis and
scapula posteriorly; Serratus Anterior, thick at this high
level, ribs and Intercostales medially; and Pectorales Major
et Minor anteriorly. There is no bone in the anterior wall.

8. The axillary sheath of areolar tissue (fig. 15), delicate and
enclosing the axillary artery and vein and the 3 cords or
fasciculi of the brachial plexus (and here an extra vein) to
form a neurovascular bundle, surrounded with axillary fat.

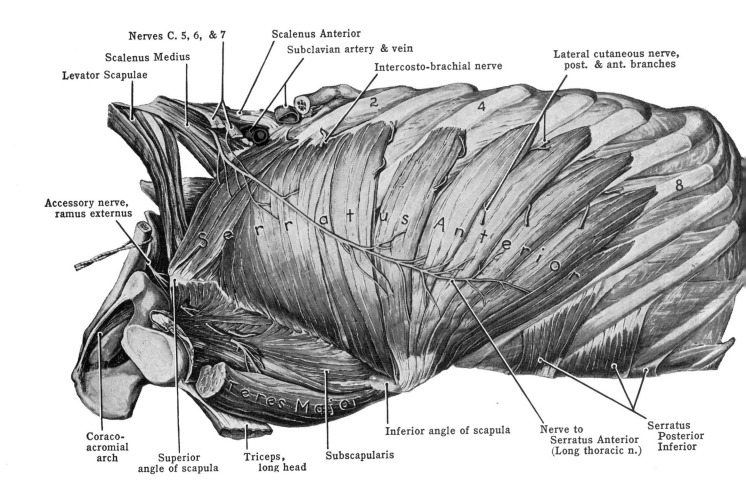

- Nerves C. 5, 6, & 7
- Scalenus Medius
- Levator Scapulae
- Scalenus Anterior
- Subclavian artery & vein
- Intercosto-brachial nerve
- Lateral cutaneous nerve, post. & ant. branches
- Accessory nerve, ramus externus
- Coraco-acromial arch
- Superior angle of scapula
- Triceps, long head
- Subscapularis
- Inferior angle of scapula
- Nerve to Serratus Anterior (Long thoracic n.)
- Serratus Posterior Inferior

23 Serratus Anterior, side view, supine position.

Observe:

1. Serratus Anterior, which forms the medial wall of the axilla, having an extensive fleshy origin from the upper 8 (here 9) ribs far forward, and an insertion into the whole length of the medial border of the scapula. The fibres from the 1st rib and from the arch between the 1st and 2nd ribs converging on the superior angle, those from the 2nd and 3rd ribs diverging to spread thinly along the medial border, and the remainder (from 4th to 9th ribs), which forms the bulk of the muscle, converging on the inferior angle and therefore having a tendinous insertion. (For bony attachments see figs. 11 & 29)

2. The nerve to Serratus Anterior, arising from C.5, 6, and 7 and applied to the whole length of the muscle. The fibres from C.5 and 6 piercing Scalenus Medius and appearing lateral to the brachial plexus; those from C.7 descending dorsal to the plexus.

3. Teres Major applied to the lateral border of Subscapularis; the nerve to Teres Major helping to supply Subscapularis.

4. The brachial plexus and the subclavian artery appearing between Scalenus Anterior and Scalenus Medius; the subclavian vein separated from the artery by Scalenus Anterior.

5. The term "Serratus Anterior" implies the existence of a "Serratus Posterior"; and the inferior part of this is seen attached to the lower 4 ribs (fig. 478).

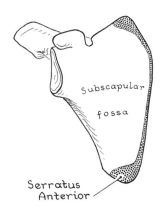

Subscapular fossa

Serratus Anterior

23.1

Diagram: Insertion of Serratus Anterior

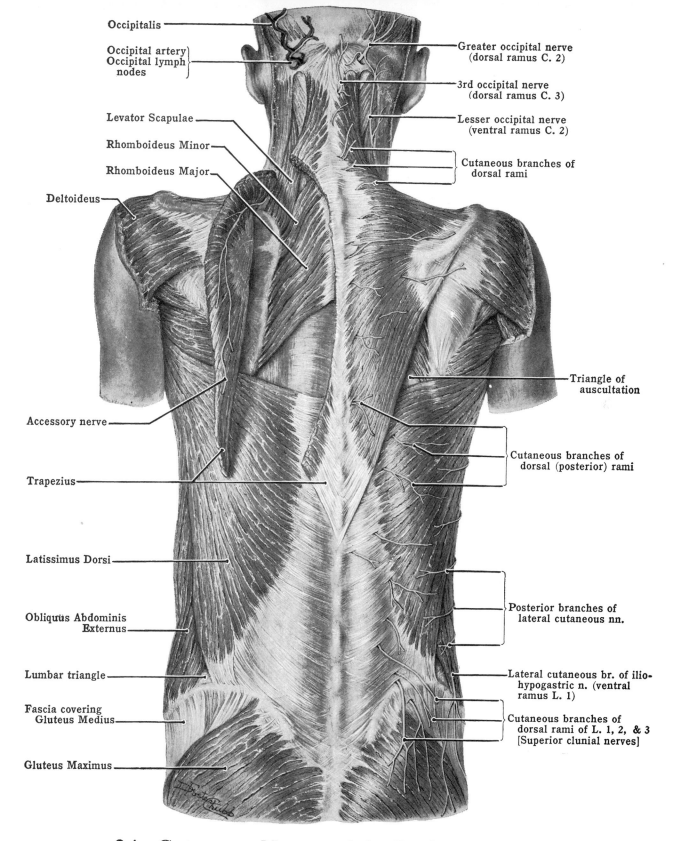

Occipitalis

Occipital artery
Occipital lymph
nodes

Levator Scapulae

Rhomboideus Minor

Rhomboideus Major

Deltoideus

Accessory nerve

Trapezius

Latissimus Dorsi

Obliquus Abdominis
Externus

Lumbar triangle

Fascia covering
Gluteus Medius

Gluteus Maximus

Greater occipital nerve
(dorsal ramus C. 2)

3rd occipital nerve
(dorsal ramus C. 3)

Lesser occipital nerve
(ventral ramus C. 2)

Cutaneous branches of
dorsal rami

Triangle of
auscultation

Cutaneous branches of
dorsal (posterior) rami

Posterior branches of
lateral cutaneous nn.

Lateral cutaneous br. of ilio-
hypogastric n. (ventral
ramus L. 1)

Cutaneous branches of
dorsal rami of L. 1, 2, & 3
[Superior clunial nerves]

24 Cutaneous Nerves of the Back: The First Two Layers of Muscles

Trapezius is severed and reflected on the left side.

Observe:

1. The cutaneous branches of the dorsal (posterior) nerve rami.

2. Trapezius and Latissimus Dorsi of the 1st layer. Levator Scapulae and Rhomboidei of the 2nd layer.

3. Two triangles: (a) the triangle of auscultation where the thoracic wall is poorly covered, and (b) the lumbar triangle.

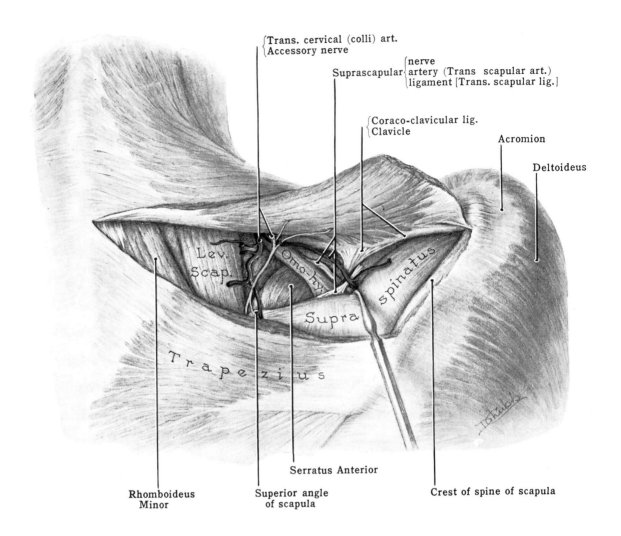

Trans. cervical (colli) art.
Accessory nerve

Suprascapular { nerve
artery (Trans scapular art.)
ligament [Trans. scapular lig.]

Coraco-clavicular lig.
Clavicle

Acromion

Deltoideus

Lev. Scap.

Omo-hy.

Supra spinatus

Trapezius

Serratus Anterior

Rhomboideus Minor

Superior angle of scapula

Crest of spine of scapula

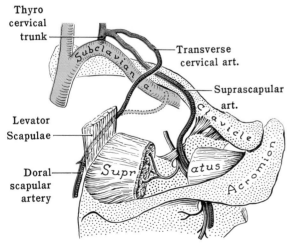

Thyro cervical trunk

Transverse cervical art.

Suprascapular art.

Levator Scapulae

Doral scapular artery

Subclavian a.

Clavicle

Supr atus

Acromion

25.1

Diagram: Source and course of suprascapular and dorsal scapular arteries, the latter having alternative origins (fig. 536).

25 Suprascapular Region

The horizontal fibres of Trapezius, at the level of the superior angle of the scapula, are separated and the incision is carried laterally along the crest of the spine of the scapula.

Observe:

1. The accessory nerve crossing the superior angle of the scapula.

2. The transverse cervical artery split by Levator Scapulae into a superficial and a deep branch, one following the accessory nerve, the other the dorsal scapular nerve (n. to Rhomboids) (not shown).

3. The finger tip, placed on the superior angle, may trace a U-shaped course— laterally along the sharp superior border of the scapula and along the sharp suprascapular ligament to the coracoid process, thence cranially along the conoid ligament to the clavicle, and thence medially behind the smooth posterior surface of the clavicle.

4. The suprascapular artery running behind the clavicle, and therefore having a retroclavicular course, before crossing above the suprascapular ligament.

5. The suprascapular nerve crossing below the ligament.

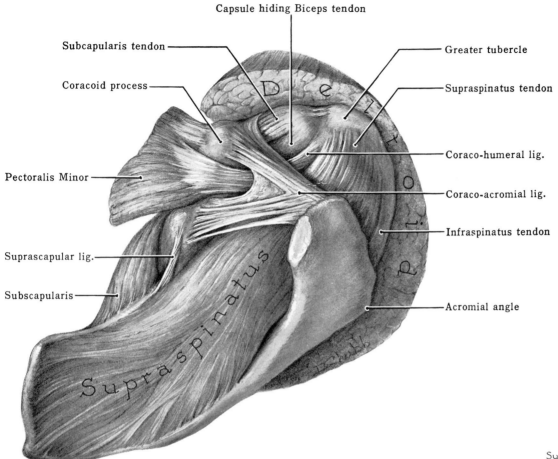

Capsule hiding Biceps tendon

Subcapularis tendon

Coracoid process

Pectoralis Minor

Suprascapular lig.

Subscapularis

Greater tubercle

Supraspinatus tendon

Coraco-humeral lig.

Coraco-acromial lig.

Infraspinatus tendon

Acromial angle

Supraspinatus

26 Supraspinous and Subdeltoid Regions

Observe:

1. The clavicular facet on the acromion. It is small, oval and obliquely set.

2. The triangular coraco-acromial ligament arching from the lateral border of the horizontal part of the coracoid process to the acromion between the facet and the tip.

3. Part of Pectoralis Minor tendon here (as commonly) dividing this ligament into 2 limbs and continuing, as the anterior part of the coraco-humeral ligament, to the greater tubercle (tuberosity) of the humerus.

4. Supraspinatus passing under the coraco-acromial arch, and then lying between Deltoid above and the capsule of the shoulder joint below. Supraspinatus and the middle fibres of Deltoid are the abductors of the joint. Though the middle part of the Deltoid is thin, it is multipennate and powerful.

(For subacromial and subdeltoid bursae see figures 35 & 38.1.)

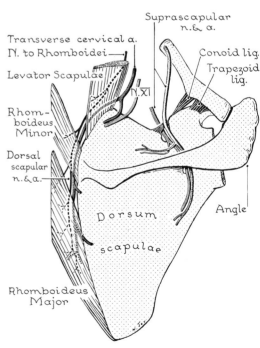

Suprascapular n.& a.

Transverse cervical a.
N. to Rhomboidei

Levator Scapulae

N. XI

Conoid lig.

Trapezoid lig.

Rhom-
boideus
Minor

Dorsal
scapular
n.& a.

Dorsum

scapulae

Angle

Rhomboideus
Major

25.2

Diagram: Medial border of scapula, showing 3 muscles and dorsal scapular nerve and artery (i.e., nerve to Rhomboids & trans. cervical art., deep branch).

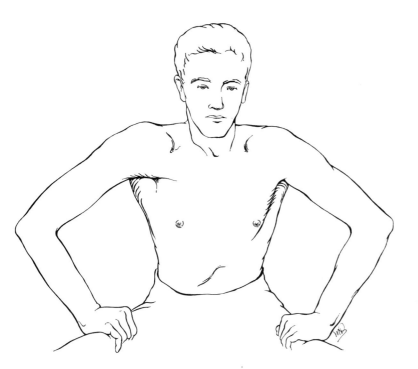

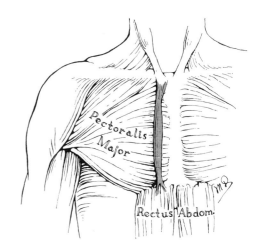

A Absence of Sternocostal Head of Right Pectoralis Major associated with compensatory hypertrophy of Latissimus Dorsi is not rare. It is revealed on pressing downwards, e.g., on the arms of a chair.

(*Courtesy of Squadron Leader David Christie.*)

B A Sternalis Muscle, in line with Rectus ~~dominis~~ Abdominis and Sternomastoid, was found in 6% 535 cadavera (R. N. Barlow).

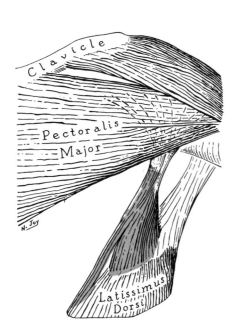

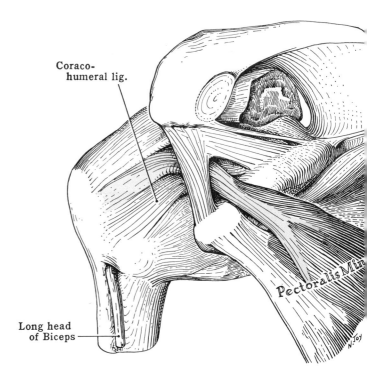

C An Axillary Arch. This occasional muscle crosses the base of the axilla superficially and joins Latissimus Dorsi to the tissues deep to Pectoralis Major.

D Pectoralis Minor inserted into Humeru. about 15% of limbs (G. A. Seib) part of the ten of the Minor passes over the coracoid process between the two limbs of the coraco-acromial ment to re-inforce the coraco-humeral ligam See figure 26.

27 Variations and Anomalies

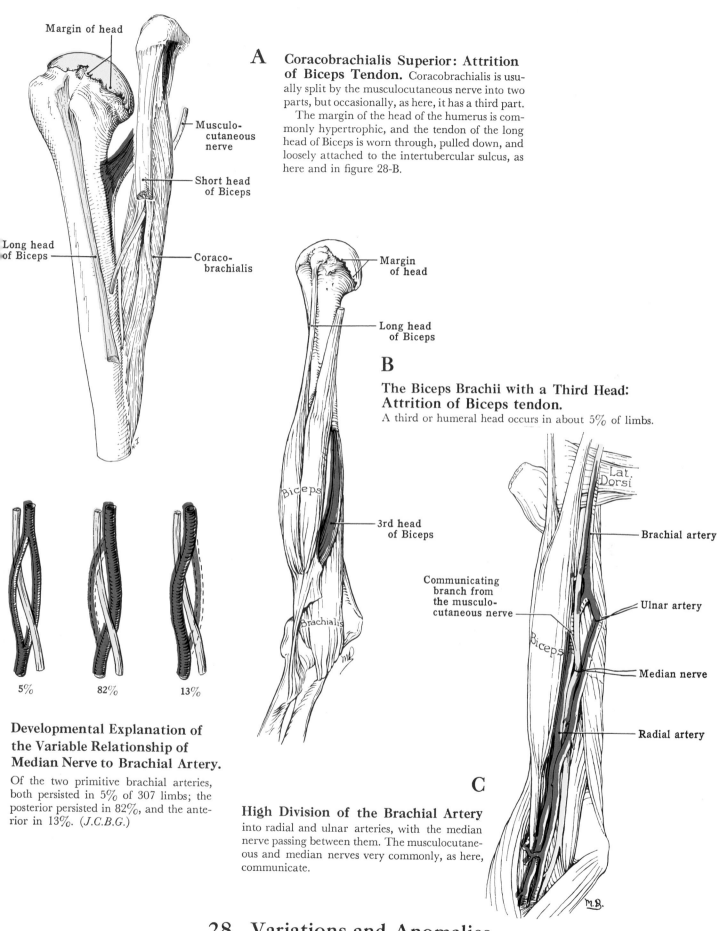

Margin of head

Musculo-
cutaneous
nerve

Short head
of Biceps

Long head
of Biceps

Coraco-
brachialis

A **Coracobrachialis Superior: Attrition of Biceps Tendon.** Coracobrachialis is usually split by the musculocutaneous nerve into two parts, but occasionally, as here, it has a third part.

The margin of the head of the humerus is commonly hypertrophic, and the tendon of the long head of Biceps is worn through, pulled down, and loosely attached to the intertubercular sulcus, as here and in figure 28-B.

Margin
of head

Long head
of Biceps

B

The Biceps Brachii with a Third Head: Attrition of Biceps tendon.
A third or humeral head occurs in about 5% of limbs.

Biceps

3rd head
of Biceps

Brachialis

Lat.
Dorsi

Brachial artery

Communicating
branch from
the musculo-
cutaneous
nerve

Biceps

Ulnar artery

Median nerve

Radial artery

5%   82%   13%

Developmental Explanation of the Variable Relationship of Median Nerve to Brachial Artery.

Of the two primitive brachial arteries, both persisted in 5% of 307 limbs; the posterior persisted in 82%, and the anterior in 13%. (*J.C.B.G.*)

C

High Division of the Brachial Artery into radial and ulnar arteries, with the median nerve passing between them. The musculocutaneous and median nerves very commonly, as here, communicate.

28 Variations and Anomalies

(Other anomalies, Figs. 40-43, 47, 48 and 97.)

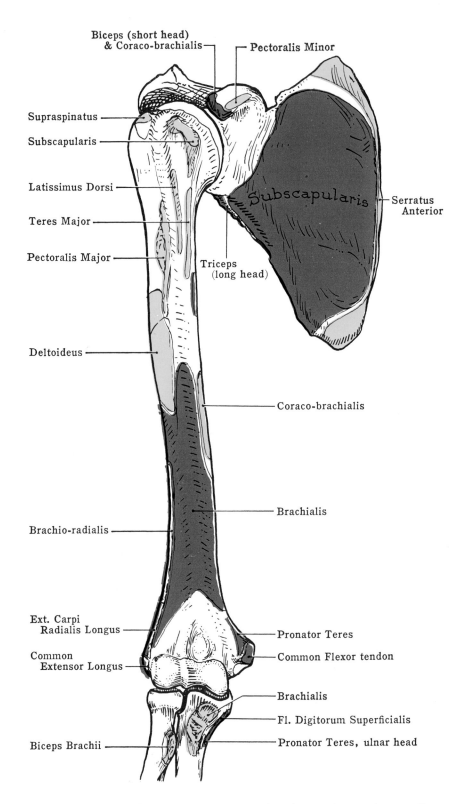

Biceps (short head)
& Coraco-brachialis

Pectoralis Minor

Supraspinatus

Subscapularis

Latissimus Dorsi

Teres Major

Pectoralis Major

Triceps
(long head)

Subscapularis

Serratus
Anterior

Deltoideus

Coraco-brachialis

Brachialis

Brachio-radialis

Ext. Carpi
Radialis Longus

Pronator Teres

Common
Extensor Longus

Common Flexor tendon

Brachialis

Fl. Digitorum Superficialis

Pronator Teres, ulnar head

Biceps Brachii

29 Bones of the Upper Limb showing Attachments of Muscles, anterior view.

Origins (red), insertions (blue)

(For Bones of Forearm, anterior view, see fig. 58.)

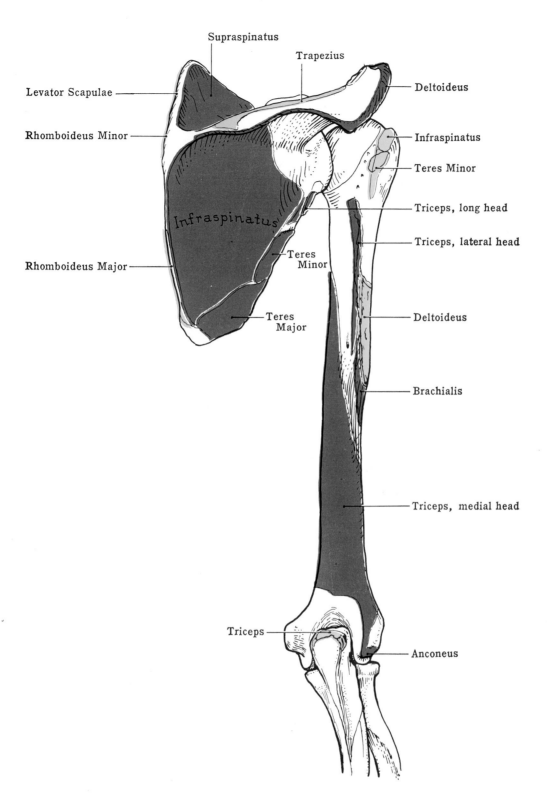

Supraspinatus

Trapezius

Levator Scapulae

Deltoideus

Rhomboideus Minor

Infraspinatus

Teres Minor

Triceps, long head

Triceps, lateral head

Infraspinatus

Rhomboideus Major

Teres
Minor

Deltoideus

Teres
Major

Brachialis

Triceps, medial head

Triceps

Anconeus

30   Bones of the Upper Limb showing Attachments of Muscles, posterior view

(For Bones of Forearm, posterior view, see fig. 77.)

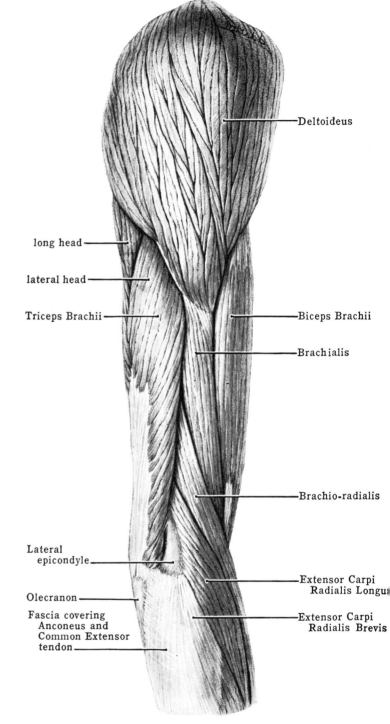

Deltoideus

long head

lateral head

Triceps Brachii

Biceps Brachii

Brachialis

Brachio-radialis

Lateral
epicondyle

Olecranon

Fascia covering
Anconeus and
Common Extensor
tendon

Extensor Carpi
Radialis Longus

Extensor Carpi
Radialis Brevis

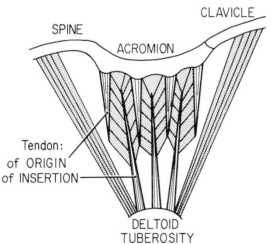

SPINE

CLAVICLE

ACROMION

Tendon:
of ORIGIN
of INSERTION

DELTOID
TUBEROSITY

31.1

Diagram: Internal structure of Deltoid, acromial part being multipennate.

31 Muscles of the Arm, lateral view

Note: The multipennate structure of the middle part of Deltoid, and the more parallel arrangement of the fibres of the anterior and posterior parts.

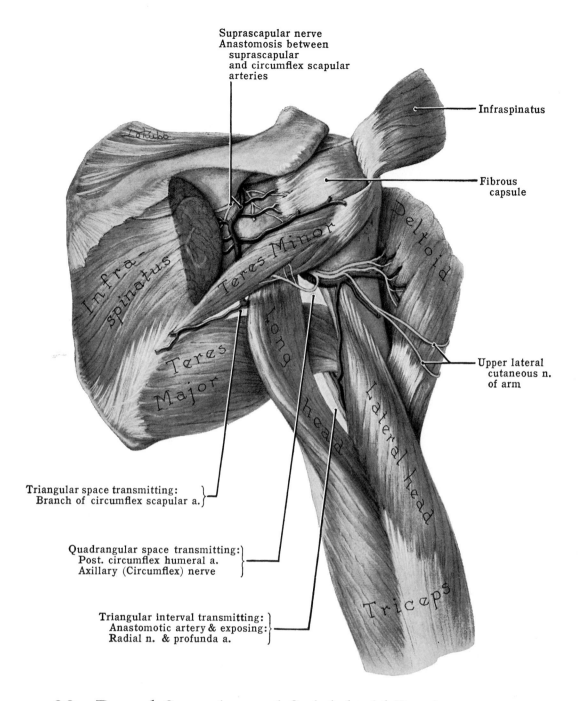

Suprascapular nerve
Anastomosis between
suprascapular
and circumflex scapular
arteries

Infraspinatus

Fibrous
capsule

Upper lateral
cutaneous n.
of arm

Triangular space transmitting:
Branch of circumflex scapular a.

Quadrangular space transmitting:
Post. circumflex humeral a.
Axillary (Circumflex) nerve

Triangular interval transmitting:
Anastomotic artery & exposing:
Radial n. & profunda a.

32 Dorsal Scapular and Subdeltoid Regions

Observe:

1. The thickness of Infraspinatus, which, aided by Teres Minor and posterior fibres of Deltoid rotates the humerus laterally.

2. Long head of Triceps passing between Teres Minor (a lateral rotator) and Teres Major (a medial rotator).

3. Long head of Triceps separating the quadrangular space from the triangular space.

4. Teres Major separating the quadrangular space from another triangular space.

5. The arterial anastomoses behind the scapula and behind the Teres Major.

6. The distribution of the suprascapular and axillary nerves. Each comes from C. 5 & 6 (fig. 10); each supplies two muscles (Supraspinatus and Infraspinatus—Teres Minor and Deltoid); each supplies the shoulder joint (figs. 32 & 39); but only one has cutaneous branches.

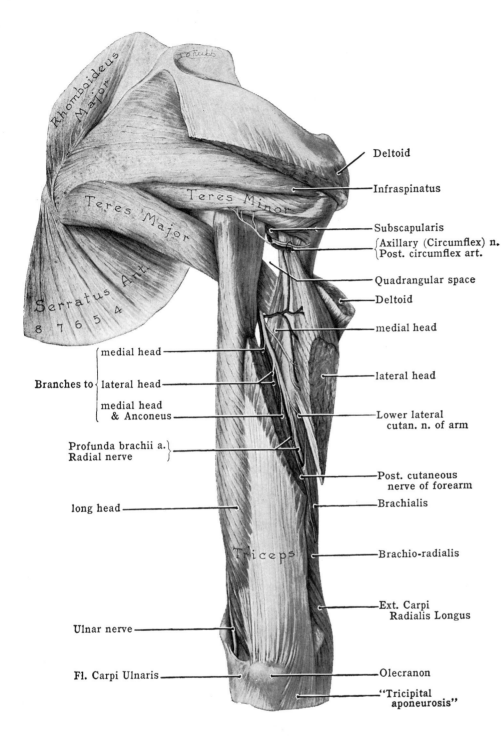

Rhomboideus Major

to rubb

Teres Major

Teres Minor

Serratus Ant.

8 7 6 5 4

Branches to { medial head
lateral head
medial head & Anconeus

Profunda brachii a.
Radial nerve }

long head

Ulnar nerve

Fl. Carpi Ulnaris

Triceps

Deltoid

Infraspinatus

Subscapularis

{ Axillary (Circumflex) n.
Post. circumflex art.

Quadrangular space

Deltoid

medial head

lateral head

Lower lateral cutan. n. of arm

Post. cutaneous nerve of forearm

Brachialis

Brachio-radialis

Ext. Carpi Radialis Longus

Olecranon

"Tricipital aponeurosis"

33 Triceps and its Three Related Nerves (axillary, radial, ulnar), posterior view

The lateral head of Triceps is divided an displaced.

Observe:

1. The long and lateral heads of Triceps lying s by side behind the medial head. The rad nerve, passing in the plane between, has l and lateral heads behind it, medial head a bone in front of it (fig. 30).

2. The lateral head of Triceps rising to the leve. Teres Minor.

3. An upward prolongation of Brachialis into spiral groove separating the radial nerve fr the insertion of Deltoid.

4. The radial nerve here supplying lateral a medial heads and Anconeus.

5. Triceps inserted into the upper aspect of olecranon and also into deep fascia of the fo arm (fig. 56).

6. Teres Major, Rhomboideus Major and Serra Anterior mainly inserted into the inferior an of the scapula, which is the end of a lever. T fibres of the two latter muscles are in alignme

34 Cross-section through the Arm, below its mid-point

(The insertion of Coraco-brachialis is seen, but no Deltoid is visible nor any Brachio-radialis; (for level consult fig. 29).

Observe:

1. The body of the humerus, nearly circular; its cortex being thickest here.

2. The 3 heads of Triceps, in the posterior compartment of the arm, i.e., behind the medial and lateral intermuscular septa.

3. The radial nerve and its companion vessels in contact with the bone.

4. The 2 heads of Biceps, the Brachialis, and the insertion of Coraco-brachialis in the anterior compartment of the arm, i.e., in front of the medial and lateral intermuscular septa.

5. The musculocutaneous nerve and its companion vessels in the septum between Biceps and Brachialis.

6. The median nerve crossing to the medial side of the brachial artery and its venae comitantes; the ulnar nerve moving posteriorly on to the side of Triceps. The basilic vein (here as 2 vessels) has pierced the deep fascia.

7. The skin and subcutaneous tissues, thicker postero-laterally where exposed to injury than antero-medially where protected.

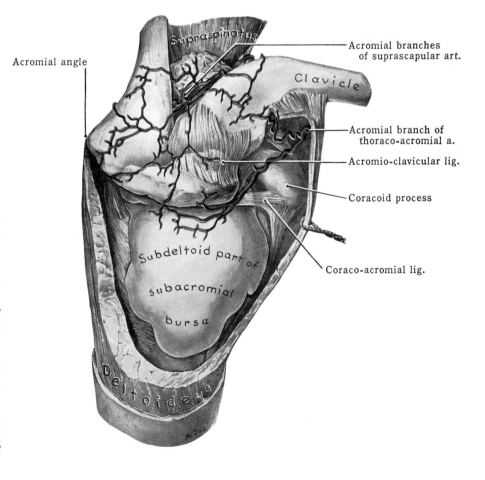

Brachial artery
Median nerve
Medial cutaneous nerve of forearm
Basilic vein
Ulnar nerve
Tributary
Superior ulnar collateral art. & ulnar collateral n. anterior to Medial intermuscular septum
Cephalic vein
Musculo-cutaneous nerve
Lateral cutaneous nerve of forearm
Coraco-brachialis
Lateral intermuscular septum
Posterior cutaneous nerve of forearm
Radial nerve
Profunda brachii artery & veins

Biceps short long
Brachialis
Humerus
medial lateral
Triceps
long

E. Blackstock

35 Subacromial Bursa, superolateral view

(Injected with yellow latex.)

Note:

1. The term "subacromial bursa" is usually understood to include the subdeltoid bursa, for the two bursae are usually combined.

2. Superficial to the bursa are parts of Deltoid, acromion, and coraco-acromial ligament and the acromio-clavicular joint.

3. Deep to the bursa are the greater tubercle of the humerus and Supraspinatus·tendon (not in view) (figs. 38.1, 39).

4. The bursa may extend more widely under the acromion, and it may through attrition (fig. 42) communicate with the shoulder joint and also with the acromioclavicular joint.

5. The acromial branches of the thoraco-acromial and suprascapular arteries are seen contributing to the acromial rete (network); the branches of the circumflex artery are destroyed.

Acromial angle
Supraspinatus
Acromial branches of suprascapular art.
Clavicle
Acromial branch of thoraco-acromial a.
Acromio-clavicular lig.
Coracoid process
Coraco-acromial lig.
Subdeltoid part of subacromial bursa
Deltoid

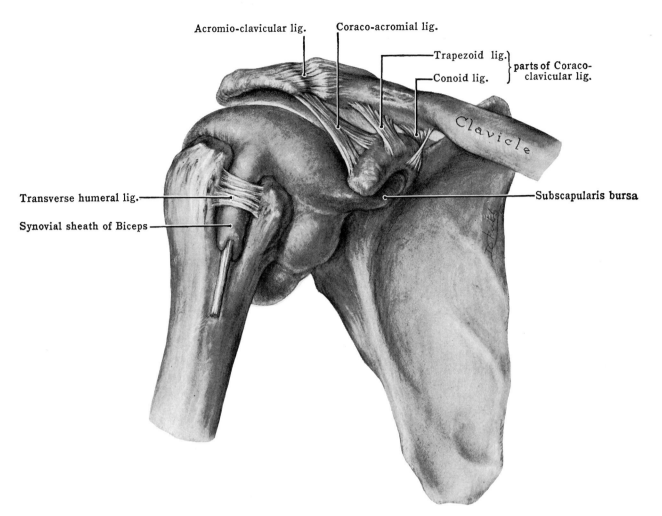

Acromio-clavicular lig. Coraco-acromial lig.

Trapezoid lig.
Conoid lig. } parts of Coraco-clavicular lig.

Clavicle

Transverse humeral lig.—

Synovial sheath of Biceps—

Subscapularis bursa

36 Synovial Capsule of the Shoulder Joint: Ligaments at the Lateral End of the Clavicle

Observe:

1. The capsule cannot extend on to the lesser and greater tubercles of the humerus, because the 4 short muscles (Sub-scapularis, Supraspinatus, Infraspinatus, and Teres Minor) are inserted there, but it can and does extend inferiorly on to the surgical neck.

2. The capsule has two prolongations: (a) where it forms a synovial sheath for the tendon of the long head of Biceps in its osseo-fibrous tunnel, and (b) below the coracoid process where it forms a bursa between Subscapularis tendon and the margin of the glenoid cavity.

3. The conoid and trapezoid ligaments are so directed that the clavicle shall hold the scapula laterally.

36.1

Demonstrating that so long as the coraco-clavicular ligament is intact, the acromion cannot be driven under the clavicle. This ligament, however, does not prevent protraction and retraction of the acromion.

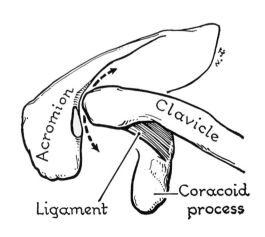

Acromion

Clavicle

Ligament

Coracoid process

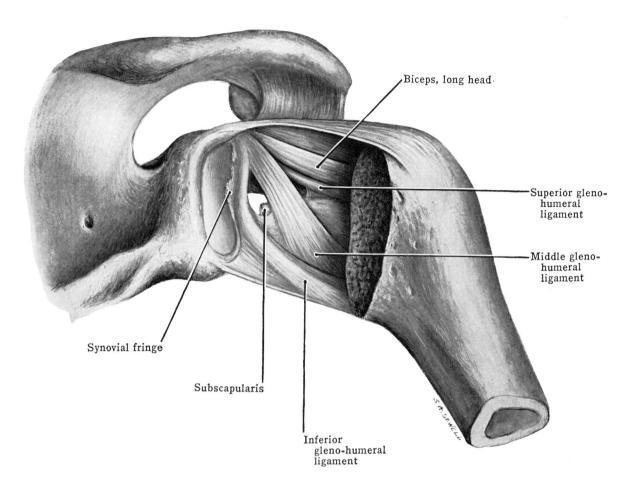

Biceps, long head

Superior gleno-
humeral
ligament

Middle gleno-
humeral
ligament

Synovial fringe

Subscapularis

Inferior
gleno-humeral
ligament

37 Interior of the Shoulder Joint

Exposed from behind by cutting away the posterior part of the capsule and sawing
off the head of the humerus.

Observe:

1. The 3 thickenings of the anterior part of the fibrous capsule,
   called the gleno-humeral ligaments, which are visible from
   within the joint, but not from without.

2. How these 3 ligaments and the long tendon of Biceps converge on the supraglenoid tubercle.

3. The slender superior ligament parallel to the Biceps tendon;

the middle ligament free medially due to the fact that the
Subscapularis bursa communicates with the joint cavity
both above this ligament and below it; the inferior ligament
contributing largely to the anterior lip of the glenoid
labrum, much as the Biceps contributes to the posterior lip
(see fig. 38).

4. The synovial fringe, constantly present, that overlies the
   anterior part of the glenoid cavity.

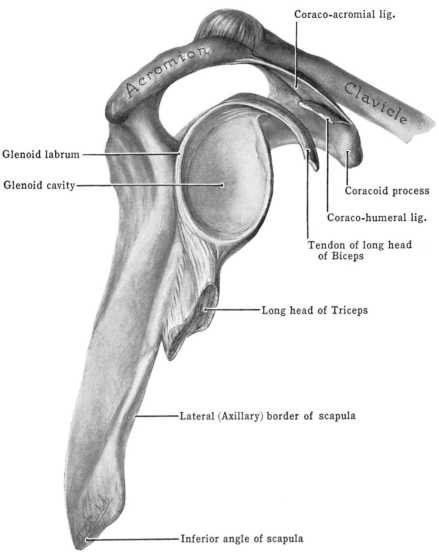

Coraco-acromial lig.

Acromion

Clavicle

Glenoid labrum

Glenoid cavity

Coracoid process

Coraco-humeral lig.

Tendon of long head
of Biceps

Long head of Triceps

Lateral (Axillary) border of scapula

Inferior angle of scapula

38 Glenoid Cavity, lateral view: Orientation of the Scapula

Observe:

1. The cavity overhung by the resilient coraco-acromial arch (i.e., coracoid process, coraco-acromial lig., and acromion), which prevents upward displacement of the head of the humerus.

2. The long head of Triceps arising just below the glenoid cavity.

3. The long head of Biceps arising just above the glenoid cavity. Proximally it is continued as the posterior lip of the glenoid labrum; distally it curves across the front of the head of the humerus—not above it.

4. The orientation of the scapula insures that should the head of the humerus be dislocated downwards it would pass on to the costal surface of the scapula.

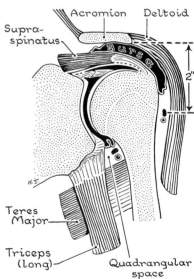

Acromion   Deltoid

Supra-spinatus

Bursa

2″

Teres Major

Triceps (long)

Quadrangular space

38.1 Diagram of the shoulder region, on coronal section, showing the relations of the subacromial bursa (fig. 35).

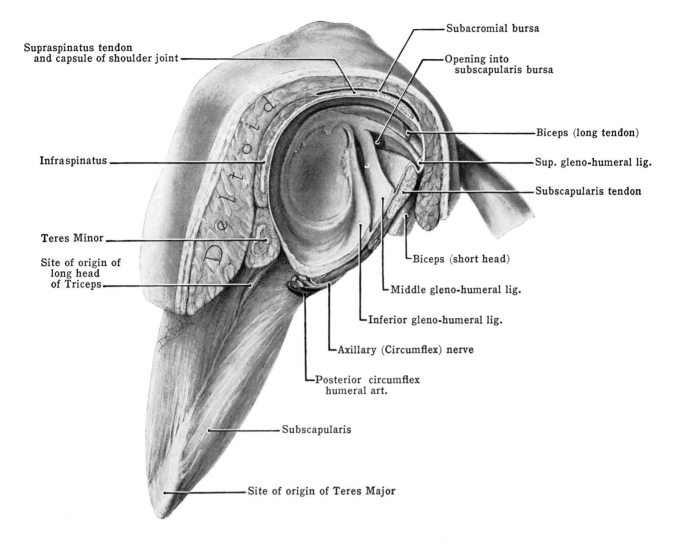

Supraspinatus tendon and capsule of shoulder joint

Infraspinatus

Teres Minor

Site of origin of long head of Triceps

Subacromial bursa

Opening into subscapularis bursa

Biceps (long tendon)

Sup. gleno-humeral lig.

Subscapularis tendon

Biceps (short head)

Middle gleno-humeral lig.

Inferior gleno-humeral lig.

Axillary (Circumflex) nerve

Posterior circumflex humeral art.

Subscapularis

Site of origin of Teres Major

Deltoid

39 Glenoid Cavity and the Relations of the Shoulder Joint, side view

Observe:

1. The fibrous capsule of the joint thickened in front by the three gleno-humeral ligaments which converge from the humerus to be attached with the long tendon of Biceps to the supraglenoid tubercle.

2. Four short muscles (Teres Minor, Infraspinatus, Supraspinatus, and Subscapularis) crossing the joint, blending with the capsule, and retaining the head of the humerus in its socket.

3. The subacromial bursa between the acromion and **Deltoid** above and the tendon of Supraspinatus below.

4. In contact with the capsule inferiorly, the **axillary nerve** and the posterior circumflex humeral artery. **The nerve** giving a twig to the capsule.

5. The Subscapularis bursa (cf. fig. 36) opening **above and** below the middle gleno-humeral ligament. Several **synovial** folds overlapping the glenoid cavity.

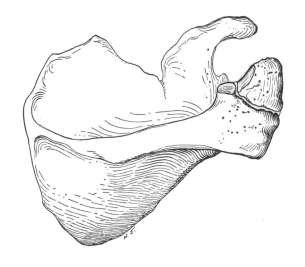

40 Unfused Acromial Epiphysis (Os acromiale)

In 16 of 194 dissecting room subjects aged over thirty years, the acromial epiphysis had failed to fuse. The epiphyseal line was transverse and passed either through or just behind the clavicular facet. The condition was bilateral in 5 subjects (10 limbs) and unilateral in 11 subjects (7 being on the right side only and 4 on the left only). (*J.C.B.G.*)

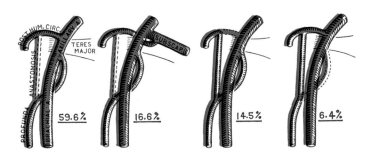

41 Circumflex and Profunda Arteries

Four types of variations in origin of the posterior humeral circumflex and profunda brachii arteries; in 2.9% the arteries were otherwise irregular. Percentages are based on 235 specimens. (*J.C.B.G.*)

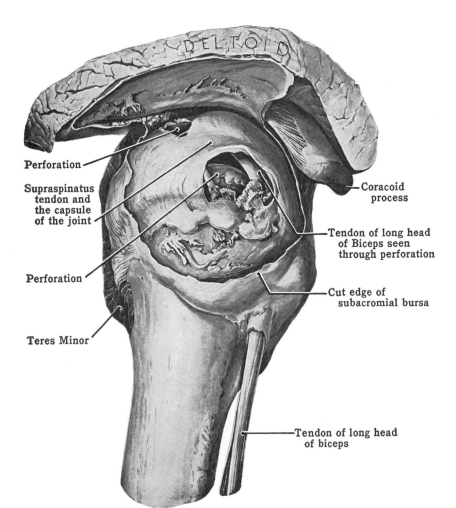

Perforation

Supraspinatus tendon and the capsule of the joint

Perforation

Teres Minor

Coracoid process

Tendon of long head of Biceps seen through perforation

Cut edge of subacromial bursa

Tendon of long head of biceps

42 Attrition of the Supraspinatus Tendon

As a result of wearing away of the Supraspinatus tendon and underlying capsule, the subacromial bursa and the shoulder joint come into wide-open communication. The intracapsular part of the long tendon of the Biceps becomes frayed—even worn away—leaving it adherent to the intertubercular sulcus, as in figures 28, A and B.

Of 95 dissecting room subjects of proved age, none of the 18 under fifty years of age had a perforation, but 4 of the 19 between fifty and sixty years, and 23 of the 57 over sixty years had perforations. The perforation was bilateral in 11 subjects (22 limbs) and unilateral in 14 subjects (8 being on the right side only and 6 on the left only). (*J.C.B.G.* and *C.G.S.*)

VARIATIONS

43 Variations in the Anterior Part of the Shoulder Joint, in older subjects

(PREPARATIONS BY DR. ROSS G. MACKENZIE.)

Observe:

I. The tendon of Subscapularis almost alone guarding the front of the shoulder joint. The middle gleno-humeral ligament in miniature and blending with the inferior glenohumeral ligament to form the anterior part of the glenoid labrum. These two ligaments making individual contributions to the thickness of the fibrous capsule. A large pouch-like subscapularis bursa, above Subscapularis and covering the root of the coracoid process.

II. The middle glenohumeral ligament broad, with free borders, and with its apex converging on the supraglenoid tubercle, largely concealing the tendon of Subscapularis. These two guarding the front of the joint. The inferior ligament forming only the lower half of the anterior part of the labrum; there is here no upper half.

III. The tendon of Subscapularis very thick. The middle and inferior glenohumeral ligaments poorly developed and contributing little to the thickness of the fibrous capsule. The joint cavity extending between the upper part of the margin of the glenoid cavity and the glenoid labrum with the result that the labrum is loosely suspended by a "synovial mesentery".

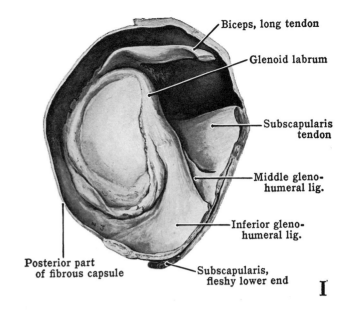

Biceps, long tendon

Glenoid labrum

Subscapularis tendon

Middle gleno-humeral lig.

Inferior gleno-humeral lig.

Posterior part of fibrous capsule

Subscapularis, fleshy lower end

I

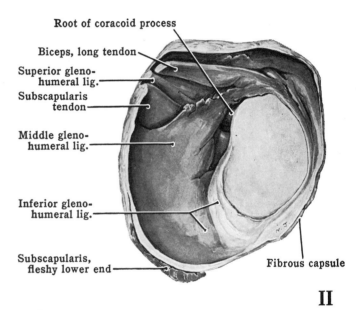

Root of coracoid process

Biceps, long tendon

Superior gleno-humeral lig.

Subscapularis tendon

Middle gleno-humeral lig.

Inferior gleno-humeral lig.

Subscapularis, fleshy lower end

Fibrous capsule

II

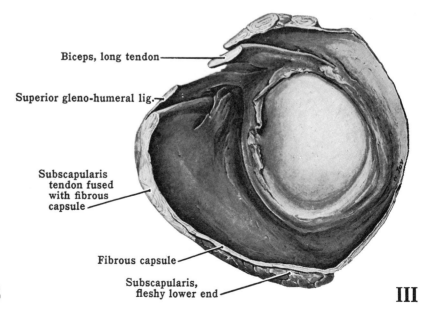

Biceps, long tendon

Superior gleno-humeral lig.

Subscapularis tendon fused with fibrous capsule

Fibrous capsule

Subscapularis, fleshy lower end

III

VARIATIONS

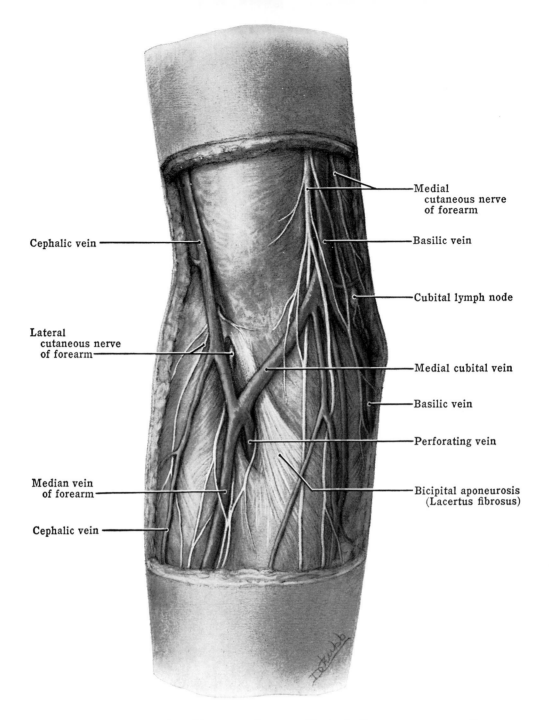

Cephalic vein

Lateral
cutaneous nerve
of forearm

Median vein
of forearm

Cephalic vein

Medial
cutaneous nerve
of forearm

Basilic vein

Cubital lymph node

Medial cubital vein

Basilic vein

Perforating vein

Bicipital aponeurosis
(Lacertus fibrosus)

44   Front of Elbow, Superficial Structures—I

Observe:

1. In the forearm, the superficial veins—cephalic, median, basilic and their connecting channels—making a (variable) M-shaped pattern.

2. The median cubital vein separated from the brachial artery (fig. 45) only by the bicipital aponeurosis.

3. A perforating vein, lateral to the bicipital aponeurosis, connecting the deep veins to the median cubital vein.

4. In the arm, the cephalic and basilic veins occupying the bicipital furrows—one on each side of Biceps.

5. In the lateral bicipital furrow, the lateral cutaneous nerve of the forearm appearing 1″ to 2″ above the elbow-crease, and piercing the deep fascia 1″ below it.

6. In the medial bicipital furrow, the medial cutaneous nerve of the forearm becoming cutaneous about the mid point of the arm.

7. Cutaneous nerves mainly on a deeper plane than superficial veins.

8. The most distal superficial lymph node of the upper limb lying about 1″ above the medial epicondyle.

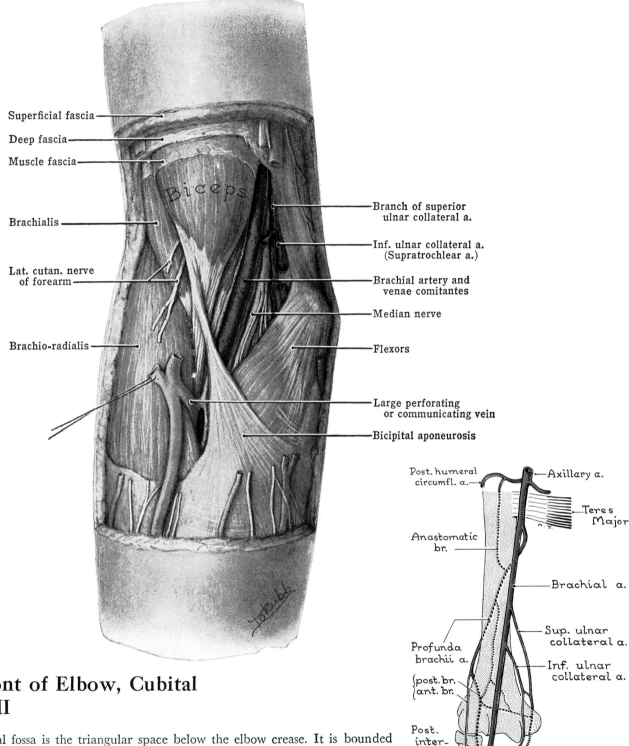

Superficial fascia —
Deep fascia —
Muscle fascia —

Biceps

Brachialis —

Lat. cutan. nerve of forearm —

Brachio-radialis —

Branch of superior ulnar collateral a.

Inf. ulnar collateral a. (Supratrochlear a.)

Brachial artery and venae comitantes

Median nerve

Flexors

Large perforating or communicating vein

Bicipital aponeurosis

Post. humeral circumfl. a.
Axillary a.
Teres Major
Anastomatic br.
Brachial a.
Profunda brachii a.
Sup. ulnar collateral a.
Inf. ulnar collateral a.
{post. br. {ant. br.
Post. inter- osseous recurr.
Ant.} Ulnar Post.} recurrent aa.
Common} Anterior} Inteross. aa. Posterior}
Radial a.   Ulnar a.

45 Front of Elbow, Cubital Fossa—II

The cubital fossa is the triangular space below the elbow crease. It is bounded laterally by the extensor muscles (represented by Brachio-radialis) and medially by the flexor muscles (represented by Pronator Teres). The apex is where these two muscles meet distally.

Observe:

1. The large perforating vein piercing the deep fascia at the apex of the fossa.
2. The 3 chief contents—Biceps tendon, brachial artery, and median nerve.
3. Biceps tendon, on approaching its insertion (fig. 29), rotating through a right angle, and the bicipital aponeurosis springing from the tendon.

45.1

Diagram: Anastomoses about the elbow joint.

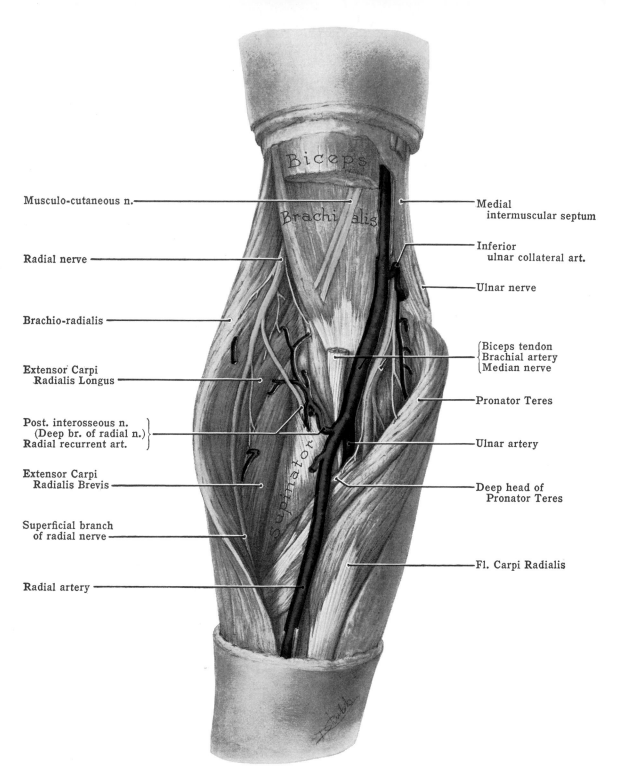

Musculo-cutaneous n.

Radial nerve

Brachio-radialis

Extensor Carpi Radialis Longus

Post. interosseous n. (Deep br. of radial n.) Radial recurrent art.

Extensor Carpi Radialis Brevis

Superficial branch of radial nerve

Radial artery

Biceps

Brachialis

Supinator

Medial intermuscular septum

Inferior ulnar collateral art.

Ulnar nerve

Biceps tendon Brachial artery Median nerve

Pronator Teres

Ulnar artery

Deep head of Pronator Teres

Fl. Carpi Radialis

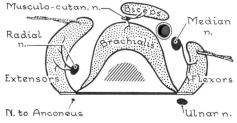

Musculo-cutan. n.

Biceps

Radial n.

Brachialis

Median n.

Extensors

Flexors

N. to Anconeus

Ulnar n.

46.1

Diagram: Motor nerves about the elbow region. (See fig. 55.)

46   Front of Elbow, Deep Structures—III

Part of Biceps is excised and the cubital fossa is opened widely.

Observe

1. The floor of the cubital fossa—Brachialis and Supinator.

2. The brachial artery lying between Biceps tendon and median nerve, and dividing into 2 nearly equal branches—the ulnar and radial arteries.

3. The median nerve supplying flexor muscles; hence its motor branches arise from its medial side,—the twig to the deep head of Pronator Teres excepted.

4. The radial nerve supplying extensor muscles; hence its motor branches arise from its lateral side,—the twig to Brachialis excepted. [The radial nerve has been displaced laterally, so its lateral branches appear in the drawing to run medially.]

5. The posterior interosseous nerve piercing Supinator.

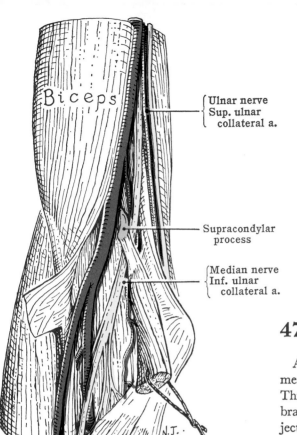

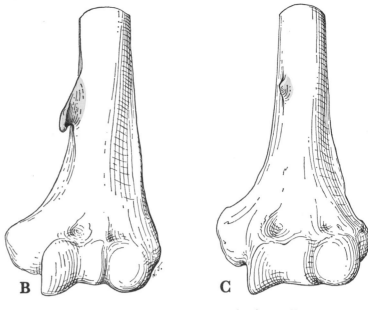

47 Supracondylar Process of the Humerus

A and B are from opposite sides of the same subject. C is a left-sided specimen. A fibrous band joins this process or spine to the medial epicondyle. Through the foramen so-formed the median nerve passes, as here, and the brachial artery may go with it. A process was found in 7 of 1000 living subjects (R. J. Terry).

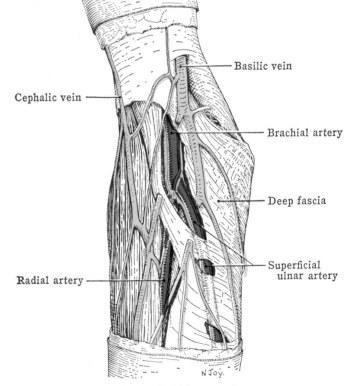

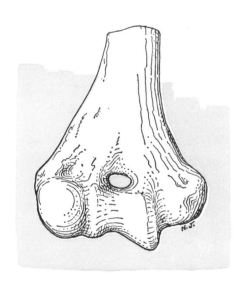

48 Supratrochlear Foramen

This hole, closed in life by membrane, was found in 4.2% of white people and 12.8% of American Negroes. It was more common on the left side than on the right, and in females than in males. (M. Trotter.)

48.1 Superficial Ulnar Artery

The ulnar artery descended superficial to the flexor muscles in 3.1% of 188 dissected limbs (paired) and in 2.7% of 542 students' limbs (paired). Of these 21 superficial arteries found in 730 limbs, 3 were present bilaterally, 8 in the right limb only, and 7 in the left only. (J. W. Hazlett.)

VARIATIONS AND ANOMALIES

(Other variations, figs. 27, 28, 97.)

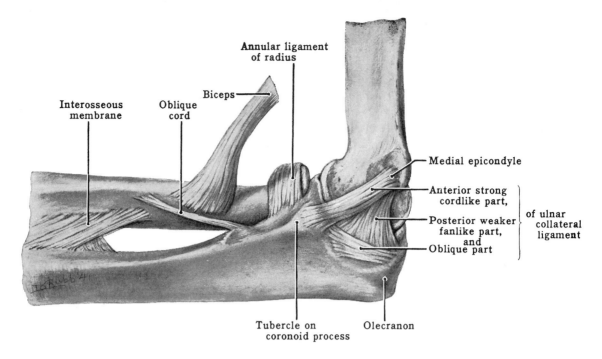

Annular ligament
of radius

Biceps

Oblique
cord

Interosseous
membrane

Medial epicondyle

Anterior strong
cordlike part,

Posterior weaker
fanlike part,
and
Oblique part

of ulnar
collateral
ligament

Tubercle on
coronoid process

Olecranon

49 Ulnar Collateral Ligament of the Elbow Joint (Medial Lig.)

The anterior part is a strong, round cord, taut in extension of the joint; the posterior part is a weak fan, taut in flexion of the joint; the oblique fibres merely deepen the socket for the trochlea of the humerus. Fl. Digitorum Superficialis arises from the cord and from an area of bone at each end of the cord; it also arises from the anterior oblique line of the radius (fig. 52).

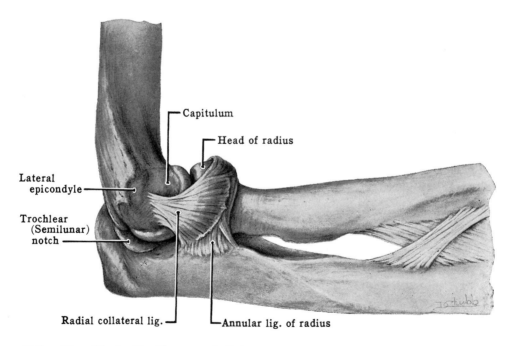

Capitulum

Head of radius

Lateral
epicondyle

Trochlear
(Semilunar)
notch

Radial collateral lig.

Annular lig. of radius

50 Radial Collateral Ligament of the Elbow Joint (Lateral Lig.)

The fan-shaped lateral ligament is attached to the annular ligament of radius, but its superficial fibres are continued onwards to the radius as Supinator—hence the ragged edge. Supinator also arises from the annular ligament and the supinator crest of the ulna, which limits the supinator fossa posteriorly.

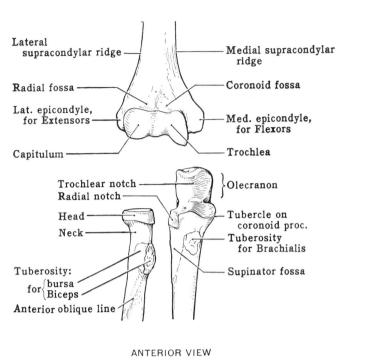

Lateral supracondylar ridge

Medial supracondylar ridge

Radial fossa

Coronoid fossa

Lat. epicondyle, for Extensors

Med. epicondyle, for Flexors

Capitulum

Trochlea

Trochlear notch

Radial notch

Olecranon

Head

Tubercle on coronoid proc.

Neck

Tuberosity for Brachialis

Tuberosity: for { bursa Biceps

Supinator fossa

Anterior oblique line

ANTERIOR VIEW

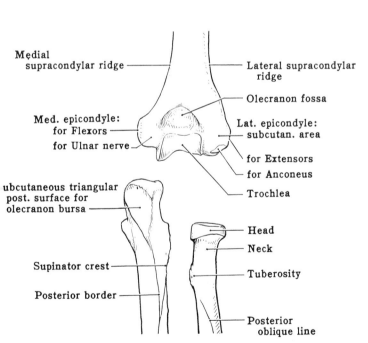

Medial supracondylar ridge

Lateral supracondylar ridge

Olecranon fossa

Med. epicondyle: for Flexors

for Ulnar nerve

Lat. epicondyle: subcutan. area

for Extensors

for Anconeus

Trochlea

ubcutaneous triangular post. surface for olecranon bursa

Head

Neck

Supinator crest

Tuberosity

Posterior border

Posterior oblique line

POSTERIOR VIEW

51 Bones of the Elbow Region

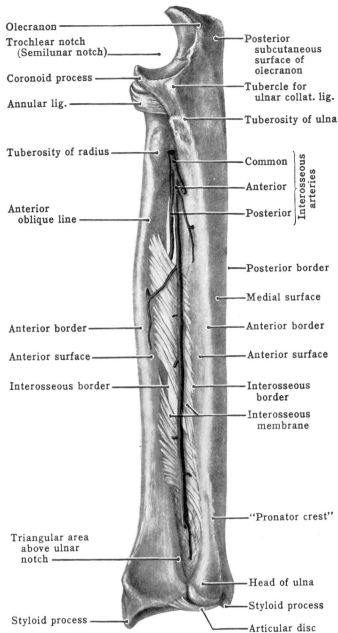

Olecranon

Trochlear notch (Semilunar notch)

Coronoid process

Annular lig.

Tuberosity of radius

Anterior oblique line

Anterior border

Anterior surface

Interosseous border

Posterior subcutaneous surface of olecranon

Tubercle for ulnar collat. lig.

Tuberosity of ulna

Common

Anterior

Posterior

} Interosseous arteries

Posterior border

Medial surface

Anterior border

Anterior surface

Interosseous border

Interosseous membrane

"Pronator crest"

Triangular area above ulnar notch

Head of ulna

Styloid process

Styloid process

Articular disc

52 Flexor Aspect of Radius and Ulna: Ligaments of the Radio-ulnar Joints: Interosseous Arteries

The ligament of the proximal radio-ulnar joint is the annular ligament; that of the distal joint is the articular disc; that of the middle joint is the interosseous membrane. The general direction of the fibres of the membrane is such that an upward thrust to the hand, and therefore received by the radius, is transmitted to the ulna. The membrane is attached to the interosseous borders of the radius and ulna, but it also spreads on to their surfaces.

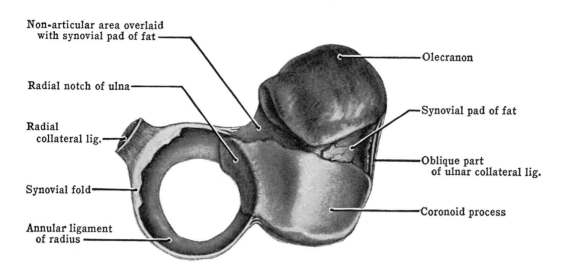

Non-articular area overlaid with synovial pad of fat

Radial notch of ulna

Radial collateral lig.

Synovial fold

Annular ligament of radius

Olecranon

Synovial pad of fat

Oblique part of ulnar collateral lig.

Coronoid process

53 Socket for Head of Radius and Trochlea of Humerus, from above

The annular ligament keeps the head of the radius applied to the radial notch of the ulna, and with it forms a cup-shaped socket (i.e. wide above, narrow below); hence the head of the radius cannot be pulled distally through its socket.

The annular ligament is bound to the humerus by the radial collateral ligament of the elbow.

A crescentic synovial fold occupies the angular space between the head of the radius and the capitulum of the humerus. Similarly, synovial folds containing fat occupy the 2 angular non-articular areas between the coronoid process and the olecranon.

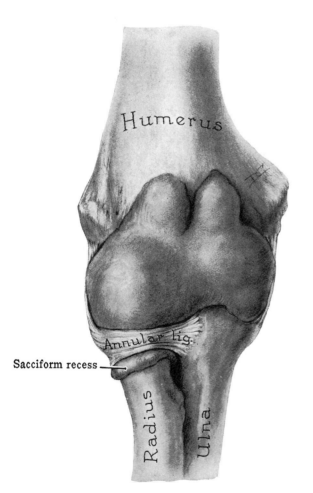

Humerus

Annular lig.

Sacciform recess

Radius

Ulna

54 Articular Cavity of the Elbow and Proximal Radio-ulnar Joints, injected with wax, anterior view

The cavity was distended with wax. The fibrous capsule has been removed; the synovial capsule remains.

The sacciform recess that encircles the neck of the radius serves a similar function to a similar recess at the distal radio-ulnar joint (fig. 90).

(For posterior view see fig. 57.)

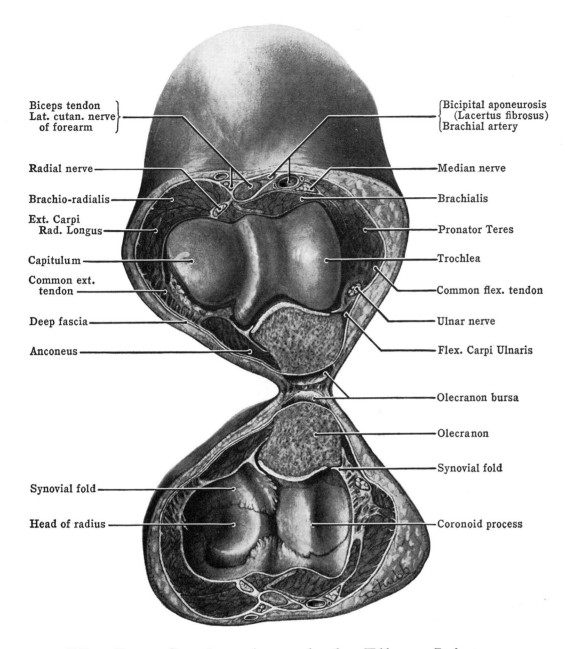

Biceps tendon
Lat. cutan. nerve
of forearm

Bicipital aponeurosis
(Lacertus fibrosus)
Brachial artery

Radial nerve

Median nerve

Brachio-radialis

Brachialis

Ext. Carpi
Rad. Longus

Pronator Teres

Capitulum

Trochlea

Common ext.
tendon

Common flex. tendon

Deep fascia

Ulnar nerve

Anconeus

Flex. Carpi Ulnaris

Olecranon bursa

Olecranon

Synovial fold

Synovial fold

Head of radius

Coronoid process

55   Cross Section through the Elbow Joint

Nerves:—The radial nerve is in direct contact with the capsule of the joint; the ulnar nerve is in contact with the ulnar collateral ligament; the median nerve is separated from the capsule by a film of fleshy fibres of Brachialis.

Synovial folds, containing fat, overlie the periphery of the head of the radius and also the non-articular indentations on the trochlear notch of the ulna.

A fracture across the olecranon would bring the subcutaneous olecranon bursa into communication with the articular cavity.

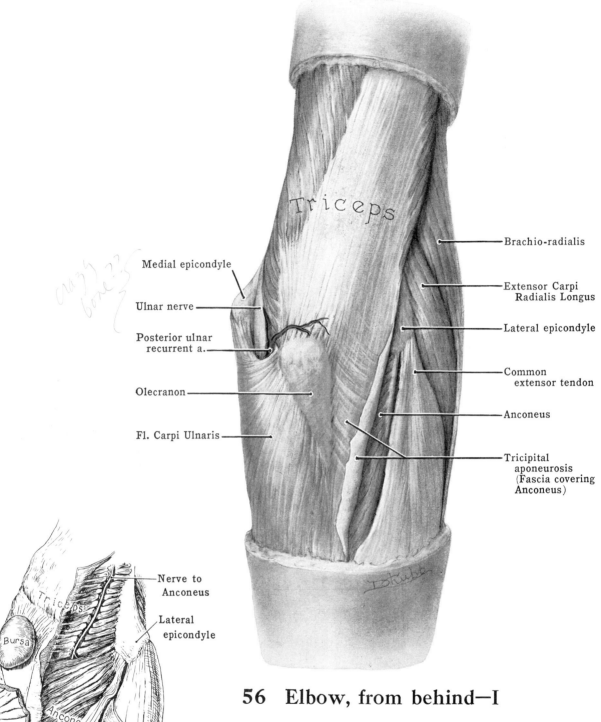

Triceps

Medial epicondyle

Ulnar nerve

Posterior ulnar recurrent a.

Olecranon

Fl. Carpi Ulnaris

Brachio-radialis

Extensor Carpi Radialis Longus

Lateral epicondyle

Common extensor tendon

Anconeus

Tricipital aponeurosis (Fascia covering Anconeus)

Nerve to Anconeus

Lateral epicondyle

Triceps

Bursa

Anconeus

Extensor

56.1

Anconeus and its nerve: Subcutaneous olecranon bursa; Interosseous recurrent artery.

56   Elbow, from behind—I

Observe:

1. Triceps inserted not only into the upper surface of the olecranon but also, via the deep fascia covering Anconeus—"tricipital aponeurosis"—into lateral border of olecranon.

2. The subcutaneous and palpable posterior surfaces of—the medial epicondyle, lateral epicondyle, and olecranon.

3. The ulnar nerve, also palpable, running subfascially behind the medial epicondyle. Distal to this point it disappears deep to the two heads of Fl. Carpi Ulnaris.

4. The two heads of Fl. Carpi Ulnaris: one arising from the common flexor tendon, the other from the medial border of the olecranon and posterior border of the shaft of the ulna.

5. The continuous linear origin from the humerus of the superficial extensor muscles. These are Brachio-radialis; Ext. Carpi Radialis Longus, common extensor tendon, and Anconeus (fig. 58).

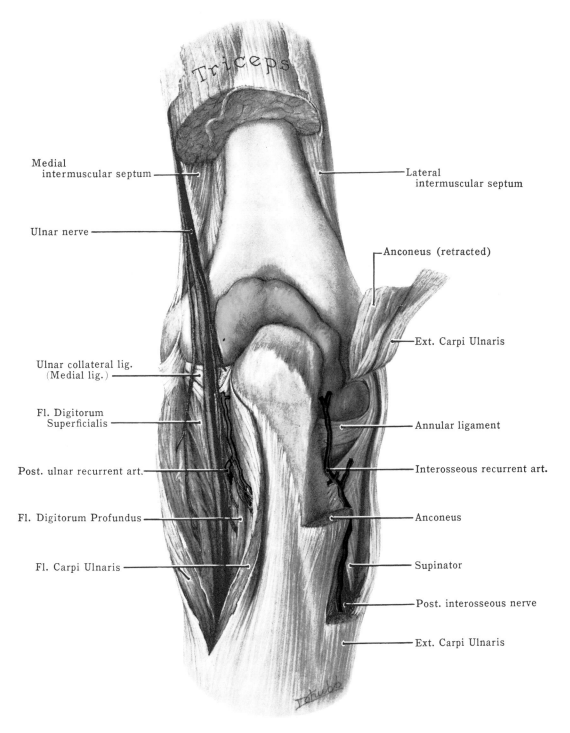

Medial intermuscular septum

Ulnar nerve

Ulnar collateral lig. (Medial lig.)

Fl. Digitorum Superficialis

Post. ulnar recurrent art.

Fl. Digitorum Profundus

Fl. Carpi Ulnaris

Lateral intermuscular septum

Anconeus (retracted)

Ext. Carpi Ulnaris

Annular ligament

Interosseous recurrent art.

Anconeus

Supinator

Post. interosseous nerve

Ext. Carpi Ulnaris

57 Elbow, from behind—II

The lower portion of Triceps is removed.

Observe:

1. The ulnar nerve descending: (1st) subfascially, within the posterior compartment of the arm, applied to the medial head of Triceps, and behind the medial epicondyle; (2nd), applied to the medial ligament of the joint; and (3rd), between Fl. Carpi Ulnaris and Fl. Digitorum Profundus.

2. The first branches of the ulnar nerve distributed to Fl. Carpi Ulnaris, half of Profundus, and the joint.

3. Laterally, the synovial membrane protruding below the annular ligament as a sacciform recess, as in fig. 54. The joint is here covered with Anconeus and the common extensor tendon, including Ext. Carpi Ulnaris.

4. The posterior interosseous nerve [deep radial n.], appearing through Supinator $2\frac{1}{2}''$ below the head of the radius.

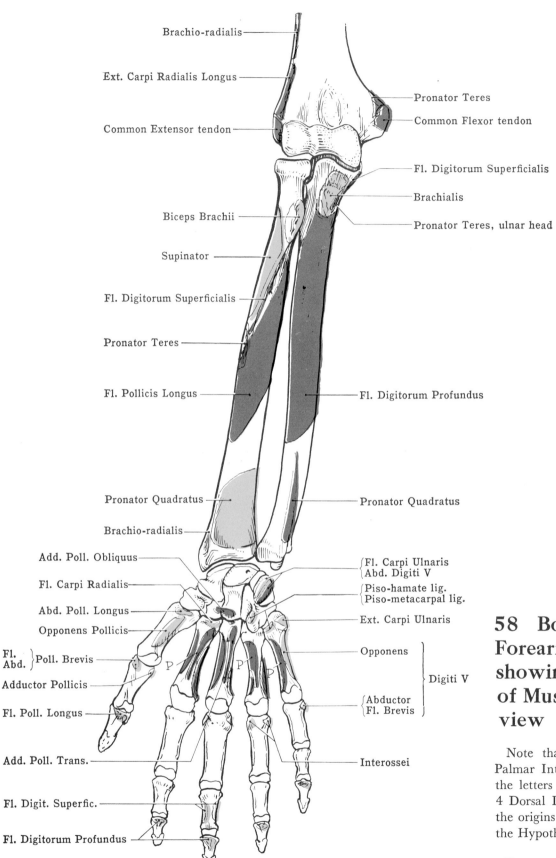

Brachio-radialis

Ext. Carpi Radialis Longus

Common Extensor tendon

Biceps Brachii

Supinator

Fl. Digitorum Superficialis

Pronator Teres

Fl. Pollicis Longus

Pronator Quadratus

Brachio-radialis

Add. Poll. Obliquus

Fl. Carpi Radialis

Abd. Poll. Longus

Opponens Pollicis

Fl.
Abd. } Poll. Brevis

Adductor Pollicis

Fl. Poll. Longus

Add. Poll. Trans.

Fl. Digit. Superfic.

Fl. Digitorum Profundus

Pronator Teres

Common Flexor tendon

Fl. Digitorum Superficialis

Brachialis

Pronator Teres, ulnar head

Fl. Digitorum Profundus

Pronator Quadratus

Fl. Carpi Ulnaris
Abd. Digiti V

Piso-hamate lig.
Piso-metacarpal lig.

Ext. Carpi Ulnaris

Opponens

} Digiti V

Abductor
Fl. Brevis }

Interossei

P   P   P

58 Bones of the Forearm and Hand showing Attachments of Muscles, anterior view

Note that the origins of the 3 Palmar Interossei are indicated by the letters P,P,P, the origins of the 4 Dorsal Interossei by colour only; the origins of the 3 Thenar and 2 of the Hypothenar muscles are omitted.

(For posterior view, see fig. 77. For humerus, see figs. 29 & 30.)

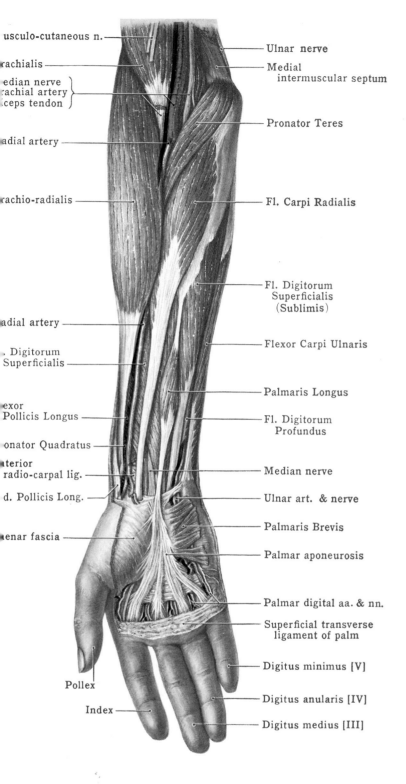

usculo-cutaneous n.
rachialis
edian nerve
rachial artery
ceps tendon
adial artery
rachio-radialis
adial artery
. Digitorum Superficialis
exor Pollicis Longus
onator Quadratus
nterior radio-carpal lig.
d. Pollicis Long.
enar fascia
Pollex
Index

Ulnar nerve
Medial intermuscular septum
Pronator Teres
Fl. Carpi Radialis
Fl. Digitorum Superficialis (Sublimis)
Flexor Carpi Ulnaris
Palmaris Longus
Fl. Digitorum Profundus
Median nerve
Ulnar art. & nerve
Palmaris Brevis
Palmar aponeurosis
Palmar digital aa. & nn.
Superficial transverse ligament of palm
Digitus minimus [V]
Digitus anularis [IV]
Digitus medius [III]

59 Superficial Muscles on the Front of the Forearm: Palmar Aponeurosis

Observe:

1. At the elbow, the brachial artery lying between Biceps tendon and median nerve, and there bifurcating into the radial and ulnar arteries.

2. At the wrist, the radial artery lateral to Fl. Carpi Radialis tendon and the ulnar artery lateral to Fl. Carpi Ulnaris tendon.

3. In the forearm, the radial artery lying between two muscle groups or two motor territories. The muscles lateral to the artery are supplied by the radial nerve; those medial to it, by the median and ulnar nerves: so, no motor nerve crosses the radial artery.

4. The lateral group of muscles, represented by Brachio-radialis, slightly overlapping the radial artery which otherwise is superficial.

5. The medial or flexor group of muscles is in three layers: superficial (shown here), middle, and deep (figs. 60 & 61).

6. The four superficial muscles, viz., Pronator Teres, Fl. Carpi Radialis, Palmaris Longus and Fl. Carpi Ulnaris, radiating from the medial epicondyle. The muscle of the middle layer Fl. Digitorum Superficialis, is partially in view.

7. Palmaris Longus continued into the palm as the palmar aponeurosis, which receives an accession of fibres from the flexor retinaculum and divides into 4 longitudinal bands, one for each finger. These bands are crossed on their deep surface by traverse fibres.

8. Palmaris Brevis arising from this aponeurosis.

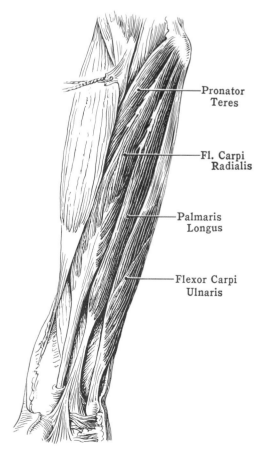

Pronator Teres
Fl. Carpi Radialis
Palmaris Longus
Flexor Carpi Ulnaris

59.1

Diagram. The fleshy fibers of Palmaris Longus usually extend proximally as far as the medial epicondyle.

(For variations, see fig. 97-D)

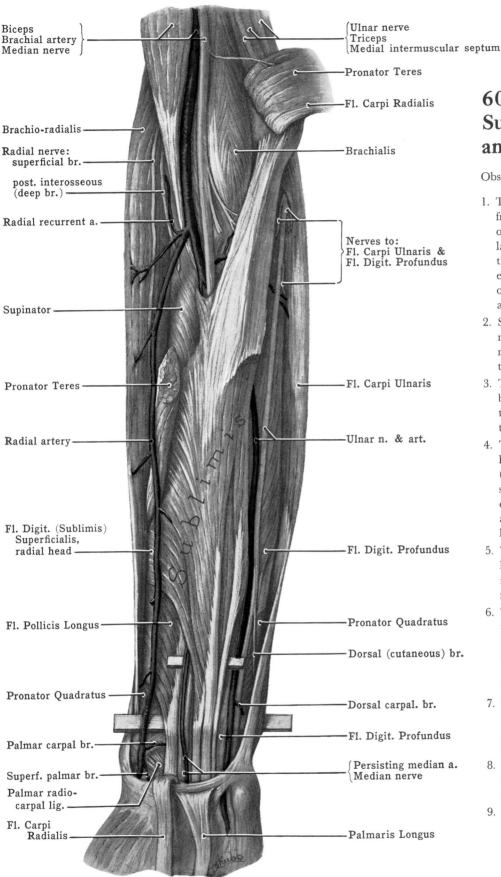

Biceps
Brachial artery
Median nerve

Brachio-radialis

Radial nerve:
superficial br.

post. interosseous
(deep br.)

Radial recurrent a.

Supinator

Pronator Teres

Radial artery

Fl. Digit. (Sublimis)
Superficialis,
radial head

Fl. Pollicis Longus

Pronator Quadratus

Palmar carpal br.

Superf. palmar br.

Palmar radio-
carpal lig.

Fl. Carpi
Radialis

Ulnar nerve
Triceps
Medial intermuscular septum

Pronator Teres

Fl. Carpi Radialis

Brachialis

Nerves to:
Fl. Carpi Ulnaris &
Fl. Digit. Profundus

Fl. Carpi Ulnaris

Ulnar n. & art.

Fl. Digit. Profundus

Pronator Quadratus

Dorsal (cutaneous) br.

Dorsal carpal. br.

Fl. Digit. Profundus

Persisting median a.
Median nerve

Palmaris Longus

Sublimis

60 Flexor Digitoru
Superficialis (Sublim
and Related Structur

Observe:

1. The oblique origin of Superficialis from—(a) the medial epicondyle of the humerus, (b) the ulnar collateral ligament of the elbow, (c) the tubercle of the coronoid process, (d) the anterior oblique line of the radius and perhaps the anterior border below it.

2. Superficialis, which like the 3 muscles in front of it and the $2\frac{1}{2}$ muscles behind it, is supplied by the median nerve.

3. The sequence of muscles crossed by the radial artery. At the wrist the artery crosses the radius and the palmar radio-carpal lig.

4. The radial artery having muscular and 3 anastomotic branches (recurrent, palmar carpal, and superficial palmar). Neither muscle nor motor nerve crosses the artery, but Brachio-radialis overlaps it.

5. The ulnar artery descending obliquely behind Superficialis to meet and accompany the ulnar nerve.

6. The ulnar nerve descending vertically near the medial border of Superficialis. It is exposed by splitting the septum between Superficialis and Fl. Carpi Ulnaris.

7. The median nerve descending vertically behind Superficialis, clinging to it, and appearing at its lateral border.

8. The digital tendons at the wrist— 3 and 4 large and side by side, 5 slender and 2 behind (fig. 64).

9. The median artery, here persisting.

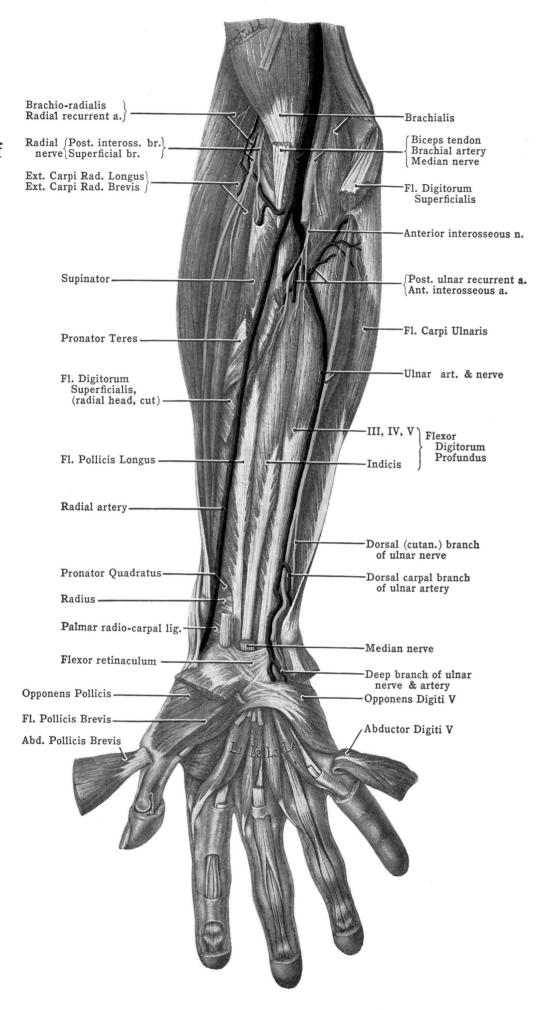

51 Deep Flexors of the Digits and the Related Structures

Observe:

The two deep, digital flexor muscles, viz., Fl. Pollicis Longus and Fl. Digitorum Profundus, forming a sheet of muscle that arises from the flexor aspects of radius, interosseous membrane, and ulna between the origin of Superficialis proximally and Pronator Quadratus distally.

The portion of Profundus for the index, here free above the wrist; the portions for digits III, IV, and V, fused.

The median nerve crossing in front of the ulnar artery at the elbow and behind the flexor retinaculum at the wrist.

The ulnar nerve is sheltered by the medial epicondyle at the elbow and by the pisiform bone at the wrist.

The ulnar nerve entering the forearm behind the medial epicondyle, descending on Profundus, joined by the ulnar artery, continuing on Profundus to the wrist, and there passing in front of the flexor retinaculum and lateral to the pisiform it enters the palm.

At the elbow it supplies Fl. Carpi Ulnaris and ½ Profundus; above the wrist it gives off its dorsal branch.

The recurrent, common interosseous, and dorsal carpal branches as well as muscular branches of the ulnar artery.

The 4 Lumbricals arising from Profundus tendons, seen better in figure 68.

Brachio-radialis
Radial recurrent a.

Radial { Post. inteross. br. } nerve { Superficial br. }

Ext. Carpi Rad. Longus
Ext. Carpi Rad. Brevis

Supinator

Pronator Teres

Fl. Digitorum Superficialis, (radial head, cut)

Fl. Pollicis Longus

Radial artery

Pronator Quadratus

Radius

Palmar radio-carpal lig.

Flexor retinaculum

Opponens Pollicis

Fl. Pollicis Brevis

Abd. Pollicis Brevis

Brachialis

Biceps tendon
Brachial artery
Median nerve

Fl. Digitorum Superficialis

Anterior interosseous n.

Post. ulnar recurrent a.
Ant. interosseous a.

Fl. Carpi Ulnaris

Ulnar art. & nerve

III, IV, V } Flexor
Indicis } Digitorum Profundus

Dorsal (cutan.) branch of ulnar nerve

Dorsal carpal branch of ulnar artery

Median nerve

Deep branch of ulnar nerve & artery
Opponens Digiti V

Abductor Digiti V

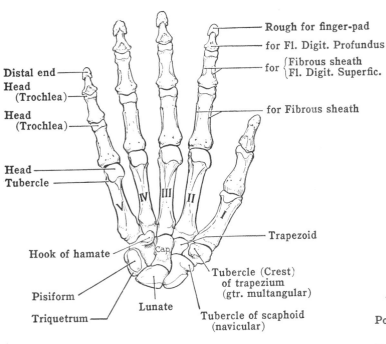

Rough for finger-pad
for Fl. Digit. Profundus
for { Fibrous sheath
      Fl. Digit. Superfic.
for Fibrous sheath

Distal end
Head
(Trochlea)

Head
(Trochlea)

Head
Tubercle

Hook of hamate
Pisiform
Triquetrum

Cap.
Lunate

Trapezoid

Tubercle (Crest)
of trapezium
(gtr. multangular)

Tubercle of scaphoid
(navicular)

V IV III II I

62 Bones of the Hand, palmar aspect

(See also fig. 95.)

(For dorsal aspect, see fig. 86.)

62.1 Muscles attached to the Anterior Aspect of the Radius and Ulna

Observe:

1. The anterior aspect of the ulna, clothed with (a) Brachialis, which is inserted into the coronoid process, (fig. 58), and distal to this with (b) Fl. Digitorum Profundus, which arises as far distally as Pronator Quadratus. Profundus also arising from the upper ⅔ of the medial aspect and with Fl. Carpi Ulnaris arising from the deep fascia.

2. The anterior aspect of the radius, clothed with (a) Supinator above the anterior oblique line and, distal to this, with (b) Fl. Pollicis Longus as far as Pronator Quadratus. Fl. Digitorum Superficialis, here removed, arises from the oblique line.

3. The 5 tendons of the deep digital flexors, side by side, converging on the carpal tunnel, and, having traversed it, diverging to the 5 terminal phalanges.

4. Biceps inserted into the medial aspect of radius, hence it can rotate laterally, i.e., supinate; whereas Pronator Teres by invading the lateral surface can rotate medially, i.e., pronate.

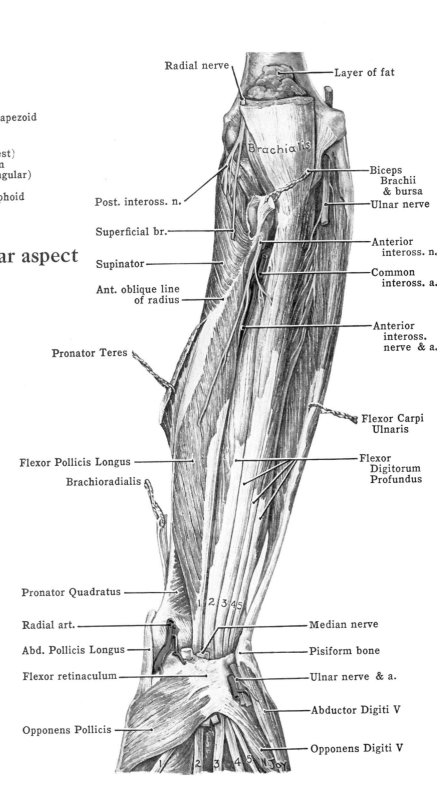

Radial nerve
Layer of fat
Brachialis
Post. inteross. n.
Superficial br.
Supinator
Ant. oblique line of radius
Pronator Teres
Flexor Pollicis Longus
Brachioradialis
Pronator Quadratus
Radial art.
Abd. Pollicis Longus
Flexor retinaculum
Opponens Pollicis

Biceps Brachii & bursa
Ulnar nerve
Anterior inteross. n.
Common inteross. a.
Anterior inteross. nerve & a.
Flexor Carpi Ulnaris
Flexor Digitorum Profundus
Median nerve
Pisiform bone
Ulnar nerve & a.
Abductor Digiti V
Opponens Digiti V

1 2 3 4 5

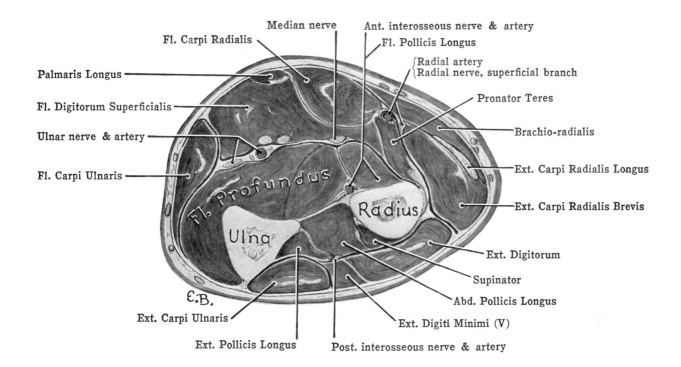

Median nerve
Fl. Carpi Radialis
Ant. interosseous nerve & artery
Fl. Pollicis Longus
Palmaris Longus
{Radial artery
Radial nerve, superficial branch
Fl. Digitorum Superficialis
Pronator Teres
Ulnar nerve & artery
Brachio-radialis
Fl. Carpi Ulnaris
Ext. Carpi Radialis Longus
Ext. Carpi Radialis Brevis
Fl. Profundus
Radius
Ulna
Ext. Digitorum
Supinator
E.B.
Abd. Pollicis Longus
Ext. Carpi Ulnaris
Ext. Digiti Minimi (V)
Ext. Pollicis Longus
Post. interosseous nerve & artery

63 Cross-section through the middle of the Forearm (at level of insertion of the Pronator Teres)

Observe:

1. The interosseous membrane stretching from the interosseous (lateral) border of the ulna to a fibro-cartilaginous labrum along the interosseous (medial) border of the radius and spreading far on to the anterior surface (fig. 52) and less far on to the posterior surface.

2. The ulnar nerve and artery and the median nerve lying in the areolar septum between the superficial and deep digital flexors, i.e., between Fl. Digitorum Superficialis and and Flexores Digitorum Profundus et Pollicis Longus. The ulnar nerve, as usual, clinging to Profundus and supplying its medial part; the median nerve clinging to Superficialis and supplying it. The anterior interosseous branch of the median nerve, placed on the skeletal plane.

3. The radial artery overlapped by Brachio-radialis.

4. The superficial branch of the radial nerve following the anterior border of Extensor Carpi Radialis Brevis; the posterior interosseous nerve lying between the superficial and deep layers of digital extensors.

5. Flexores Digitorum Profundus et Pollicis Longus wrapped around the medial and anterior surfaces of the ulna and the anterior surface of the radius—this being Flexor Territory. Pronator Teres inserted into the lateral surface of the radius—and therefore invading Extensor Territory; hence its ability to pronate.

6. Artificial Spaces, readily created: (a) The space deep to Flexor Carpi Ulnaris extending dorsally to where Fl. Carpi Ulnaris and Fl. Profundus both arise from the deep fascia and through it from the posterior border of the ulna. (b) The space deep to Ext. Carpi Ulnaris. This mucle arises slightly from the deep fascia and through it from the posterior border of the ulna. (c) The space between the superficial and deep digital flexors, noted in item 2, above. (d) The space between the long extensors of the fingers and the deep muscles of the back of the forearm. (e) The space deep to the three lateral muscles of the forearm (Brachio-radialis, Ext. Carpi Radialis Longus et Brevis).

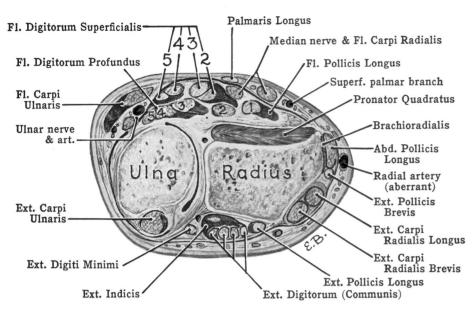

Fl. Digitorum Superficialis

Fl. Digitorum Profundus

Fl. Carpi Ulnaris

Ulnar nerve & art.

Ext. Carpi Ulnaris

Ext. Digiti Minimi

Ext. Indicis

Palmaris Longus

Median nerve & Fl. Carpi Radialis

Fl. Pollicis Longus

Superf. palmar branch

Pronator Quadratus

Brachioradialis

Abd. Pollicis Longus

Radial artery (aberrant)

Ext. Pollicis Brevis

Ext. Carpi Radialis Longus

Ext. Carpi Radialis Brevis

Ext. Pollicis Longus

Ext. Digitorum (Communis)

Ulna   Radius

64   Cross-section through the Forearm, above the wrist

Observe:

1. The synovial cavity of the distal radio-ulnar joint.
2. Fl. Carpi Radialis, Palmaris Longus and Fl. Carpi Ulnaris constituting a surface layer of flexors of the wrist.
3. Deep to these, the long flexors of the digits: (a) The 4 tendons of Fl. Digitorum Superficialis lying two deep, those to the middle and ring fingers being anterior to those to the index and little finger. (b) The 5 tendons of the deep digital flexors, lying side by side, those to the thumb (Fl. Pollicis Longus) and index being free.
4. The ulnar nerve and artery under cover of Fl. Carpi Ulnaris where the pulse of the artery could not be felt. The median nerve at the mid-point on the front of the wrist, deep to Palmaris Longus, and at the lateral border of Fl. Digitorum Superficialis. The radial artery is here aberrant (see fig. 74), so its pulse might be missed.
5. Four tendons on the dorsum of the wrist, large, because, being inserted into metacarpal bones, they work as synergists with the powerful flexors of the digits, whereas the remaining tendons being extensors of the digits, are slender (fig. 86.3).

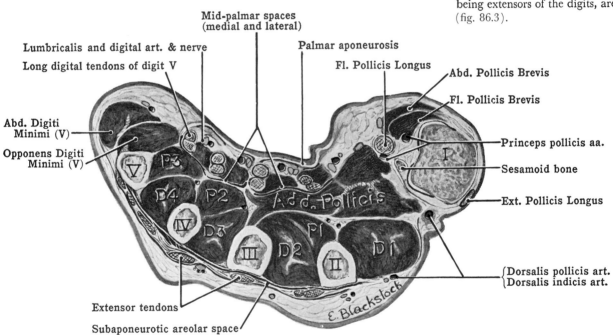

Lumbricalis and digital art. & nerve

Long digital tendons of digit V

Abd. Digiti Minimi (V)

Opponens Digiti Minimi (V)

Mid-palmar spaces (medial and lateral)

Palmar aponeurosis

Fl. Pollicis Longus

Abd. Pollicis Brevis

Fl. Pollicis Brevis

Princeps pollicis aa.

Sesamoid bone

Ext. Pollicis Longus

Dorsalis pollicis art.
Dorsalis indicis art.

Extensor tendons

Subaponeurotic areolar space

Add. Pollicis

E. Blackstock

65   Cross-section through the middle of the Palm

(The section passes through the head of the first metacarpal bone and, therefore, distal to Opponens Pollicis.)

Observe:

1. The 4 Dorsal Interossei (Abductors) filling the spaces between the 5 metacarpal bones.
2. The 3 Palmar Interossei (Adductors) arising from the palmar aspects of the 2nd, 4th and 5th metacarpal bones, and the Adductor Pollicis arising from the palmar aspects of the 3rd.

Note: All Interossei and the Adductor are supplied by the ulnar nerve.

3. Between the foregoing muscles and the palmar aponeurosis lie the long flexor tendons (superficial and deep) of the 4 fingers, the 4 Lumbricales, and the palmar digital nerves and arteries.

4. Fl. Pollicis Longus tendon, in its synovial sheath, accompanied by its palmar digital arteries and nerves, and passing anterior to the palmar ligament (palmar plate) of the metacarpo-phalangeal joint.

5. The tendons of Ext. Digitorum, flattened, and within a membrane that extends from the 2nd to the 5th metacarpal bone, and the loose areolar subaponeurotic space deep to it.

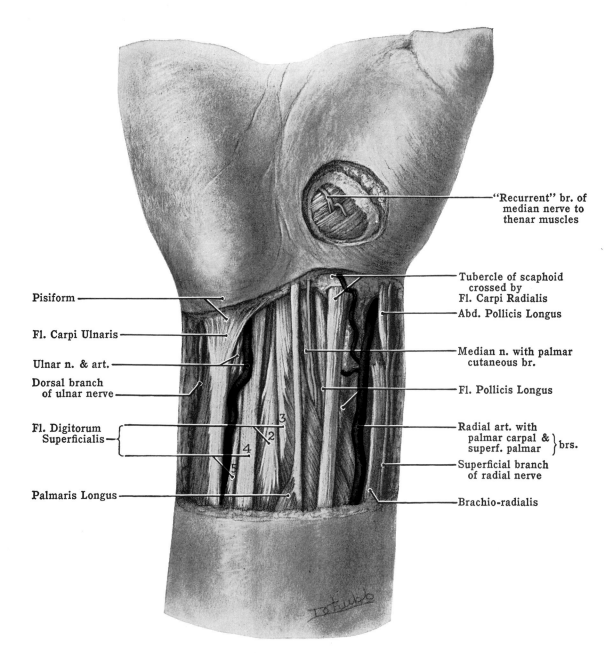

"Recurrent" br. of
median nerve to
thenar muscles

Pisiform

Fl. Carpi Ulnaris

Ulnar n. & art.

Dorsal branch
of ulnar nerve

Fl. Digitorum
Superficialis

Palmaris Longus

Tubercle of scaphoid
crossed by
Fl. Carpi Radialis

Abd. Pollicis Longus

Median n. with palmar
cutaneous br.

Fl. Pollicis Longus

Radial art. with
palmar carpal &
superf. palmar } brs.

Superficial branch
of radial nerve

Brachio-radialis

66 Structures at the Front of the Wrist

The distal transverse skin incision was made along the lowest skin-crease at the
front of the wrist. Medially this crease crosses the pisiform; and to this Fl. Carpi
Ulnaris can be followed. At the junction of its lateral one-third with its medial
two-thirds this crease crosses the tubercle of the scaphoid, and to this the conspicuous
Fl. Carpi Radialis tendon is the guide.

Observe:

. Palmaris Longus tendon bisecting the distal crease, exactly at the middle of the wrist.
  Deep to its lateral margin is the median nerve.

. Abd. Pollicis Longus and Ext. Pollicis Brevis tendons forming the lateral margin of the
  wrist. They also form the anterior margin of the "snuff-box" (figs. 73, 74).

. The radial artery disappearing deep to the Abductor.

. The ulnar nerve and artery sheltered by Fl. Carpi Ulnaris tendon and by the expansion
  this gives to the flexor retinaculum.

. Fl. Digitorum Superficialis tendons to digits 3 and 4 somewhat anterior to those to digits 2
  and 5.

. The "recurrent" branch of the median nerve to the thenar muscles lying within a circle
  whose centre is from 1″ to 1½″ below the tubercle of the scaphoid. Seek it in the proper
  plane—between deep fascia and muscle fibres.

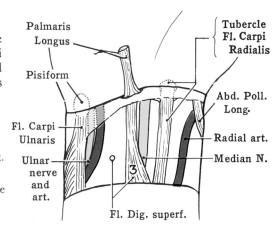

Palmaris
Longus

Pisiform

Fl. Carpi
Ulnaris

Ulnar
nerve
and
art.

Tubercle
Fl. Carpi
Radialis

Abd. Poll.
Long.

Radial art.

Median N.

Fl. Dig. superf.

66.1

Anatomy of front of wrist, simplified
by omitting the long digital flexor
tendons.

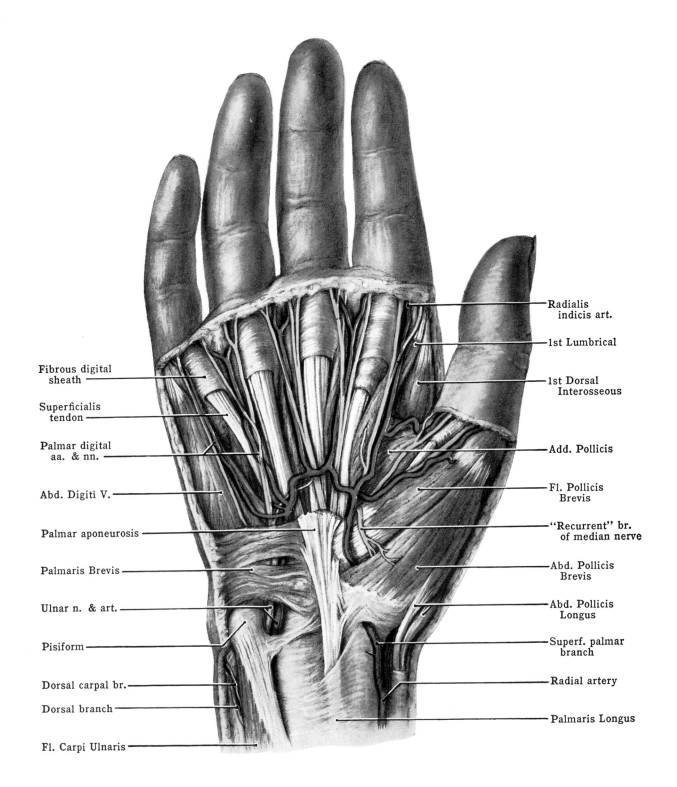

Radialis
indicis art.

1st Lumbrical

1st Dorsal
Interosseous

Add. Pollicis

Fl. Pollicis
Brevis

"Recurrent" br.
of median nerve

Abd. Pollicis
Brevis

Abd. Pollicis
Longus

Superf. palmar
branch

Radial artery

Palmaris Longus

Fibrous digital
sheath

Superficialis
tendon

Palmar digital
aa. & nn.

Abd. Digiti V.

Palmar aponeurosis

Palmaris Brevis

Ulnar n. & art.

Pisiform

Dorsal carpal br.

Dorsal branch

Fl. Carpi Ulnaris

67 Superficial Dissection of the Palm—I

The skin and the superficial fascia are removed; so are the palmar aponeurosis and the thenar and hypothenar fasciae (fig. 70).

The superficial palmar arch is formed by the ulnar artery and is completed by the superficial palmar branch of the radial artery. Only the foregoing structures and Palmaris Brevis cover the arch. It is truly superficial; so likewise are the digital vessels and nerves and the "recurrent" branch of the median nerve exposed in figure 66. The four Lumbricals lie behind digital vessels and nerves.

The prominent pisiform shelters the ulnar nerve and artery as they pass into the palm.

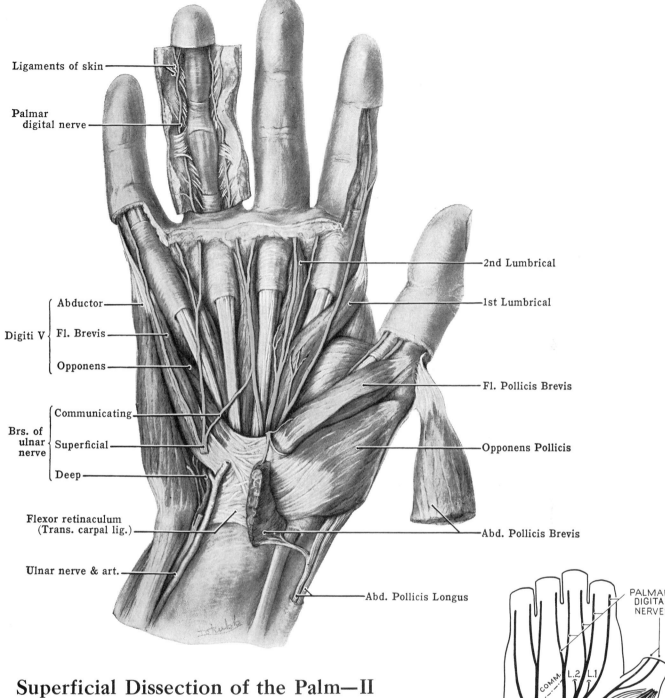

Ligaments of skin

Palmar digital nerve

Digiti V { Abductor
Fl. Brevis
Opponens

Brs. of ulnar nerve { Communicating
Superficial
Deep

Flexor retinaculum (Trans. carpal lig.)

Ulnar nerve & art.

2nd Lumbrical

1st Lumbrical

Fl. Pollicis Brevis

Opponens Pollicis

Abd. Pollicis Brevis

Abd. Pollicis Longus

PALMAR DIGITAL NERVES

COMM. L.2 L.1
DEEP
3 THENAR MUSCLES

ULNAR N. MEDIAN N.

68.1

68   Superficial Dissection of the Palm—II

The 3 thenar and 3 hypothenar muscles arise from the flexor retinaculum and from the 4 marginal carpal bones united by this retinaculum. Abd. Pollicis Brevis arises from Abd. Pollicis Longus tendon also; Abd. Digiti V arises from the pisiform only.

The 4 Lumbricals arise from the radial sides of the 4 Profundus tendons, and are inserted into the radial sides of the dorsal expansions (fig. 88) of the corresponding digits. The medial 2 Lumbricals, however, also arise from the medial sides of adjacent Profundus tendons; and the 3rd Lumbrical is commonly inserted into two extensor expansions, as here.

The median nerve is distributed in the hand to 5 muscles (3 thenar and 2 lumbrical) and to 3½ digits, including parts of their dorsal aspects (fig. 83). All other short muscles in the hand are supplied by the ulnar nerve.

The skin of the fingers cannot be pulled off like a glove, on account of the oblique fibrous strands, cutaneous ligaments, that moor it to the sides of the 1st & 2nd phalanges and front of the distal phalanges.

Diagram: Distribution of median nerve in hand—to 3 thenar & 2 lumbrical muscles, & cutaneous branches to 3½ digits. The ulnar nerve supplies all other fleshy fibers, including all Interossei, and Adductor Pollicis, and 1½ digits. There being no fleshy fibers on the dorsum of hand, radial nerve supplies none. (see fig. 83–85).

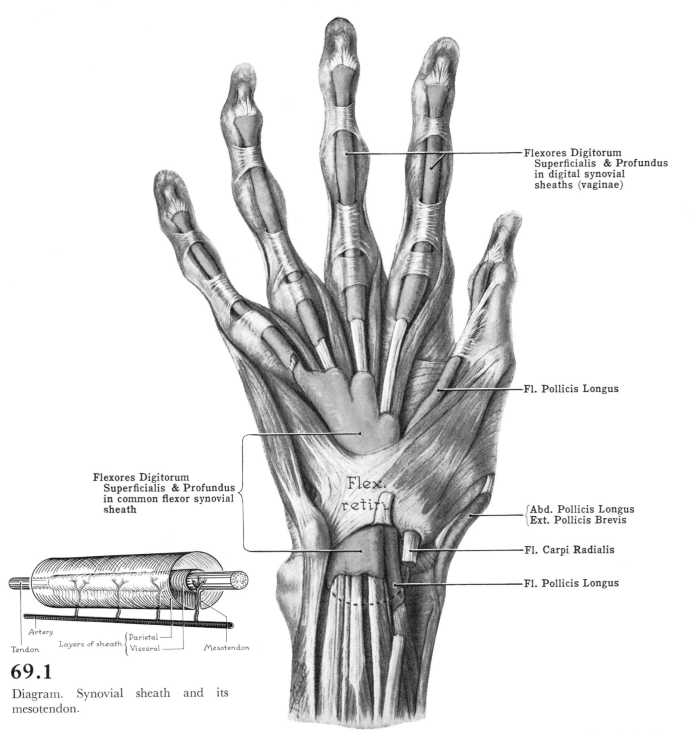

Flexores Digitorum
Superficialis & Profundus
in digital synovial
sheaths (vaginae)

Fl. Pollicis Longus

Flexores Digitorum
Superficialis & Profundus
in common flexor synovial
sheath

Flex.
retin.

Abd. Pollicis Longus
Ext. Pollicis Brevis

Fl. Carpi Radialis

Fl. Pollicis Longus

Artery

Tendon   Layers of sheath   Parietal   Mesotendon
                            Visceral

69.1

Diagram. Synovial sheath and its mesotendon.

69   Synovial Sheaths of the Long Flexor Tendons of the Digits

These sheaths or tubular bursae are lubricating devices that envelop the long digital tendons where they pass through osseofibrous tunnels. There are 2 sets: (a) proximal or carpal, behind the flexor retinaculum; (b) distal or digital, behind the fibrous sheaths of the digital flexors.

The carpal synovial sheaths of the flexors of the fingers, though developmentally separate, unite with one another to form a common flexor sheath, and the carpal sheath of the thumb tendon usually communicates with it. This common flexor sheath extends $\frac{1}{2}''$ to $1''$ proximal to and distal to the flexor retinaculum, varying distally with the extent of the site of friction and with the degree of mobility of the corresponding metacarpal bone. These are greatest in the marginal digits (thumb and little finger). Further, the marginal metacarpals being the shortest, the common flexor sheath extends to, and is continuous with, the digital sheaths of thumb and little finger.

Each digital sheath extends from the proximal end of the palmar lig. or plate (figs. 72 & 96) that covers a metacarpal head to the base of a distal phalanx.

Fluid injected into the digital sheath of the little finger will, therefore, usually flow through the common flexor sheath and on into the digital sheath of the thumb.

The flexor tendons play across the very prominent anterior border of the inferior articular surface of the radius; hence the common flexor sheath extends further behind the tendons (broken line) than in front.

The median nerve not requiring lubrication, has no sheath. Fl. Carpi Radialis tendon has a sheath, not injected in this specimen.

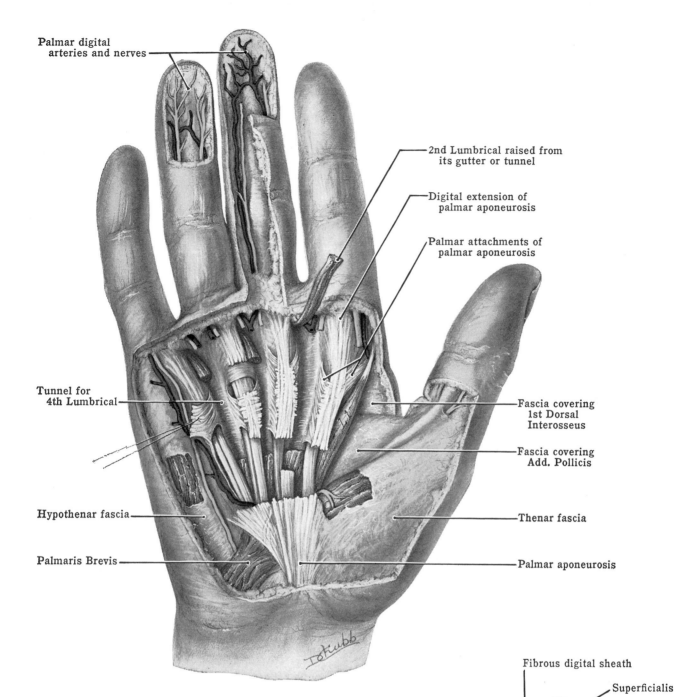

Palmar digital arteries and nerves

2nd Lumbrical raised from its gutter or tunnel

Digital extension of palmar aponeurosis

Palmar attachments of palmar aponeurosis

Tunnel for 4th Lumbrical

Fascia covering 1st Dorsal Interosseus

Fascia covering Add. Pollicis

Hypothenar fascia

Thenar fascia

Palmaris Brevis

Palmar aponeurosis

70 Attachments of the Palmar Aponeurosis: Palmar Digital Vessels and Nerves

Observe:

1. From the palmar aponeurosis a few longitudinal fibres entering the fingers where they are lost; the other fibres, forming extensive fibro-areolar septa, pass dorsally, to the palmar ligaments (fig. 72), and also, more proximally, to the fascia covering the Interossei. Thus two sets of tunnels exist in the distal half of the palm: (1) tunnels for long flexor tendons, and (2) tunnels for Lumbricals, digital vessels and digital nerves. The former are continued into the fingers; the latter open on the dorsum of the hand behind the web.

2. In a finger, the digital artery and nerve lying on the side of the fibrous digital sheath.

3. The absence of fat deep to the skin-creases of the fingers.

4. The 4 palmar spaces: (1) a "thenar", behind the thenar fascia; (2) a "hypothenar," behind the hypothenar fascia; between these (3) a "middle," behind the palmar aponeurosis; and (4) a fourth, between Adductor Pollicis and 1st Dorsal Interosseous. The middle space contains Superficialis and Profundus tendons, Lumbricals, and digital vessels and nerves. It is bounded behind by (a) the fascia covering Interossei and Add. Pollicis, (b) the palmar ligs. and (c) the deep transverse metacarpal ligs. of the palm (fig. 72).

Fibrous digital sheath

Superficialis

Profundus

nerve
artery } Palmar
vein } digital

Cutaneous lig.

Dorsal (ext.) expansion

70.1 Cross-section of a Finger, through the proximal phalanx

Observe:

1. The skin, thickest on the palmar surface.

2. The palmar digital nerve and vessels, applied to the fibrous sheath— not to the bone.

3. Ligaments, mooring skin to bone.

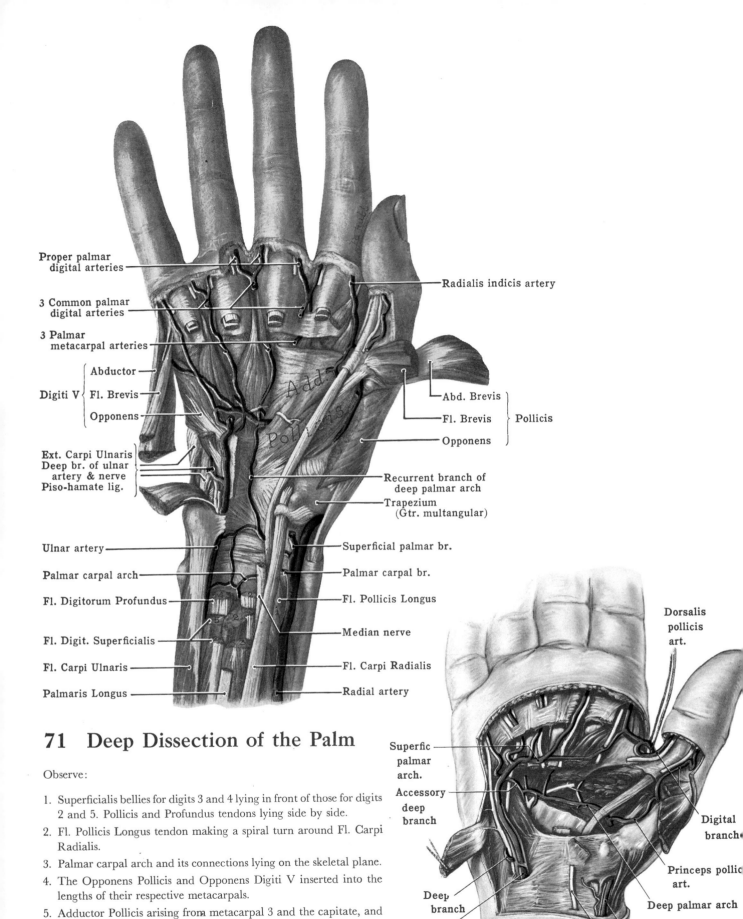

Proper palmar digital arteries

3 Common palmar digital arteries

3 Palmar metacarpal arteries

Digiti V { Abductor / Fl. Brevis / Opponens }

Ext. Carpi Ulnaris
Deep br. of ulnar artery & nerve
Piso-hamate lig.

Radialis indicis artery

Abd. Brevis / Fl. Brevis / Opponens } Pollicis

Recurrent branch of deep palmar arch

Trapezium (Gtr. multangular)

Ulnar artery

Palmar carpal arch

Fl. Digitorum Profundus

Fl. Digit. Superficialis

Fl. Carpi Ulnaris

Palmaris Longus

Superficial palmar br.

Palmar carpal br.

Fl. Pollicis Longus

Median nerve

Fl. Carpi Radialis

Radial artery

71   Deep Dissection of the Palm

Observe:

1. Superficialis bellies for digits 3 and 4 lying in front of those for digits 2 and 5. Pollicis and Profundus tendons lying side by side.

2. Fl. Pollicis Longus tendon making a spiral turn around Fl. Carpi Radialis.

3. Palmar carpal arch and its connections lying on the skeletal plane.

4. The Opponens Pollicis and Opponens Digiti V inserted into the lengths of their respective metacarpals.

5. Adductor Pollicis arising from metacarpal 3 and the capitate, and inserted, via 2 sesamoids (fig. 72), into both sides of the proximal phalanx of the thumb. Adductor divided by radial artery into a transverse and an oblique head.

6. The deep branch of the ulnar artery joining the radial artery to form the deep palmar arch.

Dorsalis pollicis art.

Superfic palmar arch.

Accessory deep branch

Deep branch

Ulnar art.

Digital branch

Princeps pollic art.

Deep palmar arch

Radial art.

Palmar cutaneous br. of median nerv

71.1

The 2 palmar arches, superficial & deep, form a circle. Section excised from Adductor Pollicis.

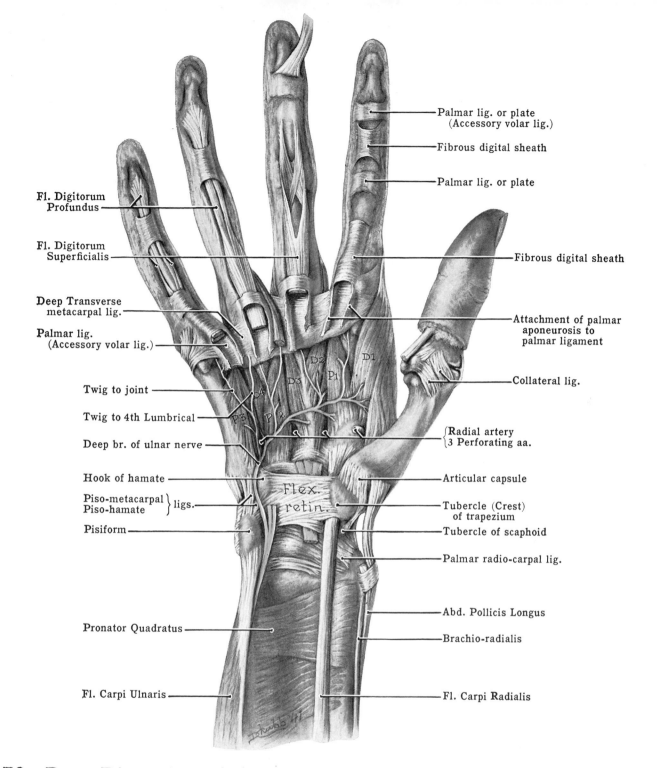

Palmar lig. or plate (Accessory volar lig.)

Fibrous digital sheath

Palmar lig. or plate

Fl. Digitorum Profundus

Fl. Digitorum Superficialis

Deep Transverse metacarpal lig.

Palmar lig. (Accessory volar lig.)

Fibrous digital sheath

Attachment of palmar aponeurosis to palmar ligament

Collateral lig.

Twig to joint

Twig to 4th Lumbrical

Deep br. of ulnar nerve

Radial artery
3 Perforating aa.

Hook of hamate

Articular capsule

Piso-metacarpal
Piso-hamate } ligs.

Flex. retin.

Tubercle (Crest) of trapezium

Pisiform

Tubercle of scaphoid

Palmar radio-carpal lig.

Abd. Pollicis Longus

Pronator Quadratus

Brachio-radialis

Fl. Carpi Ulnaris

Fl. Carpi Radialis

72 Deep Dissection of the Palm and Digits: Ulnar Nerve

Observe:

1. The flexor retinaculum (transverse carpal lig.) uniting the 4 marginal carpal bones, and having the ulnar nerve in front and the median nerve (not labelled) behind.

2. Fl. Carpi Radialis descending vertically in front of the tubercle of the scaphoid and along the groove on the trapezium to the 2nd metacarpal.

3. Fl. Carpi Ulnaris continuing beyond the pisiform as the piso-hamate and the piso-metacarpal ligament.

4. The loose capsule of the carpo-metacarpal joint of the thumb and the strong collateral ligament of its metacarpo-phalangeal joint.

5. 4 Dorsal and 3 Palmar Interossei.

6. The ulnar nerve crossing the hook of the hamate to be dis-

tributed by its deep branch to the 3 hypothenar muscles, all 7 Interossei, 2 Lumbricals, Adductor Pollicis and several joints. The superficial branch supplies Palmaris Brevis and 1½ digits.

7. The radial artery appearing in series with the 3 perforating arteries.

8. The palmar ligs., with the deep transverse metacarpal ligaments uniting them, and the septa from the palmar aponeurosis attached to them.

9. A Lumbrical passing in front of the deep transverse ligament, and Interossei passing behind.

10. On the index, a proximal and distal osseo-fibrous tunnel; on the middle finger, a Superficialis tendon spreading like a V and decussating like an X; on the ring finger, a Profundus tendon; and on the little finger, both tendons.

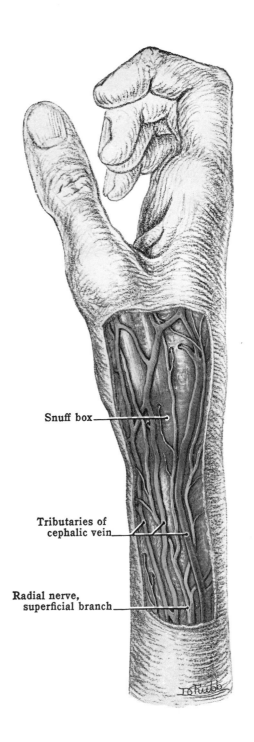

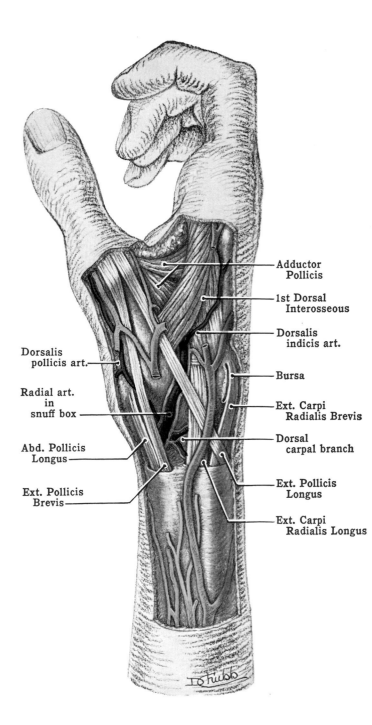

Snuff box

Tributaries of
cephalic vein

Radial nerve,
superficial branch

Adductor
Pollicis

1st Dorsal
Interosseous

Dorsalis
indicis art.

Bursa

Ext. Carpi
Radialis Brevis

Dorsal
carpal branch

Ext. Pollicis
Longus

Ext. Carpi
Radialis Longus

Dorsalis
pollicis art.

Radial art.
in
snuff box

Abd. Pollicis
Longus

Ext. Pollicis
Brevis

73 Radial Aspect of the Wrist—I

(The Anatomical Snuffbox, Dorsum of the Thumb, and First Intermetacarpal Space.)

Observe:

1. Superficial veins and nerves crossing the snuffbox.
2. Perforating veins and articular nerves piercing the deep fascia.

74 Radial Aspect of the Wrist—II

Observe:

1. Three long tendons of the thumb forming the sides of the snuffbox.
2. The radial artery and its venae comitantes crossing the floor of the snuffbox and disappearing between the two heads of the 1st Dorsal Interosseous.
3. Adductor Pollicis and 1st Dorsal Interosseous, proximal to the web between pollex and index. Both are supplied by ulnar nerve (figs. 71 and 72).

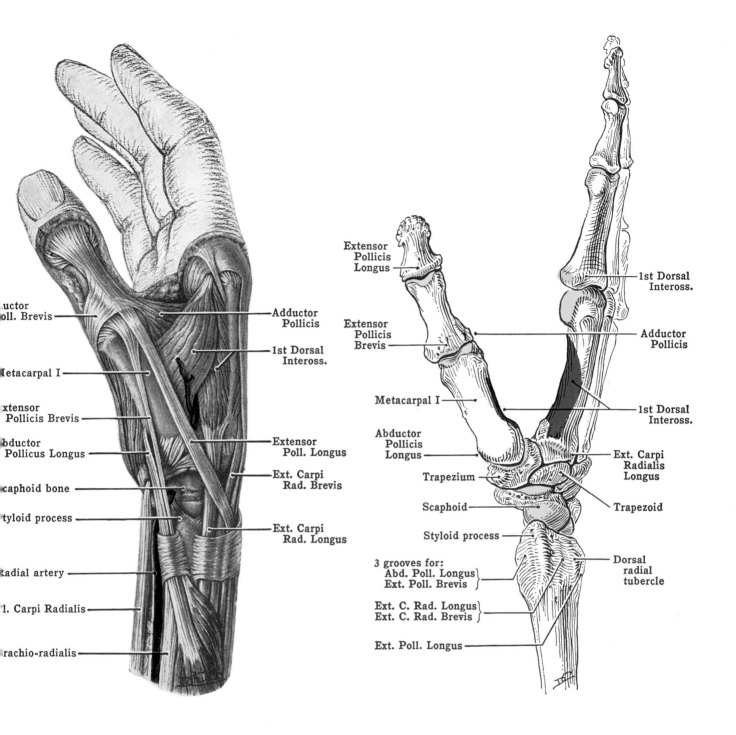

Fig. 75 labels (left figure):
- uctor oll. Brevis (Abductor Poll. Brevis)
- Metacarpal I
- Extensor Pollicis Brevis
- Abductor Pollicus Longus
- Scaphoid bone
- Styloid process
- Radial artery
- Fl. Carpi Radialis
- Brachio-radialis
- Adductor Pollicis
- 1st Dorsal Inteross.
- Extensor Poll. Longus
- Ext. Carpi Rad. Brevis
- Ext. Carpi Rad. Longus

Fig. 76 labels (right figure):
- Extensor Pollicis Longus
- Extensor Pollicis Brevis
- Metacarpal I
- Abductor Pollicis Longus
- Trapezium
- Scaphoid
- Styloid process
- 3 grooves for: Abd. Poll. Longus / Ext. Poll. Brevis
- Ext. C. Rad. Longus / Ext. C. Rad. Brevis
- Ext. Poll. Longus
- 1st Dorsal Inteross.
- Adductor Pollicis
- 1st Dorsal Inteross.
- Ext. Carpi Radialis Longus
- Trapezoid
- Dorsal radial tubercle

75 Radial Aspect of the Wrist—III

Observe:

1. The scaphoid bone; the wrist joint (and radius) proximal to the scaphoid; and the midcarpal joint (and trapezium and trapezoid) distal to it.
2. The capsule of the 1st carpo-metacarpal joint.
3. The Abductor Pollicis Brevis and Adductor Pollicis partly inserted into the dorsal (extensor) expansion.

76 Radial Aspect of the Wrist—IV

(Showing Bones and Attachment of Muscles.)

Observe:

1. The anatomical snuffbox, limited proximally by the styloid process of the radius; distally by the base of the metacarpal of the thumb.
2. The 2 lateral marginal bones of the carpus (viz., scaphoid and trapezium) forming the floor of the snuff-box.

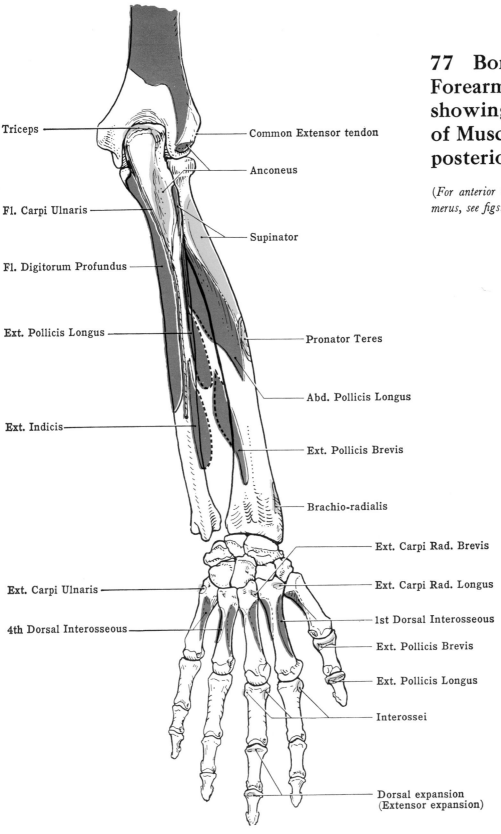

Triceps

Fl. Carpi Ulnaris

Fl. Digitorum Profundus

Ext. Pollicis Longus

Ext. Indicis

Ext. Carpi Ulnaris

4th Dorsal Interosseous

Common Extensor tendon

Anconeus

Supinator

Pronator Teres

Abd. Pollicis Longus

Ext. Pollicis Brevis

Brachio-radialis

Ext. Carpi Rad. Brevis

Ext. Carpi Rad. Longus

1st Dorsal Interosseous

Ext. Pollicis Brevis

Ext. Pollicis Longus

Interossei

Dorsal expansion
(Extensor expansion)

77 Bones of the Forearm and Hand showing Attachments of Muscles, posterior view

(For anterior view, see fig. 58. For Humerus, see figs. 29 and 30.)

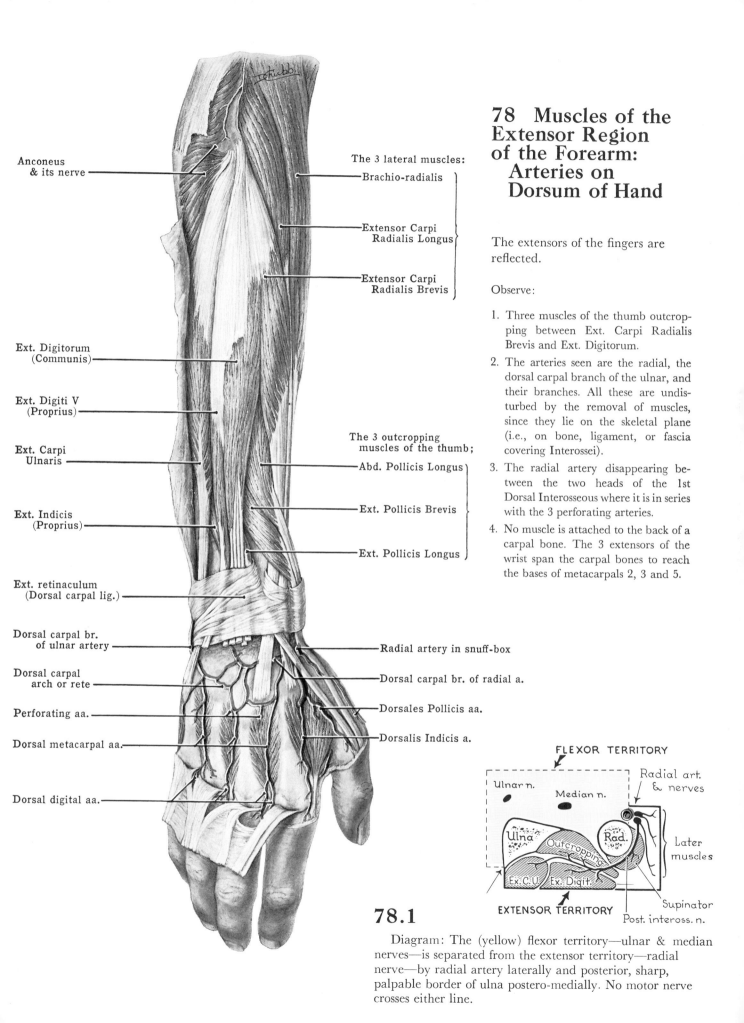

Anconeus & its nerve

The 3 lateral muscles:

Brachio-radialis

Extensor Carpi Radialis Longus

Extensor Carpi Radialis Brevis

Ext. Digitorum (Communis)

Ext. Digiti V (Proprius)

Ext. Carpi Ulnaris

Ext. Indicis (Proprius)

The 3 outcropping muscles of the thumb;

Abd. Pollicis Longus

Ext. Pollicis Brevis

Ext. Pollicis Longus

Ext. retinaculum (Dorsal carpal lig.)

Dorsal carpal br. of ulnar artery

Radial artery in snuff-box

Dorsal carpal arch or rete

Dorsal carpal br. of radial a.

Perforating aa.

Dorsales Pollicis aa.

Dorsal metacarpal aa.

Dorsalis Indicis a.

Dorsal digital aa.

78 Muscles of the Extensor Region of the Forearm: Arteries on Dorsum of Hand

The extensors of the fingers are reflected.

Observe:

1. Three muscles of the thumb outcropping between Ext. Carpi Radialis Brevis and Ext. Digitorum.

2. The arteries seen are the radial, the dorsal carpal branch of the ulnar, and their branches. All these are undisturbed by the removal of muscles, since they lie on the skeletal plane (i.e., on bone, ligament, or fascia covering Interossei).

3. The radial artery disappearing between the two heads of the 1st Dorsal Interosseous where it is in series with the 3 perforating arteries.

4. No muscle is attached to the back of a carpal bone. The 3 extensors of the wrist span the carpal bones to reach the bases of metacarpals 2, 3 and 5.

FLEXOR TERRITORY

Ulnar n. Median n. Radial art. & nerves

Ulna Outcropping Rad.

Ex.C.U. Ex. Digit.

Later muscles

EXTENSOR TERRITORY Supinator Post. inteross. n.

78.1

Diagram: The (yellow) flexor territory—ulnar & median nerves—is separated from the extensor territory—radial nerve—by radial artery laterally and posterior, sharp, palpable border of ulna postero-medially. No motor nerve crosses either line.

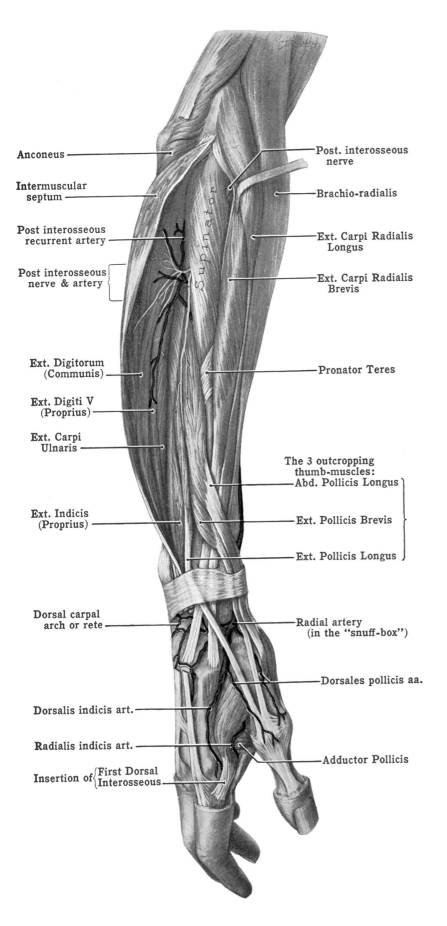

Anconeus

Intermuscular septum

Post interosseous recurrent artery

Post interosseous nerve & artery

Ext. Digitorum (Communis)

Ext. Digiti V (Proprius)

Ext. Carpi Ulnaris

Ext. Indicis (Proprius)

Dorsal carpal arch or rete

Dorsalis indicis art.

Radialis indicis art.

Insertion of {First Dorsal Interosseous}

Post. interosseous nerve

Brachio-radialis

Ext. Carpi Radialis Longus

Ext. Carpi Radialis Brevis

Pronator Teres

The 3 outcropping thumb-muscles:
Abd. Pollicis Longus

Ext. Pollicis Brevis

Ext. Pollicis Longus

Radial artery (in the "snuff-box")

Dorsales pollicis aa.

Adductor Pollicis

Supinator

79 Exposure of the Deep Structures at the Back of the Forearm: The Three Outcropping Muscles of the Thumb, postero-lateral view

The furrow from which the 3 muscles outcrop has been opened widely, up to the lateral epicondyle. It crosses Supinator and is a "line of safety" since the 3 laterally retracted muscles are supplied before the posterior interosseous nerve enters the fleshy tunnel in Supinator, whilst the others are supplied after it emerges $2\frac{1}{2}''$ below the head of the radius.

The tendons of the 3 outcropping muscles of the thumb, or pollex, pass to the epiphyses at the bases of the 3 long bones of the pollex (metacarpal, proximal phalanx, and distal phalanx) (fig. 104). Of these thumb muscles, Ext. Longus is retracted from Ext. Brevis and Abd. Longus by its pulley, the dorsal radial tubercle (figs. 92 & 94); hence the "anatomical snuffbox". No tubercle, no snuff-box.

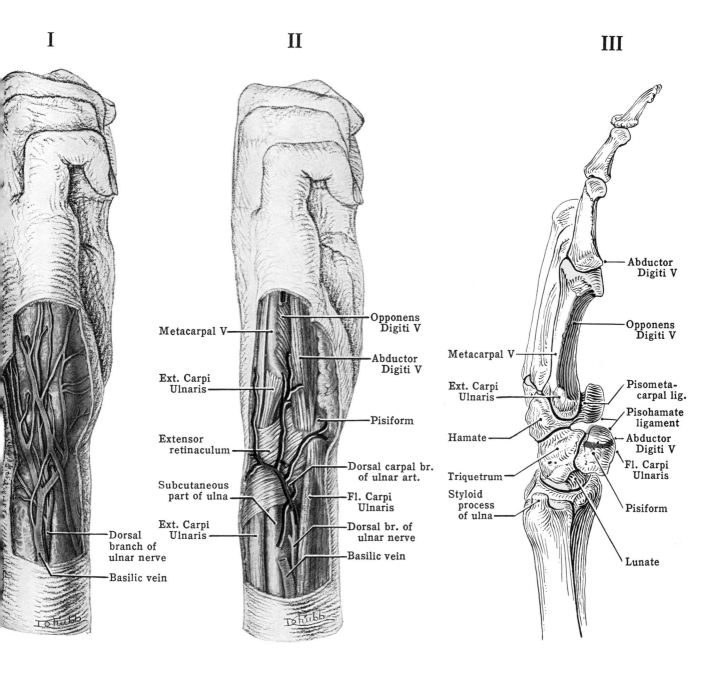

I

II

III

Metacarpal V

Ext. Carpi
Ulnaris

Extensor
retinaculum

Subcutaneous
part of ulna

Ext. Carpi
Ulnaris

Dorsal
branch of
ulnar nerve

Basilic vein

Opponens
Digiti V

Abductor
Digiti V

Pisiform

Dorsal carpal br.
of ulnar art.

Fl. Carpi
Ulnaris

Dorsal br. of
ulnar nerve

Basilic vein

Abductor
Digiti V

Opponens
Digiti V

Metacarpal V

Ext. Carpi
Ulnaris

Hamate

Triquetrum

Styloid
process
of ulna

Pisometa-
carpal lig.

Pisohamate
ligament

Abductor
Digiti V

Fl. Carpi
Ulnaris

Pisiform

Lunate

80 Ulnar Border of the Wrist—I

Observe:

1. The superficial veins and their perforating branches.
2. The superficial nerve appearing from under cover of Fl. Carpi Ulnaris.

81 Ulnar Border of the Wrist—II

Note: A vertical incision made along the medial subcutaneous surface of the ulna and along the medial border of the hand passes between two motor territories (Fl. Carpi Ulnaris, Abd. Digiti V, and Opponens Digiti V, supplied by the ulnar nerve; and Ext. Carpi Ulnaris by the post. interosseous nerve). Superficial veins, nerves, and arteries will be divided, but no motor nerves.

82 Ulnar Border of the Wrist—III

Showing Bones and Attachments of Muscle

Observe:

Ext. Carpi Ulnaris inserted directly into the base of metacarpal V; Fl. Carpi Ulnaris inserted indirectly through the medium of the pisiform bone and pisometacarpal lig.

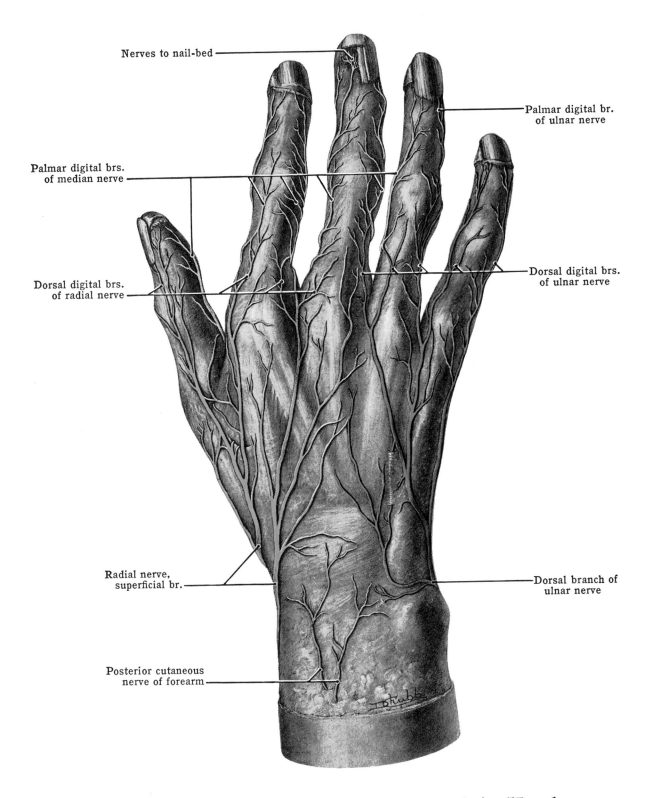

Nerves to nail-bed

Palmar digital brs.
of median nerve

Dorsal digital brs.
of radial nerve

Radial nerve,
superficial br.

Posterior cutaneous
nerve of forearm

Palmar digital br.
of ulnar nerve

Dorsal digital brs.
of ulnar nerve

Dorsal branch of
ulnar nerve

83 Cutaneous Nerves of the Dorsum of the Hand

Observe:

1. The radial nerve and the dorsal branch of the ulnar nerve distributed nearly equally and symmetrically on the dorsum of the hand and digits. The radial nerve supplies the radial half of the dorsum and extends on the 2½ digits—in fact, all the way along the first digit; the dorsal branch of the ulnar nerve behaves similarly on the ulnar half. Each distribution is almost a looking-glass distribution of the other.

2. The palmar digital branches of the median and ulnar nerves (fig. 68) alone supply the distal halves of the three middle digits, including the nail beds.

3. Communications between adjacent nerves are numerous.

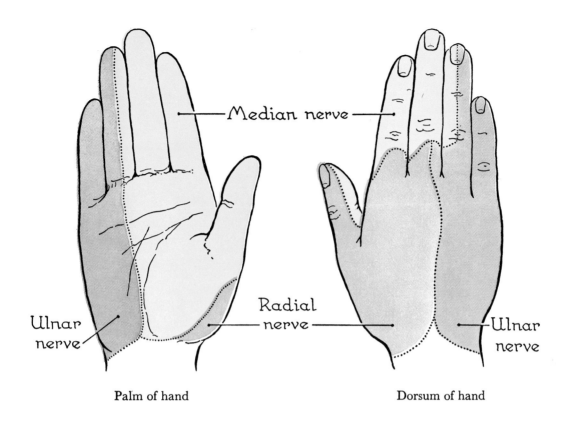

Palm of hand   Dorsum of hand

84 Distribution of the Cutaneous Nerves to the Palm and to the Dorsum of the Hand

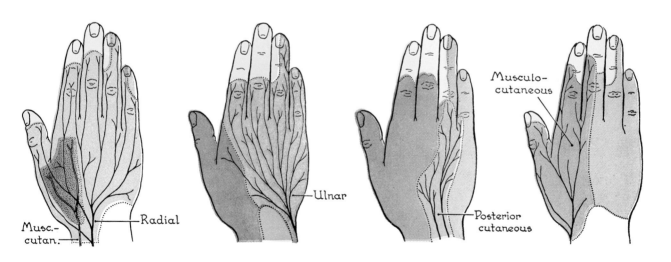

85 Variations in the Pattern of the Cutaneous Nerves in the Dorsum of the Hand

(After Learmonth, Hutton, Hutton, and Appleton respectively.)

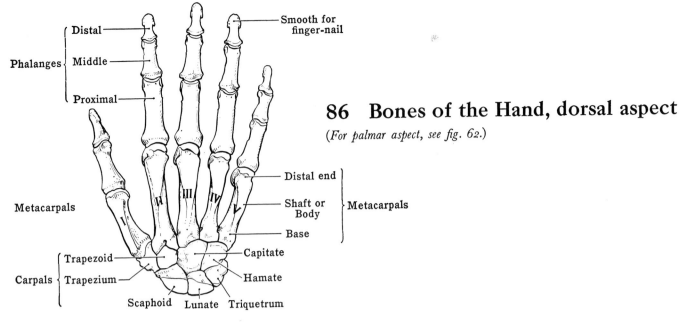

86 Bones of the Hand, dorsal aspect

(For palmar aspect, see fig. 62.)

Phalanges { Distal / Middle / Proximal

Smooth for finger-nail

Metacarpals

Distal end / Shaft or Body / Base } Metacarpals

Carpals { Trapezoid / Trapezium

Capitate / Hamate

Scaphoid   Lunate   Triquetrum

86.1 Synovial Sheaths on the Dorsum of the Wrist

Note:

These six sheaths occupy the six osseo-fibrous tunn deep to the extensor retinaculum.

They contain 9 tendons:—

3 for the thumb in sheaths (1 & 2);

3 for extensors of wrist in 2 sheaths (3 & 4);

3 for extensors of fingers in 2 sheaths (5 & 6).

They may be studied in the foregoing order after dorsal radial tubercle (figs. 2 & 94), which is the pu for Extensor Pollicis Longus, has been located.

The tendons of the three extensors of the wrist the strongest (fig. 64) because they work synergic with the flexors of the digits.

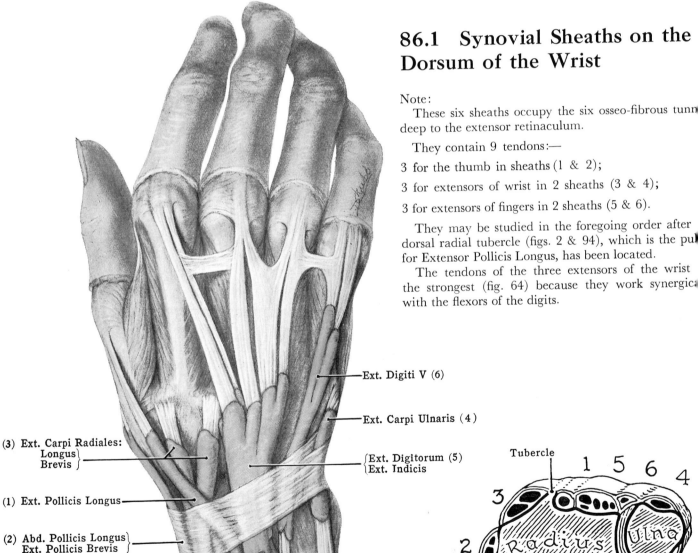

(3) Ext. Carpi Radiales: Longus / Brevis

(1) Ext. Pollicis Longus

(2) Abd. Pollicis Longus / Ext. Pollicis Brevis

Ext. Digiti V (6)

Ext. Carpi Ulnaris (4)

Ext. Digitorum (5) / Ext. Indicis

Tubercle

86.2

Diagram of a cross section of the tendo on the dorsum of the wrist.

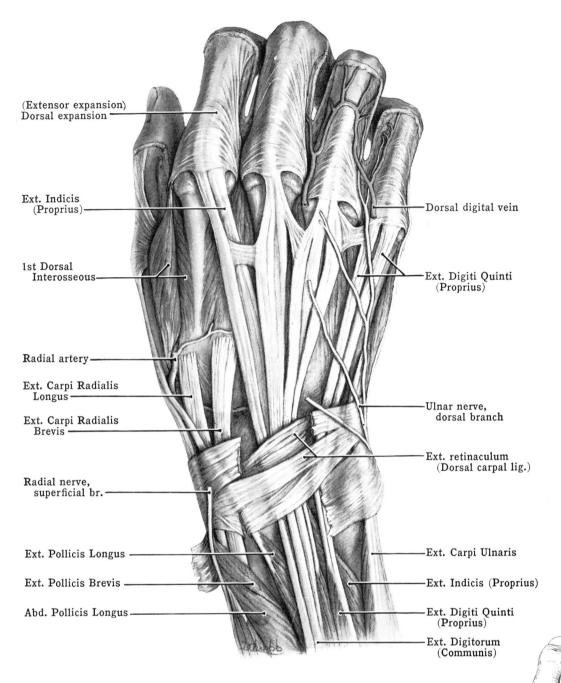

(Extensor expansion)
Dorsal expansion

Ext. Indicis
(Proprius)

1st Dorsal
Interosseous

Radial artery

Ext. Carpi Radialis
Longus

Ext. Carpi Radialis
Brevis

Radial nerve,
superficial br.

Ext. Pollicis Longus

Ext. Pollicis Brevis

Abd. Pollicis Longus

Dorsal digital vein

Ext. Digiti Quinti
(Proprius)

Ulnar nerve,
dorsal branch

Ext. retinaculum
(Dorsal carpal lig.)

Ext. Carpi Ulnaris

Ext. Indicis (Proprius)

Ext. Digiti Quinti
(Proprius)

Ext. Digitorum
(Communis)

Tendons on the Dorsum of the Hand:
xtensor Retinaculum

erve:

he disposition of the tendons of the 9 muscles at the back of the wrist and hand.

he deep fascia, here thickened and called the extensor retinaculum, stretching
bliquely from one ridge on the radius to another. Medailly it passes distal to the
lna to be attached to the pisiform and triquetrum, as depicted in figure 81.

he bands, proximal to the knuckles, that connect the tendons of the digital extensors
nd thereby restrict the independent action of the fingers.

he digital veins passing to the dorsum of the hand where they are not subjected to
ressure.

he body of the 2nd metacarpal is not covered with an extensor tendon.

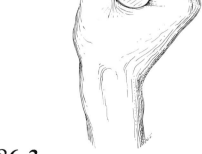

86.3

The grasping hand requires an extended
wrist.

The 3 extensors of the wrist, as synergists,
are essential to the digital flexors when grasping, hence their strength, (see fig. 64).

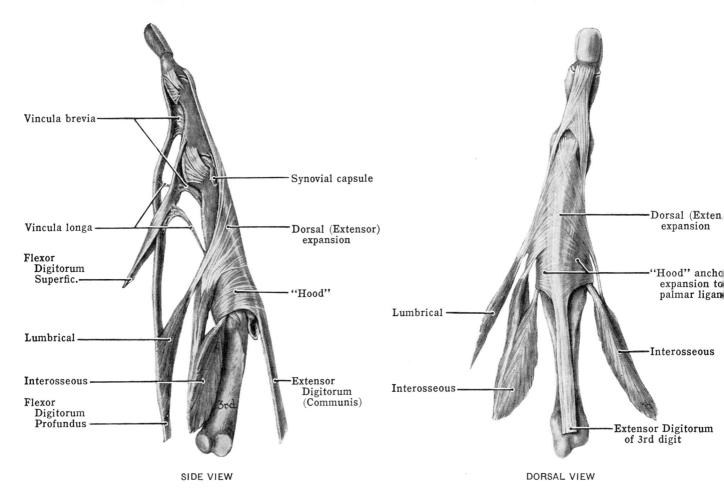

Vincula brevia

Vincula longa

Flexor
Digitorum
Superfic.

Lumbrical

Interosseous

Flexor
Digitorum
Profundus

Synovial capsule

Dorsal (Extensor)
expansion

"Hood"

3rd

Extensor
Digitorum
(Communis)

SIDE VIEW

Dorsal (Exten
expansion

"Hood" ancho
expansion to
palmar ligam

Lumbrical

Interosseous

Interosseous

Extensor Digitorum
of 3rd digit

DORSAL VIEW

88 Extensor (Dorsal) Expansion of the Middle Digit

Observe:

1. Interossei in part inserted into the bases of the proximal phalanx (figs. 76–79) and in part into the expansion.

2. Lumbrical inserted wholly into the radial side of the expansion.

3. The hood covering the head of the metacarpal. It is moored to the palmar ligament (figs. 72 and 96), hence, medial and lateral bow-stringing of the extensor tendon and expansion is prevented.

4. The expansion extending to the bases of the middle and distal phalanges, and giving a strong areolar band to the base of the proximal phalanx, here not in view, (Kaplan).

5. (On side view) the vincula longa et brevia, which are all that remain of the primitive mesotendons.

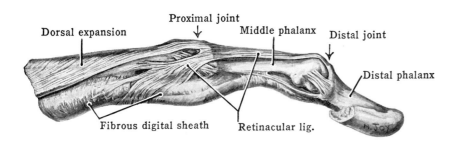

Dorsal expansion   Proximal joint   Middle phalanx   Distal joint

Distal phalanx

Fibrous digital sheath   Retinacular lig.

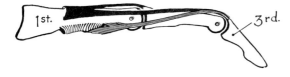

1st.   3rd.

89 Retinacular Ligament

Observe:

1. This delicate fibrous band runs from the 1st proximal phalanx and the fibrous digital she obliquely across the 2nd phalanx and the two in phalangeal joints to join the dorsal expansi and so to the 3rd or distal phalanx.

2. On flexing the distal joint either passively (as in cadaver) or voluntarily, the retinacular ligam becomes taut and pulls the proximal joint i flexion.

3. Similarly, on extending the proximal joint, distal joint is pulled by the retinacular ligam into nearly complete extension. (J. M. Landsmeer.)

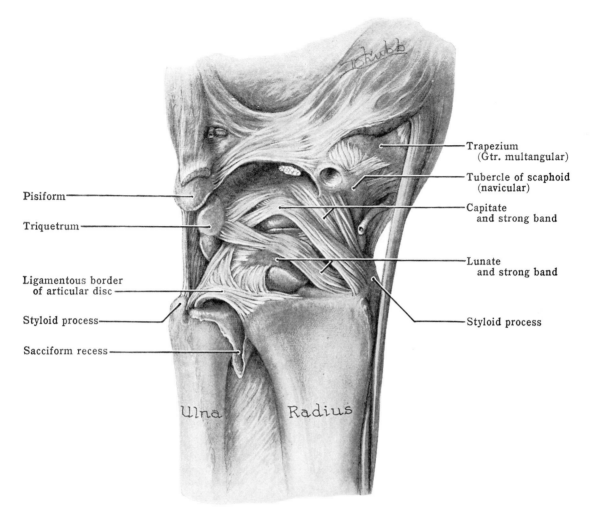

Pisiform

Triquetrum

Ligamentous border
of articular disc

Styloid process

Sacciform recess

Trapezium
(Gtr. multangular)

Tubercle of scaphoid
(navicular)

Capitate
and strong band

Lunate
and strong band

Styloid process

Ulna   Radius

90 Ligaments of the Distal Radio-ulnar, Radio-carpal and Intercarpal Joints, front view

The hand is forcibly extended.

Observe:

1. The sacciform recess of the distal radio-ulnar joint (similar to the recess of the proximal joint, fig. 54) and the ligamentous anterior border of the disc.

2. The anterior or palmar ligaments, passing from the radius to the two rows of carpal bones. It is strong, and it is so directed that the hand shall follow the radius during supination. The dorsal ligaments take the same direction, hence the hand is obedient during pronation also.

3. The proximal articular surface of the triquetrum applied to the medial ligament of the wrist.

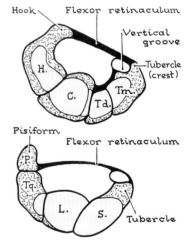

90.1

Diagram. Carpal tunnel, proximal & distal cross-sections to show thickness of flexor retinaculum and proximal articular surfaces.

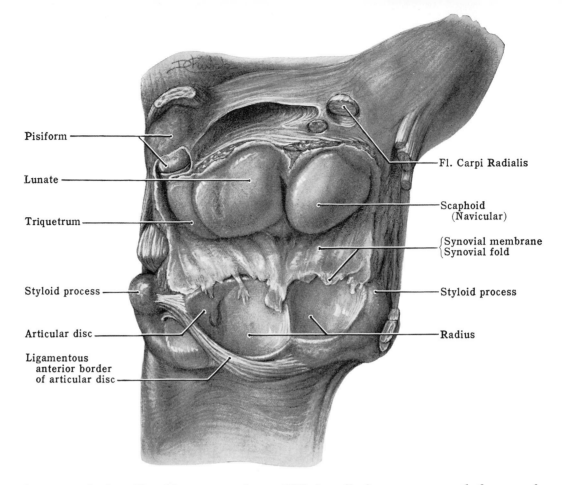

Pisiform

Lunate

Triquetrum

Styloid process

Articular disc

Ligamentous
anterior border
of articular disc

Fl. Carpi Radialis

Scaphoid
(Navicular)

{ Synovial membrane
{ Synovial fold

Styloid process

Radius

91   Surfaces of the Radio-carpal or Wrist Joint, opened from front

Observe:

1. The nearly equal proximal articular surfaces of the scaphoid and lunate.
2. The lunate articulating with the radius and the articular disc. Only during adduction of the wrist does the triquetrum come into articulation with the disc.
3. Transparent synovial folds, like cellophane, projecting between the articular surfaces.

4. The perforation in the disc and the associated roughened surface of the lunate. This is a common occurrence.
5. The pisiform joint communicating with the radio-carpal joint.
6. The interosseous ligament between the scaphoid and the lunate, partly absorbed. In such a specimen—and they are common—infection could spread widely.

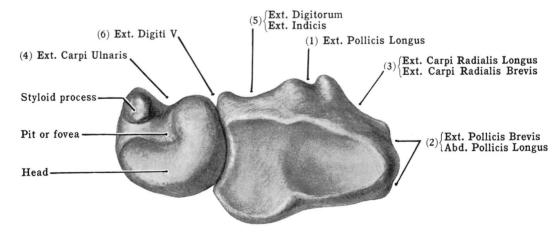

(6) Ext. Digiti V

(4) Ext. Carpi Ulnaris

Styloid process

Pit or fovea

Head

(5) { Ext. Digitorum
{ Ext. Indicis

(1) Ext. Pollicis Longus

(3) { Ext. Carpi Radialis Longus
{ Ext. Carpi Radialis Brevis

(2) { Ext. Pollicis Brevis
{ Abd. Pollicis Longus

92   Distal Ends of Radius and Ulna, from below

Observe:

1. The 4 features of the distal end of the ulna—head, fovea, styloid process, and groove for the tendon of Ext. Carpi Ulnaris.
2. The 6 grooves for the 9 tendons at the back of the wrist. Figure 86.1 shows these tendons in their synovial sheaths.

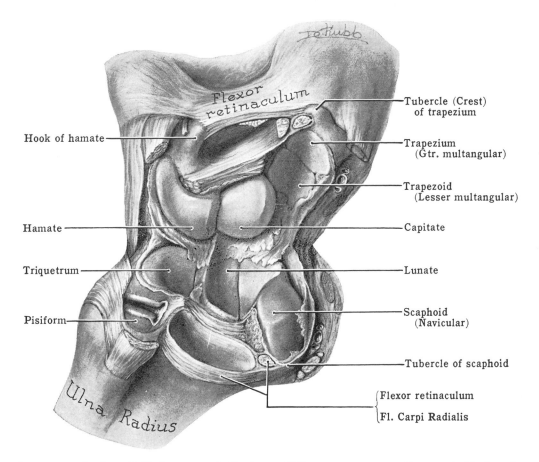

Flexor retinaculum

Hook of hamate

Hamate

Triquetrum

Pisiform

Ulna Radius

Tubercle (Crest) of trapezium

Trapezium (Gtr. multangular)

Trapezoid (Lesser multangular)

Capitate

Lunate

Scaphoid (Navicular)

Tubercle of scaphoid

Flexor retinaculum

Fl. Carpi Radialis

93   Surfaces of the Midcarpal Joint (Transverse Carpal Joint)

The flexor retinaculum (transverse carpal lig.) is divided.

Observe:

1. The sinuous surfaces of the opposed bones: the trapezium and trapezoid together presenting a concave, oval surface to the scaphoid; the capitate and hamate together presenting a convex surface to the scaphoid, lunate and triquetrum, which is slightly broken by the linear facet on the apex of the hamate for its counterpart on the lunate.

2. Synovial folds projecting into the joint.
3. The relative weakness of the proximal part of the flexor retinaculum, which stretches from the movable pisiform to the scaphoid, and the strength of the distal part, which stretches from the hook of the hamate to the tubercle (crest) of the trapezium.

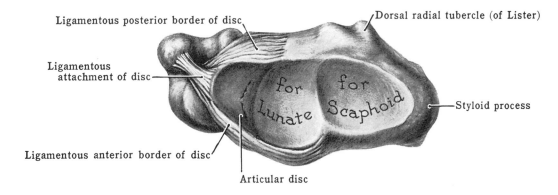

Ligamentous posterior border of disc

Dorsal radial tubercle (of Lister)

Ligamentous attachment of disc

for Lunate   for Scaphoid

Styloid process

Ligamentous anterior border of disc

Articular disc

94   Articular Disc of the Distal Radio-ulnar Joint, from below

This disc is the bond of union between the lower ends of the radius and ulna. It is fibro-cartilaginous, smooth, and stiff at the triangular area compressed between the head of the ulna and the lunate bone (figs. 52 & 91), but it is ligamentous and pliable elsewhere. The cartilaginous part is commonly fissured, as here, but the ligamentous parts are not.

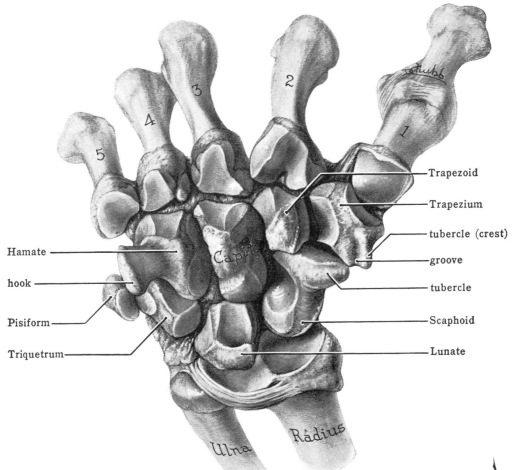

Hamate

hook

Pisiform

Triquetrum

Trapezoid

Trapezium

tubercle (crest)

groove

tubercle

Scaphoid

Lunate

95 Carpal Bones and the Bases of the Metacarpal Bones, front view

The dorsal ligaments remain as a binding allowing study of the articular facets.

Observe:

1. One bone (radius) supporting two proximal carpals (scaphoid and lunate); these in turn supporting three distal carpals (trapezium, trapezoid, and capitate) and articulating with the apex of the hamate; the four distal carpals supporting the five metacarpals. The triquetrum is unsupported.

2. The marginal projections (pisiform, hook of hamate, tubercle of scaphoid, and tubercle of trapezium) which afford attachment to the flexor retinaculum.

3. The triquetrum having an isolated facet for the pisiform.

4. Of the eight carpals only the lunate is wider in front than behind.

5. The capitate articulating with three metacarpals (2nd, 3rd, and 4th).

6. The second metacarpal articulating with three carpals (trapezium, trapezoid, and capitate).

7. The basal surfaces of the 2nd and 3rd metacarpals individually about as large as those of the 4th and 5th collectively.

8. The 2nd and 3rd carpo-metacarpal joints practically immobile; the 1st, saddle-shaped; the 4th and 5th, hinge-shaped.

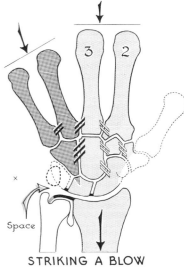

STRIKING A BLOW

95.1

Diagram. On striking a blow, trique trum being unsupported, the hamate & metacarpals 4 & 5 rely on liga ments, directed as shown, for re sistance and transmission of force

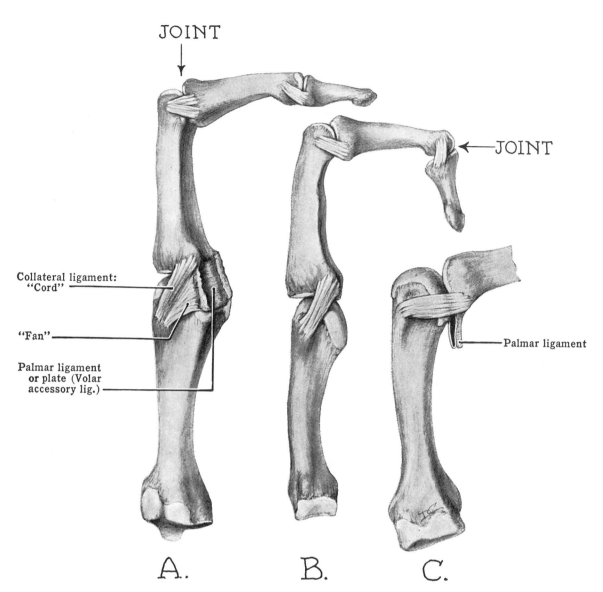

JOINT

JOINT

Collateral ligament: "Cord"

"Fan"

Palmar ligament or plate (Volar accessory lig.)

Palmar ligament

A.   B.   C.

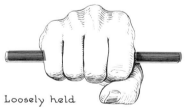

Loosely held

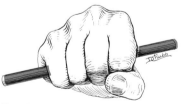

Firmly gripped

95.2

On pulling a rod or a rope, the flexion allowed at 4th & 5th carpometacarpal joints allows the grip to be more secure.

96 Metacarpo-phalangeal and Interphalangeal Joints

Observe:

1. A fibro-cartilaginous plate, the palmar ligament, hanging from the base of the proximal phalanx; fixed to the head of the metacarpal by the weaker, fanlike part, of the collateral ligament; and moving like a visor across the metacarpal head.

   Figure 72 shows the deep transverse metacarpal ligaments that unite the plates, and the insertions of the palmar aponeurosis into them.

2. The extremely strong, cordlike parts of the collateral ligaments of this joint, being eccentrically attached to the metacarpal heads. They are slack during extension and taut during flexion; hence the fingers cannot be spread (abducted) unless the hand is open.

   The interphalangeal joints have corresponding ligaments but, the distal ends of the 1st and 2nd phalanges, being flattened anteroposteriorly and having two small condyles (cf., distal end of femur), permit neither adduction nor abduction.

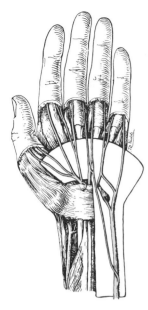

A. Long Communicating Branch from Ulnar to Median Nerve

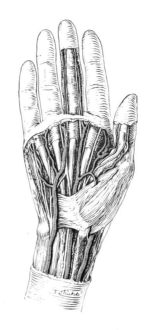

B. Persisting Median Artery

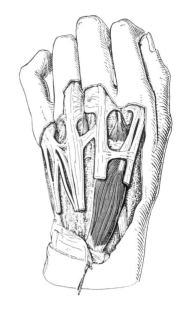

C. Extensor Digitorum Brevis

This muscle, constant on the dorsum of the foot, is found occasionally on the dorsum of the hand, usually as a single bundle.

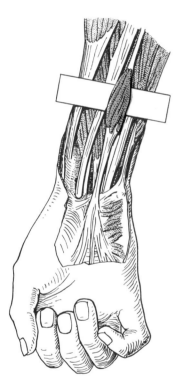
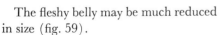

D. Palmaris Longus: misplaced or absent

The fleshy belly may be much reduced in size (fig. 59).

Palmaris Longus was absent in 98 of 716 dissected limbs (i.e., in 13.7% of 358 paired limbs, 26 times in both limbs, 26 in the right only, and 20 in the left only. (*R. K. George*).

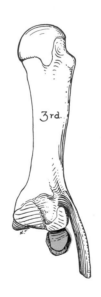

E. Separate Styloid Process of 3rd Metacarpal

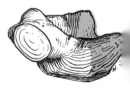

LEFT SIDE   RIGHT SIDE

F. Fused Lunate and Triquetrum

97 VARIATIONS AND ANOMALIES
of occasional occurrence

(Other variations, figs. 27-28, 40-43, 47-48.I.)

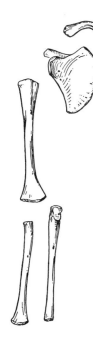

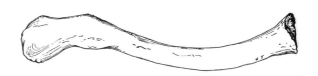

98 Bones of Upper Limb at Birth

The diaphyses of the long bones and the scapula are well ossified; but the epiphyses have not started to ossify nor have the carpal bones—except occasionally the head of the humerus and the capitate (and hamate) in the female. The coracoid process, the medial border of the scapula and the acromion are cartilaginous.

(*All ages given in figures 98—104 are for males.*)

99 Epiphysis of the Clavicle

The Clavicle has a thin epiphysis covering its sternal end. This may start to fuse at any time between the 18th and 25th years. Between the 23rd and 31st years (mostly between 26th and 29th) all undergo terminal fusion. It is the last of the long bone epiphyses to fuse. (*McKern and Stewart.*)

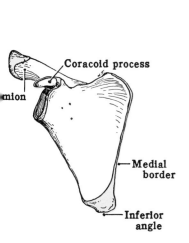

AGED ABOUT 3 YEARS.

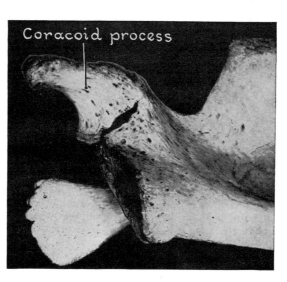

THE CORACOID PROCESS, FUSING,
AGED ABOUT 15 YEARS.

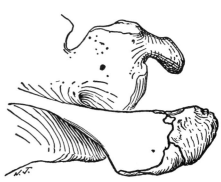

AGED ABOUT 17 YEARS.

100 Ossification of the Scapula

The **Coracoid Process.** A single ossific center appears in the coracoid during the 1st year; another center for the upper end of the glenoid cavity and adjacent part of the coracoid appears about the 10th year. These fuse with the scapula about the 15th year.

The **Acromion** has two ossific centers; the **Medial Border** and the **Inferior Angle** have separate centers.

These appear about puberty and usually start to fuse before the 17th year. Fusion of all three is usually complete between the 18th and 20th years and always by the 23rd year (McK. & S.)

(*For ununited acromial epiphysis, see fig. 40.*)

OSSIFICATION—EPIPHYSES

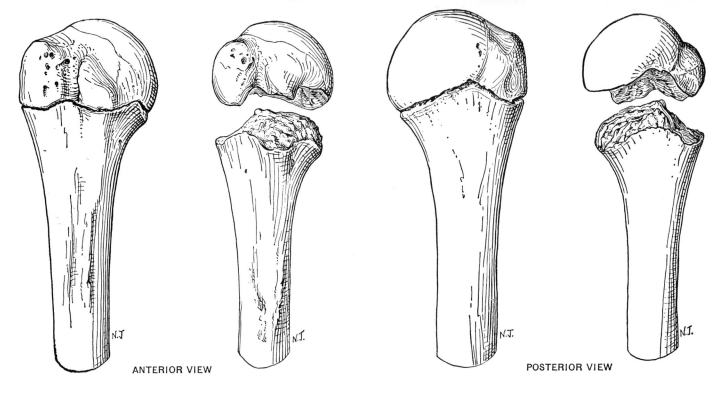

ANTERIOR VIEW   POSTERIOR VIEW

101   Humerus, proximal epiphysis

The proximal epiphysis fits on to the billowy conical end of the diaphysis. It develops from three centres, (a) one for the head during the 1st year (occasionally before birth), (b) one for the greater tubercle before the end of the 3rd year, (c) and one for the lesser tubercle before the 5th year. These have fused to form a single mass before the 7th year. This mass, or proximal epiphysis, is in some cases completely fused to the diaphysis by the 17th to 18th year and in all cases by the 24th year. (McKern and Stewart.) The centres for the head and lesser tubercle lie on the medial side of the cone; the greater tubercle lies on the lateral side. The epiphyseal plate lies well above the level of the surgical neck, and it cuts through the head medially, i.e., the articular cartilage of the head extends for 2 or 3 mm. on to the diaphysis; hence, the epiphyseal plate cuts into the shoulder joint.

102   Epiphyses at the Elbow Region

The Humerus, distal end:—The lower border of the diaphysis is oblique. It lies well below the levels of the radial, coronoid, and olecranon fossae. Its roller-like surface is ridged and pitted and the distal epiphysis fits it like a trough. There are 4 centres of ossification: for (a) lateral epicondyle, (b) capitulum and lateral part of trochlea, (c) medial part of trochlea, and (d) medial epicondyle. a, b, & c appear about the 12th, 1st, and 10th years respectively and they fuse into a single mass which is probably in all cases completely fused to the diaphysis before the end of the 17th year. It is the first of all long bone epiphyses to fuse. The epiphysis for the medial epicondyle appears about the 6th year and is completely fused to the side of the diaphysis by the end of the 19th year. (McK. & S.) It is quite independent of the main epiphysis.

The Ulna and Radius, proximal ends:—These have one centre each: for (a) olecranon, and (b) head of radius. The olecranon epiphysis is the traction epiphysis of the Triceps. It appears about the 11th year. It may be quite large, in which case it cuts into the trochlear notch (see dotted line). The centre for the head of the radius appears about the 7th year and, like the olecranon epiphysis, is usually completely fused by the 17th or 18th year and always by the 19th year. (McK. & S.) The diameters of the head and neck of a young radius are about equal; but after the 6th or 7th year the head enlarges.

OSSIFICATION—EPIPHYSES

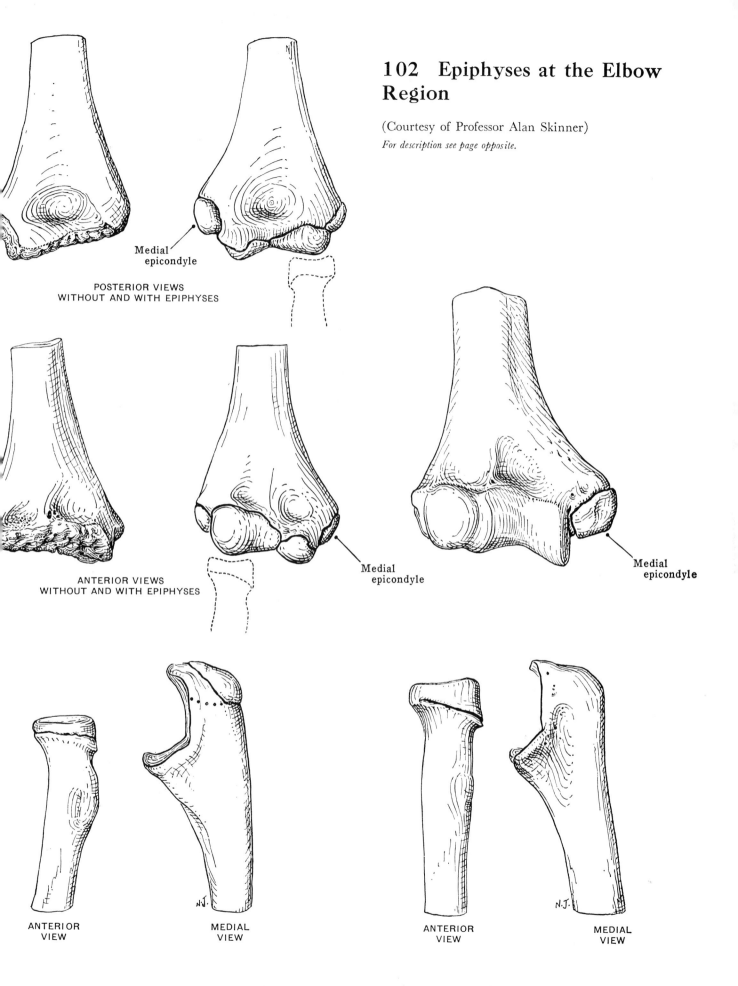

102 Epiphyses at the Elbow Region

(Courtesy of Professor Alan Skinner)

For description see page opposite.

Medial
epicondyle

POSTERIOR VIEWS
WITHOUT AND WITH EPIPHYSES

Medial
epicondyle

Medial
epicondyle

ANTERIOR VIEWS
WITHOUT AND WITH EPIPHYSES

ANTERIOR
VIEW

MEDIAL
VIEW

ANTERIOR
VIEW

MEDIAL
VIEW

OSSIFICATION—EPIPHYSES

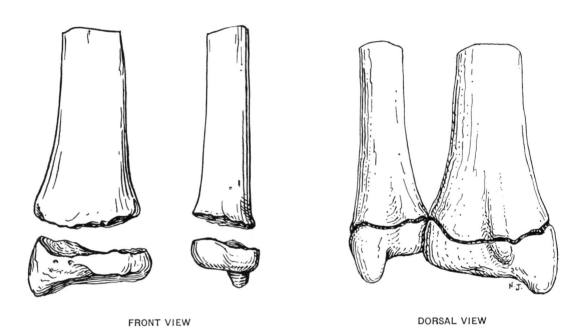

FRONT VIEW   DORSAL VIEW

103   Ulna and Radius, distal ends

The epiphyseal plates of the ulna and radius lie at the same level and cut into the distal radio-ulnar joint (fig. 90). The centre for the radius appears at the end of the 1st year; that for the ulna appears about the 7th year (C. C. Francis). Early stages of fusion occur from the 17th to 20th year; thereafter all cases are either fused or in late stages of fusion, fusion being always complete by the 23rd year (McK. & S.).

OSSIFICATION—EPIPHYSES

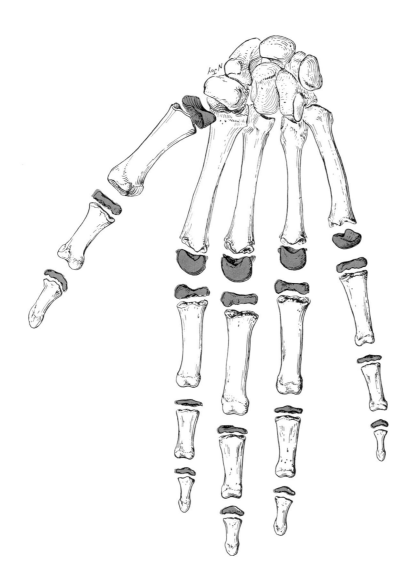

104 Bones of the Hand

Capitate starts to ossify soon after birth, or in the female at birth or even before. Is is at once followed by Hamate. Triquetrum usually starts at $2\frac{1}{2}$ years; Lunate at $3\frac{1}{2}$ years; Scaphoid, Trapezium, and Trapezoid (usually in that order) between 5 and 6 years; and Pisiform, which is the last to start, at 10 years.

Metacarpal bones and Phalanges have each one epiphysis. These epiphyses are situated at the distal ends of the metacarpals and at the proximal ends of the phalanges. The metacarpal of the thumb behaves as a phalanx.

These epiphyses usually start to ossify before the age of 3 years, and they have fused with their diaphyses before the age of 18 years—the first to fuse being the epiphyses of the distal phalanges, at $15\frac{1}{2}$ years.

(*For details consult W. W. Greulich and S. I. Pyle.*)

OSSIFICATION—EPIPHYSES

(*For epiphyses of lower limb, see figs. 350–356.*)

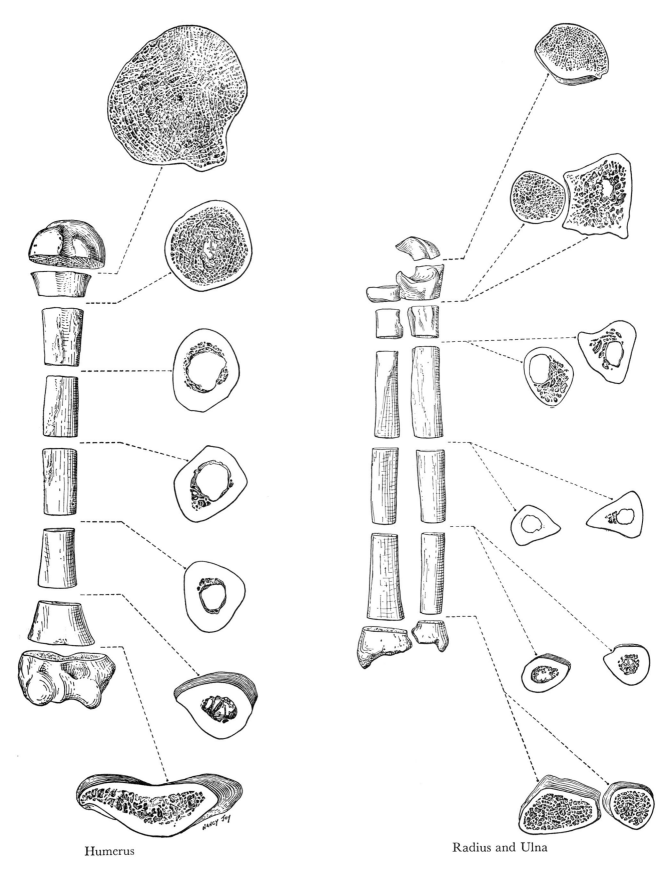

Humerus

Radius and Ulna

104.1 Cross Sections of Humerus, Radius, and Ulna

These sections demonstrate the variations in thickness of compact and spongy bone at different levels and at different parts of the same level. They demonstrate also the extent of the medullary cavity.

The Abdomen

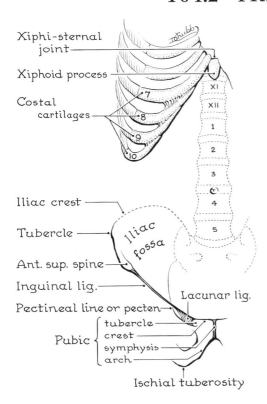

Xiphi-sternal joint

Xiphoid process

Costal cartilages

Iliac crest

Tubercle

Ant. sup. spine

Inguinal lig.

Pectineal line or pecten

Pubic { tubercle, crest, symphysis, arch

Lacunar lig.

Iliac fossa

Ischial tuberosity

A. Skeleton of abdomen.

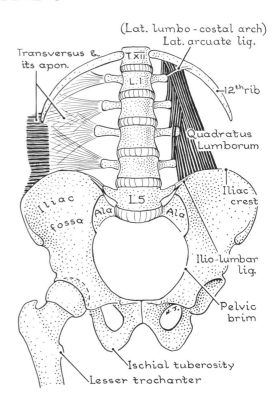

Transversus & its apon.

(Lat. lumbo-costal arch) Lat. arcuate lig.

12th rib

Quadratus Lumborum

Iliac crest

Ilio-lumbar lig.

Pelvic brim

Iliac fossa

Ischial tuberosity

Lesser trochanter

B. Two muscles of posterior abdominal wall.

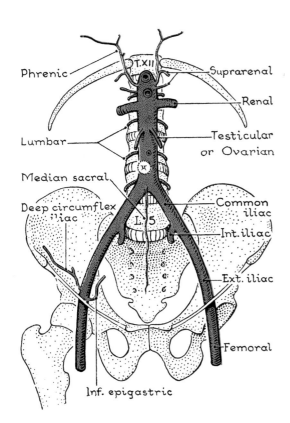

Phrenic

Lumbar

Median sacral

Deep circumflex iliac

Suprarenal

Renal

Testicular or Ovarian

Common iliac

Int. iliac

Ext. iliac

Femoral

Inf. epigastric

C. Abdominal aorta and its branches.
Note: Abdominal (lumbar) aorta begins where diaphragm rests on celiac trunk at disc between vertebrae Th.X11 and L.1. (Fig. 132.3.)

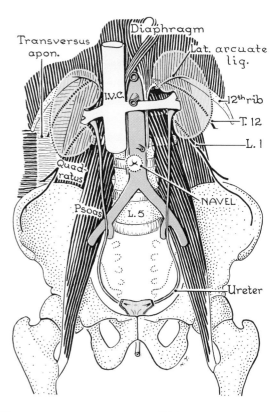

Transversus apon.

Diaphragm

Lat. arcuate lig.

12th rib

T. 12

L. 1

I.V.C.

Quadratus

Psoas

NAVEL

Ureter

D. Urinary apparatus (kidneys, ureters, bladder & urethra), which is part of the 3 paired gland composite (suprarenal, renal and genital glands fig. 210.1).

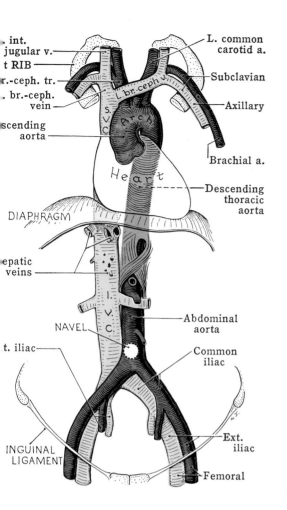

E. Great arteries and veins of the trunk.

Labels (figure E): int. jugular v.; t RIB; r.-ceph. tr.; . br.-ceph. vein; scending aorta; DIAPHRAGM; epatic veins; NAVEL; t. iliac; INGUINAL LIGAMENT; L. common carotid a.; Subclavian; Axillary; Brachial a.; Descending thoracic aorta; Abdominal aorta; Common iliac; Ext. iliac; Femoral; L. br.-ceph. v.; S.V.C.; Arch; Heart; I.V.C.

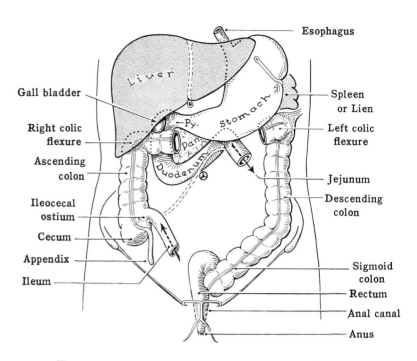

F. Gastro-intestinal tract and its 3 unpaired glands—liver, pancreas and spleen.

Labels (figure F): Esophagus; Gall bladder; Right colic flexure; Ascending colon; Ileocecal ostium; Cecum; Appendix; Ileum; Spleen or Lien; Left colic flexure; Jejunum; Descending colon; Sigmoid colon; Rectum; Anal canal; Anus; Liver; Stomach; Py.; Pan.; Duodenum

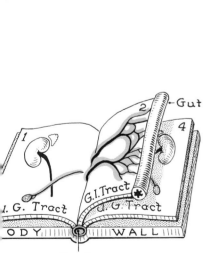

Labels (figure G): Gut; G.I. Tract; U.G. Tract; U.G. Tract; ODY; WALL; Aorta; 1; 2; 3; 4

This open book may explain the relative positions of the abdominal viscera to each other. Pages 1 & 4 represent the 3 paired glands; pages 2 & 3, the G.-1. tract and the 3 unpaired glands.

H. Vertebrae as a measuring rod— Transpyloric plane. This horizontal midway plane cuts the disc between vertebrae L.1 & 1.2. (Addison.)

Labels (figure H): "TOP" OF STERNUM; TRANSPYLORIC PLANE; "TOP" OF SYMPHYSIS

I. Table illustrating the obedience of things anatomical to biometrical laws, that is, dimensions, weights, levels, strengths, etc. attributed to structures are not absolute but average. (George.)

Frequency distribution of vertebral level of: (a) origin of celiac trunk & (b) bifurcation of aorta.

Vertebra	Class interval	Celiac trunk	Bifurcation of aorta
XII U.	1	1	
XII M.	2	1	
XII L.	3	6	
	4	18	
disc	5	20	
1	6	25	
1	7	17	
1	8	7	
disc	9	1	
2	10		
2	11	1	
2	12		
disc	13		
3	14		
3	15		
3	16		1
disc	17		8
4	18		15
4	19		20
4	20		25
disc	21		23
5	22		7
5	23		4
5	24		2
No. of cases		97	105
Mean		5.5	19.8
σ		1.59	1.64

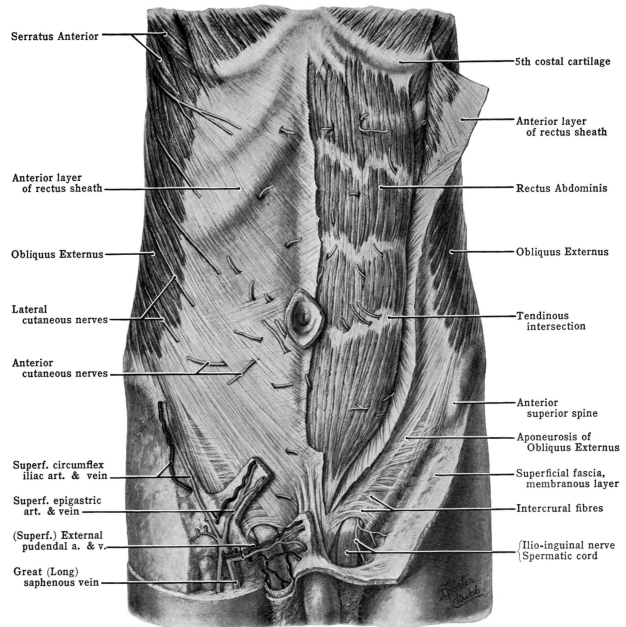

Serratus Anterior

5th costal cartilage

Anterior layer
of rectus sheath

Anterior layer
of rectus sheath

Rectus Abdominis

Obliquus Externus

Obliquus Externus

Lateral
cutaneous nerves

Tendinous
intersection

Anterior
cutaneous nerves

Anterior
superior spine

Aponeurosis of
Obliquus Externus

Superf. circumflex
iliac art. & vein

Superficial fascia,
membranous layer

Superf. epigastric
art. & vein

Intercrural fibres

(Superf.) External
pudendal a. & v.

Ilio-inguinal nerve
Spermatic cord

Great (Long)
saphenous vein

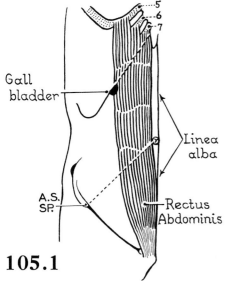

5
6
7

Gall
bladder

Linea
alba

A.S.
SP.

Rectus
Abdominis

105.1

Diagram. Rectus Abdominis is 3 times
as wide cranially, where fleshy, as it is
caudally, where tendinous. Its lateral
border passes midway between navel and
a. s. spine, and crosses the gall bladder.

105 Anterior Abdominal Wall—I

Anterior layer of Rectus sheath is reflected, on the right side.

Observe:

1. Obliquus Externus, aponeurotic medial to a line that curves upwards from a point 1″ lateral
   to the ant. sup. iliac spine to the 5th rib. The aponeurosis gives origin to a slip of Pectoralis
   Major.
2. The lateral border of Rectus Abdominis curving from the pubic tubercle, through the mid-
   point between the navel and the ant. sup. spine, and across the chest margin to the 5th rib.
3. The anterior cutaneous nerves (Th. 7–12) piercing Rectus and the anterior layer of its
   sheath. T. 10 supplies the region of the umbilicus or navel.
4. In the superficial fascia (of Camper), the three superficial inguinal branches of the femoral
   artery and the three superficial inguinal tributaries of the great saphenous vein. Of these, the
   external pudendal artery and vein cross the spermatic cord.
5. The membranous layer of the superficial fascia (of Scarpa) blending with the fascia lata a
   finger's breadth below the inguinal ligament and thereby forming a gutter that empties into
   the superficial perineal pouch (of Colles).
6. The spermatic cord and the ilio-inguinal nerve issuing through the superficial. (subcutaneous) inguinal ring.

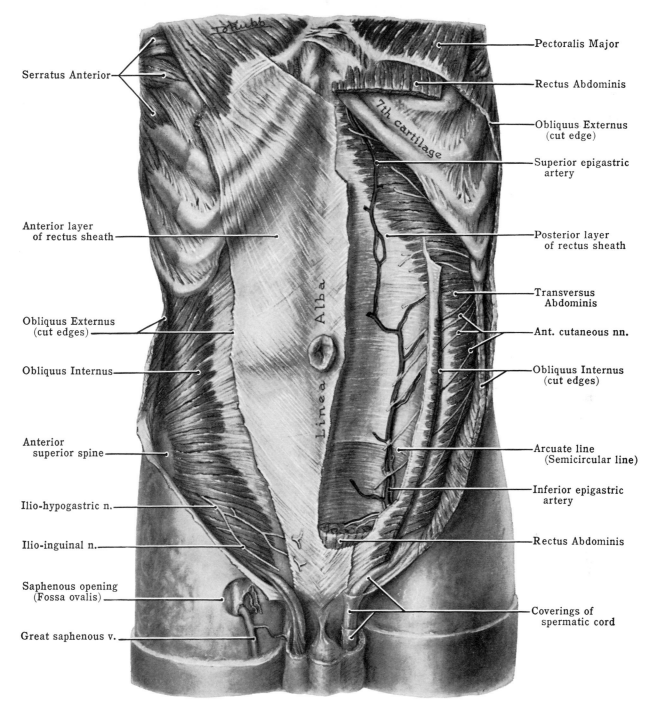

Serratus Anterior

Pectoralis Major

Rectus Abdominis

Obliquus Externus
(cut edge)

Superior epigastric
artery

7th cartilage

Anterior layer
of rectus sheath

Posterior layer
of rectus sheath

Linea Alba

Transversus
Abdominis

Obliquus Externus
(cut edges)

Ant. cutaneous nn.

Obliquus Internus

Obliquus Internus
(cut edges)

Anterior
superior spine

Arcuate line
(Semicircular line)

Ilio-hypogastric n.

Inferior epigastric
artery

Ilio-inguinal n.

Rectus Abdominis

Saphenous opening
(Fossa ovalis)

Coverings of
spermatic cord

Great saphenous v.

106 Anterior Abdominal Wall—II

On the left side, most of Obliquus Externus is excised. On the right, Rectus Abdominis
is excised and Obliquus Internus divided.

Observe:

1. Obliquus Internus fibers running horizontally at the level of the ant. sup. spine; running
   obliquely upwards above this level, and obliquely downwards below it.

2. The two anterior branches of nerve L. 1 piercing Obliquus Internus infero-medial to the
   ant. sup. spine and running forwards and medially; the upper branch then piercing Obliquus Externus aponeurosis; the lower lying within ½″ of the inguinal lig. and passing
   through the superficial inguinal ring with the spermatic cord.

3. The arcuate line at the level of the ant. sup. iliac spine.

4. The anastomosis between the superior and inferior epigastric arteries which indirectly
   unites the arteries of the upper limb to those of the lower. (viz., subclavian to ext. iliac).

5. Nerves Th. 7–12, but not L. 1, entering the Rectus sheath. Of these nerves, the upper ones
   ascend, the lower ones descend.

6. Obliquus Externus attached a hand's breadth above the costal margin; Obliquus Internus
   to the margin; and Transversus within the margin.

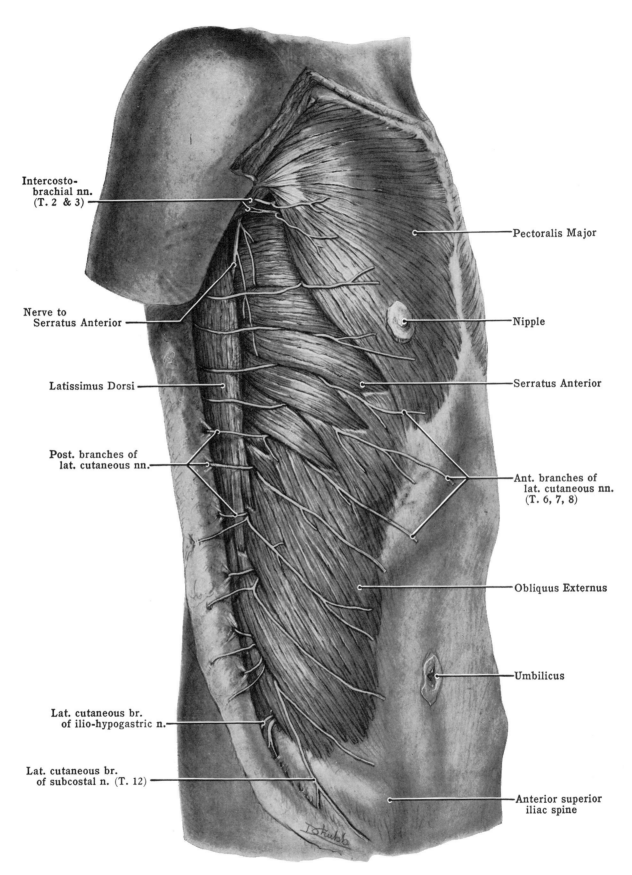

Intercosto-
brachial nn.
(T. 2 & 3)

Nerve to
Serratus Anterior

Latissimus Dorsi

Post. branches of
lat. cutaneous nn.

Lat. cutaneous br.
of ilio-hypogastric n.

Lat. cutaneous br.
of subcostal n. (T. 12)

Pectoralis Major

Nipple

Serratus Anterior

Ant. branches of
lat. cutaneous nn.
(T. 6, 7, 8)

Obliquus Externus

Umbilicus

Anterior superior
iliac spine

107   Lateral Cutaneous Nerves

Note twigs supplying Obliquus Externus. The shoulder is pushed forwards, hence
the nerve to Serratus is partly concealed by Latissimus.

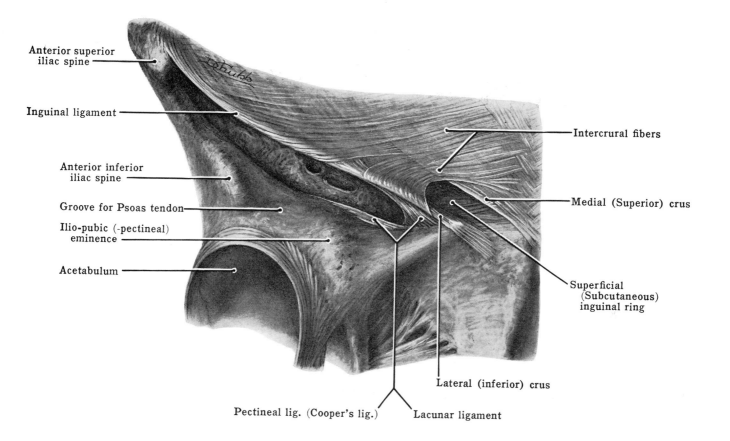

Anterior superior
iliac spine

Inguinal ligament

Anterior inferior
iliac spine

Groove for Psoas tendon

Ilio-pubic (-pectineal)
eminence

Acetabulum

Intercrural fibers

Medial (Superior) crus

Superficial
(Subcutaneous)
inguinal ring

Lateral (inferior) crus

Pectineal lig. (Cooper's lig.)   Lacunar ligament

108 Inguinal Ligament, antero-inferior view

Observe:

1. The inguinal ligament extending from the anterior superior iliac spine to the pubic tubercle and receiving accessions of fibres from the External Oblique aponeurosis.

2. The fibres of the ligament that, falling short of the pubic tubercle, find attachment to the pecten pubis as the lacunar ligament. This ligament forms the medial border of the lacuna, or space, called the femoral ring (fig. 258).

3. Unnamed fibers, extending beyond the pubic tubercle, find attachment to the body of the pubis.

4. The pectineal ligament whose fibres run along the pecten pubis (pectineal line).

5. The lateral crus of the superficial inguinal ring formed by the inguinal ligament, which is rounded; the medial crus formed by the aponeurosis of External Oblique, which is sharp.

6. The space between the inguinal ligament and the hip bone. The lateral part transmits:—Iliacus, Psoas, femoral nerve, and lateral cutaneous nerve of the thigh. The medial part transmits:—femoral artery, vein, and lymph vessels and femoral branch of the genitofemoral nerve (figs. 110, 256).

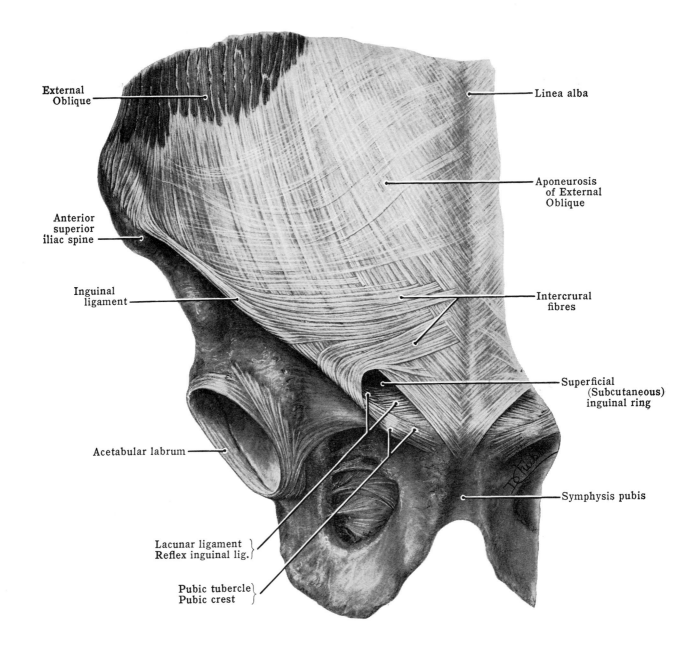

External Oblique

Linea alba

Aponeurosis of External Oblique

Anterior superior iliac spine

Inguinal ligament

Intercrural fibres

Superficial (Subcutaneous) inguinal ring

Acetabular labrum

Symphysis pubis

Lacunar ligament
Reflex inguinal lig.

Pubic tubercle
Pubic crest

109 Inguinal Region—I

Aponeurosis of External Oblique: Superficial Inguinal Ring.

Observe:

1. The linea alba to be not an unyielding ligament uniting the sternum to the symphysis pubis, but a line across which fibres decussate in bias and therefore extensible.

2. The intercrural fibres, well developed in this specimen, preventing the crura of the inguinal ring from spreading. (See also fig. 105.)

3. The superficial inguinal ring to be triangular in shape, its central point being above the pubic tubercle, its base being the lateral half of the pubic crest, its lateral crus being the inguinal ligament, and its medial crus being fibres of External Oblique aponeurosis that cross the pubic crest at its mid point.

4. Behind the ring, some fibres of External Oblique aponeurosis from the opposite side passing to the pubic crest and pecten pubis are called the reflected inguinal ligament.

5. Most fleshy fibres, here shown, of External Oblique sending their tendinous fibres to reinforce the inguinal ligament.

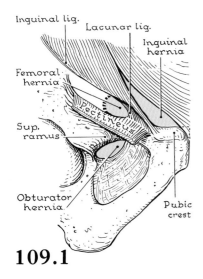

Inguinal lig.

Lacunar lig.

Inguinal hernia

Femoral hernia

Sup. ramus

Obturator hernia

Pubic crest

109.1

Diagram. Three hernial sites and their boundaries.

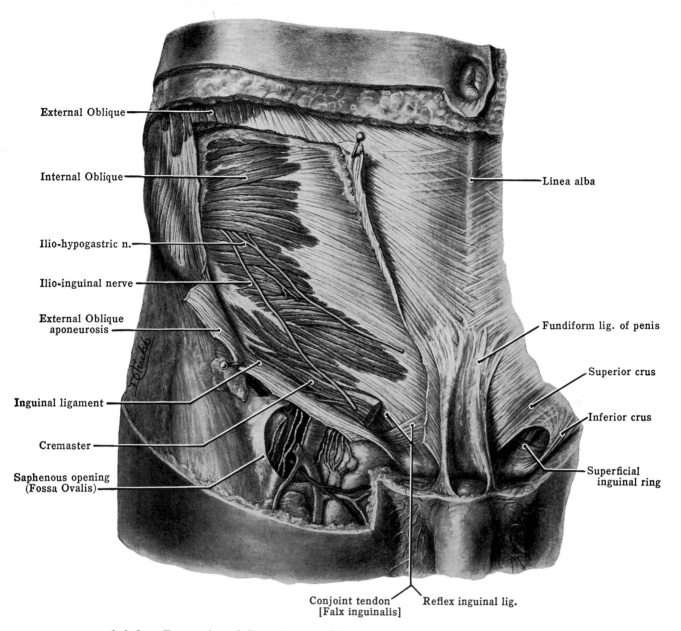

External Oblique

Internal Oblique

Ilio-hypogastric n.

Ilio-inguinal nerve

External Oblique
aponeurosis

Inguinal ligament

Cremaster

Saphenous opening
(Fossa Ovalis)

Linea alba

Fundiform lig. of penis

Superior crus

Inferior crus

Superficial
inguinal ring

Conjoint tendon
[Falx inguinalis]

Reflex inguinal lig.

110   Inguinal Region—II

Internal Oblique and Cremaster Muscles.
(External Oblique aponeurosis is partly cut away; spermatic cord is cut short.)

Observe:

1. The laminated, fundiform (suspensory) lig. of the penis descending to the junction of the fixed and mobile parts of the organ.

2. The reflex inguinal lig., which represents External Oblique, lying anterior to the conjoint tendon [falx inguinalis] which represents Internal Oblique and Transversus.

3. The only two structures that course between External and Internal Obliques, namely, the ilio-hypogastric and ilio-inguinal branches of the 1st lumbar nerve segment. They are sensory from this point to their terminations.

4. The fleshy fibres of Internal Oblique at the level of the anterior superior spine running horizontally; those from the iliac crest passing medio-cranially; and those from the inguinal ligament arching medio-caudally.

5. The Cremaster muscle covering the cord and filling the arched space between conjoint tendon and inguinal ligament.

6. At the level of the navel, the aponeurosis of External Oblique blending with the aponeurosis of Internal Oblique near the lateral border of the Rectus, but in the suprapubic region free as far as the median plane.

7. Numerous lymph vessels (not labelled) streaming cranially around the femoral vessels.

(For femoral sheath see fig. 256.)

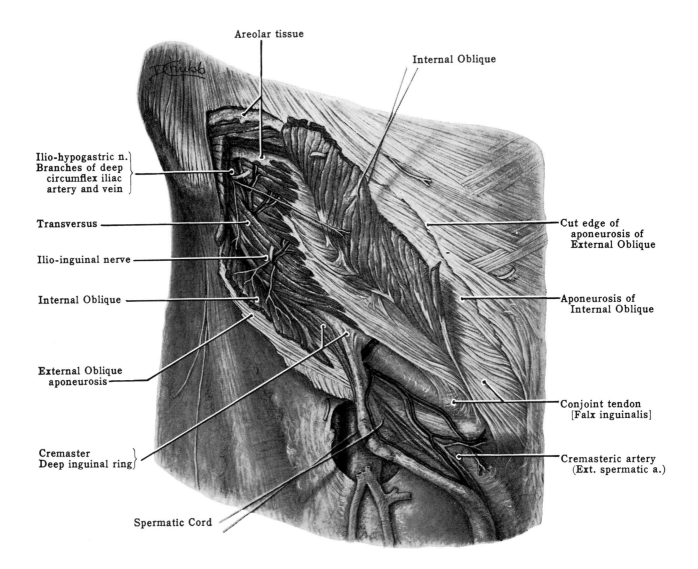

Areolar tissue

Internal Oblique

Ilio-hypogastric n.
Branches of deep
circumflex iliac
artery and vein

Transversus

Ilio-inguinal nerve

Internal Oblique

External Oblique
aponeurosis

Cremaster
Deep inguinal ring

Spermatic Cord

Cut edge of
aponeurosis of
External Oblique

Aponeurosis of
Internal Oblique

Conjoint tendon
[Falx inguinalis]

Cremasteric artery
(Ext. spermatic a.)

111   Inguinal Region—III

(Internal Oblique is reflected and the spermatic cord is retracted.)

Observe:

1. Transversus fibres taking, in this region, the same common medio-caudal direction as the fibres of External Oblique aponeurosis and Internal Oblique.

2. Transversus having a less extensive origin from the inguinal ligament than Internal Oblique.

3. The Internal Oblique portion of the conjoint tendon attached to the pubic crest; Transversus portion extending laterally along the pecten pubis (pectineal line).

4. Conjoint tendon not sharply defined from fascia transversalis, but blending with it.

5. Segment lumbar I, via the ilio-hypogastric and ilio-inguinal nerves, supplying the fibres of Internal Oblique and Transversus that control the conjoint tendon.

6. Fascia transversalis evaginated to form the tubular internal spermatic fascia. The mouth of the tube, called the deep (abdominal) inguinal ring, situated lateral to the inferior epigastric vessels.

7. The cremasteric artery (a branch of the inf. epigastric art.) which in figure 119 is seen to anastomose with the testicular artery and the artery to the deferent duct (vas deferens).

8. The Cremaster muscle arising from the inguinal ligament.

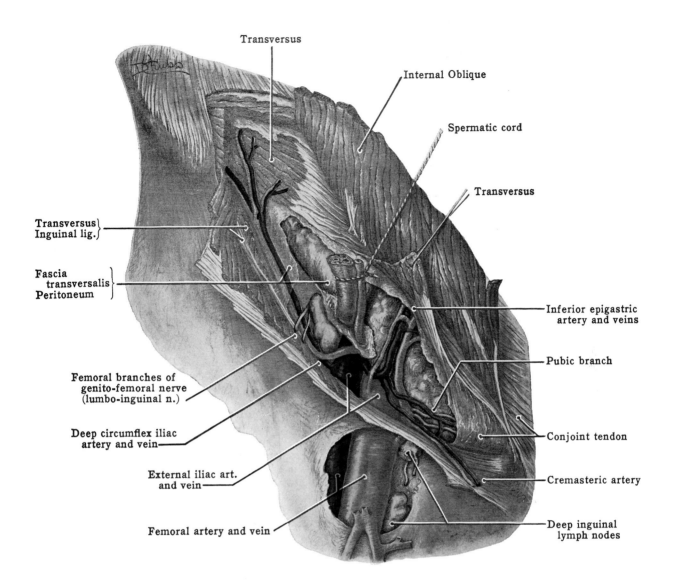

Transversus

Internal Oblique

Spermatic cord

Transversus

Transversus Inguinal lig.

Fascia transversalis Peritoneum

Inferior epigastric artery and veins

Pubic branch

Femoral branches of genito-femoral nerve (lumbo-inguinal n.)

Deep circumflex iliac artery and vein

Conjoint tendon

Cremasteric artery

External iliac art. and vein

Deep inguinal lymph nodes

Femoral artery and vein

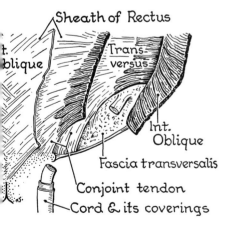

Sheath of Rectus

t. blique

Trans-versus

Int. Oblique

Fascia transversalis

Conjoint tendon

Cord & its coverings

111.1

Demonstrating the continuity of Rectus sheath with conjoint tendon.

112 Inguinal Region—IV

(The inguinal part of Transversus and fascia transversalis are partly cut away and the spermatic cord is excised.)

Observe:

1. The lower limit of the peritoneal sac. It lies some distance above the inguinal ligament laterally but close to it medially.

2. The location of the deep (abdominal) inguinal ring—a finger's breadth above the inguinal ligament at the midpoint between the anterior superior spine and the pubic tubercle.

3. The testicular vessels and the deferent duct (retracted) starting to part company at the deep inguinal ring.

4. The proximity of the external iliac artery and vein to the inguinal canal.

5. The only 2 branches of the external iliac artery:—the deep circumflex iliac and inferior epigastric arteries; note also the cremasteric and pubic branches of the latter.

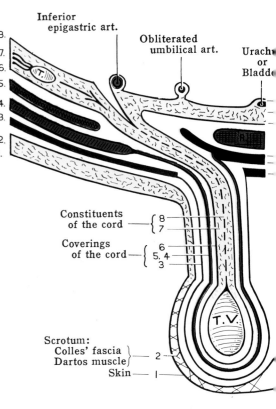

Peritoneum	— 8.
Subperitoneal fat	— 7.
Fascia transversalis	— 6.
Transversus	— 5.
Internal Oblique	— 4.
External Oblique aponeurosis	— 3.
Subcutaneous fat	— 2.
Skin	— I.

Inferior epigastric art.

Obliterated umbilical art.

Urach or Bladd

Constituents of the cord { 8 7

Coverings of the cord { 6 5, 4 3

Scrotum:
Colles' fascia } — 2 —
Dartos muscle }
Skin — I —

113   Scheme of the Inguinal Canal

The Eight Layers of the Abdominal Wall and their Evaginations.

(In this schematic horizontal section, the scrotum and testis are assumed to have been raised to the level of the superficial inguinal ring.)

The evaginations become:—(a) the scrotum, (b) the coverings of the spermatic cord, and (c) the constituents of that cord.

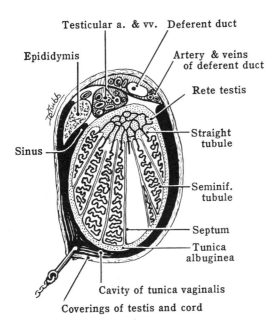

Testicular a. & vv.   Deferent duct

Epididymis

Artery & veins of deferent duct

Rete testis

Straight tubule

Seminif. tubule

Septum

Tunica albuginea

Sinus

Cavity of tunica vaginalis

Coverings of testis and cord

114   Testis on Cross Section

(RIGHT TESTIS, VIEWED FROM ABOVE.)

Observe:

1. The cavity of the tunica vaginalis testis surrounding the testis in front and at the sides and extending between testis and epididymis as the sinus of the epididymis.
2. The epididymis lying postero-lateral to the testis. It indicates to which side a testis belongs, for it is on the right side of a right testis and on the left side of a left testis.
3. The deferent duct with its fine lumen and thick wall lying postero-medial to the testis.
4. The 3 groups of longitudinal veins (a) around the testicular artery, (b) medial to the duct with the artery of the duct, and (c) lateral to it.
5. The pyramidal compartments for the seminiferous tubules, shown semi-diagrammatically. Each of the 250 compartments contains two or three hair-like seminiferous tubules which join in the mediastinum testis to form a rete.

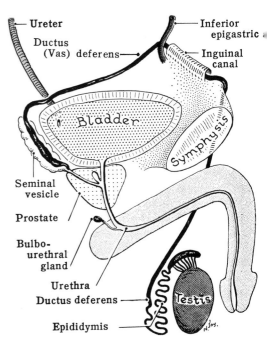

Ureter

Ductus (Vas) deferens

Inferior epigastric

Inguinal canal

Bladder

Symphysis

Seminal vesicle

Prostate

Bulbo-urethral gland

Urethra

Ductus deferens

Testis

Epididymis

115   Diagram of the Male Genital System

indicating the course of the deferent duct (The ejaculatory ducts and the utriculus, both within the prostate, see fig. 207.1.)

(For urinary system, see fig. 182.)

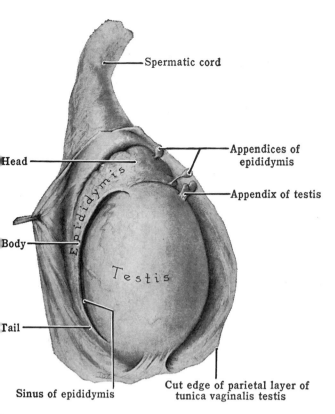

- Spermatic cord
- Head
- Body
- Tail
- Sinus of epididymis
- Appendices of epididymis
- Appendix of testis
- Cut edge of parietal layer of tunica vaginalis testis

Epididymis

Testis

116 Testis, lateral view

The tunica vaginalis testis has been incised longitudinally.

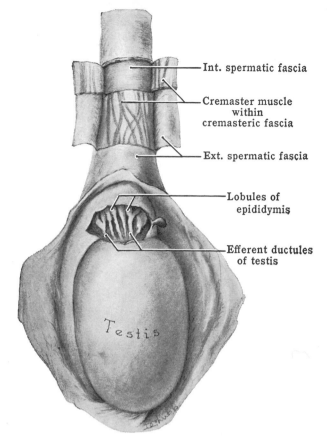

- Int. spermatic fascia
- Cremaster muscle within cremasteric fascia
- Ext. spermatic fascia
- Lobules of epididymis
- Efferent ductules of testis

Testis

117 Coverings of Spermatic Cord. Efferent Ductules

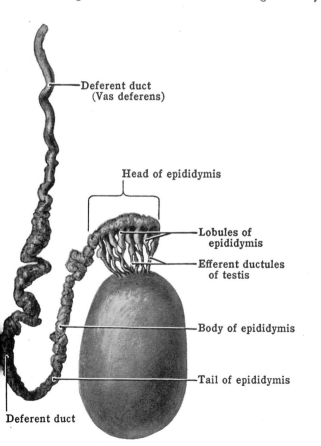

- Deferent duct (Vas deferens)
- Head of epididymis
- Lobules of epididymis
- Efferent ductules of testis
- Body of epididymis
- Tail of epididymis
- Deferent duct

18 Epididymis

Note the eight efferent ductules uniting the epididymis to the upper pole of the testis.

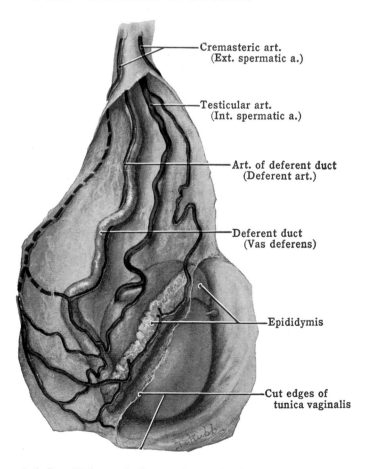

- Cremasteric art. (Ext. spermatic a.)
- Testicular art. (Int. spermatic a.)
- Art. of deferent duct (Deferent art.)
- Deferent duct (Vas deferens)
- Epididymis
- Cut edges of tunica vaginalis

119 Blood Supply of the Testis

The epididymis is displaced slightly to the lateral side. Note the free anastomosis between the three arteries.

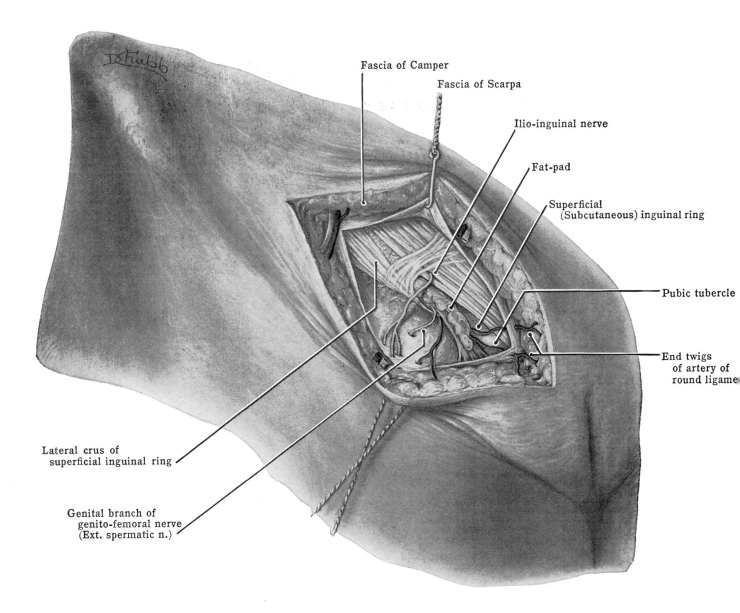

Fascia of Camper

Fascia of Scarpa

Ilio-inguinal nerve

Fat-pad

Superficial
(Subcutaneous) inguinal ring

Pubic tubercle

End twigs
of artery of
round ligame[...]

Lateral crus of
superficial inguinal ring

Genital branch of
genito-femoral nerve
(Ext. spermatic n.)

120, 121, 122, and 123 Female Inguinal Canal, progressive dissections

Observe:

1. In 120, the superficial inguinal ring, small and its crura prevented by the intercrural fibres from spreading.

2. Issuing from the superficial inguinal ring: (a) the round ligament of the uterus [lig. teres uteri], (b) a closely applied pad of fat, (c) the genital branch of the genito-femoral nerve, and (d) the artery of the round ligament of the uterus. This artery is homologous with the cremasteric artery in the male, shown in figure 112.

3. The ilio-inguinal nerve, here, perforating the medial crus of the superficial inguinal ring.

4. In 121, the Cremaster muscle, not extending beyond the ring.

5. In 122, the round ligament breaking up into strands as it leaves the inguinal canal and approaches the labium majus.

6. In 123, the close relationship of the external iliac artery and vein to the inguinal canal.

Fig. 121

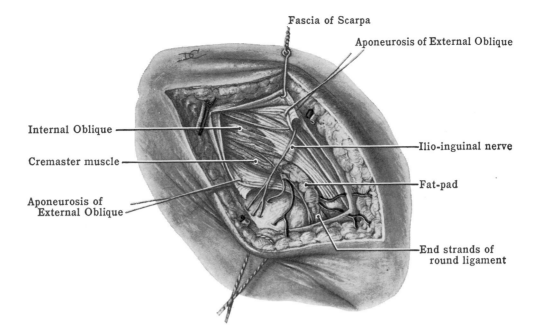

Fascia of Scarpa

Aponeurosis of External Oblique

Internal Oblique

Cremaster muscle

Aponeurosis of
External Oblique

Ilio-inguinal nerve

Fat-pad

End strands of
round ligament

Fig. 122

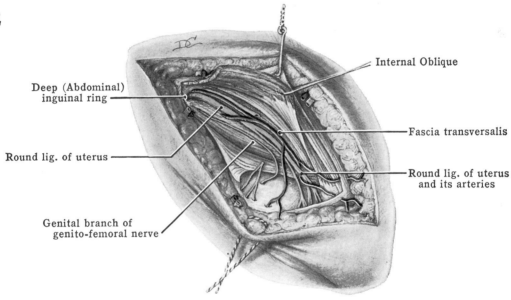

Deep (Abdominal)
inguinal ring

Round lig. of uterus

Genital branch of
genito-femoral nerve

Internal Oblique

Fascia transversalis

Round lig. of uterus
and its arteries

Fig. 123

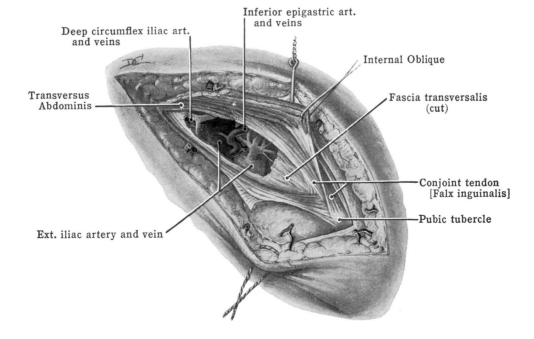

Deep circumflex iliac art.
and veins

Inferior epigastric art.
and veins

Internal Oblique

Transversus
Abdominis

Fascia transversalis
(cut)

Conjoint tendon
[Falx inguinalis]

Pubic tubercle

Ext. iliac artery and vein

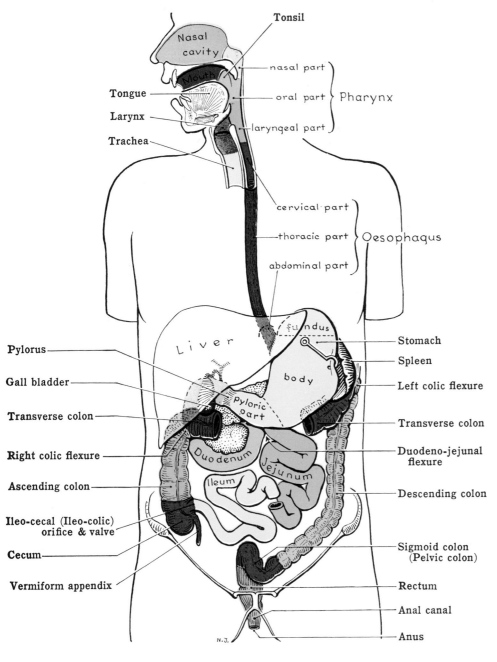

Tonsil

Nasal cavity

Mouth

nasal part

oral part — Pharynx

Tongue

Larynx

laryngeal part

Trachea

cervical part

thoracic part — Oesophagus

abdominal part

fundus

Liver

Stomach

Spleen

body

Pylorus

Gall bladder

Transverse colon

pyloric part

Left colic flexure

Transverse colon

Right colic flexure

Duodenum

Jejunum

Duodeno-jejunal flexure

Ascending colon

Ileum

Descending colon

Ileo-cecal (Ileo-colic) orifice & valve

Cecum

Sigmoid colon (Pelvic colon)

Vermiform appendix

Rectum

Anal canal

N.J.

Anus

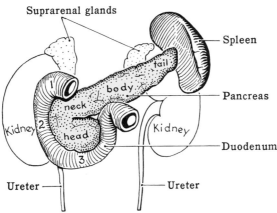

Suprarenal glands

Spleen

tail

body

Pancreas

neck

Kidney 1 2

head

Kidney

Duodenum

3

Ureter

Ureter

124 Diagram of the Digestive System

In the lower figure, 3 organs—spleen, pancreas, and duodenum—are uncovered by removal of the stomach and the transverse colon.

Digestive System c
Apparatus

This system extends from the lip to the anus.

Here is a list of its chief parts:

CAVITY OF THE MOUTH OR CAVUM ORIS
Vestibule of mouth
Lips or labia
Cheeks or buccae
Gums or gingivae
Teeth or dentes
Cavity proper of mouth
Palate
hard
soft
Tongue or lingua
Salivary glands
Parotid
Sublingual
Submandibular
Palato-glossal arch

CAVITY OF THE PHARYNX
Oral part
Palatine tonsil
Laryngeal part
Entrance, or aditus, to larynx

ALIMENTARY CANAL
Esophagus
Cervical part
Thoracic part
Abdominal part
Stomach or Ventriculus or Gaster
Cardiac orifice
Incisura cardiaca
Greater curvature
Lesser curvature
Incisura angularis
Fundus
Body
Pyloric part
Pyloric antrum
Pyloric canal
Pylorus
Pyloric orifice
Small intestine
Duodenum
1st or superior part
2nd or descending part
3rd or inferior part
horizontal part
ascending part (4th)
Duodeno-jejunal flexure
Jejunum
Ileum
Ileo-cecal orifice and valve
Large intestine
Vermiform appendix
Cecum
Ascending colon
Right colic flexure
(Hepatic flexure)
Transverse colon
Left colic flexure
(Splenic flexure)
Descending colon
Sigmoid colon
Rectum
Anal canal
Anus

ASSOCIATED ORGANS
Liver or Hepar
Gall bladder
fundus, body, and neck
Biliary passages
Pancreas
head, neck, body, tail, and duct
Spleen or Lien

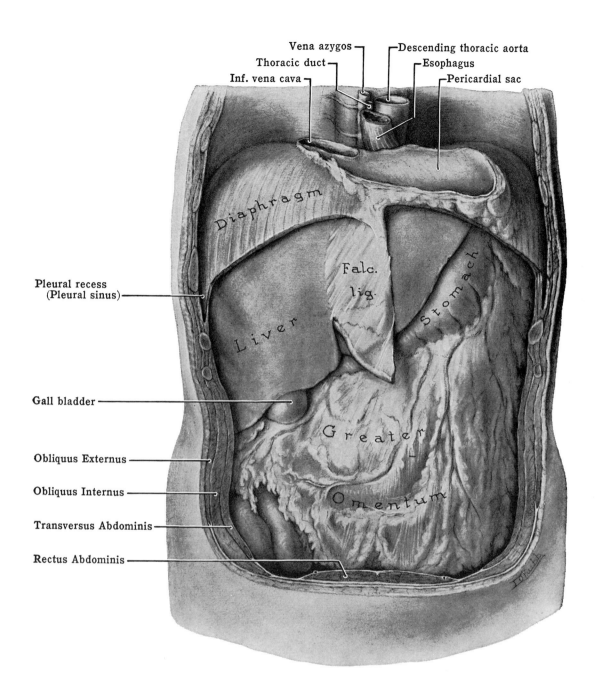

Vena azygos — ⌐Descending thoracic aorta
Thoracic duct — ⌐Esophagus
Inf. vena cava — ⌐Pericardial sac

Diaphragm

Falc. lig.

Stomach

Pleural recess
(Pleural sinus)

Liver

Gall bladder

Greater

Obliquus Externus

Omentum

Obliquus Internus

Transversus Abdominis

Rectus Abdominis

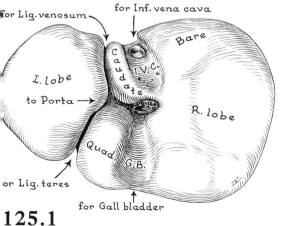

for Lig. venosum   for Inf. vena cava

Bare

l. lobe

Caudate

I.V.C.

to Porta →

R. lobe

Quad. G.B.

or Lig. teres

125.1

for Gall bladder

Liver (Hepar), postero-inferior view, not visible until removed from the body. Note the porta.

125   Abdominal Contents, undisturbed

The anterior abdominal and thoracic walls are cut away.

Observe:

1. The falciform lig., with the lig. teres hepatis, or round ligament of liver, in its free edge, severed at its attachment to the abdominal wall and Diaphragm in the median plane. Its attachment to the liver is its own width to the right of the median plane. It resists displacement of the liver to the right.

2. The gall bladder projecting below the sharp, inferior border of the liver.

3. The two Recti meeting in the median plane above the pubis.

4. Obliquus Internus, the thickest of the three flat abdominal muscles.

5. The pleural cavities separating the upper abdominal viscera from the body wall.

6. Two thirds of the pericardial sac lying to the left of the median plane; its apex, i.e. the lowest and leftmost point, overlying the stomach.

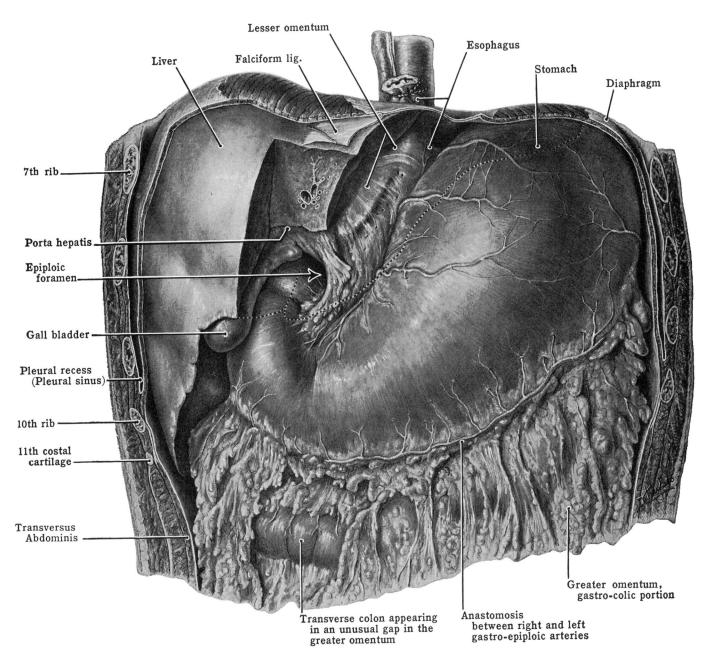

Lesser omentum

Esophagus

Liver

Falciform lig.

Stomach

Diaphragm

7th rib

Porta hepatis

Epiploic foramen

Gall bladder

Pleural recess (Pleural sinus)

10th rib

11th costal cartilage

Transversus Abdominis

Transverse colon appearing in an unusual gap in the greater omentum

Anastomosis between right and left gastro-epiploic arteries

Greater omentum, gastro-colic portion

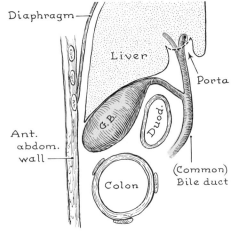

Diaphragm

Liver

Porta

Ant. abdom. wall

G.B.

Duod.

(Common) Bile duct

Colon

126.1

Diagram. The 4 contact relations of the gall bladder.

126 Stomach and the Omenta, front view

The stomach is inflated with air; the left part of the liver is cut away.

Observe:

1. The pyloric end of the stomach which has moved to the right and has come to lie below, or rather infero-posterior to, the gall bladder; the 1st or superior part of the duodenum—placed behind the arrow head—almost occluding the epiploic foramen (mouth of the lesser sac).

2. The gall bladder, followed cranially, leading to the free margin of the lesser omentum, and hence acting as a guide to the epiploic foramen, which lies behind that free margin.

3. The lesser omentum passing from the lesser curvature of the stomach and first inch of the duodenum to the fissure for the lig. venosum and porta hepatis. This omentum, thickened at its free margin but elsewhere like gossamer, much perforated, and caudate lobe of the liver visible through it.

4. The greater omentum hanging from the greater curvature of the stomach.

5. The right cupola of the diaphragm rising higher than the left cupola, which is usual.

6. The relative thinness of the Transversus Abdominis. The pleural recess, about two fingers breadth above the costal margin in the mid-lateral line.

127 Stomach, front view

The cardiac notch and the angular notch [incisura angularis] are here well marked. The pyloric antrum is here not demarcated from the tubular pyloric canal.

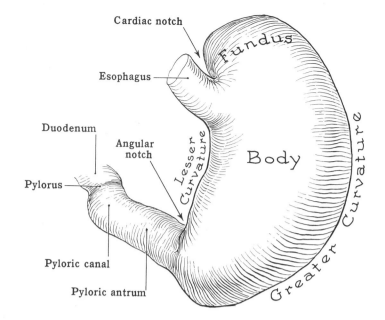

128 Mucous Membrane of the Stomach

Along the lesser curvature several longitudinal ridges extend from esophagus to pylorus, elsewhere the mucous membrane is rugose when the stomach is empty.

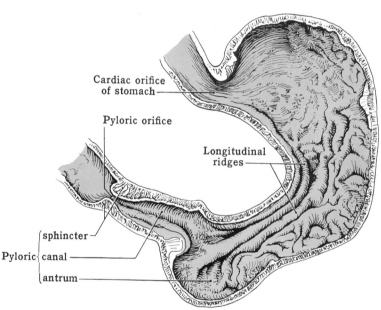

129 Muscular Coat of the Stomach, from within

The stomach is cut along the greater curvature and the loosely adherent mucous and submucous coats are dissected off.

The fibres of the innermost or oblique muscle layer form ∩-shaped loops that extend over the fundus and down both surfaces of the stomach as far as the antrum. Their medial limit is at the cardiac notch, hence the fibres of the middle or circular layer become the innermost layer along the lesser curvature and in the pyloric region; at the pylorus they are thickened to form the pyloric sphincter. They are present everywhere except at the fundus. The fibres of the outermost or longitudinal layer (not seen) are best marked along the curvatures.

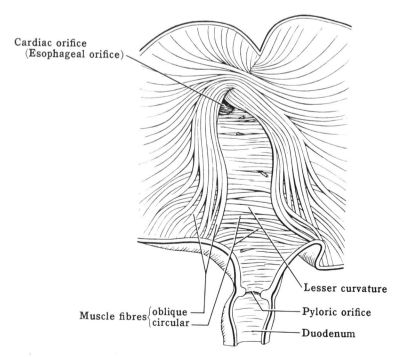

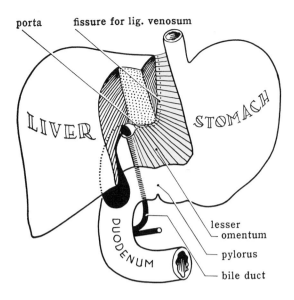

130 Diagram: Attachments of the Lesser Omentum

Two sagittal cuts have been made through the liver—one at the fissure for the lig. venosum; the other at the right limit of the porta hepatis. These two cuts have been joined by a coronal cut.

Note:

1. The lesser omentum may be regarded as the "mesentery" of the bile passages, seeing they occupy its free edge (fig. 147).
2. The lesser omentum extends from the lesser curvature of the stomach and first inch of the duodenum to the fissure for the lig. venosum and to the porta. The part attached to the body of the stomach passes to the fissure; the part attached to the pyloric part of the stomach and duodenum passes to the porta.

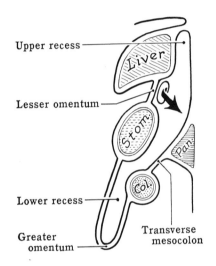

130.1 Diagram: Vertical Extent of the Omental Bursa (Lesser Sac) in the median plane

The arrow passes from the greater sac of peritoneum through the epiploic foramen (mouth of the lesser sac) into the omental bursa (lesser sac).

Note the 3 approaches to the bursa: it may be opened by tearing through (a) the lesser omentum, (b) the greater omentum, or (c) the transverse mesocolon.

130.2 Diagram: Horizontal Extent of the Omental Bursa at the Level of the Epiploic Foramen (Mouth of Sac). Pedicle of the Spleen

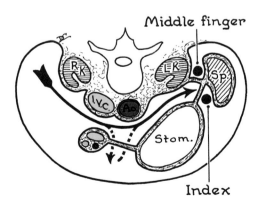

Instructions:

1. While standing on the right side of the body, run your right middle finger upwards between the left kidney and the spleen, and your right index upwards between the stomach and the spleen. The 'pedicle or stalk' of the spleen now lies in the cleft between these two fingers, as though in a clamp. The pedicle has a free lower border (and a free upper border), or you could not grasp it as you are doing. Its linear site of attachment to the spleen is around the hilus.
2. Clamped between your index and middle finger are four layers of peritoneum. Of this you can satisfy yourself by passing your left index through the epiploic foramen and across the abdomen, behind the stomach, till it touches the spleen between your two right fingers. If your left index will not reach all the way, pass it as far as it will go, tear through the lesser omentum over its tip, withdraw the finger, and reinsert it at the half-way opening just made. The hilus of the spleen, which you are palpating, is situated at the left extremity of the omental bursa.

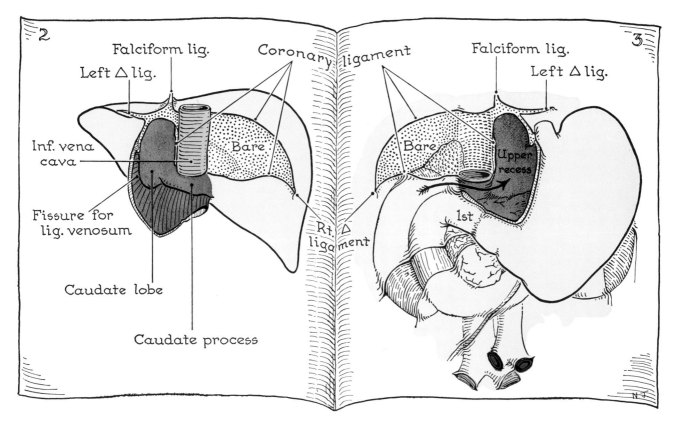

Falciform lig.
Left △ lig.
Coronary ligament
Falciform lig.
Left △ lig.

Bare

Inf. vena cava

Bare

Upper recess

Fissure for lig. venosum

Rt. △ ligament

1st

Caudate lobe

Caudate process

N͡J

131 Diagram of the Peritoneal Ligaments of the Liver

(The attachments of the liver are cut through and the liver is turned to the right side of the cadaver, as you would turn the page of a book. Hence, the posterior aspect of the liver is shown on page 2 and its posterior relations on page 3.

Note:

1. The arrow passing from the greater sac of peritoneum (yellow) into the lesser sac (orange).

2. The upper recess of the lesser sac, or omental bursa occupies the median plane of the body. Dorsally lies the descending thoracic aorta, diaphragm intervening (fig. 131.1). Ventrally is the lesser omentum. On the left is esophagus, and on the right is inf. vena cava, both of which lie bare on the diaphragm.

3. The inferior vena cava occupies the left or medial limit of the bare area of the liver.

4. The bare area is triangular; hence, the so-called coronary ligament, which surrounds it, is not a corona, but is three-sided. Its left side or base is between the i.v. cava and the caudate lobe; it is palpated when the right index is inserted into the upper recess.

5. Its apex is at the right triangular ligament, where the cranial and caudal layers of the coronary ligament meet.

6. The lower or caudal layer of the ligament is reflected from the liver on to: diaphragm, right kidney, and right suprarenal gland. It is called the hepato-renal ligament by the surgeon. Followed medially this layer crosses the i.v. cava at the epiploic foramen, and turning cranially becomes the left or basal layer of the ligament (fig. 177).

7. The lesser omentum is divided close to the stomach. It is not labelled, nor is the kidney, nor the suprarenal gland.

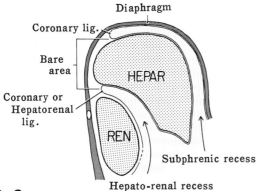

Diaphragm

Coronary lig.

Bare area

Coronary or Hepatorenal lig.

HEPAR

REN

Subphrenic recess

Hepato-renal recess

130.3

Diagram. Paramedian section through diaphragm, liver & right kidney to show the bare area of liver to be situated between the dorsal ends of 2 peritoneal recesses or pouches.

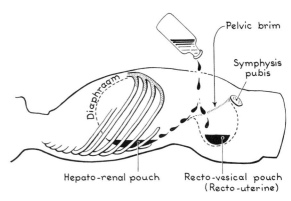

Pelvic brim

Symphysis pubis

Diaphragm

Hepato-renal pouch

Recto-vesical pouch (Recto-uterine)

130.4

Diagram. The two lowest (most dorsal) parts of peritoneal cavity, when subject lies recumbent.

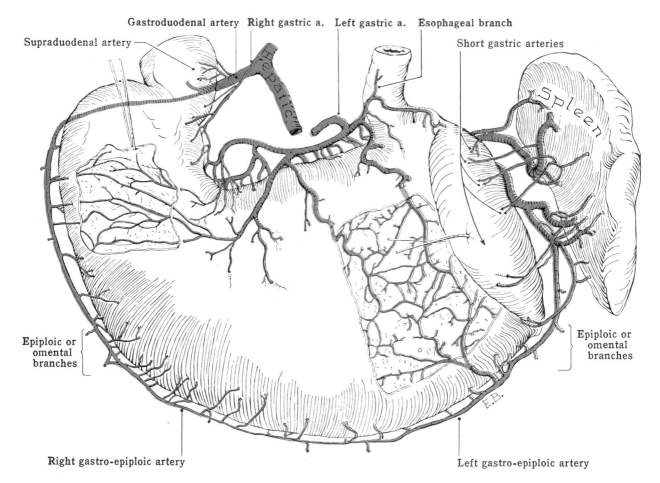

Supraduodenal artery — Gastroduodenal artery — Right gastric a. — Left gastric a. — Esophageal branch — Short gastric arteries

Epiploic or omental branches

Epiploic or omental branches

Right gastro-epiploic artery

Left gastro-epiploic artery

132   Arteries of the Stomach and Spleen

The serous and muscular coats are removed from two areas of the stomach, thereby revealing the anasto-motic networks in the submucous coat.

Observe:

1. The arterial arch on the lesser curvature formed by the larger left gastric artery and completed by the much smaller right gastric artery.
2. The arterial arch on the greater curvature formed equally by the right and the left gastro-epiploic artery. The anas-

tomosis between their two trunks is attenuated; commonly it is absent.

3. The anastomoses between the branches of the two foregoing arterial arches taking place in the submucous coat two-thirds of the distance from lesser to greater curvature.
4. Four or five tenuous short gastric arteries leaving the terminal branches of the splenic artery close to the spleen; and the left gastro-epiploic artery, belonging to the short gastric artery series, arising within 2.5 cm. of the hilus of the spleen.

(*For details consult Michels, N. A.*)

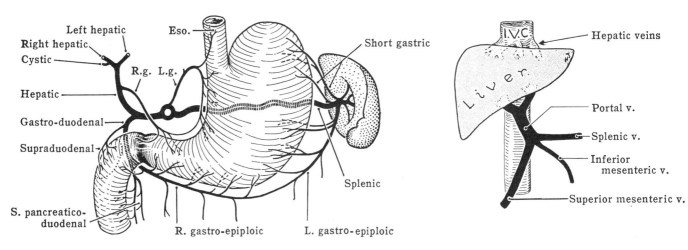

Left hepatic — Right hepatic — Cystic — R.g. L.g. — Eso. — Short gastric

Hepatic —

Gastro-duodenal —

Supraduodenal —

S. pancreatico-duodenal —

R. gastro-epiploic   L. gastro-epiploic   Splenic

I.V.C — Hepatic veins — Portal v. — Splenic v. — Inferior mesenteric v. — Superior mesenteric v.   Liver

132.1   Scheme of the distribution of the celiac trunk (artery).

132.2   Diagram of the blood from the gastro-intestinal apparatus entering the liver via the portal vein and leaving it via the hepatic veins to enter the inf. vena cava.

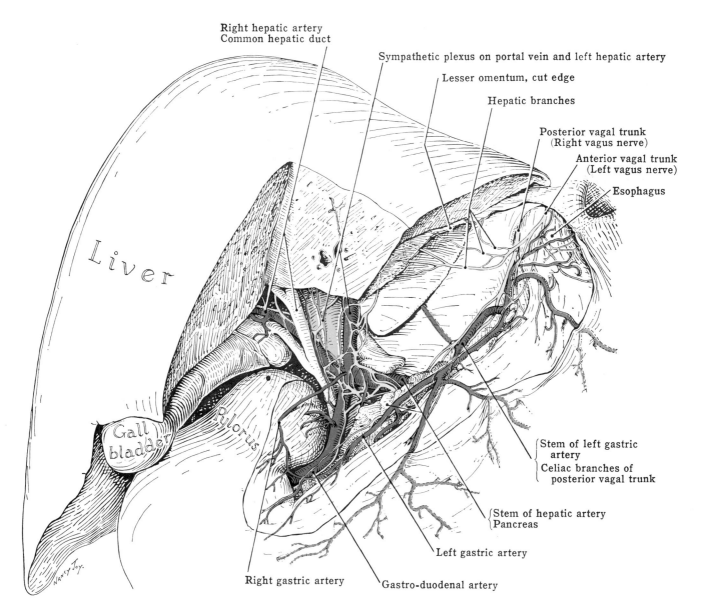

Right hepatic artery
Common hepatic duct

Sympathetic plexus on portal vein and left hepatic artery

Lesser omentum, cut edge

Hepatic branches

Posterior vagal trunk
(Right vagus nerve)

Anterior vagal trunk
(Left vagus nerve)

Esophagus

Liver

Gall bladder

Pylorus

Stem of left gastric artery

Celiac branches of posterior vagal trunk

Stem of hepatic artery
Pancreas

Left gastric artery

Right gastric artery

Gastro-duodenal artery

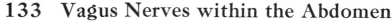

133 Vagus Nerves within the Abdomen

The liver is divided, as in fig. 126. The lesser omentum is removed. The lesser curvature and both ends of the stomach are in view.

Observe:

1. The posterior and anterior vagal trunks entering the abdomen, applied to the esophagus.

2. Gastric branches of these two trunks running near each other along the lesser curvature, communicating with each other, supplying the respective surfaces of stomach, and extending to pyloric antrum.

3. The celiac branch of the post. vagal trunk, descending along the stem of the left gastric artery to the celiac ganglia (fig. 180). Thence it is distributed mostly with the sympathetic plexuses along the blood vessels to the abdominal viscera (spleen, pancreas, kidneys, and intestines as far as the left colic flexure fig. 660).

4. The hepatic branches of the ant. vagal trunk running in the lesser omentum to the liver, and there joining sympathetic fibres from the celiac plexus that are ascending with the hepatic artery to the liver.

5. A lower branch (not shown), in series with the hepatic branches, turns downwards in the lesser omentum from near the porta and sends twigs (a) to the pylorus and 1st part of duodenum, (b) with the right gastric artery to the pyloric canal, (c) with the gastroduodenal artery to the 2nd part of the duodenum and the head of the pancreas, and (d) a branch turns upwards on the hepatic artery to communicate with the sympathetic fibres passing to the gall bladder (E. D. McCrea)

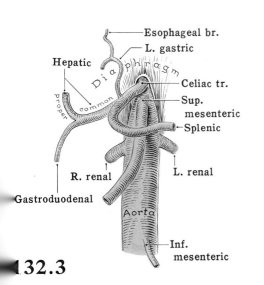

Esophageal br.

L. gastric

Hepatic

Diaphragm

proper

common

Celiac tr.

Sup. mesenteric

Splenic

R. renal

L. renal

Gastroduodenal

Aorta

Inf. mesenteric

132.3

Stems of the 3 arteries (celiac, sup. mesenteric & inf. mesenteric) supplying G.I. tract and its 3 unpaired glands (liver, pancreas & spleen).

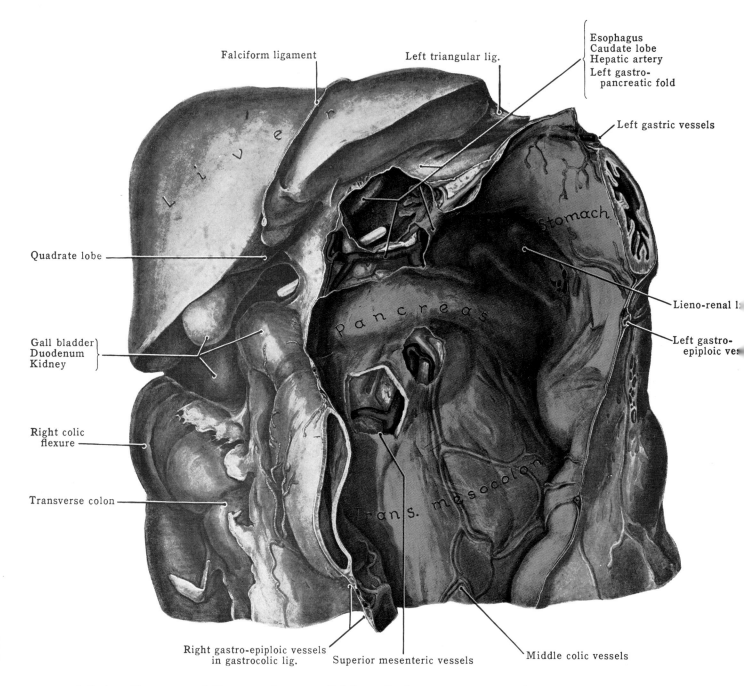

Falciform ligament

Left triangular lig.

Esophagus
Caudate lobe
Hepatic artery
Left gastro-
pancreatic fold

Left gastric vessels

Quadrate lobe

Lieno-renal l

Left gastro-
epiploic ve

Gall bladder
Duodenum
Kidney

Right colic
flexure

Transverse colon

Right gastro-epiploic vessels
in gastrocolic lig.

Superior mesenteric vessels

Middle colic vessels

134   Omental Bursa in an Older Subject, opened—I

The anterior wall of the bursa, consisting of the stomach with its two omenta and the vessels along its two curvatures, has been divided vertically and the two parts have been turned to the left and the right.

Observe:

1. The esophagus and the body of the stomach on the left side of the cadaver, and the pyloric part and the superior (1st) part of the duodenum on the right side. The 1st part of the duodenum running backwards, upwards and to the right, and having the gall bladder and quadrate lobe in contact with it above.

2. The right kidney forming the posterior wall of the hepato-renal pouch, and the white rod passed from that pouch, through the epiploic foramen, into the omental bursa.

3. The pancreas on the posterior wall of the bursa, moulded on the vertebral column, and lying roughly horizontally. Below this, the transverse mesocolon, the root of which has slipped caudally from its attachment to the pancreas.

4. Above the pancreas, the left gastro-pancreatic fold, which is the "mesentery" of the arch of the left gastric vessels, separates the upper recess, into which the caudate lobe projects, from the splenic recess, which lies to the left.

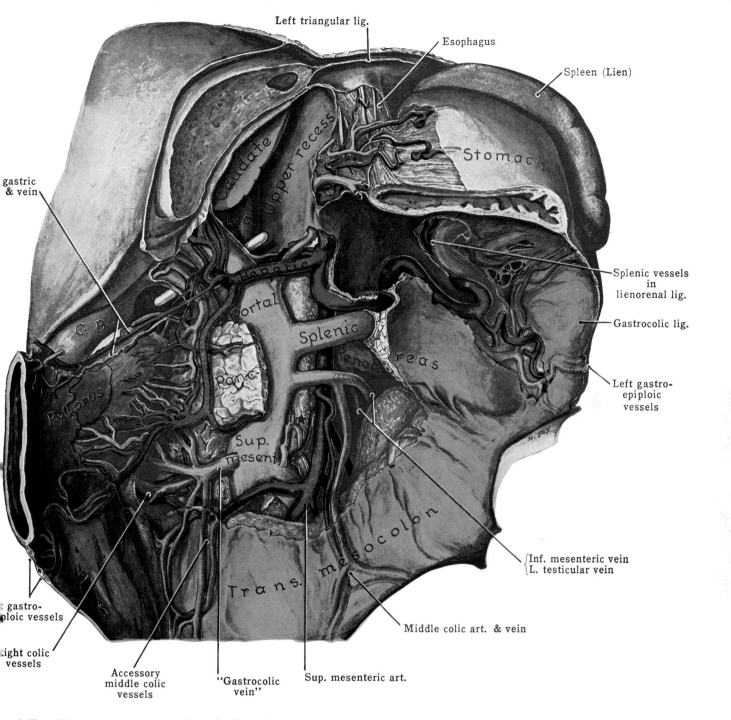

Left triangular lig. — **Esophagus** — **Spleen (Lien)**

gastric & vein

Caudate

Lv c Upper recess

Stomach

Hepatic

Portal

Splenic

Renal reas

Pancreas

Splenic vessels in lienorenal lig.

Gastrocolic lig.

Left gastro-epiploic vessels

G.B.

Pylorus

Sup. mesent

Trans. mesocolon

Inf. mesenteric vein
L. testicular vein

Middle colic art. & vein

gastro-ploic vessels

ight colic vessels

Accessory middle colic vessels

"Gastrocolic vein"

Sup. mesenteric art.

135 Posterior Wall of the Omental Bursa in an Older Subject—II

The peritoneum of the posterior wall has largely been removed and a section of pancreas has been excised.

Observe:

1. The white rod passed through the epiploic foramen.

2. The esophagus and the left gastro-pancreatic fold (fig. 134) bounding the left side of the upper recess.
The esophageal branches of the left gastric vessels and the ant. and post. vagal trunks applied to the esophagus.

3. The celiac trunk (not labelled) from which (a) the left gastric art. arches upwards, (b) the splenic art. runs tortuously to the left, and (c) the hepatic art. runs straight to the right to the front of the portal vein where it bifurcates like the letter Y or T set horizontally.

4. The right hepatic artery here arising early and passing dorsal to the portal vein (fig. 144 C). This was not obvious

in figure 134.

5. The portal vein formed behind the neck of the pancreas by the union of the superior mesenteric and splenic veins, with the inferior mesenteric vein joining at or near the angle of union. Here, the left gastric vein joins it. Usually, it is joined by:—right gastric vein (fig. 145), post. sup. pancreatico-duodenal vein (fig. 148) and one or two small duodenal or pancreatic veins.

6. The sup. mesenteric vein to be joined by the gastro-colic trunk (Falconer and Griffiths) which is formed by:—(a) ant. sup. pancreatico-duodenal vein, (b) right gastro-epiploic vein, (c) a right colic vein, and (d) here two middle colic veins. The middle colic vein accompanying the middle colic artery here ends in the inferior mesenteric vein.

7. The left renal vein receiving the left testicular vein on a plane dorsal to the splenic vein.

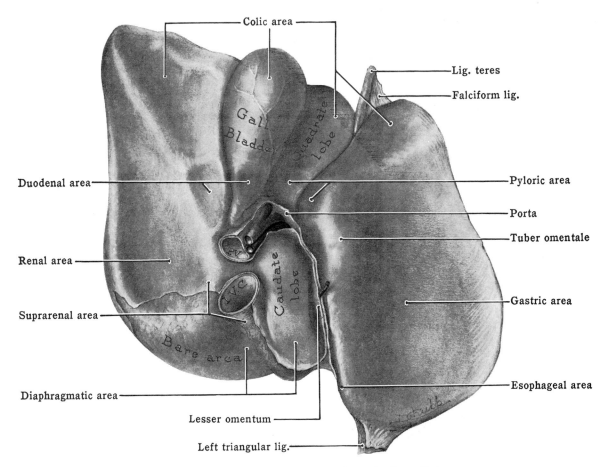

The Inferior and Posterior Surfaces of the Liver labels:
- Colic area
- Lig. teres
- Falciform lig.
- Gall Bladder
- Quadrate lobe
- Duodenal area
- Pyloric area
- Porta
- Tuber omentale
- Renal area
- IVC
- Caudate lobe
- Gastric area
- Suprarenal area
- Bare area
- Diaphragmatic area
- Esophageal area
- Lesser omentum
- Left triangular lig.

136 The Inferior and Posterior Surfaces of the Liver

You are standing on the right side of the cadaver and facing the head. The attachments of the liver are divided and the sharp, inferior border is raised.

Observe:

1. The visceral areas: (a) for esophagus, stomach, pylorus, and duodenum; (b) for transverse colon; and (c) for right kidney and right suprarenal gland. The gall bladder rests on the transverse colon and on the duodenum (fig. 126).

2. The posterior surface comprising: (a) the bare area, occupied on its left by the inf. vena cava, (b) the caudate lobe, and (c) the groove for the esophagus.

3. The caudate lobe separated from the quadrate lobe by the porta, and joined to the right lobe by the caudate process (not labelled) which is squeezed between the inf. vena cava and the portal vein.

4. The cut edge of the peritoneum: At the right end of the bare area the right triangular lig. (not labelled) bifurcates into the upper and the lower layer of the coronary lig. The lower layer crosses the renal and suprarenal areas, and, after passing in front of the inf. vena cava, turns cranially as the left layer, or base, of the coronary lig. Followed to the left this layer of peritoneum forms the upper limit of the upper recess and then turns caudally as the posterior layer of the lesser omentum. This omentum is attached to the fissure for the lig. venosum and to the porta. In this specimen it contains an accessory hepatic artery, a branch of the left gastric artery.

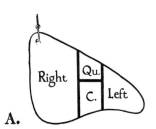

A.

The 4 lobes of the liver— right, quadrate, caudate, and left.

Labels: Right, Qu., C., Left

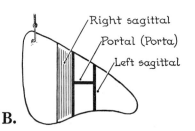

B.

The H-shaped deep fissures and wide sulci, defining the lobes.

Labels: Right sagittal, Portal (Porta), Left sagittal

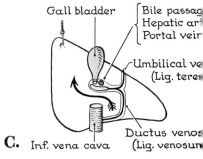

C.

The occupants of the fissures and sulci.

Labels: Gall bladder, Bile passage, Hepatic ar[tery], Portal vein, Umbilical ve[in] (Lig. teres), Ductus venos[us] (Lig. venosum), Inf. vena cava

136.1 In C, the arrow traverses the epiploic foramen. Behind it lies the inf. vena cava; in front, the portal vein; and above (at the roof) a narrow isthmus, the caudate process, joins the caudate lobe to the right lobe.

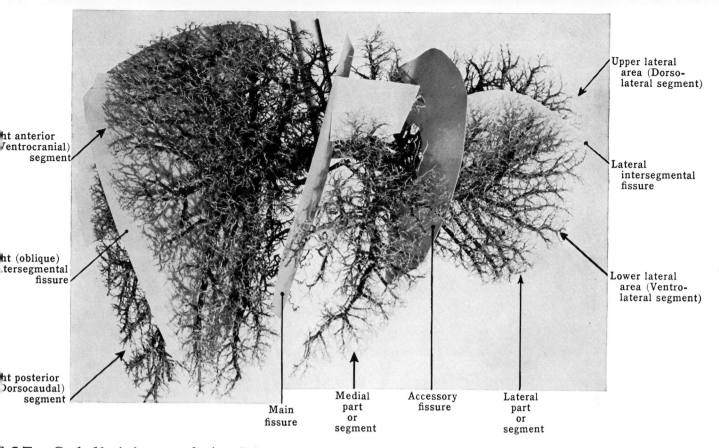

ht anterior
(Ventrocranial)
segment

ht (oblique)
tersegmental
fissure

ht posterior
(Dorsocaudal)
segment

Main
fissure

Medial
part
or
segment

Accessory
fissure

Lateral
part
or
segment

Upper lateral
area (Dorso-
lateral segment)

Lateral
intersegmental
fissure

Lower lateral
area (Ventro-
lateral segment)

137 Subdivisions of the Liver, anterior view (Courtesy of Douglas Bilbey.)

Corrosion specimen of the portal structures.

The main fissure divides the liver into almost equal halves, "the right and left portal lobes", served by right and left portal veins, hepatic arteries, and bile passages. Its surface markings are the right sagittal sulci and an imaginary line, 3 or 4 cmm from the falciform lig.

The right half is divided into an anterior and a posterior segment; the left half is divided into a medial and

a lateral segment by the accessory fissure, whose surface markings are the left sagittal fissures and the attachment of the falciform lig.

Each of these 4 segments is subdivisible into an upper and a lower area (segment), as revealed by the inserted slips of paper and the branches seen in figs. 138 & 140. Notable are the upper and lower lateral areas.

137.1 Large Hepatic Veins, anterior view

These 3 veins are intersegmental, as re pulmonary veins. They occupy the main, the right and the accessory and lateral intersegmental fissures. (The portal vein is injected white.)

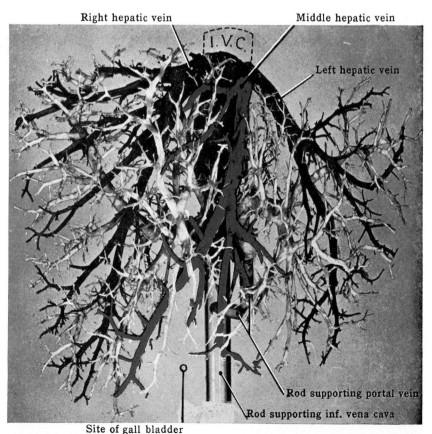

Right hepatic vein

Middle hepatic vein

I.V.C.

Left hepatic vein

Rod supporting portal vein

Rod supporting inf. vena cava

Site of gall bladder

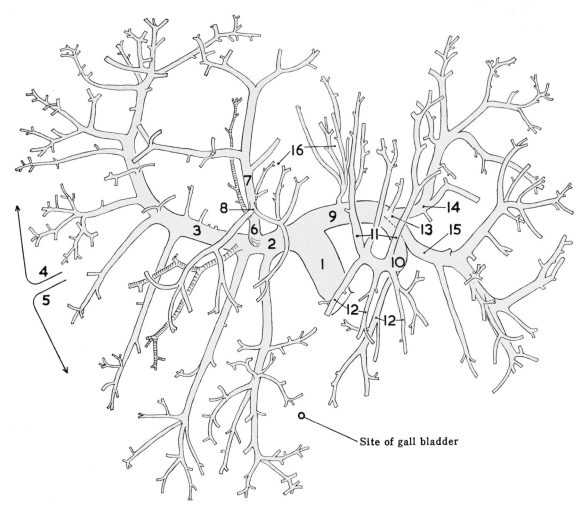

Site of gall bladder

138 Portal Vein and its Branches, left antero-inferior view

(Figures 138 & 140 were traced from a projected koda-chrome of a corrosion specimen. Photograph by Professor Duckworth. The specimen was tilted slightly in various directions to bring structures more fully into view.)

Perhaps it is simplest to regard the portal vein as branching and re-branching dichotomously. If branches 10 & 15 were split back to where 14 arises (broken line), branch 13 would be created. This figure of the portal vein would then serve equally as a plan of the hepatic artery and of the bile passages, as figure 140 shows.

1 = portal vein; 2 & 9—right & left portal veins; 16—caudate veins.
3 = Posterior (Dorso-caudal), 13 = Lateral ⎫ Segmental
6 = Anterior (Ventro-cranial), 10 = Medial ⎭ veins

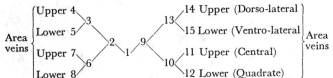

(Numbering is after Healey, Schroy and Sorensen. Terminology is after J. E. Healey et al.; and C. H. Hjortsjo who should be consulted for details and variations.)

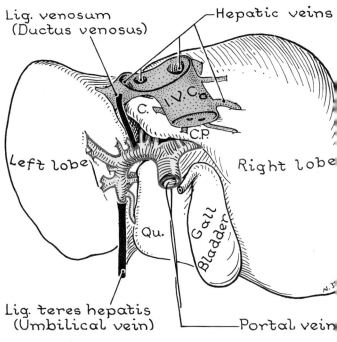

Lig. venosum (Ductus venosus) — Hepatic veins

I.V.C.

C.

C.P.

Left lobe

Right lobe

Qu.

Gall Bladder

Lig. teres hepatis (Umbilical vein) — Portal vein

139 Veins of the Liver, posterior view

Note the branches of the portal vein (yellow) entering the liver, and 3 large and several small hepatic veins (blue) leaving it to join the inf. vena cava. (C. = caudate lobe C.P. = caudate process.)

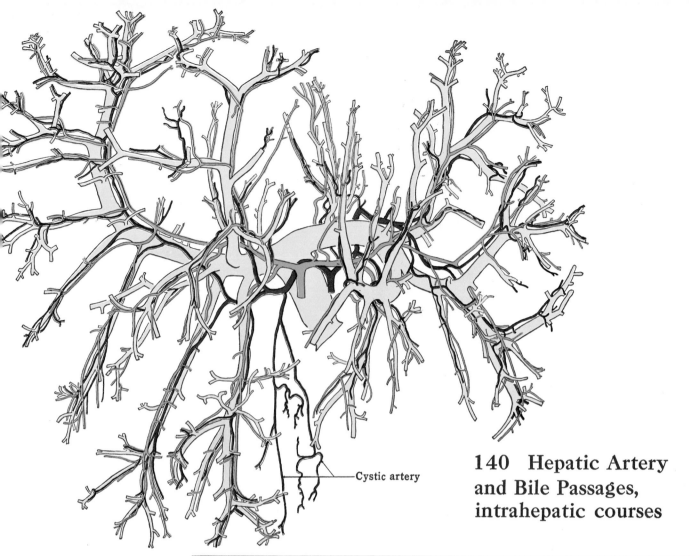

Cystic artery

**140 Hepatic Artery
and Bile Passages,
intrahepatic courses**

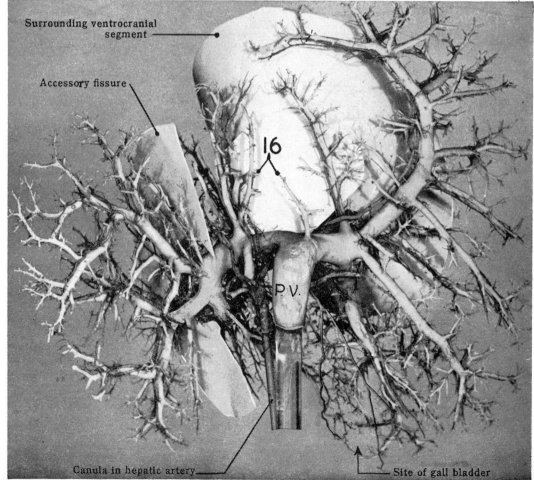

Surrounding ventrocranial
segment

Accessory fissure

16

P.V.

**Portal Structures,
ahepatic courses,
erior view**

m same specimen as used for
140. A lens may aid you.)

Canula in hepatic artery

Site of gall bladder

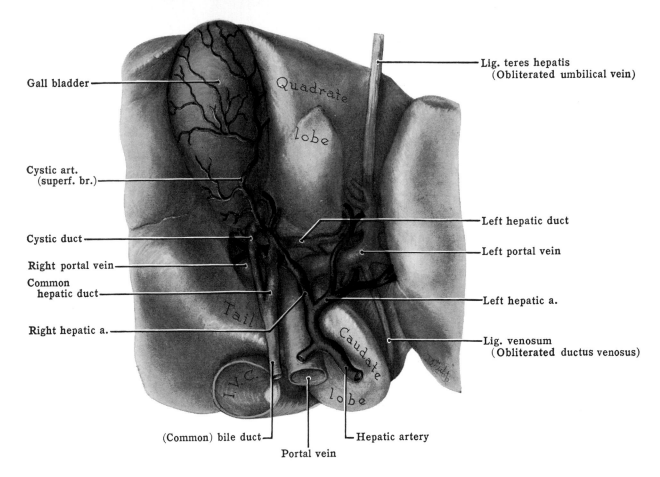

Gall bladder

Cystic art.
(superf. br.)

Cystic duct

Right portal vein

Common
hepatic duct

Right hepatic a.

Quadrate
lobe

Tail

Caudate
lobe

I.V.C.

(Common) bile duct

Portal vein

Hepatic artery

Lig. teres hepatis
(Obliterated umbilical vein)

Left hepatic duct

Left portal vein

Left hepatic a.

Lig. venosum
(Obliterated ductus venosus)

142 Porta Hepatis and the Cystic Artery

1. The tail of the caudate lobe forming the roof of the epiploic foramen, and lying between the upper end of the portal vein, and the inf. vena cava.

2. The relation of structures as they ascend to the porta—duct to the right, artery to the left, vein behind.

3. The order of structures at the porta—duct, artery, vein—from before backwards.

4. The left portal vein and left hepatic artery supplying the quadrate and caudate lobes en route to the left lobe, and accompanied by tributaries of the left hepatic duct.

5. The lig. teres hepatis passing to the left portal vein, and the lig. venosum arising opposite it and ascending to the inf. vena cava (as in fig. 139).

6. The cystic artery springing from the right hepatic artery and dividing into a superficial and a deep branch which arborise on the respective surfaces of the bladder.

7. The cystic duct, sinuous at its origin.

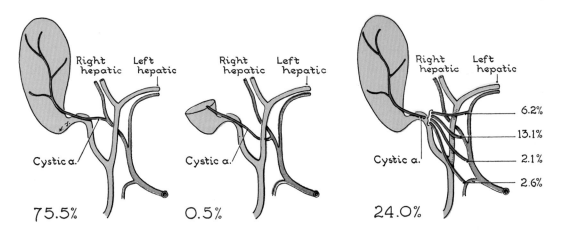

Right hepatic   Left hepatic

Cystic a.

75.5%

Right hepatic   Left hepatic

Cystic a.

0.5%

Right hepatic   Left hepatic

6.2%

13.1%

2.1%

2.6%

Cystic a.

24.0%

143 Variations in the Origin and Course of the Cystic Artery

The cystic art. usually arises from the right hepatic art. in the angle between the common hepatic duct and the cystic duct, and has no occasion to cross the common hepatic duct, as in figures 144 and 147. When, however, it arises on the left of the bile passages, it almost always crosses anterior to the passages, as in figure 142, and only rarely (3 in 580 cases) does it cross behind. (Diagrams based on 580 cases by Daseler, Anson, Hambley and Reimann.)

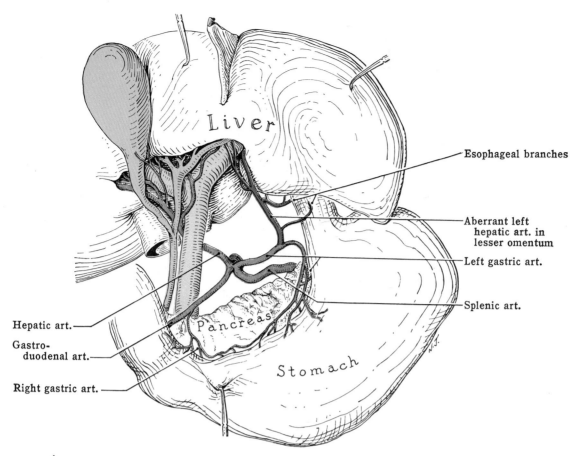

A. Aberrant Left Hepatic Artery.

The left hepatic artery was entirely replaced by a branch of the left gastric artery, as in this specimen, in 11.5% of 200 cadavera, and in another 11.5% it was partially replaced. (Michels, N. A.)

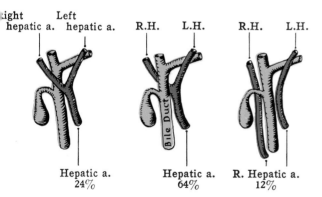

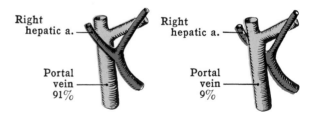

C. Right Hepatic Artery and Portal Vein.

The artery crossed ventral to the portal vein in 91% of 165 specimens and dorsal in 9%. (*J.C.B.G.*)

Right Hepatic Artery and Bile Passages: Aberrant Right Hepatic Artery.

The right hepatic artery crossed ventral to the bile passages in 24% of 165 specimens, and dorsal in 64%, whereas in 12% it was aberrant, arising from the superior mesenteric artery. (*J.C.B.G.*)

144 **Variations in the Hepatic Arteries**

VARIATIONS

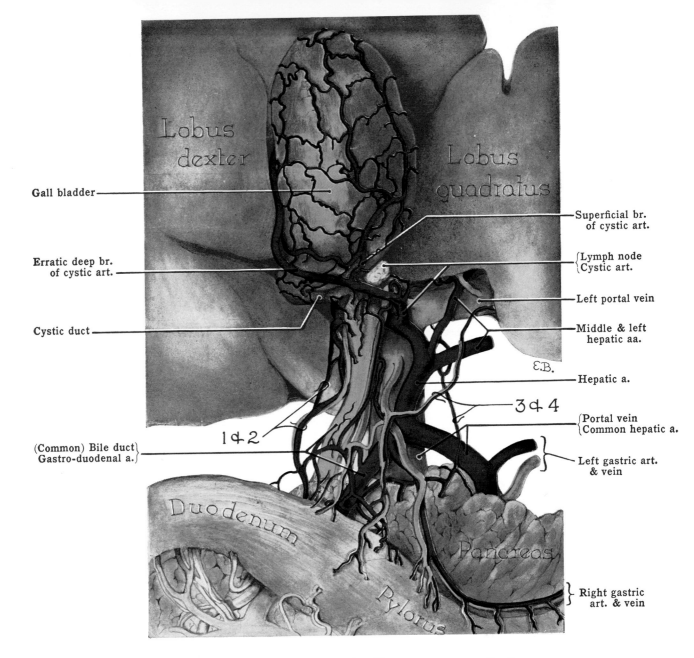

Gall bladder

Erratic deep br. of cystic art.

Cystic duct

(Common) Bile duct
Gastro-duodenal a.

Lobus dexter

Lobus quadratus

Superficial br. of cystic art.

Lymph node
Cystic art.

Left portal vein

Middle & left hepatic aa.

E.B.

Hepatic a.

3 & 4

1 & 2

Portal vein
Common hepatic a.

Left gastric art. & vein

Duodenum

Pancreas

Pylorus

Right gastric art. & vein

145 Gall Bladder, the Bile Passages, and the related Blood Vessels

The liver is turned up and the duodenum is pulled down. (*Preparation by Dr. A. J. A. Noronha.*)

Observe:

1. The network of arteries on the gall bladder. Most of the smaller arteries lying on a deeper plane than the larger arteries.

2. A large erratic, deep branch of the cystic artery, crossing superficial to the neck of the gall bladder.

3. The cystic lymph node.

4. Many fine sinuous arterial twigs supplying the bile passages and springing from nearby arteries.

5. The right gastric artery, here arising very low—indeed, from the gastro-duodenal artery.

6. The right gastric vein, here ending high in the portal vein.

7. Several, here 5, anastomotic arteries capable of bringing blood from various gastric and pancreatic arteries to the porta hepatis. 4 of these have been retracted, 1 of them passing to the left lobe.

8. Veins (not all shown), accompanying faithfully most arteries.

9. A middle hepatic artery, seen here, passing to the quadrate lobe is common (Michels).

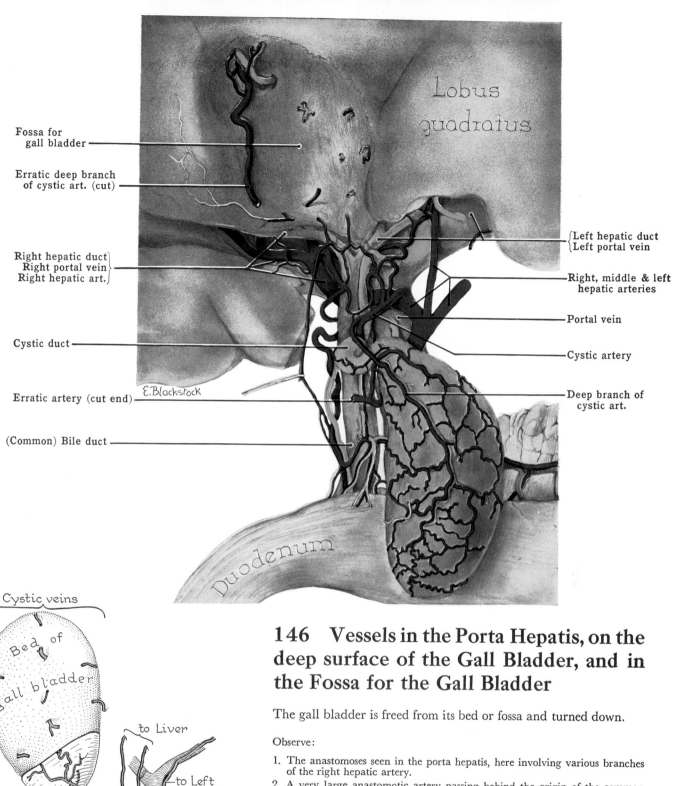

Fossa for gall bladder

Erratic deep branch of cystic art. (cut)

Right hepatic duct
Right portal vein
Right hepatic art.

Cystic duct

Erratic artery (cut end)

E. Blackstock

(Common) Bile duct

Lobus quadratus

Left hepatic duct
Left portal vein

Right, middle & left hepatic arteries

Portal vein

Cystic artery

Deep branch of cystic art.

Duodenum

Cystic veins

Bed of gall bladder

to Liver

to Left portal v.

Ant. cystic v.

Post. cystic v.

Common hepatic duct

R. gastric v.

Cystic duct

Bile duct

Post. sup. pancreatico-duodenal v.

146 Vessels in the Porta Hepatis, on the deep surface of the Gall Bladder, and in the Fossa for the Gall Bladder

The gall bladder is freed from its bed or fossa and turned down.

Observe:

1. The anastomoses seen in the porta hepatis, here involving various branches of the right hepatic artery.
2. A very large anastomotic artery passing behind the origin of the common hepatic duct; several smaller arteries forming a network (rete) in front of the ducts. From the network, twigs passing to the subcapsular arterial plexus.
3. The deep branch of the cystic artery, aided by a branch of the erratic deep cystic artery, ramifying on the deep or attached surface of the gall bladder, anastomosing with twigs of the superficial branch of the cystic artery, and sending twigs into the bed of the gall bladder. (The cut ends of the arterial and venous twigs can be seen.)
4. The erratic artery plunging into the bed.

146.1 Veins of the Extrahepatic Bile Passages and Gall bladder

Note: The venous twigs draining the passages and the neck of the bladder join veins which, clinging to the passages, connect gastric, duodenal and pancreatic veins partly to the liver directly and partly via a portal vein. The veins of the fundus and body, here 8, plunge directly into the liver.

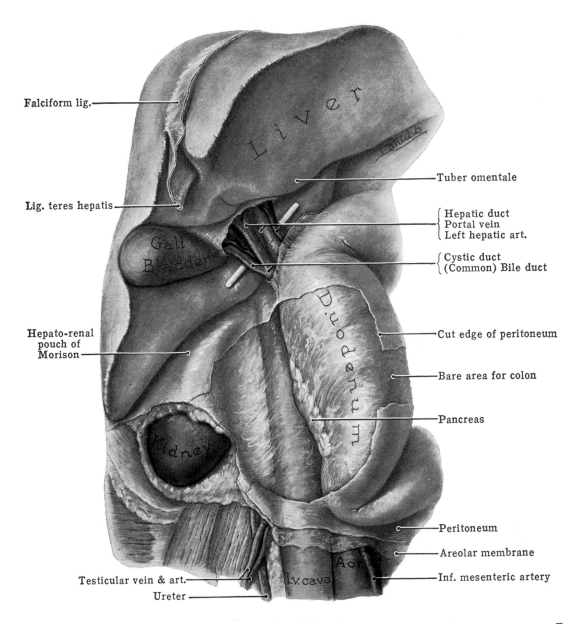

Falciform lig.

Lig. teres hepatis

Gall Bladder

Hepato-renal pouch of Morison

Kidney

Liver

Tuber omentale

Hepatic duct
Portal vein
Left hepatic art.

Cystic duct
(Common) Bile duct

Cut edge of peritoneum

Bare area for colon

Pancreas

Duodenum

Testicular vein & art.

Ureter

I.v. cava

Ao.

Peritoneum

Areolar membrane

Inf. mesenteric artery

147   Exposure of the (Common) Bile Duct, posterior aspect—I

A white rod is passed through the epiploic foramen. The lesser omentum is removed. The transverse colon is separated from the front of the descending, or 2nd, part of the duodenum and thrown down; the peritoneum is cut along the right or convex border of the 2nd part of the duodenum, and this part of the duodenum is swung forwards like a door on a hinge.

Note:

1. The space opened up is virtually a bursal space, comparable to the retropubic space where two smooth areolar membranes are applied to each other. Here one membrane covers the posterior aspect of the 2nd part of the duodenum and the head of the pancreas; the other covers the aorta, inf. vena cava, renal vessels and perinephric fat.

   The duodenum can expand and contract, but, being suspended from the liver by the structures entering the porta, it cannot descend unless the liver either alters its shape or descends with it.

2. To find the epiploic foramen either: (a) follow the liver, at the upper limit of the hepato-renal pouch, medially to the caudate process (tail of the caudate lobe), which forms the roof of the foramen and which lies in front of the inf. vena cava, which forms the posterior wall; or (b) follow the gall bladder to the cystic duct, which occupies the free edge of the lesser omentum, which forms the anterior wall of the foramen.

3. Of the three main structures in the anterior wall—the portal vein is posterior, the hepatic artery ascends from the left, and the bile passages descend to the right (fig. 142).

4. In this specimen the right hepatic artery springs from the superior mesenteric artery. (For data on this common variant, see fig. 144 B.)

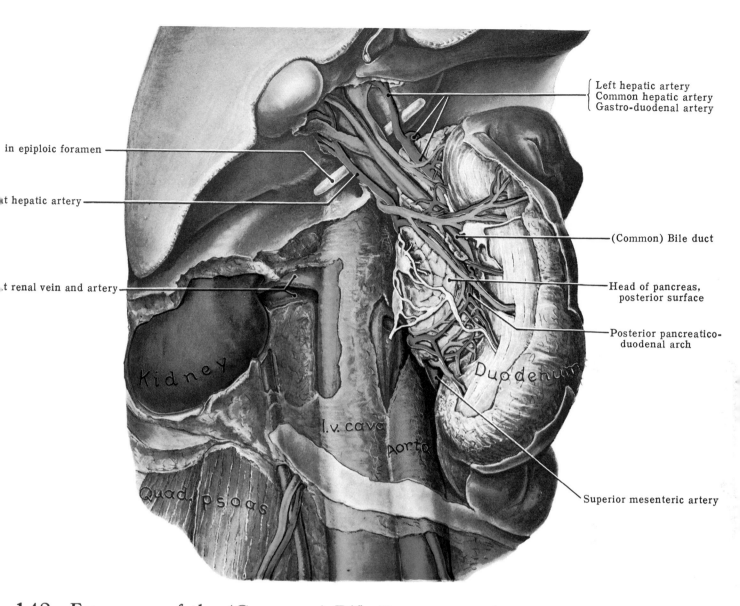

in epiploic foramen ——

t hepatic artery ——

t renal vein and artery ——

Kidney

Quad. psoas

I.v. cava

Aorta

{ Left hepatic artery
Common hepatic artery
Gastro-duodenal artery

—— (Common) Bile duct

—— Head of pancreas,
posterior surface

—— Posterior pancreatico-
duodenal arch

Duodenum

—— Superior mesenteric artery

148   Exposure of the (Common) Bile Duct, posterior aspect—II

The duodenum is swung still further forwards and to the left, taking the head of the pancreas with it. In effect, the epiploic foramen has been enlarged caudally. The areolar membrane covering these two organs is largely removed; that covering the great vessels is in part removed.

Observe:

1. The right renal vein to be short, and the right artery, which passes behind the inf. vena cava, to be long.
2. The bile duct descending in a groove on the head of the pancreas, and a tongue of that head (reflected) lying behind the end of the duct.
3. Vasa recta, accompanied by veins and lymph vessels,

passing from the posterior pancreatico-duodenal arch to the duodenum.

4. Of the two posterior pancreatico-duodenal arteries that form the posterior arch, the inferior springing from the superior mesenteric artery, and the superior here springing from the right hepatic artery, but usually from the gastro-duodenal artery, as in figure 159.
5. The posterior superior pancreatico-duodenal vein ending in the portal vein.
6. The very close posterior relationship of the inf. vena cava to the portal vein and the bile duct.
7. The duct ending at the level of the hilus of the kidney, and the ureter beginning at the same level.

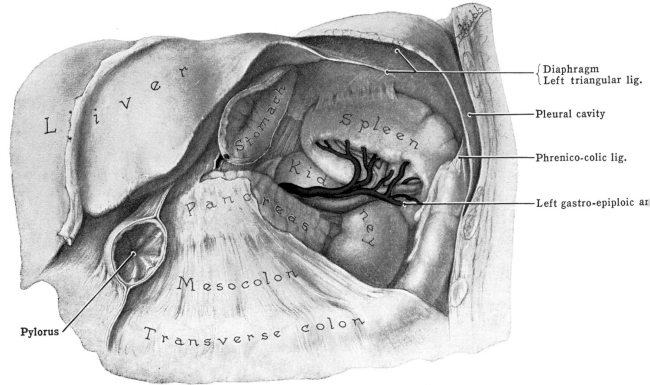

149 Stomach Bed

The stomach is excised. The peritoneum of the omental bursa, or lesser sac, covering the stomach bed is largely removed; so is the peritoneum of the greater sac covering the lower part of the kidney and pancreas.

The pancreas is unusually short; the adhesions binding the spleen to Diaphragm are pathological but not unusual.

Unlabelled are:—1. The branch of the posterior vagal trunk that descends on the right side of the left gastric artery to the celiac plexus (fig. 180). 2. The left suprarenal gland. 3. Three short gastric branches of the splenic artery, cut short (see fig. 132). 4. The tuber omentale of the liver and that of the pancreas, which fit into the lesser curvature of the stomach. 5. The lesser omentum attached to the upper border of the pylorus and the greater omentum to the lower border.

Note the pleural cavity separating the spleen and Diaphragm from the thoracic wall.

150 Spleen or Lien, visceral surfac

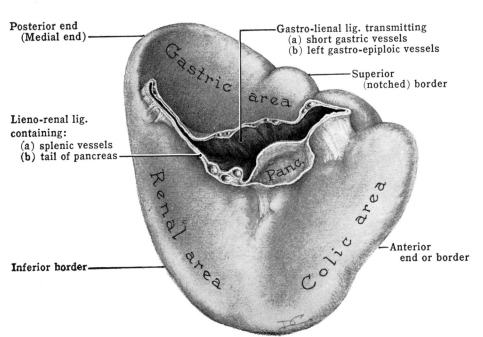

For orientation see figure 149.

Observe:

1. A "circumferential border" comprising th⟨ ⟩ferior, superior, and anterior borders, separating the visceral surface from the phragmatic surface.

2. The notches characteristic of the sup⟨ ⟩border.

3. The left limit of the omental bursa at the ⟨ ⟩of the spleen, between the lieno-renal and ⟨ ⟩trolienal ligs.

4. The spleen taking the impressions of the s⟨ ⟩tures in contact with it. The large colic area here is reduced in figure 152—presumab⟨ ⟩the one case the colon was full (of gas), a⟨ ⟩the other it was empty.

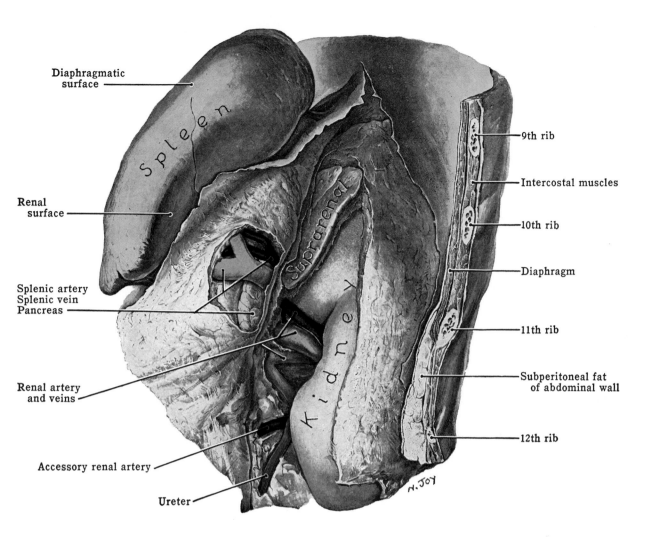

Diaphragmatic
surface

Renal
surface

Splenic artery
Splenic vein
Pancreas

Renal artery
and veins

Accessory renal artery

Ureter

9th rib

Intercostal muscles

10th rib

Diaphragm

11th rib

Subperitoneal fat
of abdominal wall

12th rib

151 Reflexion of the Spleen: Exposure of the Left Kidney and Suprarenal Gland, front view

The spleen and the lieno-renal ligament are turned forwards to the right, like the page of a book, taking the splenic vessels and the tail of the pancreas with them. Part of the fatty capsule of the kidney is cut away.

Observe:

The exposed left kidney, renal vessels, and ureter, also the left suprarenal gland, separated from the kidney by a thin layer of fat.

When in situ, the splenic vessels lie ventral to the renal vessels (fig. 149); but two areolar membranes, closely applied to each other, and some fatty capsule are seen to intervene. There are two comparable membranes on the right side (figs. 147 & 148).

The subperitoneal fat of the abdominal wall stopping on reaching the diaphragm.

Note that this exposure is, in effect, a restoration to the embryological state.

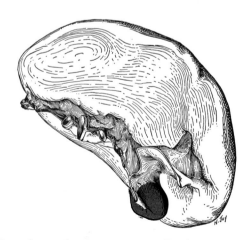

152 An Accessory Spleen

Accessory spleens resemble lymph nodes, about 1 cm. in diameter, but they are usually covered with peritoneum, as is the spleen itself. They lie along the course of the splenic artery or its gastro-epiploic branch, but they may be elsewhere. The commonest location is at or near the hilus of the spleen, but 1 in 6 are partially (or wholly) embedded in the tail of the pancreas. At 3000 necropsies on male veteran patients, 311, or 10%, had accessory spleens. Of these, 272 were solitary and 39 were multiple. (B. Halpert & F. Gyorkey; G. M. Curtis & D. Movitz.)

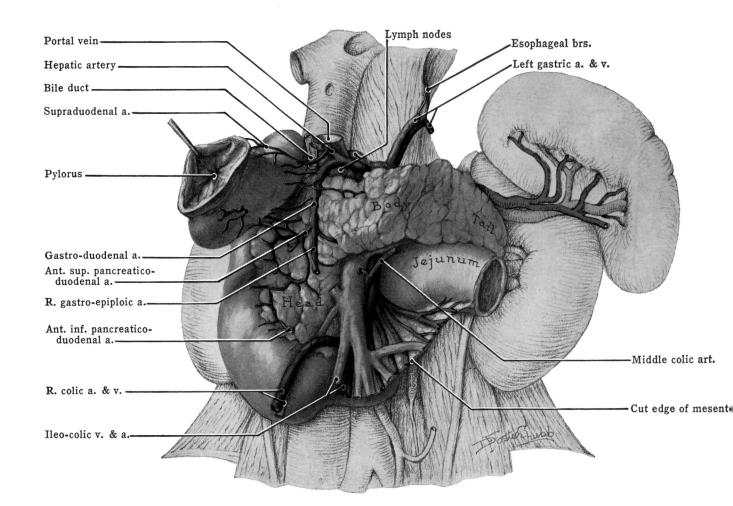

Portal vein

Hepatic artery

Bile duct

Supraduodenal a.

Pylorus

Gastro-duodenal a.

Ant. sup. pancreatico-duodenal a.

R. gastro-epiploic a.

Ant. inf. pancreatico-duodenal a.

R. colic a. & v.

Ileo-colic v. & a.

Lymph nodes

Esophageal brs.

Left gastric a. & v.

Body

Tail

Jejunum

Head

Middle colic art.

Cut edge of mesent

153   Duodenum and Pancreas in situ, front view

Observe:

1. *The duodenum* moulded around the head of the pancreas. Its 1st or superior part (retracted) overlapping the pancreas and passing backwards, upwards, and to the right. The remaining parts (2nd, 3rd & 4th) overlapped by the pancreas. Near the junction of its 3rd and 4th parts the duodenum is crossed by the superior mesenteric vessels. These appearing from under cover of the neck of the pancreas, descending in front of the uncinate process, and entering the root of the mesentery, may, as here, by constricting the duodenum, causes the 1st, 2nd & 3rd parts to be dilated.

2. *The pancreas*, here very short—its tail usually abuts on the spleen and is blunt (fig. 150). It is arched forwards because it crosses the vertebral column and aorta.

3. *The celiac trunk*, which lies behind the upper border of the pancreas, sending (a) the left gastric a. upwards on the diaphragm towards the cardiac orifice of the stomach to enter the lesser omentum: (b) the splenic a. to the left; and (c) the hepatic a. to the right. The hepatic a. passing on to the front of the portal vein and giving off the gastro-duodenal a., which descends between the duodenum and pancreas, less than an inch from the pylorus, and divides into the right gastroepiploic a. and the superior pancreatico-duodenal a. Note the single supraduodenal a. and the several retroduodenal aa. supplying the first inch of the duodenum.

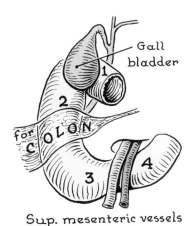

Gall bladder

for COLON

Sup. mesenteric vessels

153.1

Diagram. The 3 notable, ventral contact relations of the duodenum.

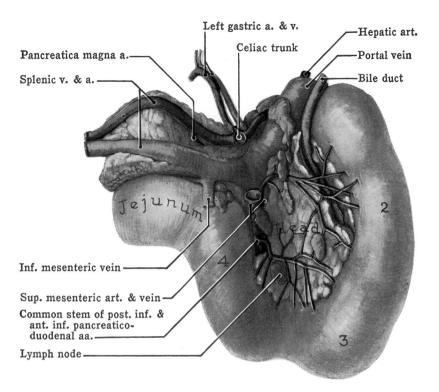

Pancreatica magna a.

Splenic v. & a.

Left gastric a. & v.

Celiac trunk

Hepatic art.

Portal vein

Bile duct

Jejunum

head

2

4

3

Inf. mesenteric vein

Sup. mesenteric art. & vein

Common stem of post. inf. & ant. inf. pancreatico-duodenal aa.

Lymph node

154 Duodenum, Pancreas and Bile Duct, from behind

This is the reverse of the specimen depicted in figure 153.

Observe:

1. Only the end of the 1st or superior part of the duodenum is in view.
2. The bile duct here descending in a long fissure (opened up) in the posterior part of the head of the pancreas—contrast figure 148.
3. Arteries: In the absence of the usual posterior superior pancreatico-duodenal artery, the vasa recta that pass behind the duct springing from an accessory branch of the superior mesenteric artery—compare figure 159.

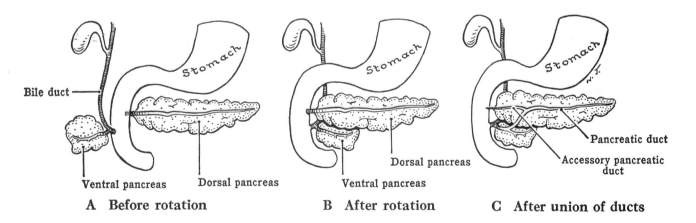

Bile duct

Stomach

Ventral pancreas   Dorsal pancreas

A Before rotation

Stomach

Dorsal pancreas

Ventral pancreas

B After rotation

Stomach

Pancreatic duct

Accessory pancreatic duct

C After union of ducts

155 Developmental Explanation of Variability of Pancreatic Ducts

Note:

(a) A smaller primitive ventral bud arises in common with the bile duct, and a larger primitive dorsal bud arises independently from the duodenum, cranial to this.

(b) The 2nd or descending part of the duodenum rotates on its long axis, which brings the ventral bud and the bile duct behind the dorsal bud.

(c) A connecting segment unites the dorsal duct to the ventral duct, whereupon the duodenal end of the dorsal duct tends to atrophy and the direction of flow within it is reversed.

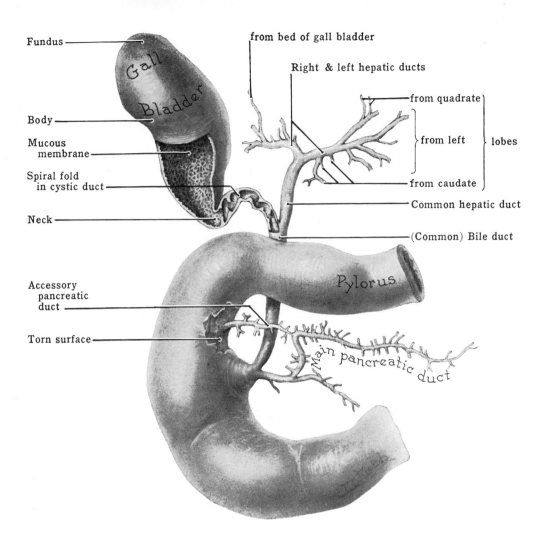

Fundus

Gall Bladder

Body

Mucous membrane

Spiral fold in cystic duct

Neck

Accessory pancreatic duct

Torn surface

from bed of gall bladder

Right & left hepatic ducts

from quadrate
from left } lobes
from caudate

Common hepatic duct

(Common) Bile duct

Pylorus

Main pancreatic duct

156 Extra-hepatic Bile Passages and the Pancreatic Ducts

Note: The right hepatic duct collects from the right lobe of the liver; the left hepatic duct collects from the left, quadrate and caudate lobes. The common hepatic duct unites with the cystic duct close above the duodenum. The mucous membrane of the gall bladder has a low honeycomb surface. The cystic duct is sinuous; its mucous membrane forms a spiral fold (spiral valve).

The bile duct, after descending behind the 1st part of the duodenum and the accessory pancreatic duct, is joined by the main pancreatic duct; these open on the duodenal papilla (fig. 168).

The main pancreatic duct with its tributaries bears semblance to a herring bone, and differs from the common hepatic duct with its tributaries which resembles a deciduous tree. The accessory pancreatic duct retains its anastomosis with the main duct. The pancreas invades the duodenal wall around the accessory duct, and cannot be removed without lacerating the duodenum.

157 Comments on the Pancreatic Ducts

Dimensions: The average length of 27 pancreases is 8.2″. The main duct begins 1″ from the tip of the tail and there the internal diameter is 0.5 mm.; at 2″ from the tip it ranges from 0.5 mm. to 1.5 mm.; at 4″ it ranges from 1.5 mm. to 3.0 mm.; and in the head the average diameter is 3.5 mm. The primary ductules narrow at their entrances to the main duct, and they approach it from all sides. Branches are fewest where the gland is narrowest, i.e., where it crosses the sup. mesenteric vessels, indeed, it may there be bald. (Horsey W. J. and Paul W. M.)

Connections with Duodenum: In about 9% the primitive dorsal duct (fig. 155) persists, usually quite uncon-

nected with the primitive ventral duct, as in fig. 157-D In about 44% the accessory duct loses its connection with the duodenum (fig. 157-A); or in 8% ends blindly at the duodenum; or in 9% retains only a negligibly small opening into the duodenum. In about 10%, however, the accessory duct is large enough to relieve an obstructed main duct (fig. 157-B), and in 20% it could probably substitute for it (fig. 157-C). Further in about 5% the bile and main pancreatic ducts open separately on the duodenal papilla (fig. 157-B). (Data based on radiograms of 200 specimens injected with radio-opaque material. E. Millbourn, 1950.)

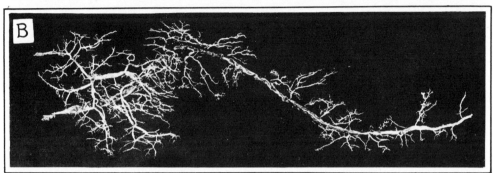

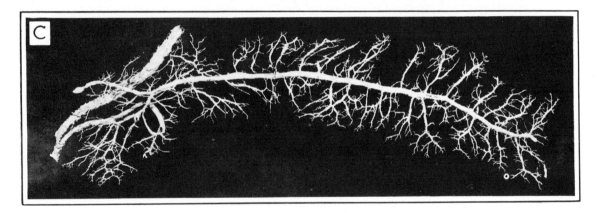

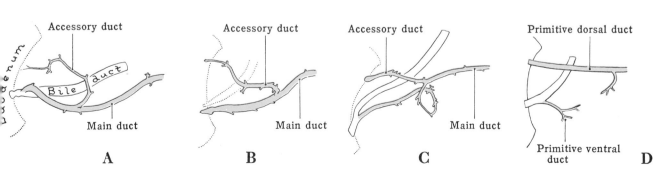

157   Corrosion Preparations of the Pancreatic Ducts

(Prepared by W. J. Horsey and W. M. Paul, photographed by C. E. Storton.)

The pancreatic ducts were injected with plastic by retrograde flow, via the bile duct, and then corroded with acid. In specimens where the bile duct and the main pancreatic duct (of Wirsung) opened separately on to the duodenal papilla (of Vater) injection was made directly into the main duct.

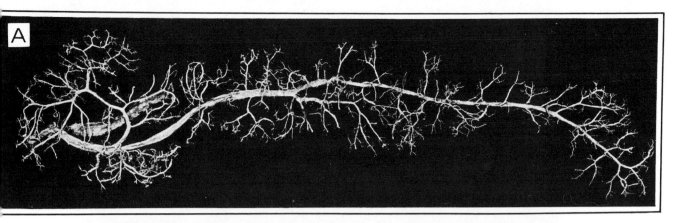

KEY TO FIGURE 157

For comments see opposite page.

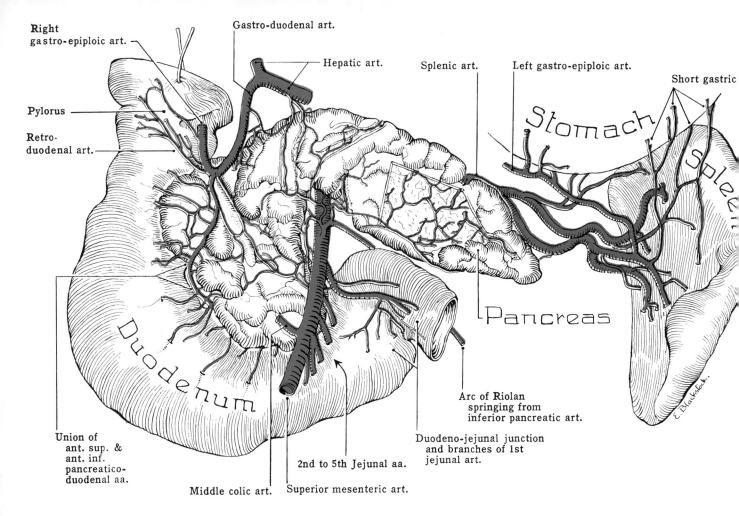

Right
gastro-epiploic art.

Gastro-duodenal art.

Hepatic art.

Splenic art.

Left gastro-epiploic art.

Short gastric

Pylorus

Stomach

Spleen

Retro-
duodenal art.

Pancreas

Duodenum

Arc of Riolan
springing from
inferior pancreatic art.

Duodeno-jejunal junction
and branches of 1st
jejunal art.

Union of
ant. sup. &
ant. inf.
pancreatico-
duodenal aa.

E. Blackstock.

2nd to 5th Jejunal aa.

Middle colic art.

Superior mesenteric art.

158 Blood Supply to the Pancreas, Duodenum, and Spleen, front view

Two or three short slices have been removed from the pancreas.

Observe:

1. This territory to be supplied by the hepatic, splenic, and superior mesenteric arteries.

2. Several retroduodenal branches springing from the right gastro-epiploic artery.

3. The anterior superior pancreatico-duodenal branch of the gastro-duodenal artery and the anterior inferior pancreatico-duodenal branch of the superior mesenteric artery forming an

continued on facing page

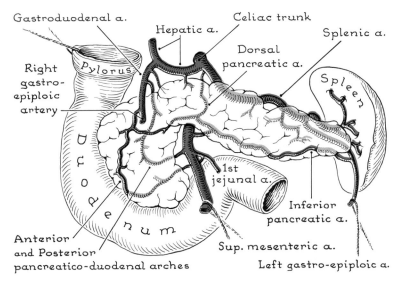

Gastroduodenal a.

Celiac trunk

Hepatic a.

Splenic a.

Right
gastro-
epiploic
artery

Pylorus

Dorsal
pancreatic a.

Spleen

Duodenum

1st
jejunal a.

Inferior
pancreatic a.

Anterior
and Posterior
pancreatico-duodenal arches

Sup. mesenteric a.

Left gastro-epiploic a.

158.1

Diagram of blood supply to pancreas. The excellent supply to this cellular organ lies at the junction of celiac trunk and sup. mesenteric artery.

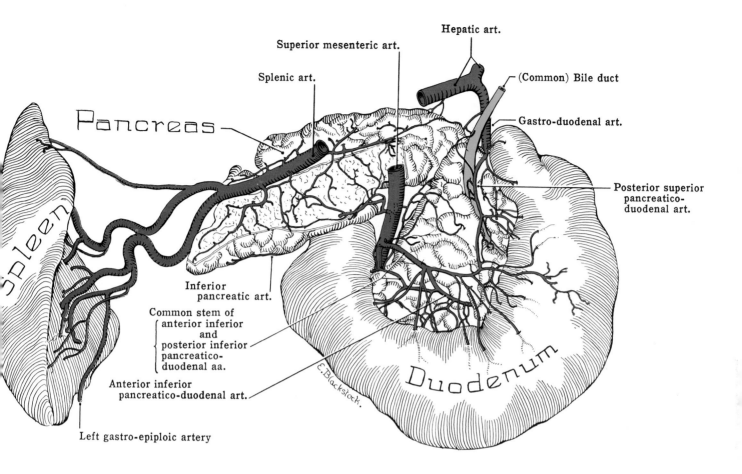

Hepatic art.

Superior mesenteric art.

Splenic art.

(Common) Bile duct

Pancreas

Gastro-duodenal art.

Posterior superior
pancreatico-
duodenal art.

Spleen

Inferior
pancreatic art.

Common stem of
{ anterior inferior
and
posterior inferior
pancreatico-
duodenal aa.

Anterior inferior
pancreatico-duodenal art.

C. Blackstock.

Duodenum

Left gastro-epiploic artery

159 Blood Supply to the Pancreas, Duodenum, and Spleen, dorsal view

continued from facing page

arch in front of the head of the pancreas. The posterior superior and posterior inferior branches of the same two arteries forming another arch behind the pancreas. The 2 inferior arteries here, as usually, spring from a common stem. From each arch thus formed straight vessels, called vasa recta duodeni, passing to the anterior and posterior surfaces respectively of the 2nd, 3rd and 4th parts of the duodenum. The duodeno-jejunal junction supplied by the large branching vessel depicted.

4. The fine network of arteries that pervades the pancreas to be derived from:—common (stem of) hepatic artery, the gastro-duodenal artery, the pancreatico-duodenal arches, the splenic artery, and also from the superior mesenteric artery.

5. The arc of Riolan, an occasional artery on the posterior abdominal wall, which connects the superior mesenteric artery to a branch of the inferior mesenteric artery.

(For more details see Michels; Woodburne.)

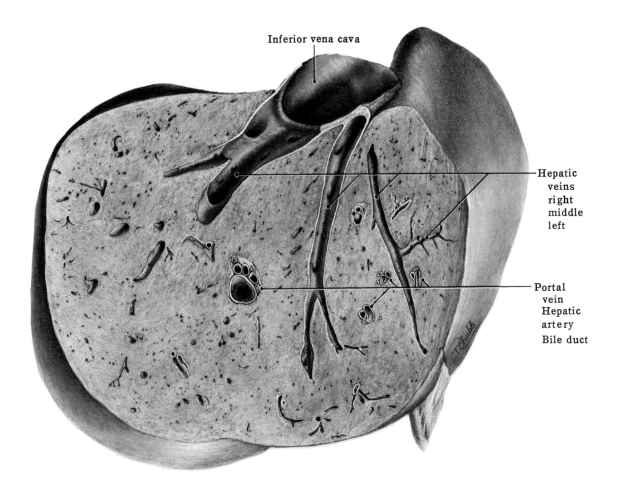

Inferior vena cava

Hepatic
veins
right
middle
left

Portal
vein
Hepatic
artery
Bile duct

160   Section of Liver,
approximately horizontal

Observe:

1. Perivascular fibrous capsules (Glisson's capsule), each containing a branch
   (or branches) of the portal vein, hepatic artery, bile ductules and lymph
   vessels cut across throughout the section (cf. fig. 140).
2. Interdigitating with these are branches of the three main hepatic veins
   which, unaccompanied and having no capsules, converge fanwise on the inf.
   vena cava (cf. fig. 137.1).

160.1   Porta-Caval System

Diagram. Collateral Portal Circulation
(by-pass in case of obstruction in liver or portal vein).

Blue = portal tributaries, Striped = systemic tributaries,
Black = communicating veins.

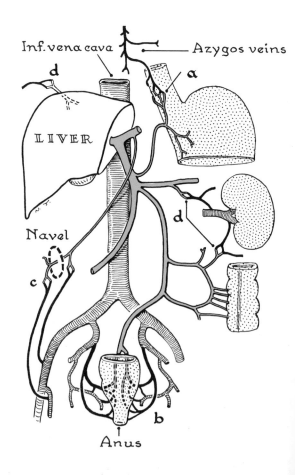

Inf. vena cava   Azygos veins

d

LIVER

a

Navel

d

c

b

Anus

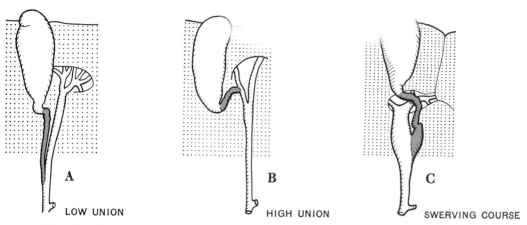

LOW UNION   HIGH UNION   SWERVING COURSE

A—Variations in the Length and Course of the Cystic Duct

The cystic duct usually lies on the right of the common hepatic duct and joins it just above the 1st part of the duodenum, but this varies as in a, b, c.

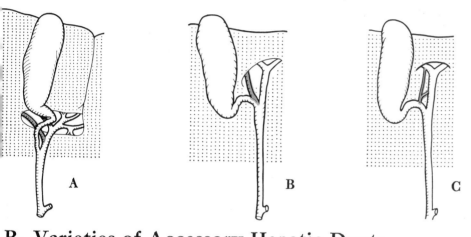

B—Varieties of Accessory Hepatic Ducts

Accessory right hepatic ducts are common. Thus, of 95 gall bladders and bile passages injected in situ with melted paraffin wax and then dissected, 7 had accessory hepatic ducts in positions of surgical danger. Of these:—(A) 4 joined the common hepatic duct near the cystic duct; (B) 2 joined the cystic duct; and (C) 1 was an anastomosing duct (*J.C.B.G.*) "Accessory" ducts are now known to be not additional ducts but either area or segmental ducts that arise early.

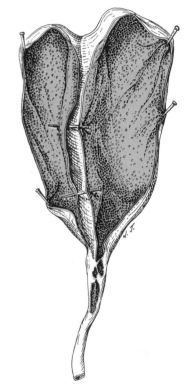

D—Double Gall Bladder

(Courtesy of Professor William Boyd.)

The gall bladder was rarely double with two cystic ducts and very rarely was it bilobed. (Boyden, E. A.)

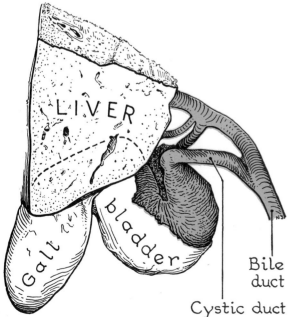

LIVER

Gall

bladder

Bile duct

Cystic duct

C—Folded Gall Bladder

Radiologically, the body of the gall bladder was found to be folded, or kinked, upon itself in 14.5% of 165 persons. The fundus was folded upon the bladder in 3.5%, as in fig. A above. (Boyden, E. A.)

161   **Variations in the Bile Passages and Gall Bladder**

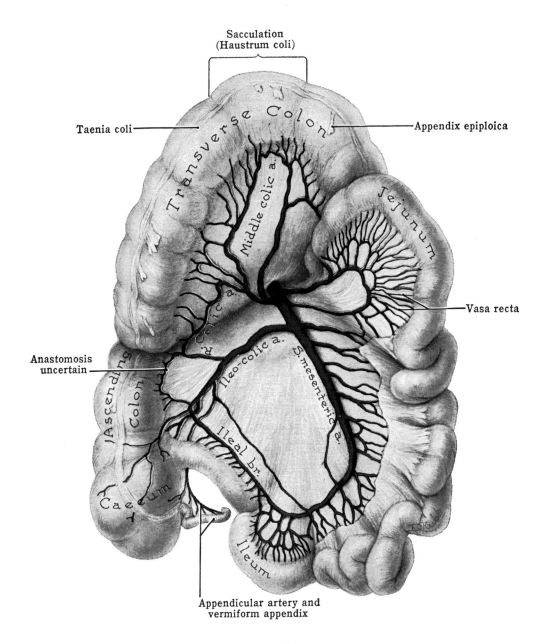

Sacculation
(Haustrum coli)

Taenia coli

Transverse Colon

Appendix epiploica

Middle colic a.

Jejunum

R. Colic a.

Vasa recta

Anastomosis
uncertain

Ascending Colon

Ileo-colic a.

S. mesenteric a.

Ileal br.

Caecum

Ileum

Appendicular artery and
vermiform appendix

162 Superior Mesenteric Artery

The peritoneum is in part stripped off.

Observe:

1. The sup. mesenteric artery ending by anastomosing with one of its own branches, viz., the ileal branch of the ileo-colic artery.

2. Its branches:
   (a) From its left side, twelve or more jejunal and ileal branches. These anastomose to form arcades from which vasa recta pass to the small gut.
   (b) From its right side, the middle colic, the ileo-colic, and commonly, but not here, an independent right colic artery. These anastomose to form a marginal artery (labelled in fig. 163) from which vasa recta pass to the large gut.
   (c) The two inferior pancreatico-duodenal arteries (not in view, but seen in fig. 154) arise from the main artery either directly or in conjunction with the 1st jejunal branch.

3. Teniae coli, sacculations, and appendices epiploicae which distinguish the large gut from the smooth walled small gut.

(For variations in patterns of arteries see J. V. Basmajian.)

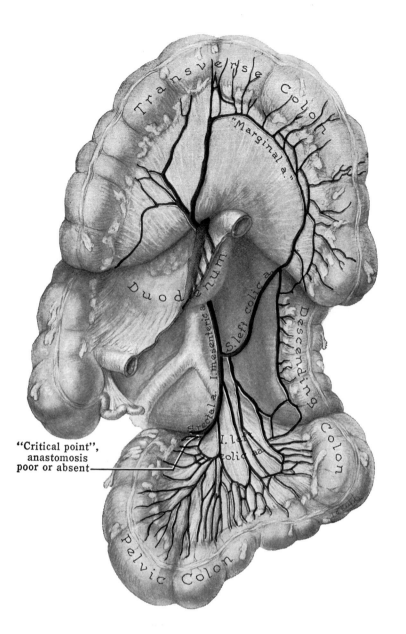

"Critical point", anastomosis poor or absent —

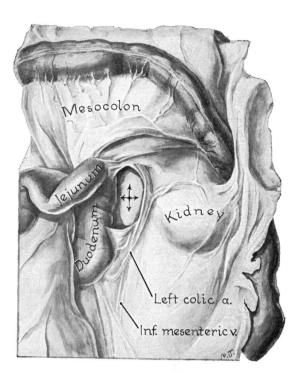

163.1 Duodenal Recesses

These occasional peritoneal fossae may pass either upwards or downwards or to the right or to left. The lower fold is bloodless. When present, the left fold does, and the upper fold may, contain the inferior mesenteric vein. The right recess is retro-duodenal.

163 Inferior Mesenteric Artery

The mesentery has been cut at its root and discarded with the jejunum and ileum. (Pelvic colon = Sigmoid colon.)

Observe:

1. The inf. mesenteric artery arising behind the duodenum, $1\frac{1}{2}''$ above the bifurcation of the aorta. On crossing the left common iliac artery, it becomes the superior rectal (haemorrhoidal) artery.

2. Its branches:
    (a) a single (superior) left colic artery and
    (b) several sigmoid arteries (inf. left colic aa.) springing from its left side. In this specimen the two lowest sigmoid arteries spring from the superior rectal artery. The point at which the last artery to the colon leaves the artery to the rectum is known as the critical point of Sudeck.

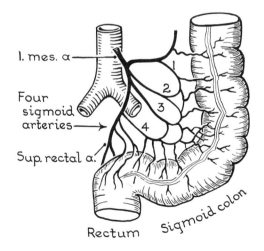

163.2

Diagram. A common pattern of the two to four sigmoid arteries. (Based on Goligher.)

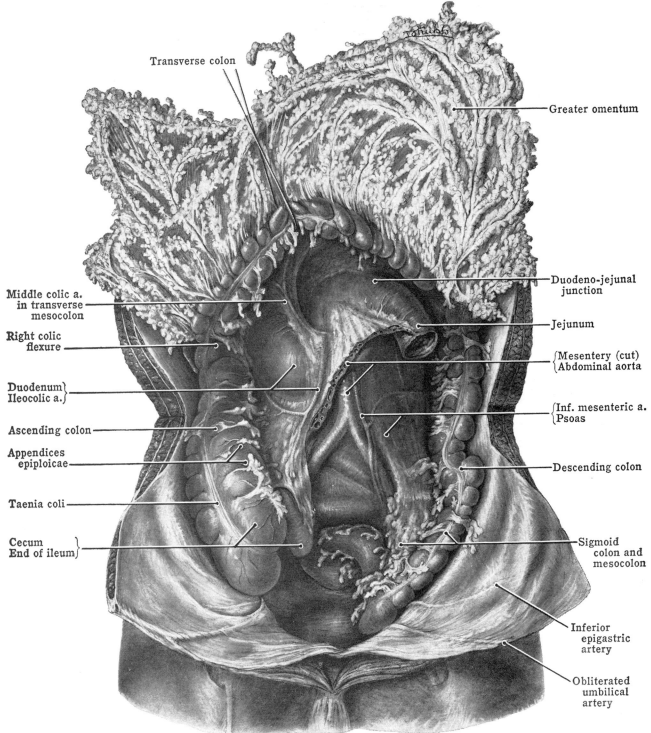

Transverse colon

Greater omentum

Middle colic a.
in transverse
mesocolon

Right colic
flexure

Duodenum}
Ileocolic a.}

Ascending colon

Appendices
epiploicae

Taenia coli

Cecum
End of ileum}

Duodeno-jejunal
junction

Jejunum

{Mesentery (cut)
{Abdominal aorta

{Inf. mesenteric a.
{Psoas

Descending colon

Sigmoid
colon and
mesocolon

Inferior
epigastric
artery

Obliterated
umbilical
artery

164 Intestines

The greater omentum is thrown upwards and with it go the transverse colon and transverse mesocolon. The jejunum and ileum are cut away, excepting their end pieces, and the mesentery is cut short. Examine in conjunction with figure 165 facing.

Observe:

1. The duodeno-jejunal junction, situated to the left of the median plane and immediately below the root of the transverse mesocolon.

2. The first few inches of the jejunum descending infero-sinistrally anterior to the left kidney. The last few inches of the ileum ascending supero-dextrally out of the pelvic cavity. Of these two parallel pieces of gut, the former being much larger.

3. The root of the mesentery directed infero-dextrally and crossing in turn—the junction of the 3rd and 4th parts of the duodenum, the inferior vena cava, the right ureter, and the right Psoas (fig. 165).

4. The large gut forming $3\frac{1}{2}$ sides of a square, or picture frame, around the jejunum and ileum (removed); the missing $\frac{1}{2}$ side being infero-dextral, between the cecum and the sigmoid colon.

5. The distinguishing features of the large gut: (a) its position around the small gut, (b) the teniae coli or longitudinal muscle bands, (c) the sacculations or haustra, and (d) the appendices epiploicae.

6. The right colic flexure, which lies below the liver, placed at a lower level than the left colic flexure which lies below the spleen.

7. The vermiform appendix had been removed at operation.

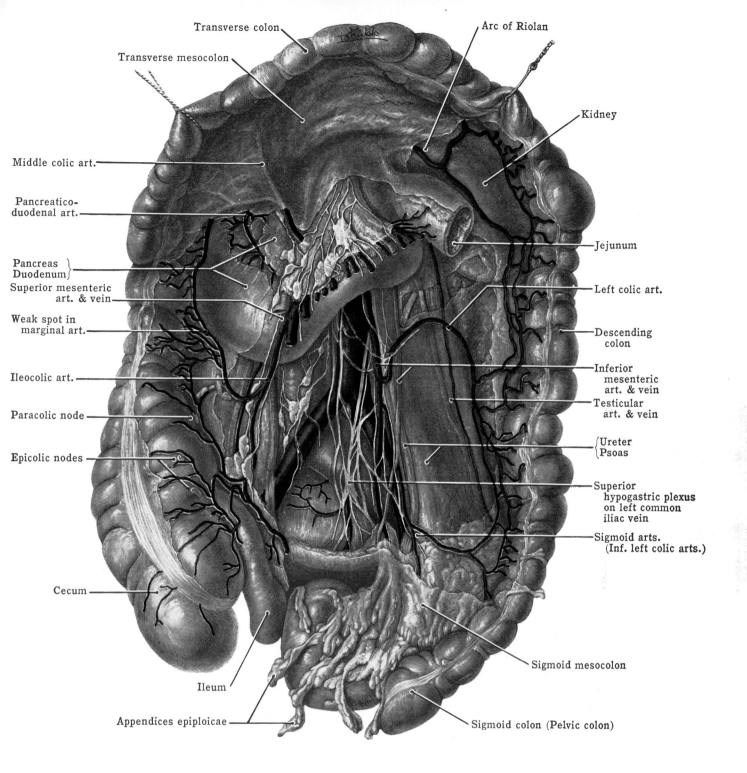

Transverse colon

Transverse mesocolon

Arc of Riolan

Kidney

Middle colic art.

Pancreatico-
duodenal art.

Pancreas
Duodenum

Superior mesenteric
art. & vein

Jejunum

Left colic art.

Weak spot in
marginal art.

Descending
colon

Ileocolic art.

Inferior
mesenteric
art. & vein

Paracolic node

Testicular
art. & vein

Ureter
Psoas

Epicolic nodes

Superior
hypogastric plexus
on left common
iliac vein

Sigmoid arts.
(Inf. left colic arts.)

Cecum

Sigmoid mesocolon

Ileum

Appendices epiploicae

Sigmoid colon (Pelvic colon)

165   Structures on the Posterior Abdominal Wall

This is figure 164 enlarged and with much peritoneum removed.

Observe:

1. The duodenum, of large diameter before the site of crossing
of the superior mesenteric vessels, and narrow beyond. It is,
indeed, much wider than the descending colon.

2. The jejunal and ileal branches (cut) passing from the left
side of the superior mesenteric artery; the right colic artery,
here as commonly, being a branch of the ileocolic artery.

3. An accessory artery, called the arc of Riolan, which connects
the superior mesenteric artery to the left colic artery.

4. On the right side: small (epicolic) lymph nodes on the colon;

small (paracolic) nodes beside the colon; nodes along the
ileo-colic artery which drain into main nodes ventral to the
pancreas.

5. (a) The intestines and the intestinal vessels lying on a plane
anterior to (b) that of the testicular vessels, and these in turn
lying (c) anterior to the plane of the kidney, its vessels, and
the ureter.

6. The right and left ureters asymmetrically placed, in this
specimen.

7. The superior hypogastric plexus (presacral nerve) lying
within the fork of the aorta and ventral to the left common
iliac vein, the body of the 5th lumbar vertebra and the 5th
disc.

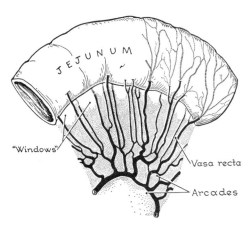

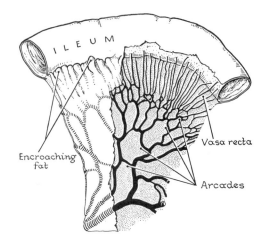

166 Jejunum contrasted with Ileum

Note whether: large diameter or small; thick wall or thin; one or two arterial arcades or several; long vasa recta or short; and translucent (fat-free) areas at the mesenteric border or fat encroaching on the wall of the gut.

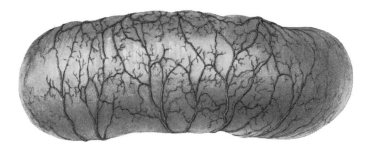

Antimesenteric border of gut

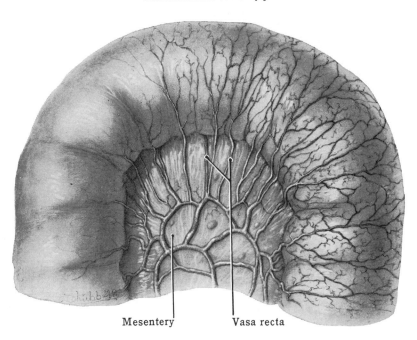

Segment of Intestinum Jejunum with Mesentery and Arteries.

167 Blood Supply of the Small Intestine

Observe:

1. The series of anastomotic arterial arches in the mesentery.

2. The vasa recta that proceed from the arches to the mesenteric border of the gut and then pass more or less alternately to opposite sides of the gut.

3. The arborisations of the vasa in the wall of the gut and the fine anastomoses effected between adjacent arborisations.

4. The efficient anastomoses across the anti-mesenteric border.

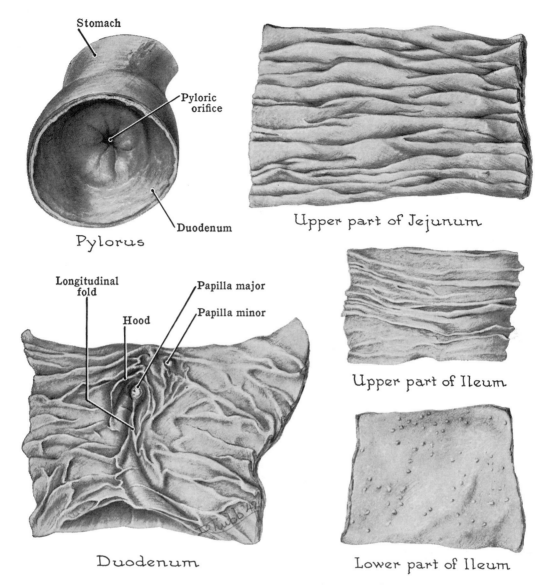

Stomach

Pyloric orifice

Duodenum

Pylorus

Upper part of Jejunum

Longitudinal fold

Hood

Papilla major

Papilla minor

Duodenum

Upper part of Ileum

Lower part of Ileum

168 Interior of the Small Intestine

Pylorus: The pylorus pouts into the 1st (superior) part of the duodenum and, having a fornix around it, resembles the cervix projecting into the vagina. The first $1\frac{1}{2}''$ of the duodenum has no plicae circulares, but the mucous membrane may be rugose.

Duodenum: The larger duodenal papilla (of Vater) projects into the 2nd (descending) part of the duodenum on the concave border $3\frac{1}{2}''$ from the pylorus (in fig. 156 it is at the apex of a conical evagination). On its tip is the orifice of the bile duct and, below this, the orifice of the pancreatic duct, but usually these 2 ducts open together (see fig. 157). A hood is thrown over the larger papilla, a longitudinal fold descends from it, and the smaller duo-

denal papilla, of the accessory pancreatic duct, lies $\frac{1}{4}''$–$\frac{3}{4}''$ antero-superior to it. Plicae circulares are pronounced.

Jejunum, upper part: The plicae circulares are tall, closely packed, and commonly branched.

Ileum, upper part: The plicae circulares are low and becoming sparse. The calibre of the gut is reduced and the wall is thinner.

Ileum, lower part: Plicae are now absent. Solitary lymph nodules stud the wall. [In youth, aggregated lymph nodules, up to $1\frac{1}{2}''$ long and $\frac{3}{4}''$ wide, are scattered along the antimesenteric border.]

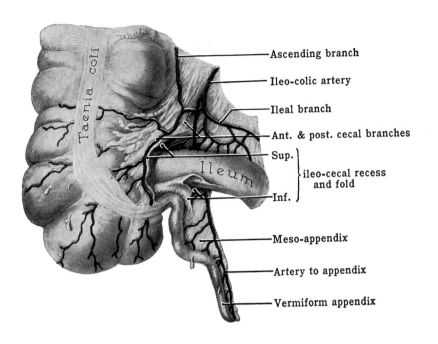

- Ascending branch
- Ileo-colic artery
- Ileal branch
- Ant. & post. cecal branches
- Sup.
  ileo-cecal recess and fold
- Inf.
- Meso-appendix
- Artery to appendix
- Vermiform appendix

169 Ileo-cecal Region

Observe:

1. The appendix in one free border of the mesoappendix and the artery in the other.
2. The anterior tenia coli leading to the appendix.
3. The inferior ileocecal (bloodless) fold extending from ileum to meso-appendix.
4. The vascular cecal fold is the official name for the superior ileocecal fold.

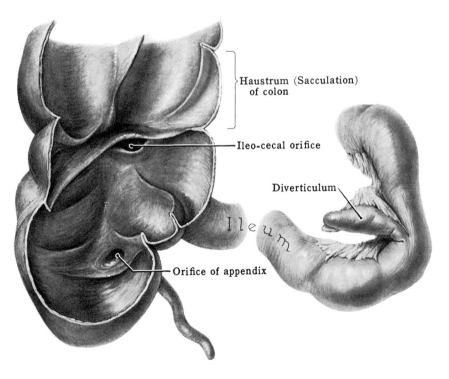

- Haustrum (Sacculation) of colon
- Ileo-cecal orifice
- Diverticulum
- Orifice of appendix

170   Interior of a Dried Cecum

This cecum was filled with air until dry, opened and varnished.

Observe:

1. The ileocecal valve guarding the ileocecal orifice; its pouting upper lip overhanging the lower lip; and the folds or frenula running horizontally from the commissures of the lips.
2. The slight fold closing the upper part of the orifice of the appendix.

170.1   Diverticulum Ilei (Meckel's)

Meckel's diverticulum, found in 2% of persons, is the remains of the prenatal vitello-intestinal duct. It projects from the side of the ileum (theoretically, from the antimesenteric border) and it is attached to it by a short peritoneal fold. Usually less than 2 inches in length, it may attain ten inches. About 75% of diverticula are located within $3\frac{1}{2}$ feet of the ileocecal orifice, and 25% from $3\frac{1}{2}$ to $5\frac{1}{2}$ feet. (*G. D. Jay et al.*).

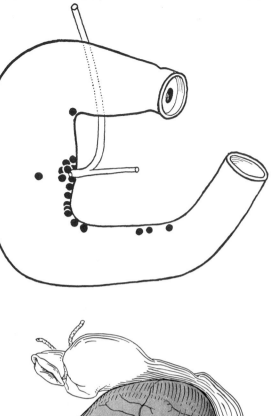

171 Duodenal Diverticula

A.

Sites of 20 diverticula found in 15 of 133 duodena investigated. Melted wax, poured into the duodena, fills any diverticula that may be present; these are revealed when the wax hardens. (*J.C.B.G.*)

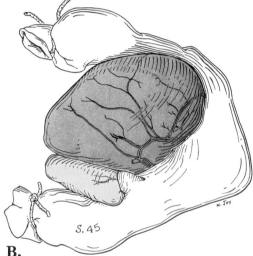

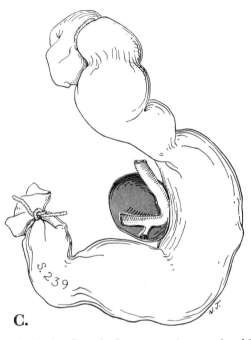

B.

Two diverticula, posterior to the bile and pancreatic ducts, posterior view.

C.

A single diverticulum, anterior to the bile and pancreatic ducts, posterior view.

Note that the mucous and submucous coats are herniated through the muscular coats.

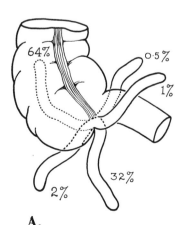

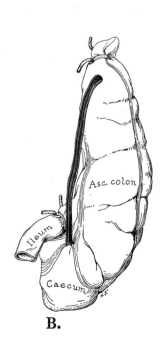

172 Vermiform Appendix

A.

Locations and their Approximate Frequencies. (After Wakeley.) Like the hands of a clock, the appendix may be long or short, and it may occupy any position consistent with its length.

B.

A Retrocolic Appendix seven inches long.

VARIATIONS AND ANOMALIES

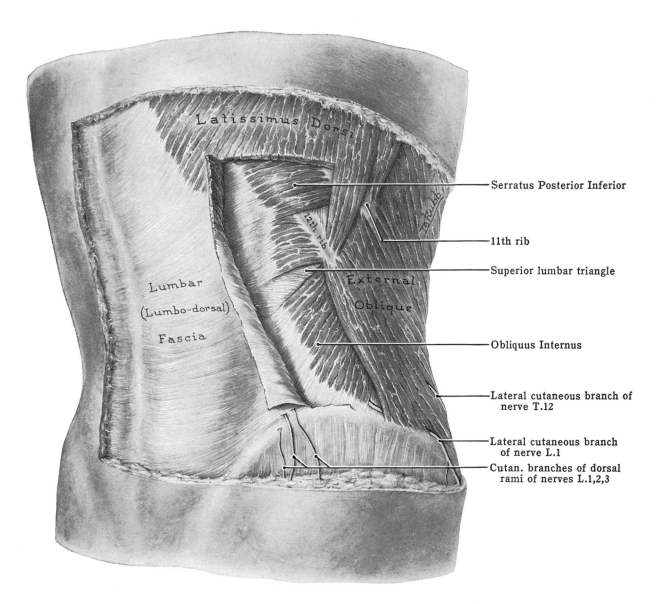

Latissimus Dorsi

Serratus Posterior Inferior

12th rib

11th rib

Superior lumbar triangle

Lumbar
(Lumbo-dorsal)
Fascia

External
Oblique

Obliquus Internus

Lateral cutaneous branch of
nerve T.12

Lateral cutaneous branch
of nerve L.1

Cutan. branches of dorsal
rami of nerves L.1,2,3

173 Posterior Abdominal Wall,
postero-lateral view—I

Latissimus Dorsi is in part reflected.

Observe:

1. External Oblique having an oblique, free, posterior border which extends from the tip of
   the 12th rib to the mid-point of the iliac crest.

2. The small, triangular space between External Oblique, Latissimus Dorsi, and the iliac
   crest. This is the (inferior) lumbar triangle (fig. 24).

3. Internal Oblique extending behind External Oblique. It forms the floor of the lumbar triangle, creeps up on to the lumbar fascia, and has a triangle between it and Serratus
   Posterior Inferior. This is the "superior lumbar triangle".

   (In N. A. P. lumbo-dorsal fascia reads thoraco-lumbar fascia.)

4 Posterior Abdominal
all—II

hen External Oblique has been incised
turned laterally, and Internal Oblique
ed and turned medially, Transversus Ab-
inis and its posterior aponeurosis are ex-
d where pierced by the subcostal (T.12)
ilio-hypogastric (L.1) nerves. These
es give off motor twigs and lateral cuta-
us (iliac) branches, and continue forwards
een Internal Oblique and Transversus.

5 Posterior Abdominal
all—III

n dividing the posterior aponeurosis of
nsversus between the subcostal and ilio-
ogastric nerves, and lateral to the oblique
ral border of Quadratus Lumborum, the
operitoneal fat surrounding the kidney
posed. The renal fascia is within this fat.
portion of fat inside the renal fascia is
ed fatty renal capsule (perinephric fat);
fat outside is paranephric fat.

Quadratus Lumborum, ventral view, see
190.)

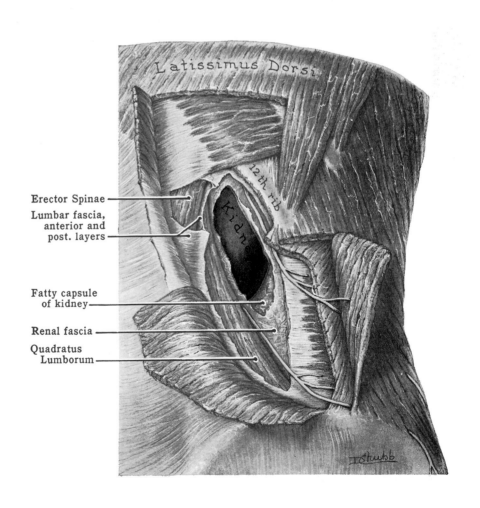

Serratus Posterior
Inferior

11th rib

Subcostal nerve
(Nerve T.12)

Obliquus Externus

Obliquus Internus

Transversus
and its aponeurosis

Ilio-hypogastric n.
(Nerve L.1)

Erector Spinae

Lumbar fascia,
anterior and
post. layers

Fatty capsule
of kidney

Renal fascia

Quadratus
Lumborum

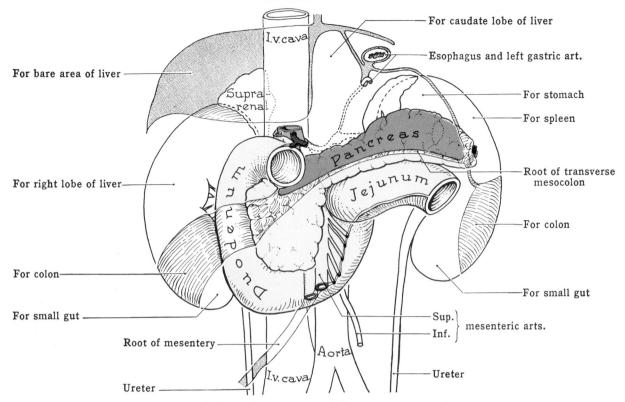

For bare area of liver

For caudate lobe of liver

Esophagus and left gastric art.

I.v.cava

Supra-renal

Pancreas

For stomach

For spleen

For right lobe of liver

Duodenum

Jejunum

Root of transverse mesocolon

For colon

For colon

For small gut

For small gut

Root of mesentery

Sup.
Inf. } mesenteric arts.

Aorta

Ureter

I.v.cava

Ureter

176   Duodenum and Pancreas, in situ

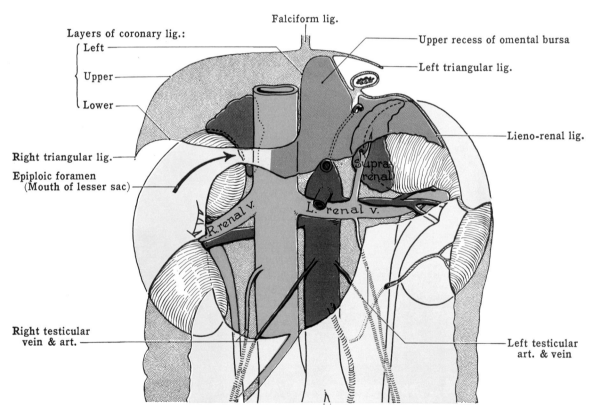

Falciform lig.

Layers of coronary lig.:

Left

Upper recess of omental bursa

Left triangular lig.

Upper

Lower

Lieno-renal lig.

Right triangular lig.

Epiploic foramen
(Mouth of lesser sac)

Supra-renal

R.renal v.

L. renal v.

Right testicular
vein & art.

Left testicular
art. & vein

177   Duodenum and Pancreas, removed

176 & 177   Posterior Abdominal Viscera and their Ventral Relations

Observe:

1. The peritoneal covering (yellow) of pancreas and duodenum.

2. The colic area of right kidney, second part of duodenum, and head of pancreas; the line of attachment of the transverse mesocolon to the body and tail of the pancreas and the colic area of the left kidney.

4. The ventral relations of the kidneys and suprarenal glands.

5. The right suprarenal gland at the epiploic foramen.

6. The three parts of the coronary ligament attached to the diaphragm except where—inf. vena cava, suprarenal gland, and kidney—intervene.

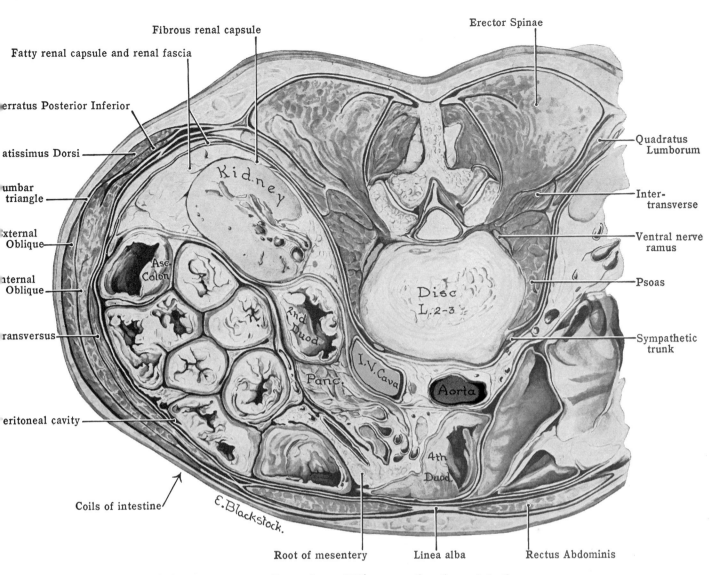

Labels (clockwise from upper left):

Fatty renal capsule and renal fascia

Fibrous renal capsule

Erector Spinae

[S]erratus Posterior Inferior

[L]atissimus Dorsi

[L]umbar triangle

[E]xternal Oblique

[I]nternal Oblique

[T]ransversus

[P]eritoneal cavity

Quadratus Lumborum

Inter-transverse

Ventral nerve ramus

Psoas

Sympathetic trunk

Kidney

Asc. Colon

Disc L.2-3

2nd Duod.

I.V. Cava

Panc.

Aorta

4th Duod.

Coils of intestine

E. Blackstock.

Root of mesentery

Linea alba

Rectus Abdominis

178   Transverse Section Through the Abdomen

at the level of the disc between the 2nd and 3rd lumbar vertebrae and between their transverse processes.

Observe:

1. The anterior aspect of the vertebral column, nearer to the ventral surface of the body than to the dorsal surface in this thin recumbent subject.

2. The coils of small intestine, not circular as seen at operation, but mutually compressed.

3. The mucous membrane of the small intestine—which in life is much more moist and succulent than in this hardened specimen—in loose folds which almost completely occlude the lumen.

4. The ascending colon with an appendix epiploica, having no mesentery but being bare posteriorly.

5. The anterior and posterior surfaces of the kidney facing not ventrally and dorsally but ventro-laterally and dorso-medially.

6. The adipose renal capsule (perinephric fat) massed along the borders of the kidney and leaving the anterior surface close to the peritoneum.

7. The kidney projecting lateral to Quadratus Lumborum.

8. The 2nd or descending part of the duodenum overlapping this surface of the kidney.

9. The sympathetic trunk lying along the anterior border of Psoas; and on the right side behind the inferior vena cava

10. The lipping at the epiphyseal plate of the vertebral body which first begins to show itself before the age of 30 years.

11. The linea alba, band-like above the navel, though linear below it.

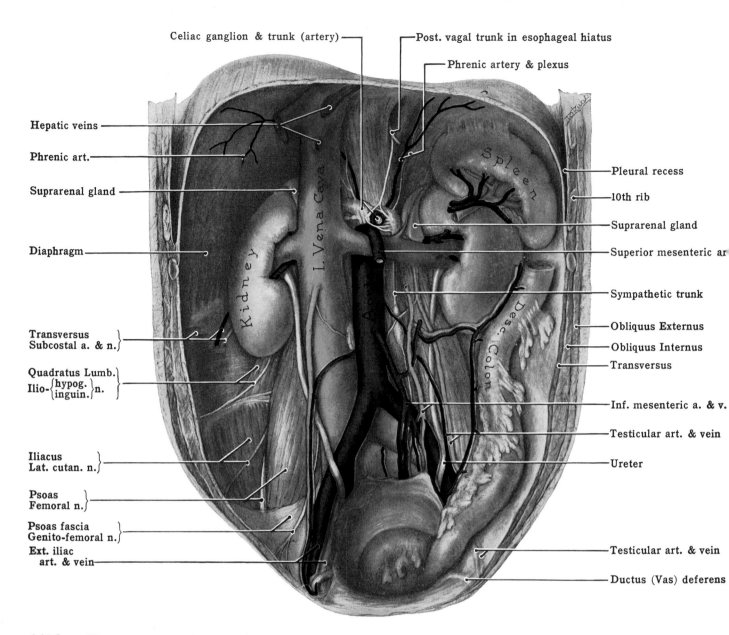

Celiac ganglion & trunk (artery) —

Post. vagal trunk in esophageal hiatus

Phrenic artery & plexus

Hepatic veins —

Phrenic art.—

Suprarenal gland —

Diaphragm—

Transversus
Subcostal a. & n.

Quadratus Lumb.
Ilio-{hypog.
inguin.}n.

Iliacus
Lat. cutan. n.

Psoas
Femoral n.

Psoas fascia
Genito-femoral n.

Ext. iliac
art. & vein—

Pleural recess

10th rib

Suprarenal gland

Superior mesenteric ar

Sympathetic trunk

Obliquus Externus

Obliquus Internus

Transversus

Inf. mesenteric a. & v.

Testicular art. & vein

Ureter

Testicular art. & vein

Ductus (Vas) deferens

179   Great vessels: Kidneys: Suprarenal Glands

The abdominal aorta is shorter than the combined common and external iliac arteries.

The celiac trunk, straddled by crura and the median arcuate lig. (figs. 133.1 & 191), appears above the pancreas (158.1).

The superior mesenteric artery arises just below the celiac trunk.

The inferior mesenteric artery arises $1\frac{1}{2}''$ above the aortic bifurcation and crosses the left common iliac vessels to become the superior rectal artery.

The kidneys lie ventral to—Diaphragm, Transversus aponeurosis, Quadratus Lumborum and Psoas. (fig. 190).

The ureter crosses the external iliac artery just beyond the common iliac bifurcation.

The testicular vessels cross ventral to the ureter and join the ductus deferens at the deep inguinal ring (fig. 202).

179.1

Diagram. The aorta and the sup. mesenteric art., like nutcrackers, the weight of the gut being the force, may compress left renal vein and duodenum (fig. 153).

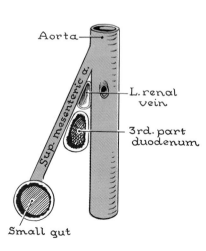

Aorta

L. renal vein

3rd. part duodenum

Sup. mesenteric a.

Small gut

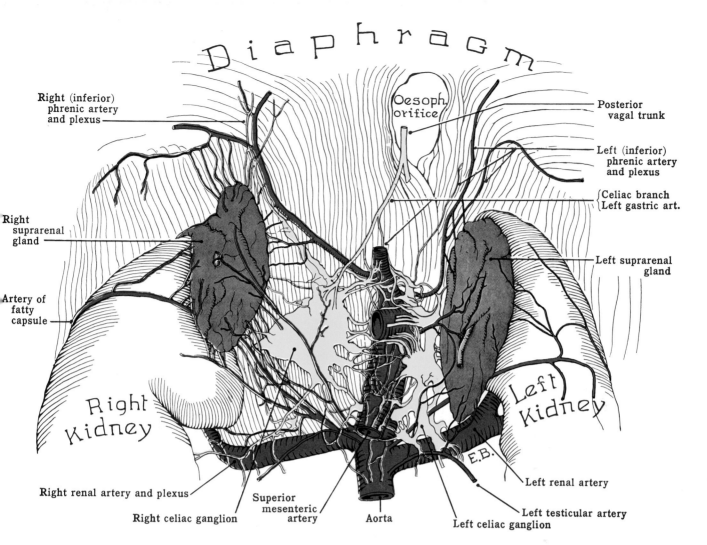

Right (inferior) phrenic artery and plexus

Oesoph. orifice

Posterior vagal trunk

Left (inferior) phrenic artery and plexus

{Celiac branch
Left gastric art.

Right suprarenal gland

Left suprarenal gland

Artery of fatty capsule

Right Kidney

Left Kidney

E.B.

Left renal artery

Right renal artery and plexus

Superior mesenteric artery

Aorta

Left testicular artery

Right celiac ganglion

Left celiac ganglion

180   Celiac Trunk, Plexus, and Ganglia, and the Suprarenal Glands

(Dissection by Ian B. MacDonald.)

Observe:

1. The celiac plexus of nerves surrounding the celiac trunk (not labelled) and connecting the right and the left celiac ganglion.

2. A stout branch from the posterior vagal trunk descending along the stem of the left gastric artery and conveying vagal (parasympathetic) fibres to the celiac ganglia.

3. Nerves extending along the arteries to the viscera, and down the aorta. The nerves to the suprarenal glands are mostly preganglionic.

4. The suprarenal glands, abreast of the celiac trunk, two inches apart, but not equidistant from the medial plane. (For relations, see fig. 177.)

5. The right suprarenal vein, about 5 mm long, ascending to join the i.v. cava (fig. 188.2): the left vein descending to join the left renal vein.

6. The very numerous thread-like branches of the phrenic art. aorta, renal art. and artery of the fatty capsule of the kidney convering on the periphery of the suprarenal gland.

(For variations on the blood vessels of the gland, see Kenneth Clark.)

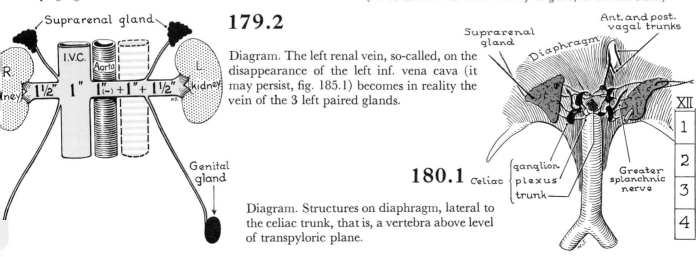

179.2

Diagram. The left renal vein, so-called, on the disappearance of the left inf. vena cava (it may persist, fig. 185.1) becomes in reality the vein of the 3 left paired glands.

Suprarenal gland

I.V.C.

Aorta

R ney

L kidney

1½"   1"   1"(-) + 1" + 1½"

Genital gland

Suprarenal gland

Ant. and post. vagal trunks

Diaphragm

180.1 Celiac

{ganglion
plexus
trunk

Greater splanchnic nerve

XII
1
2
3
4

Diagram. Structures on diaphragm, lateral to the celiac trunk, that is, a vertebra above level of transpyloric plane.

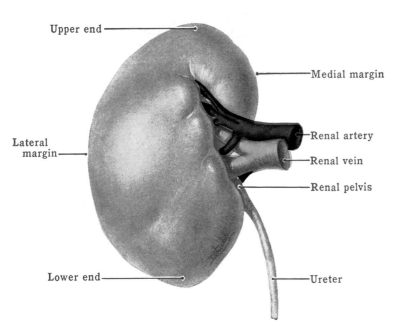

Upper end

Medial margin

Lateral margin

Renal artery

Renal vein

Renal pelvis

Lower end

Ureter

181   Right Kidney, front view

The order of structures at the hilus (entrance to the renal sinus) from before backwards is—vein, artery, duct (pelvis or ureter), and a branch of the artery crosses behind the pelvis.

The upper end of the kidney is usually wider than the lower, and closer to the median plane, as in figure 183.

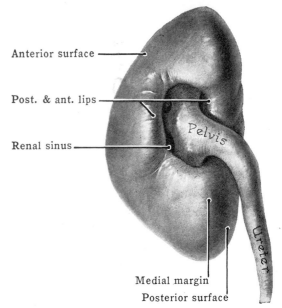

Anterior surface

Post. & ant. lips

Renal sinus

Pelvis

Ureter

Medial margin

Posterior surface

181.1   Sinus of the Kidney

The anterior surface has an upper and a lower incli plane.

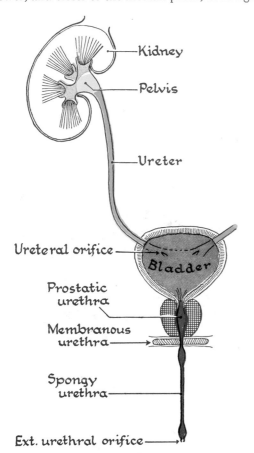

Kidney

Pelvis

Ureter

Ureteral orifice

Bladder

Prostatic urethra

Membranous urethra

Spongy urethra

Ext. urethral orifice

182   Diagram of the Male Urinary System

(For genital system, see fig. 115.)

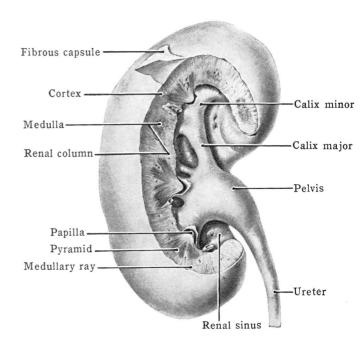

Fibrous capsule

Cortex

Medulla

Renal column

Calix minor

Calix major

Pelvis

Papilla

Pyramid

Medullary ray

Ureter

Renal sinus

183   Structure of the Kidney

The anterior lip of the sinus is cut away. The outer $\frac{1}{3}$ of the renal substance is cortex; the inner $\frac{2}{3}$ is medulla. Cortical tissue (glomeruli, convoluted tubules) is granular on section and extends, as renal columns (of Bertin), through the medulla to the sinus. The medullar contains 7 to 14 pyramids which are striated because they consist of converging tubules (collecting, loops of Henle). Each pyramid sends finger-like rays into the cortex and each ends as a papilla on which a dozen or more ducts open. One or two (or more) papillae project into each calix minor; several calices minores unite to form a calix major. Of calices majores there are usually two, an upper and a lower, but not uncommonly there are also one or two middle.

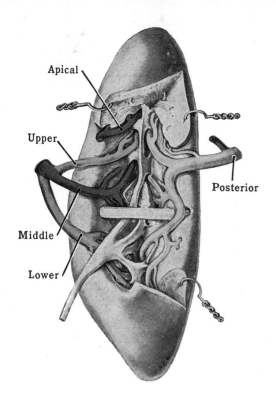

Apical

Upper

Posterior

Middle

Lower

183.1 Branches of the Renal Artery within the Sinus

Typically, as shown, there are 5 such segmental arteries. The posterior lip of the sinus has been incised, above and below, near the limits of the territory of the posterior segmental artery. (Riches; Graves; and Roberts.)

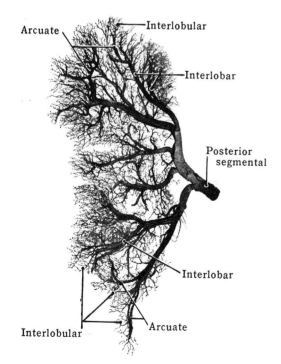

Arcuate — Interlobular

Interlobar

Posterior segmental

Interlobar

Interlobular — Arcuate

183.2 A Segmental Artery

Segmental arteries are end arteries, whereas segmental veins anastomose freely.

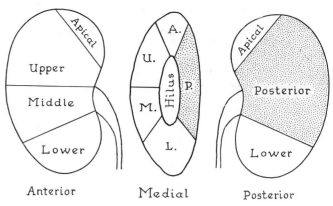

Apical

Upper

Middle

Lower

A.

U.

Hilus

P.

M.

L.

Apical

Posterior

Lower

Anterior   Medial   Posterior

184

Diagram. **Segments of the Kidney,** (after Graves, modified).

According to its arterial supply the kidney:—5 segments:—has 1. apical [superior]; 2. superior [antero-superior]; 3. middle [antero-inferior]; 4. lower or inferior; and 5. posterior.

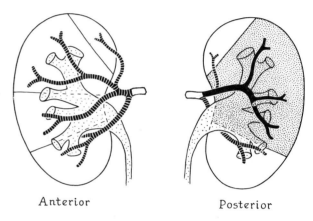

Anterior   Posterior

184.1

Diagram. **Segmental Arteries of the Kidney**

Only the apical and inferior arteries supply the whole thickness of the kidney. The posterior artery crosses cranial to the renal pelvis to reach its segment.

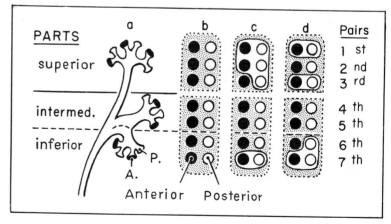

PARTS	a	b	c	d	Pairs
superior					1 st
					2 nd
					3 rd
intermed.					4 th
					5 th
inferior	P.				6 th
	A.				7 th

Anterior   Posterior

184.2

Scheme explaining the **Variation in the Number of Pyramids and Calices Minores,** (after Lofgren, modified).

Of the 7 paired (anterior & posterior) primitive pyramids, each dips into its own calix minor, there being 14 in all. Some of those at the upper and lower ends of the kidney, being crowded, coalesce; hence, the maximum number of 14 (see b) is almost always reduced to about 9 or 10 compound pyramids and calices minores (see c and d).

An intermediate (or middle) calix major commonly splits off the lower calix major, as shown.

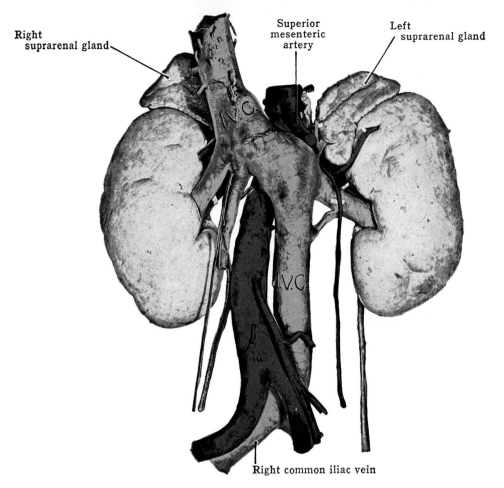

Right
suprarenal gland

Superior
mesenteric
artery

Left
suprarenal gland

Right common iliac vein

185   Left Postrenal Inferior Vena Cava

[Courtesy of Dr. J. E. Anderson.]

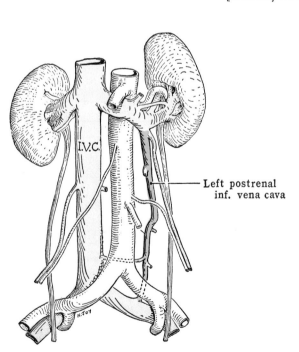

Left postrenal
inf. vena cava

185.1   Persisting Left Inferior Vena Cava

joins the left common iliac vein to the left renal vein. This occasional vessel may be small, as in this specimen, or it may be large.

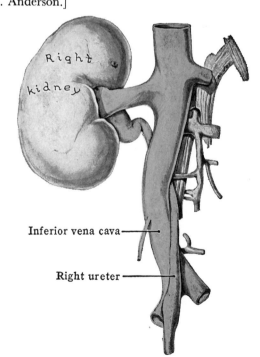

Inferior vena cava

Right ureter

186   Retrocaval Ureter

There were only 34 isolated cases of retrocaval ureter re ported up to the year 1946 (Lowsley).

Anomalies of the Inferior Vena Cava

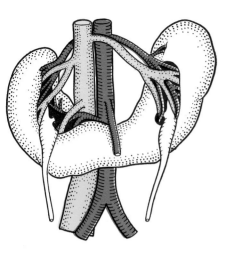

Horseshoe Kidney

"In our 35,329 postmortems there were 94 cases, 1:376." (Bell, E. T.)

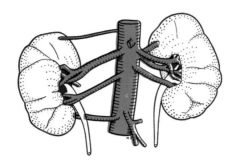

Multiple Renal Arteries and Fetal Lobulation

About 25% of kidneys receive directly from the aorta 2nd, 3rd, and even 4th branches. These enter either through the renal sinus or at the upper or lower pole. (Data from Adachi; Lloyd, L. W.)

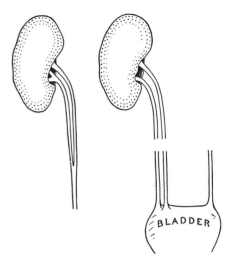

Duplicated or Bifid Ureters

These may be either unilateral or bilateral, and either complete or incomplete.

In 32,360 postmortems 205 cases were found, 1:157. The incidence is probably higher. Of these, 167 were unilateral, 37 being complete; and 38 were bilateral, 11 being complete on both sides, and 3 on one side. (Bell, E. T.; also Campbell, M.)

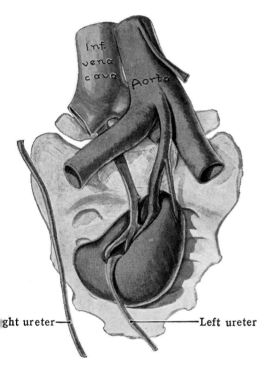

Ectopic Pelvic Kidney

Pelvic kidneys have no fatty capsule. During childbirth, they may both cause obstruction and suffer injury. Of 112 recorded cases, 97 were unilateral (mostly left), 10 were bilateral (either fused or separate), and 5 were solitary. (Anderson, Rice and Harris.)

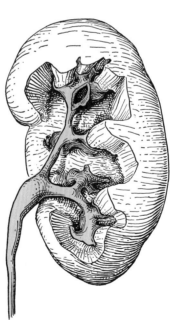

Bifid Pelves

(*Dissections by Dr. C. A. Armstrong.*)

The pelves are almost replaced by two long calyces majores, which lie entirely within the sinus (left), and partly within and partly without (right).

187   Anomalies of the Kidney and Ureter

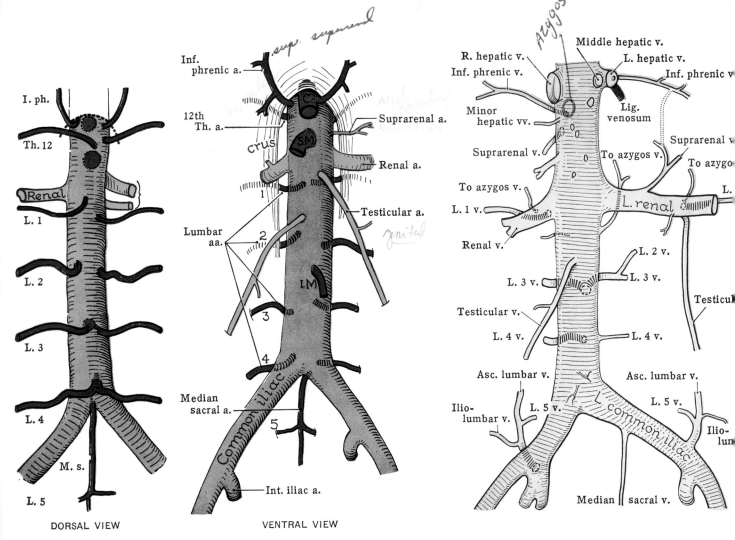

I. ph.

Th. 12

Renal

L. 1

L. 2

L. 3

L. 4

M. s.

L. 5

DORSAL VIEW

Inf. phrenic a.

sup. segmental

12th Th. a.

crus

Lumbar aa.

Median sacral a.

Int. iliac a.

VENTRAL VIEW

Suprarenal a.

Renal a.

Testicular a.

genital

Common iliac

R. hepatic v.
Inf. phrenic v.

Azygos

Middle hepatic v.

L. hepatic v.
Inf. phrenic v

Minor hepatic vv.

Lig. venosum

Suprarenal v

Suprarenal v.

To azygos v.

To azygos

To azygos v.

L. renal

L.

L. 1 v.

Renal v.

L. 2 v.

L. 3 v.

L. 3 v.

Testicul

Testicular v.

L. 4 v.

L. 4 v.

Asc. lumbar v.

Asc. lumbar v.

Iliolumbar v.

L. 5 v.

common iliac

L. 5 v.

Iliolun

Median sacral v.

188   Abdominal Aorta and its Branches

(The dorsal and ventral views are of different specimens.)
(*Thoracic aorta & branches, also entire aorta, see fig. 457.1.*)

188.2   Inferior Vena Cava and its Tributaries

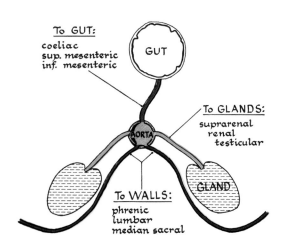

To GUT:
coeliac
sup. mesenteric
inf. mesenteric

GUT

To GLANDS:
suprarenal
renal
testicular

AORTA

GLAND

To WALLS:
phrenic
lumbar
median sacral

188.1   Its Branches Classified

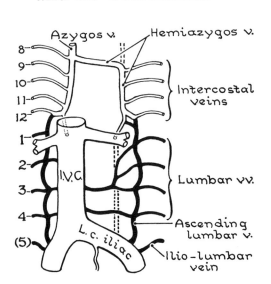

Azygos v.

Hemiazygos v.

8
9
10
11
12

Intercostal veins

I.V.C.

1
2
3
4

Lumbar vv.

Ascending lumbar v.

(5)

L. c. iliac

Ilio-lumbar vein

188.3   Diagram of Ascending Lumbar Vein

This intersegmental vein, which lies on the transverse processes, is interrupted in about 15% of cases (Seib, G. A.).

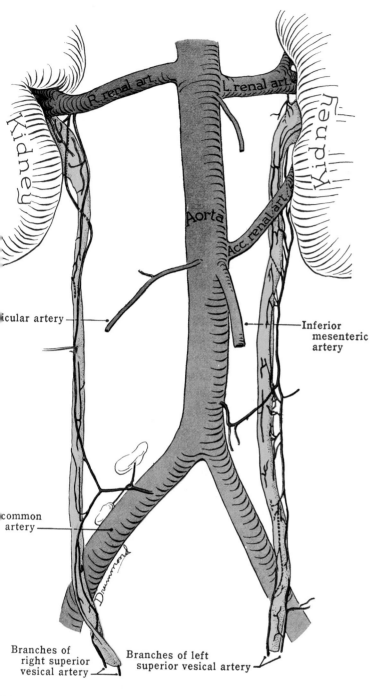

R. renal art.

L. renal art.

Kidney

Kidney

Aorta

Acc. renal art.

…icular artery

Inferior mesenteric artery

…common artery

Drummond

Branches of right superior vesical artery

Branches of left superior vesical artery

'9   Blood Supply to the Ureter

… arterial system was injected with latex by way of the
…oral artery. (*Dissection by W. R. Mitchell.*)

…rve:

…he blood supply to the ureter coming from 3 main sources: (a) from the
…nal artery above, (b) from a vesical artery below, and (c) about the
…iddle of its course either from the common iliac artery or from the aorta.

…hese branches approaching the ureter from the medial side. **In this
…ecimen an accessory renal artery also supplies branches. The testicular
…tery may also contribute a branch.**

…he excellent anastomotic chain made by these long, tenuous branches.

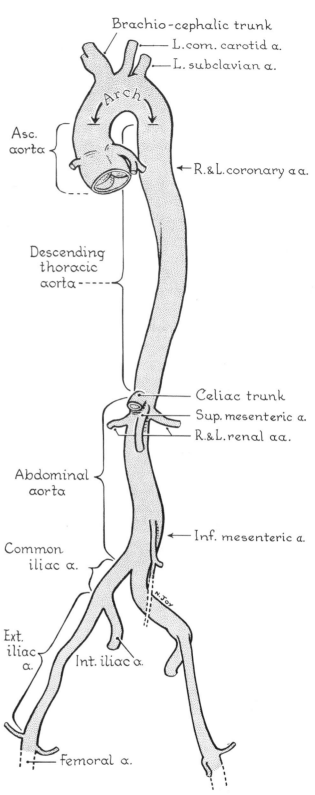

Brachio-cephalic trunk

L. com. carotid a.

L. subclavian a.

Arch

Asc. aorta

R. & L. coronary a a.

Descending thoracic aorta

Celiac trunk

Sup. mesenteric a.

R. & L. renal a a.

Abdominal aorta

Inf. mesenteric a.

Common iliac a.

Ext. iliac a.

Int. iliac a.

N. Joy

Femoral a.

189.1

The Aorta and its Larger Branches, from an older person.

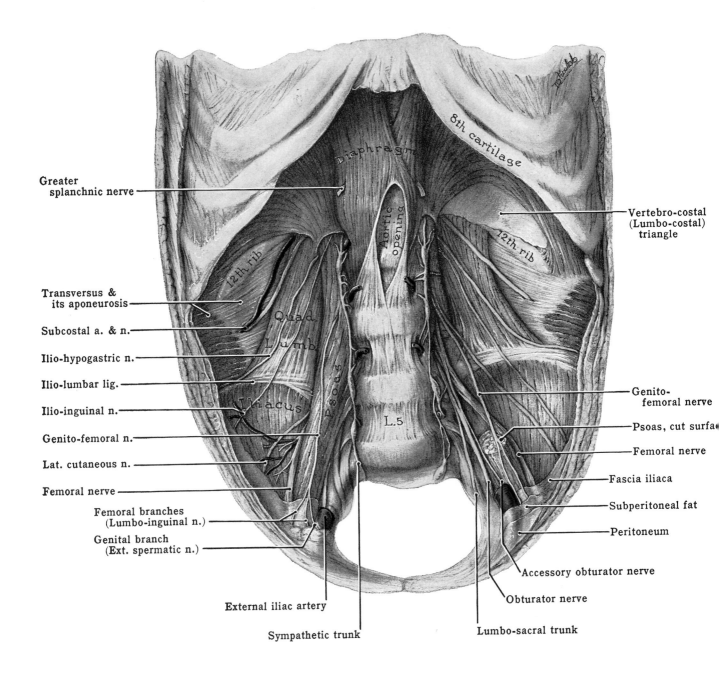

Greater
splanchnic nerve

8th cartilage

Diaphragm

Aortic opening

Vertebro-costal
(Lumbo-costal)
triangle

12th rib

12th rib

Transversus &
its aponeurosis

Quad

Lumb

Subcostal a. & n.

Iliacus

Psoas

Ilio-hypogastric n.

Ilio-lumbar lig.

Ilio-inguinal n.

Genito-femoral n.

L.5

Genito-
femoral nerve

Lat. cutaneous n.

Psoas, cut surface

Femoral nerve

Femoral nerve

Fascia iliaca

Femoral branches
(Lumbo-inguinal n.)

Subperitoneal fat

Genital branch
(Ext. spermatic n.)

Peritoneum

Accessory obturator nerve

External iliac artery

Obturator nerve

Sympathetic trunk

Lumbo-sacral trunk

190 Posterior Abdominal Wall: Lumbar Plexus

Muscles. Transversus Abdominis becomes aponeurotic on a line dropped from the tip of the 12th rib. Quadratus Lumborum has an oblique lateral border; its fascia is thickened to form the lateral arcuate lig. above, and the ilio-lumbar lig. below. Iliacus lies below the iliac crest. Psoas rises above the crest and extends above the medial arcuate lig. which is thickened Psoas fascia.

Nerves. The subcostal nerve (T.12) passes behind the lateral arcuate lig. and runs at some distance below the 12th rib (with its artery). The next four nerves appear at the lateral border of Psoas. Of these, the ilio-hypogastric (T.12, L.1) takes the characteristic course here shown; the ilio-inguinal (L.1) and the lateral cutaneous of the

thigh (L.2, 3) are variable; the femoral (L.2, 3, 4) descends in the angle between Iliacus and Psoas. The genito-femoral nerve (L.1, 2) pierces Psoas and its fascia anteriorly. The obturator nerve (L.2 3, 4) and a branch of L.4 that joins with L.5 to form the lumbo-sacral trunk appear at the medial border of Psoas, and, crossing the ala of the sacrum, enter the pelvis.

The Sympathetic Trunk enters the abdomen with Psoas from behind the medial arcuate lig. It descends on vertebral bodies and intervertebral discs, following closely the attached border of Psoas to enter the pelvis. Its rami communicantes run dorsally with, or near, the lumbar arteries to join the lumbar nerves.

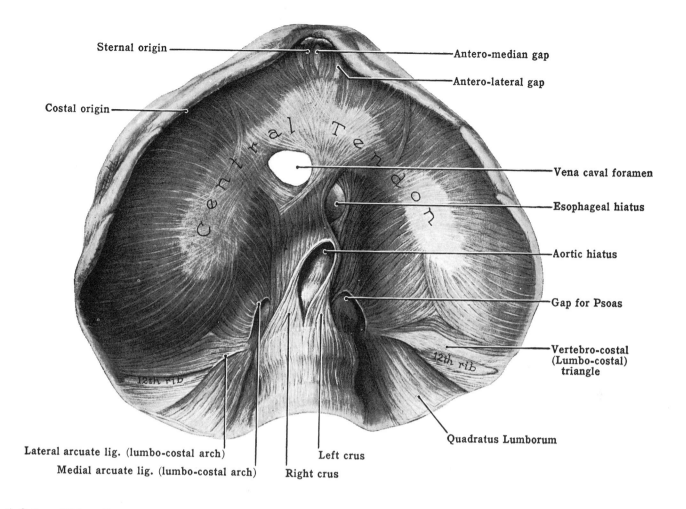

Sternal origin —————————————— Antero-median gap

————————————————— Antero-lateral gap

Costal origin —————

Central Tendon

——————————— Vena caval foramen

——————————— Esophageal hiatus

——————————— Aortic hiatus

——————————— Gap for Psoas

——————————— Vertebro-costal
(Lumbo-costal)
triangle

12th rib

12th rib

Quadratus Lumborum

Lateral arcuate lig. (lumbo-costal arch)

Medial arcuate lig. (lumbo-costal arch)

Left crus

Right crus

191   Diaphragm, viewed from below

Observe:

1. The trefoil-shaped, aponeurotic insertion called the central tendon; and the fleshy fibres of the sternal, costal, and vertebral origins (crura) that converge on this tendon.

2. Three large openings—(a) foramen for the inferior vena cava in the central tendon; (b) esophageal hiatus, which is almost a canal, surrounded by fibres of one or both crura aortic hiatus lying medianly behind the diaphragm.

3. The right and left crura, on the sides of the aortic hiatus, and united above by a fibrous arch, the *median arcuate ligament*. Also, thickenings of the Psoas and Quadratus Lumborum fasciae, called the medial and lateral arcuate ligaments. These structures afford origin to the Diaphragm.

4. The Diaphragm, in this specimen, failing to arise from the left arcuate lig., hence the vertebrocostal triangle, where only an areolar membrane separates kidney and surrounding fat from the pleura.

191.1

Diagram of Nerve Supply to Diaphragm. Each phrenic nerve (C.3, 4, 5) is the sole motor nerve to its own half of the diaphragm. It is also sensory to its own half, including the pleura above and the peritoneum below, but — the lower intercostal nerves are sensory to the peripheral fringe.

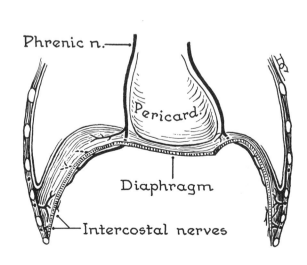

Phrenic n. —

Pericard.

Diaphragm

Intercostal nerves

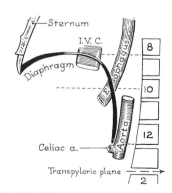

Sternum

I.V.C.

Diaphragm

Esophagus

Aorta

Celiac a. —

Transpyloric plane

8

10

12

2

191.2

Diagram. The 3 large openings in the diaphragm and their vertebral levels.

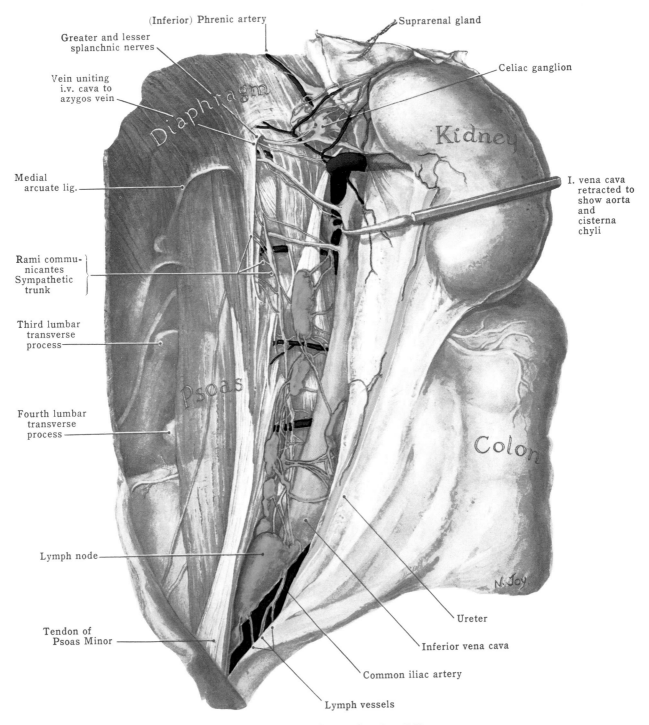

(Inferior) Phrenic artery

Greater and lesser
splanchnic nerves

Vein uniting
i.v. cava to
azygos vein

Diaphragm

Suprarenal gland

Celiac ganglion

Kidney

Medial
arcuate lig.

I. vena cava
retracted to
show aorta
and
cisterna
chyli

Rami communi-
nicantes
Sympathetic
trunk

Third lumbar
transverse
process

Psoas

Fourth lumbar
transverse
process

Colon

N. Joy

Lymph node

Ureter

Tendon of
Psoas Minor

Inferior vena cava

Common iliac artery

Lymph vessels

191.3 Right Celiac Ganglion, Splanchnic Nerves, and Sympathetic Trunk

The right suprarenal gland, kidney, ureter, and colon are reflected; the inferior vena cava is pulled medially; and the third and fourth lumbar veins are removed.

Observe:

1. In this specimen a Psoas Minor.

2. A wide cleft in the right crus (not labelled) of the diaphragm through which pass both splanchnic nerves, the sympathetic trunk, and a communicating vein. This unusually wide cleft is present on the left side also.

3. The greater splanchnic nerve ending in the celiac ganglion; the lesser splanchnic nerve here ending in the renal plexus (aortico-renal ganglion). Usually, as in figure 190, the greater splanchnic nerve pierces the crus at the level of the celiac trunk; the lesser nerve infero-lateral to this: and the sympathetic trunk enters with the Psoas.

4. The sympathetic trunk lying on the bodies of the vertebrae, the lumbar vessels alone intervening, and descending along the anterior border of the Psoas. The trunk is slender where it enters the abdomen; its ganglia are ill-defined: about eleven rami communicantes join it postero-laterally; and about six visceral branches, or lumbar splanchnic nerves, leave it antero-medially.

5. The 4 right lumbar arteries and cranial 2 veins (not labelled); the tip of the 3rd lumbar transverse process projecting further than the other transverse processes; and the right lumbar lymph nodes and vessels draining into the cisterna chyli.

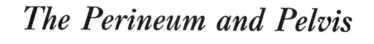

The Perineum and Pelvis

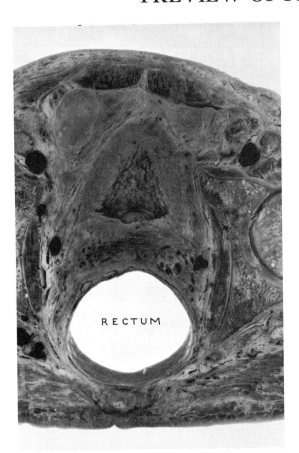

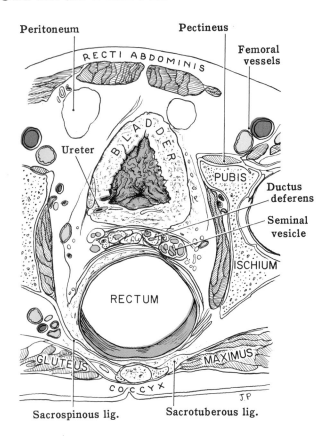

A. At Level of Bladder

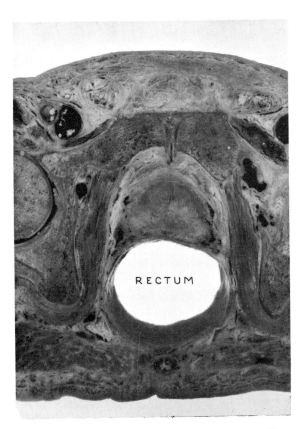

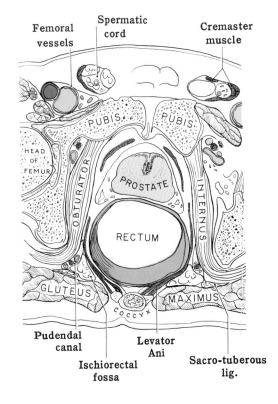

B. At Level of Prostate

191.6 Male Pelvis, on Horizontal Section

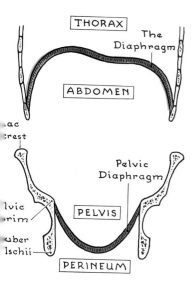

THORAX

The Diaphragm

ABDOMEN

ac crest

Pelvic Diaphragm

lvic rim

PELVIS

uber Ischii

PERINEUM

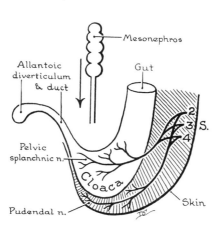

Mesonephros

Allantoic diverticulum & duct

Gut

2. 3 S. 4

Pelvic splanchnic n.

Cloaca

Pudendal n.

Skin

D.

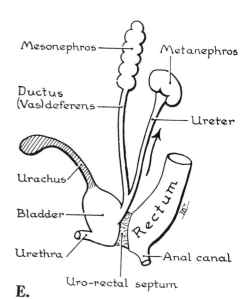

Mesonephros

Metanephros

Ductus (Vas) deferens

Ureter

Urachus

Rectum

Bladder

Urethra

Anal canal

Uro-rectal septum

E.

finitions. Diaphragm and Pelvic Dia-ragm. These partitions might more rmatively be called "The thoraco-ominal & pelvi-perineal diaphragms". e perineum is the region caudal (inferior) he pelvic diaphragm.

The embryonic cloaca about to receive the mesonephric duct (paired) from which springs the ureter (paired). The nerve supply to the whole region.

Diagram. The cloaca later split by a meso-dermal septum into bladder and rectum. This uro-rectal septum is occupied by internal genital organs — male or female. The nerve supply is retained.

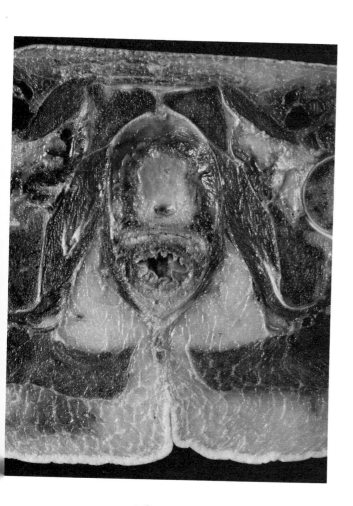

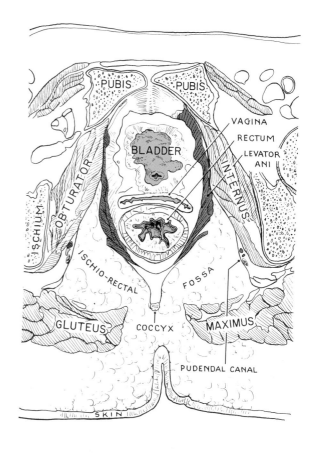

PUBIS PUBIS

VAGINA

RECTUM

BLADDER

LEVATOR ANI

ISCHIUM

OBTURATOR

INTERNUS

ISCHIO-RECTAL

FOSSA

GLUTEUS

COCCYX

MAXIMUS

PUDENDAL CANAL

SKIN

191.7   Female Pelvis, on Horizontal Section

(Courtesy of Professor C. H. Sawyer, Department of Anatomy, University of California, at Los Angeles.)

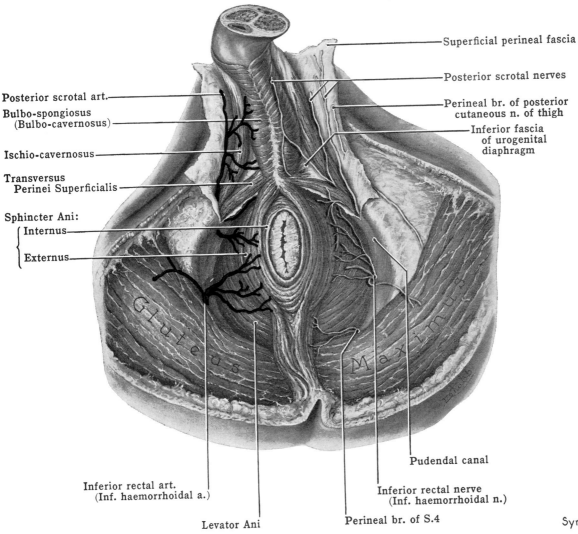

Posterior scrotal art.
Bulbo-spongiosus
(Bulbo-cavernosus)
Ischio-cavernosus
Transversus
   Perinei Superficialis
Sphincter Ani:
   { Internus
   { Externus

Superficial perineal fascia
Posterior scrotal nerves
Perineal br. of posterior
   cutaneous n. of thigh
Inferior fascia
   of urogenital
   diaphragm

Pudendal canal

Inferior rectal art.
(Inf. haemorrhoidal a.)

Levator Ani

Perineal br. of S.4

Inferior rectal nerve
(Inf. haemorrhoidal n.)

192   Male Perineum

Observe in the anal region or triangle:

1. The anal orifice at the center of the anal triangle, surrounded by Sphincter Ani
   Externus, and an ischio-rectal fossa on each side.

2. The superficial fibres of Sphincter Ani Externus anchoring the anus in front to the
   perineal body, or central tendon of the perineum, and behind to the coccyx—here
   to the skin.

3. The ischio-rectal fossa, filled with fat, bounded medially by Levator Ani and Sphincter
   Ani Externus; laterally by Obturator Internus fascia; behind by Gluteus Maximus
   overlying the sacro-tuberous ligament; in front by the base of the perineal membrane.
   (figs. 193 & 193.1). The apex or roof is where the medial and lateral walls meet. The
   base or floor, formed by tough skin and deep fascia, is removed.

4. The inferior rectal nerve leaving the pudendal canal and, with the perineal branch of
   S.4, supplying Sphincter Ani Externus. Its cutaneous twigs to the anus are removed.
   The branch turning round Gluteus Maximus is replacing the perforating cutaneous
   nerve.

Observe in the urogenital region or triangle:

5. The superficial perineal fascia (of Colles) incised in the midline, freed from its attachment to the base of the perineal membrane, and reflected.

6. The cutaneous nerves and artery in the superficial perineal space (pouch).

7. The three paired superficial perineal muscles—Bulbospongiosus, Ischiocavernosus,
   and Transversus Perinei Superficialis.

8. The exposed triangular portion of the perineal membrane or inferior fascia of urogenital diaphragm.

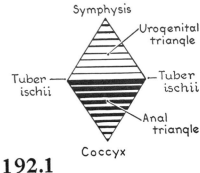

Symphysis
Urogenital
   triangle
Tuber
ischii
Tuber
ischii
Anal
triangle
Coccyx

192.1

Diagram. The 4 angles of the diamo
shaped perineal region, from below.

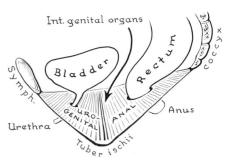

Int. genital organs
Bladder
Rectum
coccyx
Symph.
Anus
Urethra
Tuber ischii

192.2

Diagram. The 2 halves of the diam
face different directions, side view.

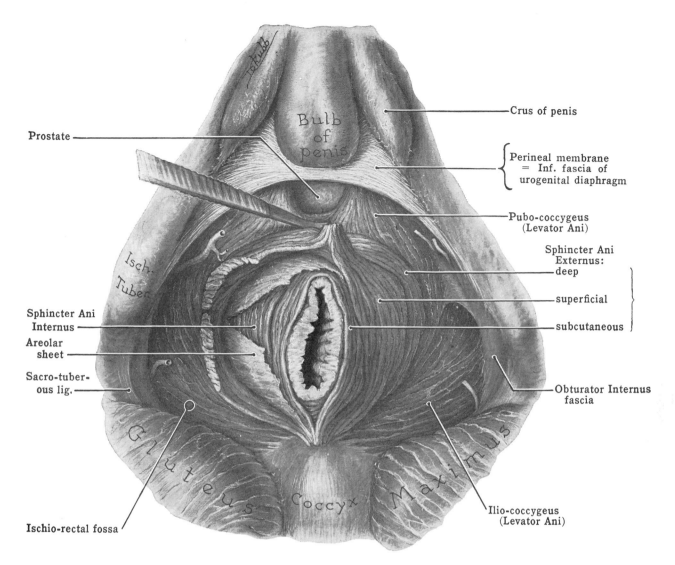

Prostate

Crus of penis

Perineal membrane
= Inf. fascia of
urogenital diaphragm

Pubo-coccygeus
(Levator Ani)

Sphincter Ani
Externus:
deep

superficial

subcutaneous

Isch. Tuber.

Sphincter Ani
Internus

Areolar
sheet

Sacro-tuber-
ous lig.

Obturator Internus
fascia

Ischio-rectal fossa

Ilio-coccygeus
(Levator Ani)

193 Dissection of Sphincter Ani Externus

Observe:

1. The 3 parts of this voluntary sphincter: (a) subcutaneous—encircling the anàl orifice;
   (b) superficial—anchoring the anus in the median plane, to perineal body in front and
   to the coccyx behind (fig. 192); and (c) deep—forming a wide encircling band (fig.
   204).

2. On left of figure: the superficial and deep parts of the sphincter are reflected, and the
   underlying sheet, consisting of areolar tissue, Levator Ani fibres, and outer longitudinal
   muscular coat of the gut, is cut, in order to reveal the inner circular muscular coat of
   the gut, which is thickened to form an involuntary Sphincter Ani Internus. (fig. 196).

3. The anterior free borders of Levatores Ani meeting in front of the anal canal, and
   pressed backwards in order to expose the prostate.

4. On right of figure: the remains of the "false roof" of the ischio-rectal fossa, i.e., a
   layer of fascia that stretches from Obturator Internus fascia to the thin fascia covering
   Levator Ani.

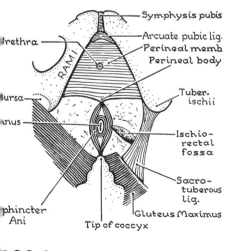

193.1

Diagram. Boundaries of perineal region, also perineal membrane.

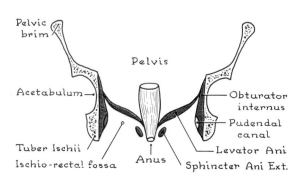

193.2

Diagram. Anal region on coronal section.

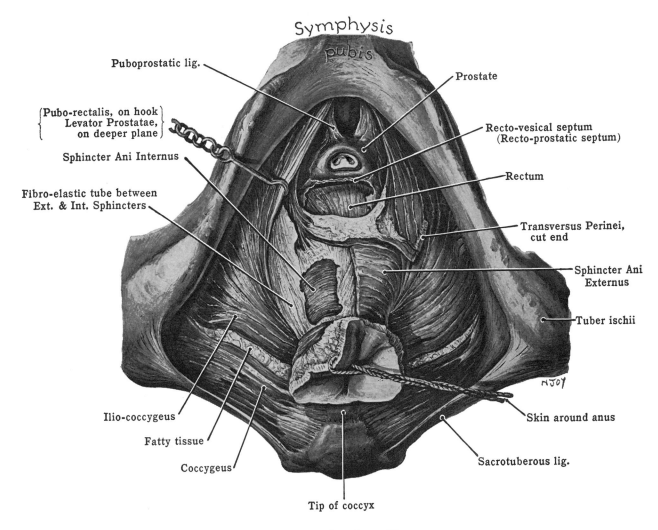

Symphysis pubis

Puboprostatic lig.

{Pubo-rectalis, on hook
Levator Prostatae,
on deeper plane}

Sphincter Ani Internus

Fibro-elastic tube between
Ext. & Int. Sphincters

Prostate

Recto-vesical septum
(Recto-prostatic septum)

Rectum

Transversus Perinei,
cut end

Sphincter Ani
Externus

Tuber ischii

Skin around anus

Ilio-coccygeus

Fatty tissue

Coccygeus

Sacrotuberous lig.

Tip of coccyx

194 Levatores Ani and Coccygei, the Exposure of the Prostate, from perineum.

(Urogenital diaphragm and its fasciae have been removed.)

Observe:

1. The anal canal guarded by two sphincters: Sphincter Ani Internus being a continuation of the circular muscle coat of the gut; it is smooth muscle. Sphincter Ani Externus extending below Sphincter Internus and having three parts; it is skeletal muscle.

2. Puborectalis, the sling-like muscle uniting with Sphincter Externus behind and at the sides. (It is better shown in figures 203 & 204).

3. The anal columns united half way down the Internal Sphincter by semilunar anal valves.

4. The pecten, or smooth zone of simple stratified epithelium, between the anal valves above and the lower border of the Internal Sphincter below. It is transitional between intestinal mucosa above and skin having dermal papillae and appendages below.

5. The longitudinal muscle coat of the rectum and its fascia blending with the Levator Ani and its fasciae to form a fibroelastic tube which descends between the two Sphincters. From this tube septa pass through the Internal Sphincter to the submucous coat, through the External Sphincter to the skin, and, as the anal intermuscular septum, below the Internal Sphincter. (*Wilde, F. R.*)

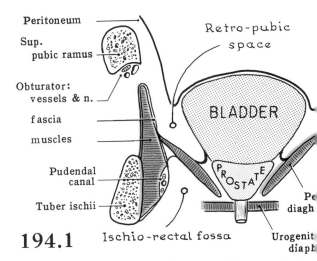

Peritoneum

Sup. pubic ramus

Obturator:
vessels & n.

fascia

muscles

Pudendal canal

Tuber ischii

Retro-pubic space

BLADDER

PROSTATE

Pe
diaph

Urogenit
diaph

194.1   Ischio-rectal fossa

Diagram. Only the pelvic diaphragm (Levator Ani po̶—tion) intervenes between ischio-rectal fossa and ret̶—pubic space,

(*For pelvic aspect of Levatores Ani, see figs. 209 male & 231 female.*)

195 Arteries of the Rectum and Anal Canal, front view

(The Levatores Ani are semidiagrammatic.)

Observe:

1. The branches of the right and left divisions of the superior rectal artery obliquely encircling the rectum, much as the branches of the dorsal arteries of the penis encircle the penis (fig. 199).

2. The middle rectal arteries (branches of the int. iliac arteries) are usually small. In this specimen the right artery is small, but the left one is large and partly replaces the left division of the superior rectal artery.

3. The inferior rectal arteries (branches of the int. pudendal arteries) are largely expended on the anal canal.

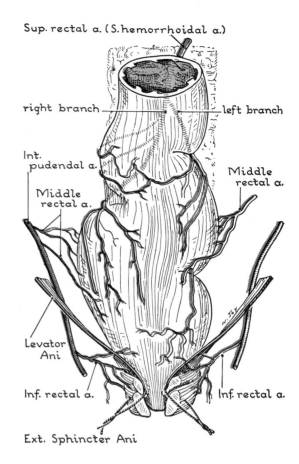

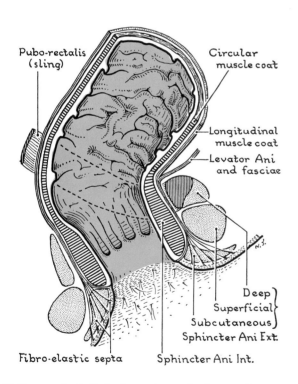

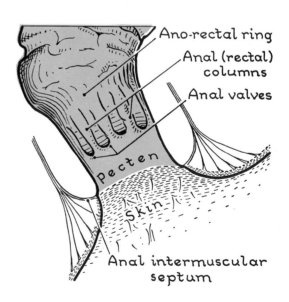

196 and 196.1   Anal Canal, on median section, semidiagrammatic

(*partly after Wilde*)

(See text of fig. 194.)

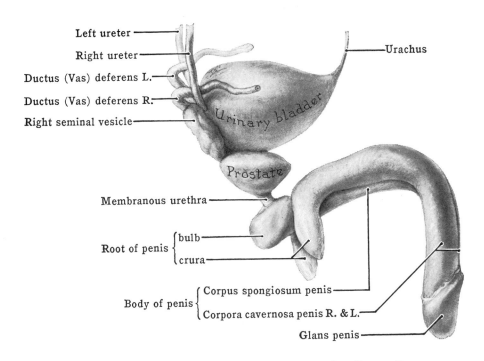

Left ureter

Right ureter

Ductus (Vas) deferens L.

Ductus (Vas) deferens R.

Right seminal vesicle

Urachus

Urinary bladder

Prostate

Membranous urethra

Root of penis { bulb
{ crura

Body of penis { Corpus spongiosum penis
{ Corpora cavernosa penis R. & L.

Glans penis

197 Lower Parts of Male Genital and Urinary Tracts

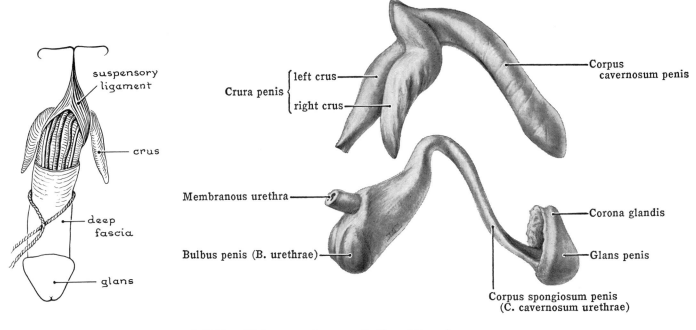

suspensory ligament

crus

deep fascia

glans

Crura penis { left crus
{ right crus

Corpus cavernosum penis

Membranous urethra

Bulbus penis (B. urethrae)

Corona glandis

Glans penis

Corpus spongiosum penis
(C. cavernosum urethrae)

198.1

Diagram. Suspensory ligament of penis. For fundiform ligament of penis, see fig. 110.

198 Dissection of the Penis

The corpus spongiosum is separated from the corpora cavernosa penis. The natural flexures are preserved.

Observe:

1. The corpora cavernosa penis bent where that organ is slung by the suspensory ligament of the penis, and grooved by encircling vessels.

2. The corpus spongiosum penis massed (a) below the urethra posteriorly to form the bulb of the penis, and (b) above the urethra anteriorly to form the glans which fits like a cap on the blunt ends of the corpora cavernosa penis.

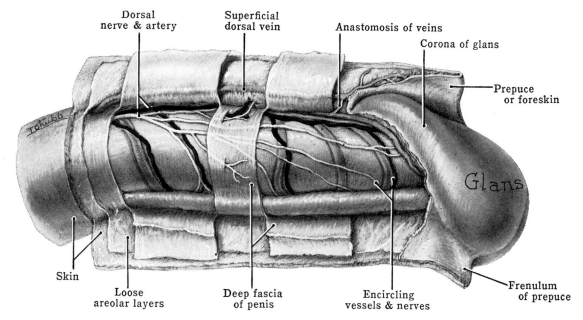

Dorsal nerve & artery

Superficial dorsal vein

Anastomosis of veins

Corona of glans

Prepuce or foreskin

Glans

Skin

Loose areolar layers

Deep fascia of penis

Encircling vessels & nerves

Frenulum of prepuce

199 Penis, side view

The three tubular envelopes of the penis are reflected, so also is the prepuce.

Observe:

1. The skin carried forward as the prepuce.
2. The loose, laminated, subcutaneous, areolar tissue (Dartos and Colles' fascia), called the superficial fascia of the penis, carried forward into the prepuce, and containing the superficial dorsal vein. This vein begins in the prepuce, anastomoses with the deep dorsal vein from the glans, and ends in the superficial inguinal veins.
3. The deep fascia penis (Buck's fascia). It ends at the glans penis.
4. Large encircling tributaries of the deep dorsal vein; thread-like companion arteries; numerous oblique nerves.
5. The vessels and nerves at the neck plunging into the glans penis.

199.1 Interior of the Spongy (Penile) Urethra

A longitudinal incision was made on the urethral surface of the penis and carried through the floor of the urethra; so, the view is of the dorsal surface of the interior of the urethra. The prepuce is retracted.

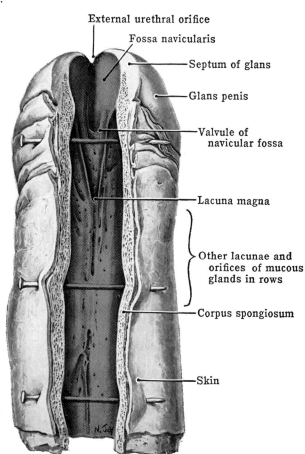

External urethral orifice

Fossa navicularis

Septum of glans

Glans penis

Valvule of navicular fossa

Lacuna magna

Other lacunae and orifices of mucous glands in rows

Corpus spongiosum

Skin

200 Section across the Root of the Penis

Observe that the urethra is dilated within the bulb of the penis.

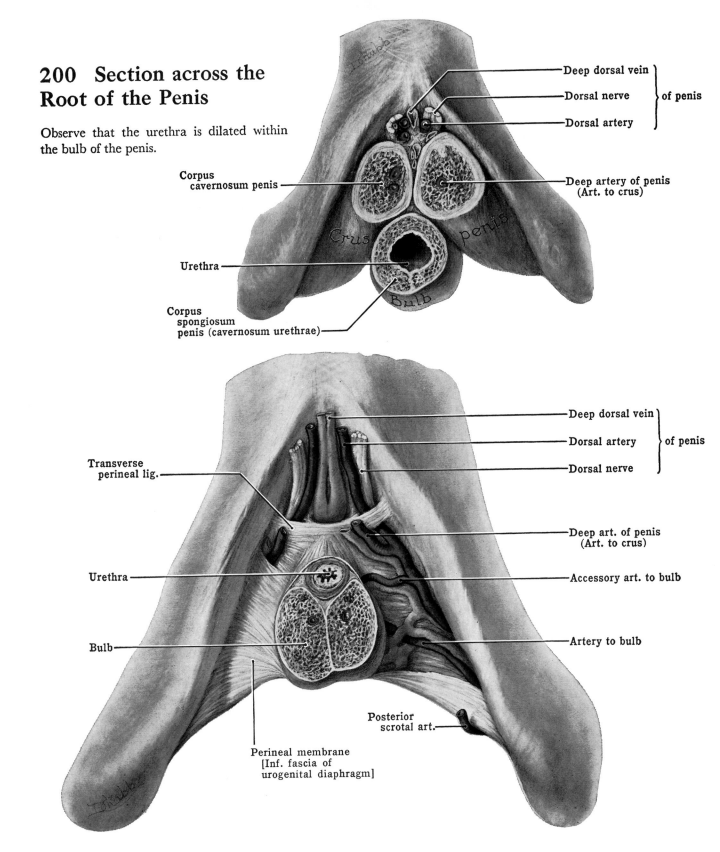

Deep dorsal vein ⎫
Dorsal nerve ⎬ of penis
Dorsal artery ⎭

Corpus cavernosum penis

Deep artery of penis (Art. to crus)

Urethra

Corpus spongiosum penis (cavernosum urethrae)

Deep dorsal vein ⎫
Dorsal artery ⎬ of penis
Dorsal nerve ⎭

Transverse perineal lig.

Deep art. of penis (Art. to crus)

Urethra

Accessory art. to bulb

Bulb

Artery to bulb

Posterior scrotal art.

Perineal membrane [Inf. fascia of urogenital diaphragm]

201 Deep Perineal Space

Enclosed by the two layers of the urogenital diaphragm.

The crura are removed and the bulb is cut shorter than in figure 200 and viewed more from below.

On right of page, the perineal membrane is in part removed and the deep perineal space is thereby opened.

Observe:

1. The fibres of the perineal membrane converging on the bulb and mooring it to the pubic arch.
2. The urethra, still membranous and bound to the dorsum of the bulb.
3. The septum in the bulb indicating its bilateral origin.
4. The artery to the bulb (here double); the artery to the crus, called the deep artery; and the dorsal artery which ends in the glans penis. The deep dorsal vein, originally double, which ends in the prostatic plexus.

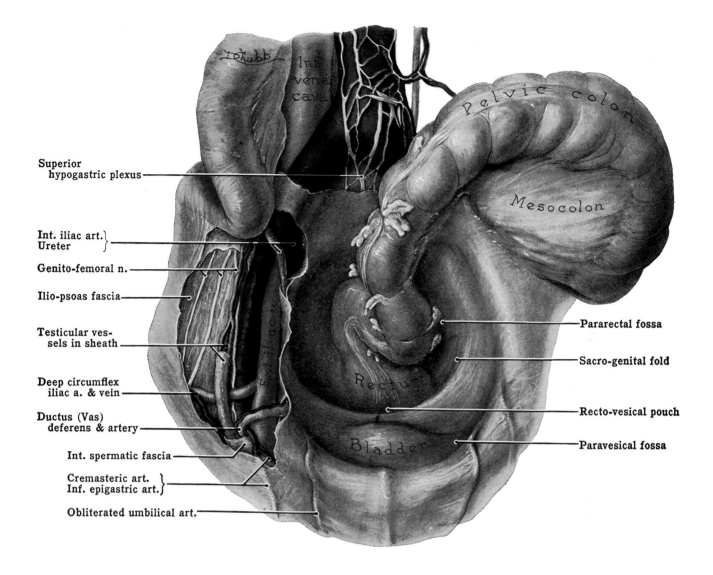

Superior hypogastric plexus——

Int. iliac art.⎫
Ureter   ⎬——

Genito-femoral n.——

Ilio-psoas fascia——

Testicular vessels in sheath——

Deep circumflex iliac a. & vein——

Ductus (Vas) deferens & artery——

Int. spermatic fascia——

Cremasteric art.⎫
Inf. epigastric art.⎭——

Obliterated umbilical art.——

——Pararectal fossa

——Sacro-genital fold

——Recto-vesical pouch

——Paravesical fossa

Labels within image: Inf. vena cava, Pelvic colon, Mesocolon, Rectum, Bladder

202 Male Pelvis and Surroundings, antero-superior view

Observe:

1. One limb of the inverted V-shaped root of the sigmoid (pelvic) mesocolon ascending near the external iliac vessels; the other descending to the third piece of the sacrum. At the apex is the mouth of the intersigmoid recess, and behind the mouth lies the left ureter.

2. The teniae coli forming two wide bands; one in front of the rectum, the other behind.

3. The crescentic fold of peritoneum called the sacro-genital fold.

4. The superior hypogastric plexus (presacral nerve) lying in the fork of the aorta and in front of the left common iliac vein.

5. The ureter adhering to the peritoneum, crossing the external iliac vessels, and descending in front of the internal iliac artery. The ductus deferens and its artery also adhering to peritoneum, crossing the external iliac vessels, and then hooking round the inferior epigastric artery to join the other constituents of the spermatic cord.

6. The genito-femoral nerve on the Psoas fascia. Its two lateral (femoral) branches become cutaneous; its medial (genital) branch supplies Cremaster and becomes cutaneous.

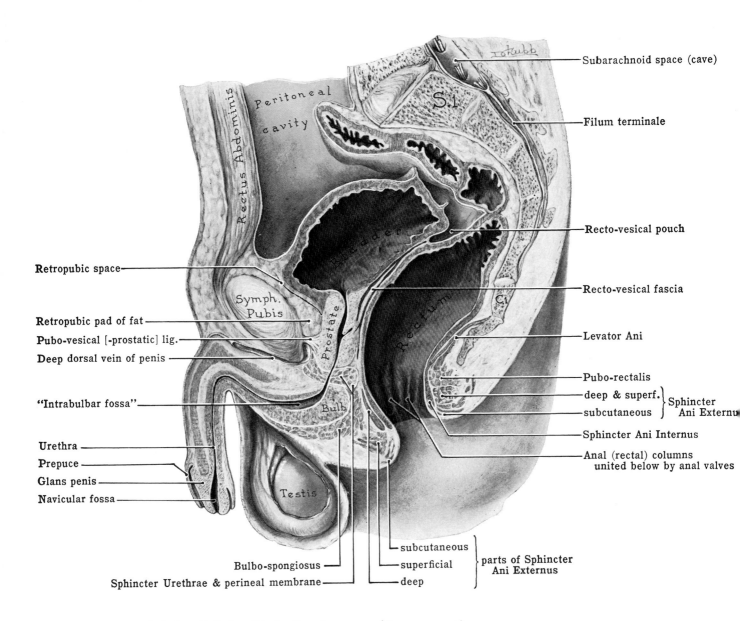

Subarachnoid space (cave)

Filum terminale

Peritoneal cavity

Rectus Abdominis

S.1

Recto-vesical pouch

Retropubic space

Recto-vesical fascia

Symph. Pubis

Bladder

Prostate

Rectum

C.1

Retropubic pad of fat

Pubo-vesical [-prostatic] lig.

Deep dorsal vein of penis

Levator Ani

Pubo-rectalis

deep & superf. } Sphincter Ani Externus
subcutaneous }

"Intrabulbar fossa"

Bulb

Sphincter Ani Internus

Urethra

Prepuce

Glans penis

Navicular fossa

Anal (rectal) columns
united below by anal valves

Testis

Bulbo-spongiosus

Sphincter Urethrae & perineal membrane

subcutaneous
superficial
deep

} parts of Sphincter
Ani Externus

203 Male Pelvis, in median section

Observe:

1. The urinary bladder slightly distended and resting on the rectum; the prostatic urethra descending vertically through a somewhat elongated prostate and showing the prostatic utricle opening on to its posterior wall; the short membranous urethra passing through the deep perineal space; the spongy urethra with a low lying dilatation in the bulb and another in the glans; and the Bulbo-spongiosus which by contracting empties the urethra.

2. The involuntary Sphincter Ani Internus not descending so far as the voluntary Sphincter Ani Externus, and separated from it by an areolar layer.

3. The two layers of recto-vesical fascia in the median plane between bladder and rectum. On each side it contains the deferent duct, seminal vesicle, and vesical vessels (figs. 204, 205).

4. The peritoneum passing from the abdominal wall above the symphysis to the distended bladder, over the bladder to the bottom of the recto-vesical pouch, and up the anterior aspect of the rectum.

5. The tunica vaginalis (not labelled), opened in order to expose the testis, which here happens to be rotated so that the epididymis is to the front.

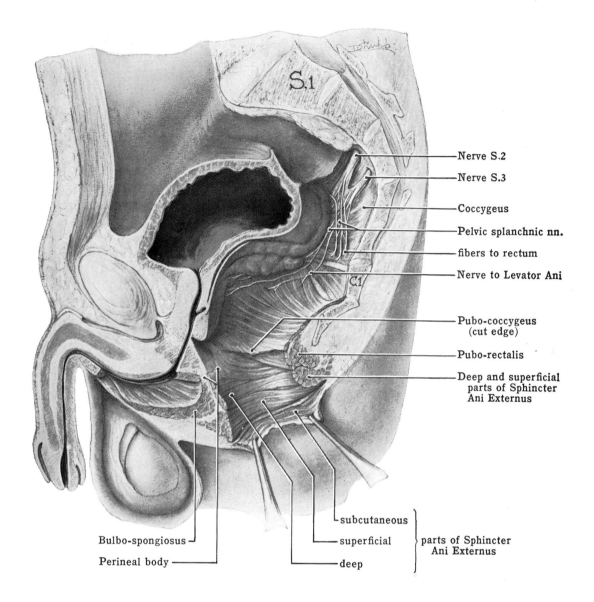

Nerve S.2
Nerve S.3
Coccygeus
Pelvic splanchnic nn.
fibers to rectum
Nerve to Levator Ani
Pubo-coccygeus (cut edge)
Pubo-rectalis
Deep and superficial parts of Sphincter Ani Externus

Bulbo-spongiosus
Perineal body

subcutaneous
superficial
deep
} parts of Sphincter Ani Externus

204 Sphincter Ani Externus and Levator Ani

This is figure 203 from which the rectum, anal canal, and bulb of the penis are removed.

Observe:

1. The subcutaneous fibres of Sphincter Ani Externus held reflected with forceps; the superficial fibres mingling posteriorly with deep fibres; and deep fibres mingling posteriorly with Pubo-rectalis (inferior fibres of Pubo-coccygeus) which forms a sling that occupies the angle between the rectum and the anal canal (fig. 194).

2. Pubo-coccygeus divided to allow of the removal of the anal canal to which it is in part attached (fig. 209).

3. The ampulla of the deferent duct and seminal vesicle curving to fit the cylindrical rectum.

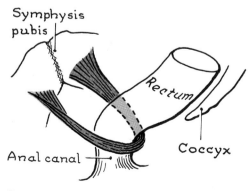

Symphysis pubis

Rectum

Anal canal

Coccyx

204.1

Diagram. Pubo-rectalis (puborectal sling)

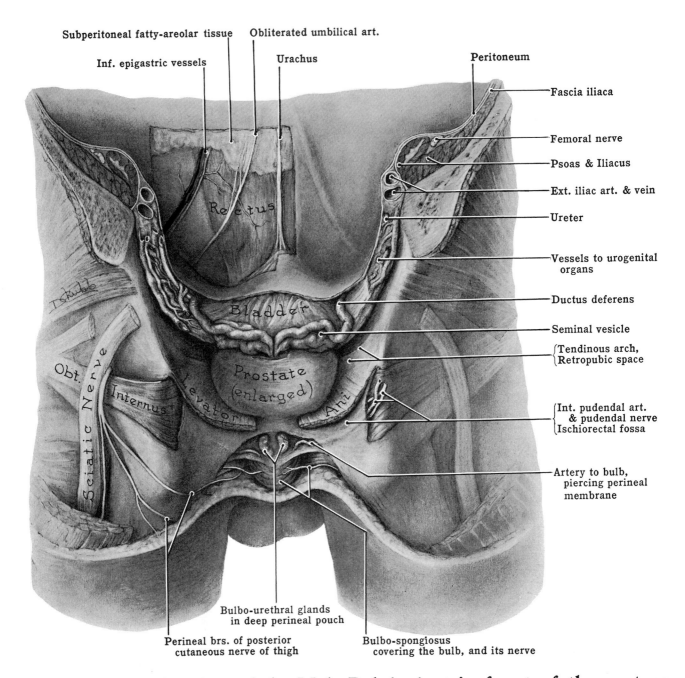

Subperitoneal fatty-areolar tissue

Obliterated umbilical art.

Inf. epigastric vessels

Urachus

Peritoneum

Fascia iliaca

Femoral nerve

Psoas & Iliacus

Ext. iliac art. & vein

Ureter

Vessels to urogenital organs

Ductus deferens

Seminal vesicle

Tendinous arch, Retropubic space

Int. pudendal art. & pudendal nerve Ischiorectal fossa

Artery to bulb, piercing perineal membrane

Rectus

Bladder

Prostate (enlarged)

Obt. Nerve

Internus

Levator Ani

Sciatic Nerve

Ischium

Bulbo-urethral glands in deep perineal pouch

Perineal brs. of posterior cutaneous nerve of thigh

Bulbo-spongiosus covering the bulb, and its nerve

205 Coronal Section of the Male Pelvis, just in front of the rectum. View of the anterior portion from behind

Observe:

1. The inferior epigastric artery and venae comitantes entering the Rectus sheath, whilst the obliterated umbilical artery and the urachus, like the bladder, remain subperitoneal. *Terminology.* The peritoneal folds having these 3 structures in their free edges are called:—lateral, medial, and median umbilical folds.

2. The femoral nerve lying between Psoas and Iliacus outside the Psoas fascia, which is attached to the pelvic brim, whilst the external iliac art. and vein lie inside.

3. The ductus deferens and ureter, both subperitoneal. Near the bladder, the ureter accompanying a leash of vesical vessels enclosed in recto-vesical fascia.

4. Levator Ani and its fascial coverings separating the retro-pubic (prevesical) space from the ischio-rectal fossa.

5. The free, anterior borders of Levatores Ani. They are the width of the handle of a scalpel apart.

6. The bulbo-urethral glands (Cowper's) and the artery to the bulb lying above the perineal membrane [inf. fascia of the urogenital diaphragm], i.e. in the deep perineal space.

7. Obturator Internus making a right-angled turn as it escapes from its osseo-fascial pocket (fig. 281).

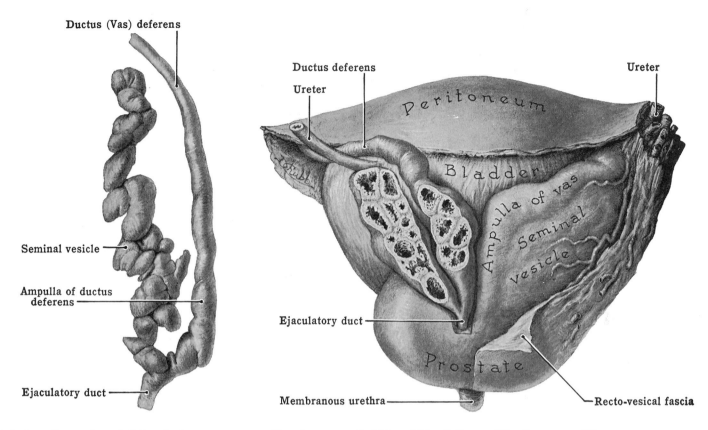

Ductus (Vas) deferens

Seminal vesicle

Ampulla of ductus
deferens

Ejaculatory duct

Ductus deferens

Ureter

Peritoneum

Bladder

Ampulla of vas

Seminal
vesicle

Ureter

Ejaculatory duct

Prostate

Membranous urethra

Recto-vesical fascia

206   Seminal Vesicle, unravelled

The vesicle is a tortuous tube with numerous outpouchings. The lower end of the ampulla of the ductus
deferens has similar outpouchings.

207   Bladder, Deferent Ducts, Seminal Vesicles, and Prostate, from behind

The left vesicle and ampulla are dissected free and
sliced open. (For X-section, see fig. 191.6 A.)

207.1   Prostate, dissected from behind.

(Courtesy of G. F. Lewis)

Observe:

1. The right and the left ejaculatory
   duct, each formed where the duct
   of a seminal vesicle joins the
   ampullary end of a deferent duct.

2. The prostatic utricle (uterus masculinus), lying in between the ends
   of the two ejaculatory ducts, and
   all three flattened from side to
   side. All three opened into the
   prostatic urethra (fig. 208).

3. The prostatic ductules, in all
   about 63 in number and mostly
   opening on to the prostatic sinus
   (fig. 208, Lowsley).

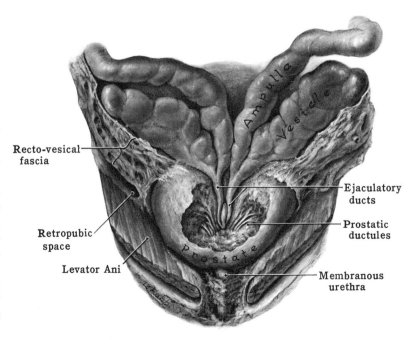

Recto-vesical
fascia

Retropubic
space

Levator Ani

Ampulla

Vesicle

Ejaculatory
ducts

Prostatic
ductules

Prostate

Membranous
urethra

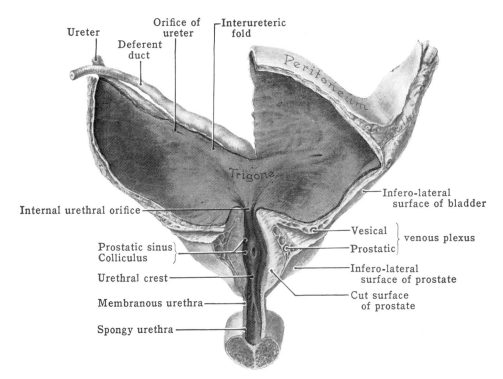

208 Interior of the Male Urinary Bladder and Prostatic Urethra

The anterior parts of the bladder, prostate and urethra were cut away. The knife was then carried through the posterior wall of the bladder, at the upper border of the right ureter and interureteric fold, which unites the two ureters along the upper limit of the smooth trigone.

Observe:

1. The right ureter not joining the bladder wall but traversing it obliquely as far as its slitlike orifice, which is situated 1″ to 1½″ from the left orifice.

2. The mucous membrane, smooth over the trigone, but rugose elsewhere—especially when the bladder is empty.

3. The slight fulness behind the internal urethral orifice, which, when exaggerated, becomes the uvula vesicae.

4. The mouth of the prostatic utricle (not labelled) at the summit of the colliculus, on the urethral crest, and the orifice of an ejaculatory duct on each side of the utricle.

5. The urethral crest extending rather higher than usual and bifurcating rather lower than usual.

6. The prostatic fascia enclosing a venous plexus.

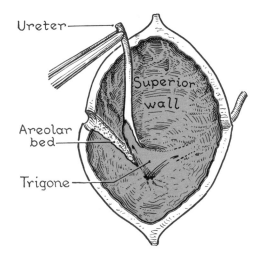

208.1

Sketch of the ureter being raised from its areolar bed as it passes obliquely through the muscular coat of the bladder to blend with the trigonal muscle.

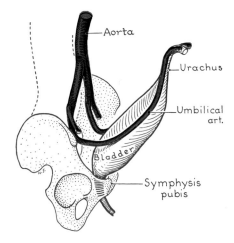

208.2

At birth the bladder is abdominal in position and fusiform in shape and the two umbilical arteries lie along its sides.

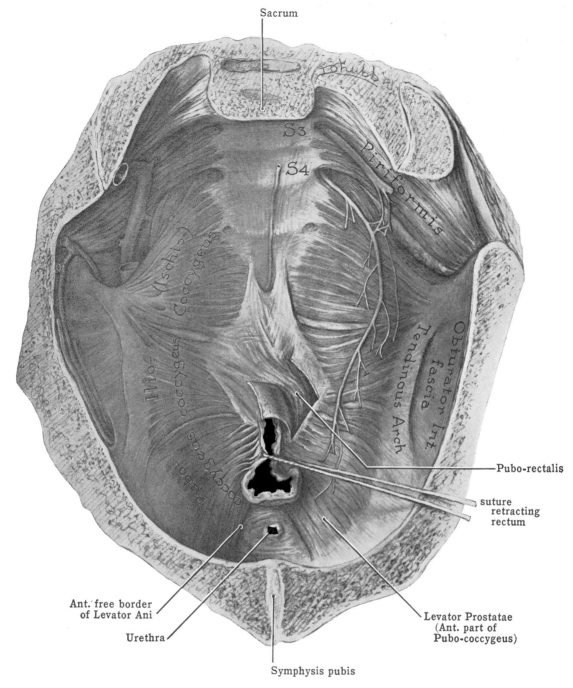

Sacrum

S3

S4

Piriformis

(Ischio-)Coccygeus

Ilio-coccygeus

Pubo-coccygeus

Obturator Int. fascia

Tendinous Arch

Pubo-rectalis

suture retracting rectum

Ant. free border of Levator Ani

Urethra

Levator Prostatae (Ant. part of Pubo-coccygeus)

Symphysis pubis

209 Levatores Ani and Coccygei, male, from above

The pelvic viscera are removed and the bony pelvis is sawn through transversely.

Observe:

1. Pubo-coccygeus arising mainly from the pubic bone, Ischio-coccygeus from the ischial spine, and Ilio-coccygeus from the tendinous arch in between. Pubo-coccygeus is strong (fig. 216); Ilio-coccygeus is weak; Ischio-coccygeus is largely transformed into the sacrospinous ligament (fig. 217). Pubo- and Ilio-coccygei together constitute Levator Ani.
2. The anterior free border of Pubo-coccygeus; the posterior free border of Ischio-coccygeus; the clefts at the borders of Ilio-coccygeus closed by areolar membranes.
3. The urethra passing between the anterior borders of Pubo-coccygei. The rectum perforating Pubo-coccygeus, thus: (a) the anterior fibres of the muscles of opposite sides meet and unite in the central tendon of the perineum (perineal body) in front of the rectum; (b) the posterior fibres unite behind the rectum in an aponeurosis that extends backwards to the anterior sacro-coccygeal ligament; (c) the middle fibres blend with the outer wall of the anal canal and pass between Internal and External Sphincters of the anus (fig. 194); (d) on the right hand, this aponeurosis is reflected to show Pubo-rectalis; (fig. 204).

4. Branches of S.3 & 4 supplying Levator Ani and Coccygeus. (The pudendal nerve, via its perineal branch, fig. 215, also supplies Levator Ani.)

(For perineal aspect of Levatores Ani see figure 194.)

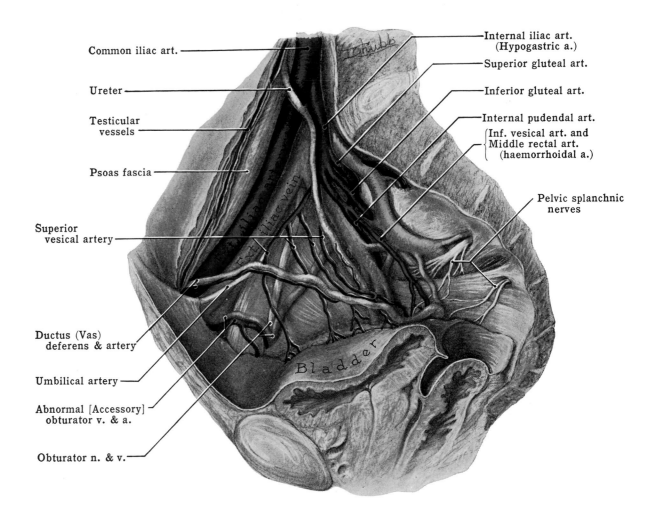

Common iliac art. —

Ureter —

Testicular
vessels —

Psoas fascia —

Superior
vesical artery —

Ductus (Vas)
deferens & artery —

Umbilical artery —

Abnormal [Accessory]
obturator v. & a. —

Obturator n. & v. —

Internal iliac art.
(Hypogastric a.)

Superior gluteal art.

Inferior gluteal art.

Internal pudendal art.

Inf. vesical art. and
Middle rectal art.
(haemorrhoidal a.)

Pelvic splanchnic
nerves

Bladder

210   Side Wall of the Male Pelvis

Observe:

1. The ureter and ductus deferens running a strictly subperitoneal course across the external iliac vessels, umbilical artery, obturator nerve and vessels, and each receiving a branch from a vesical artery.

    The ureter crosses ext. iliac art. at its origin (at common iliac bifurcation); the ductus crosses it at its termination (at the deep inguinal ring). (Also fig. 179)

2. The umbilical artery, obliterated beyond the origin of the last superior vesical artery and creating a peritoneal fold.

3. The obturator artery here springing from the inferior epigastric artery, i.e., the artery is "abnormal". There are here both a normal and an "abnormal" obturator vein.

4. The veins forming an open network through which the arteries are threaded.

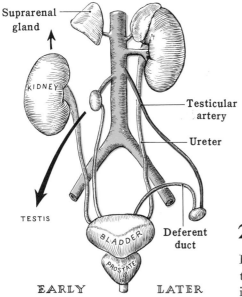

Suprarenal
gland

KIDNEY

Testicular
artery

Ureter

TESTIS

BLADDER

PROSTATE

Deferent
duct

EARLY   LATER

210.1

Diagram of the 3 paired glands. Explaining how the ureter comes to be crossed by testicular vessels in the abdomen and deferent duct in the pelvis

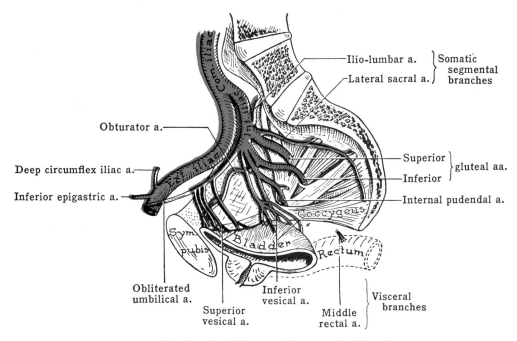

Ilio-lumbar a. } Somatic segmental branches
Lateral sacral a. }

Obturator a.

Deep circumflex iliac a.

Inferior epigastric a.

Superior } gluteal aa.
Inferior }

Internal pudendal a.

Obliterated umbilical a.

Superior vesical a.

Inferior vesical a.

Middle rectal a. } Visceral branches

211 Iliac Arteries and their Branches, side view

Observe:

1. The common iliac artery having two terminal branches, but no collateral branches.
2. The external iliac artery having two collateral branches, and ending as the femoral artery.
3. The internal iliac (hypogastric) artery ending as an anterior and a posterior division. From these, branches arise variably. Commonly, as here, the ilio-lumbar a., lateral sacral a., and superior gluteal a. spring from the posterior division; the others spring from the anterior division.
4. Of the 10 branches of the internal iliac artery, the obliterated umbilical, which in the fetus passed to the placenta, and 3 others are visceral; 2 supply the 5th lumbar and the sacral segments and are somatic segmental; 3 enter the gluteal region; and one passes to the front of the thigh.

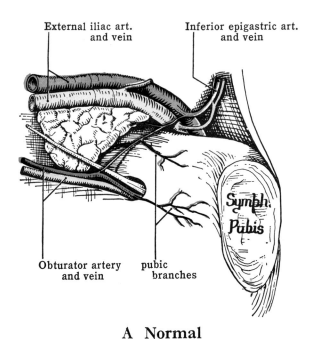

External iliac art. and vein

Inferior epigastric art. and vein

Obturator artery and vein

pubic branches

Symph. Pubis

A Normal

Inferior epigastric art.

External iliac art. and vein

pubic branch

Symph. pubis

pubic branch

Obturator art. and vein

B Abnormal [Accessory]

212 Normal and Abnormal [Accessory] Obturator Arteries

A. The pubic branch of the obturator artery anastomoses behind the body of the pubis with the pubic branch of the inferior epigastric artery.
B. The obturator artery sprang from the internal iliac artery in 70.0% of 283 limbs; from the inferior epigastric via the pubic anastomoses in 25.4%; and nearly equally from both internal iliac and inferior epigastric in 4.6%. (*J.C.B.G.*)

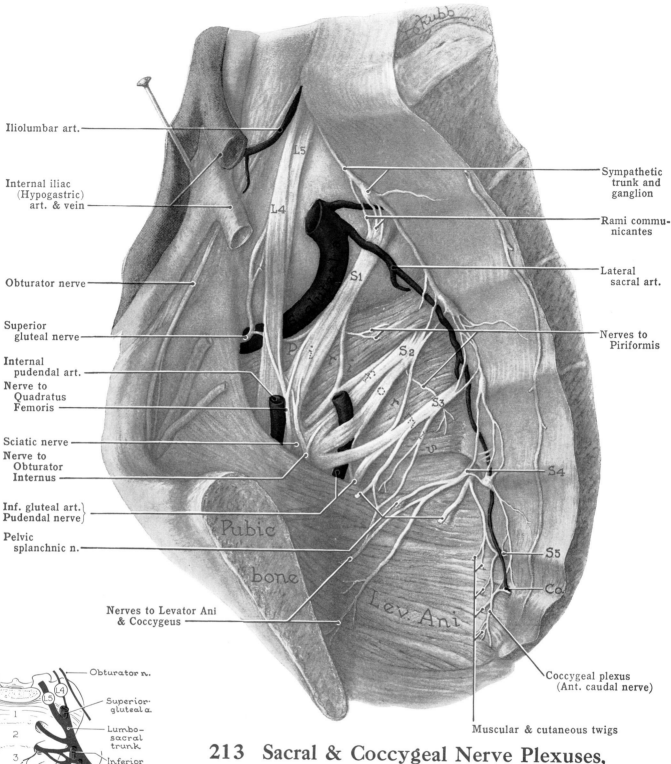

Iliolumbar art.

Internal iliac (Hypogastric) art. & vein

Obturator nerve

Superior gluteal nerve

Internal pudendal art.

Nerve to Quadratus Femoris

Sciatic nerve

Nerve to Obturator Internus

Inf. gluteal art. } Pudendal nerve }

Pelvic splanchnic n.

Nerves to Levator Ani & Coccygeus

Sympathetic trunk and ganglion

Rami communicantes

Lateral sacral art.

Nerves to Piriformis

Coccygeal plexus (Ant. caudal nerve)

Muscular & cutaneous twigs

L5

L4

S1

S2

S3

S4

S5

Co.

Pubic bone

Lev. Ani

Obturator n.

Superior gluteal a.

Lumbo-sacral trunk

Inferior gluteal a.

Int. pudendal n. and a.
Anterior caudal n.

Pelvic splanchnic n.

213.1

Diagram. The sacral plexus is pierced by the sup. and inf. gluteal arteries which turn dorsally; whereas the pudendal artery, continues downward and forward towards the ischial spine.

213 Sacral & Coccygeal Nerve Plexuses,

Observe:

1. Either the sympathetic trunk or its ganglia sending gray rami communicantes to each sacral nerve and the coccygeal nerve.

2. The branch from L.4 joining L.5 to form the lumbo-sacral trunk.

3. The roots of S.1, 2 supplying Piriformis; S.3, 4 supplying Coccygeus and Levator Ani; S.(2), 3, 4 each contributing a branch to the formation of the pelvic splanchnic nerve.

4. The sciatic nerve springing from segments L.4, 5, S.1, 2, 3; the pudendal nerve from S.2, 3, (4); the coccygeal plexus from S.4, 5, Co.

5. The ilio-lumbar artery accompanying nerve L.5; the branches of the lateral sacral artery accompanying the sacral nerves; the superior gluteal artery passing backwards between L.5 and S.1—its position is not constant.

214 Diagram of the Nerve Supply to the Bladder and Urethra

(Broken lines indicate afferent fibres.)

Parasympathetic: The pelvic splanchnic nerves (nervi erigentes; S.2, 3, 4) are the motor nerves to the bladder; when they are stimulated the bladder empties, the blood vessels dilate, and the penis becomes erect. They are also the sensory nerves of the bladder.

Sympathetic, through the superior hypogastric plexus (presacral nerve; Th. lower, L. 1, 2, 3) is motor to a continuous muscle sheet comprising the ureteric musculature, the trigonal muscle, and the muscle of the urethral crest. It also supplies the muscle of the epididymis, ductus deferens, seminal vesicle, and prostate. When the plexus is stimulated, the seminal fluid is ejaculated into the urethra but is hindered from entering the bladder perhaps by the muscle sheet which is drawn towards the internal urethral orifice. The sympathetic is also vaso-constrictor and to some slight extent it is sensory to the trigonal region.

The pudendal nerve is motor to the sphincter urethrae and sensory to the glans penis and the urethra.

It would seem that the sympathetic supply to the bladder has a vaso-constrictor and a sexual effect and that as regards micturition it is not antagonistic to the parasympathetic supply. (Learmonth; Langworthy; and Mitchell.)

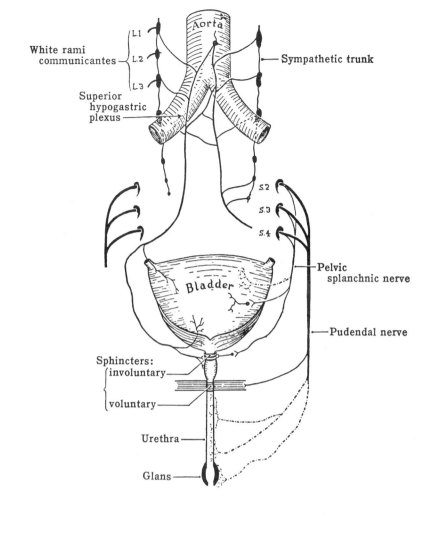

215 Diagram of the Pudendal Nerve

Note:

(1) the 5 regions in which it runs, and

(2) the 3 divisions into which it divides.

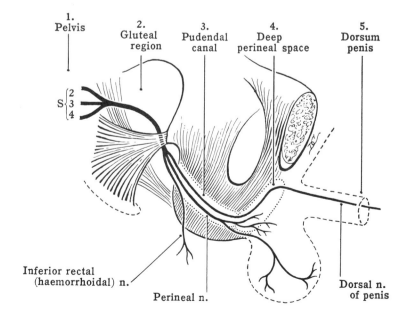

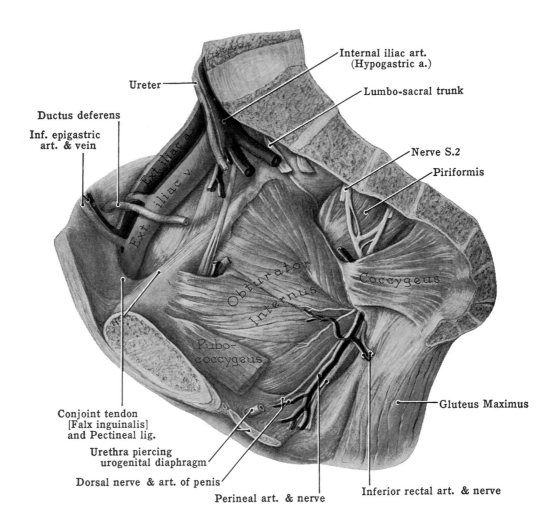

Internal iliac art.
(Hypogastric a.)

Ureter

Lumbo-sacral trunk

Ductus deferens

Inf. epigastric
art. & vein

Nerve S.2

Piriformis

Ext. iliac a.

Ext. iliac v.

Obturator Internus

Coccygeus

Pubo-coccygeus

Gluteus Maximus

Conjoint tendon
[Falx inguinalis]
and Pectineal lig.

Urethra piercing
urogenital diaphragm

Dorsal nerve & art. of penis

Perineal art. & nerve

Inferior rectal art. & nerve

216 Muscles of the Pelvis Minor (male specimen)

Observe:

1. Obturator Internus padding the side wall of the pelvis and escaping through the lesser sciatic foramen; its nerve is seen. Piriformis padding the posterior wall and escaping through the greater sciatic foramen. Coccygeus concealing the sacro-spinous lig. Pubococcygeus, which is the chief and strongest part of Levator Ani, springing from the body of the pubis.

2. The obturator nerve, artery and vein escaping through the obturator foramen. The internal pudendal artery and the pudendal nerve making an exit through the greater foramen, and a re-entry through the lesser foramen, and taking a forward course (in the pudendal canal) within the Obturator Internus fascia to the urogenital diaphragm.

3. In the pelvis major, the deferent duct and the ureter descending across the external iliac artery and vein, the Psoas fascia, and the pelvic brim to enter the pelvis minor or true pelvis.

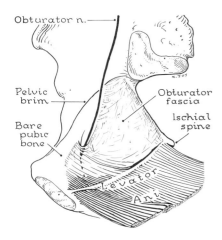

Obturator n.

Pelvic
brim

Bare
pubic
bone

Obturator
fascia

Ischial
spine

Levator Ani

216.1

Diagram. Origin of Levator Ani: from body of pubis, ischial spine and the tendinous arch in between, compare fig. 209.

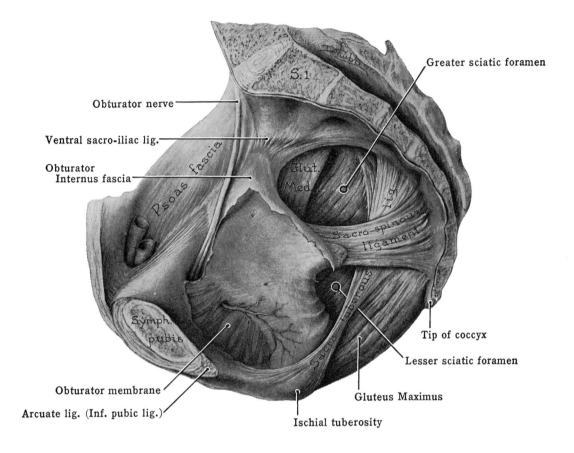

Obturator nerve

Ventral sacro-iliac lig.

Obturator
Internus fascia

Greater sciatic foramen

Psoas fascia

Glut. Med.

S.1

Sacro-spinous ligament

Sacro-tuberous lig.

Symph. pubis

Obturator membrane

Arcuate lig. (Inf. pubic lig.)

Ischial tuberosity

Gluteus Maximus

Lesser sciatic foramen

Tip of coccyx

217 Bony and Ligamentous Walls of the Pelvis Minor (female specimen)

In front is the pubis; behind are the sacrum and coccyx. Postero-laterally, the coccyx and lower part of the sacrum are fastened to the ischial tuberosity by the sacro-tuberous lig. and to the ischial spine by the sacro-spinous lig., whilst the upper part of the sacrum is joined to the ilium by the ventral sacro-iliac lig. Anterior to the sacro-tuberous lig. are the greater and lesser sciatic foramina, the one being above, and the other below, the sacro-spinous lig.

Antero-laterally, the fascia covering Obturator Internus is snipped away and Obturator Internus removed from its osseo-fascial pocket, thereby exposing the ischium and obturator membrane. The mouth of this pocket is the lesser sciatic foramen. Through it Obturator Internus escapes from the pelvis, and the grooves made by its tendon are conspicuous.

Obturator Internus fascia is attached along the line of the obturator nerve above; to the sacro-tuberous lig. below; and to the posterior border of the body of the ischium behind.

(For interosseous lig. see fig. 223.1, dorsal ligs. fig. 273, and ilio-lumbar lig. fig. 190.)

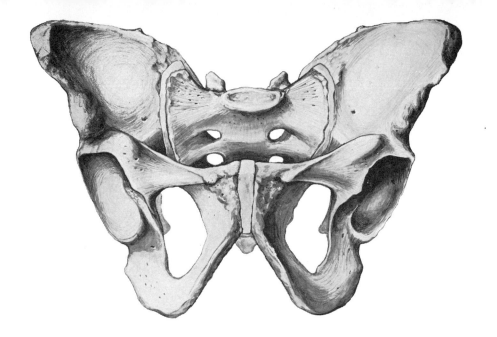

218 Male Pelvis, from the front

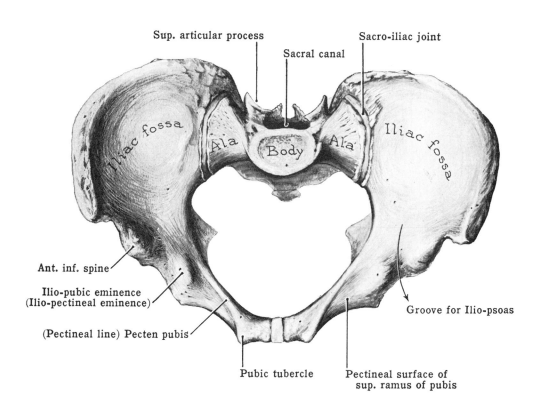

Sup. articular process

Sacral canal

Sacro-iliac joint

Iliac fossa

Ala

Body

Ala

Iliac fossa

Ant. inf. spine

Ilio-pubic eminence
(Ilio-pectineal eminence)

(Pectineal line) Pecten pubis

Groove for Ilio-psoas

Pubic tubercle

Pectineal surface of
sup. ramus of pubis

219 Male Pelvis, from above

The iliac fossae and the alae (of the base) of the sacrum constitute the false or greater pelvis. The groove between the anterior inferior iliac spine and the ilio-pubic eminence conducts Ilio-psoas from the false pelvis to the thigh. The pectineal (anterior) surface of the superior ramus of the pubis is part of the thigh. It gives **origin** to Pectineus and is limited behind by the pecten pubis.

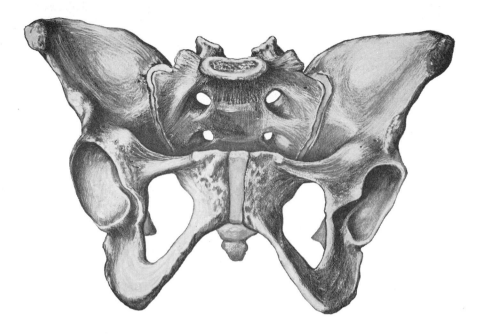

220   Female Pelvis, from the front

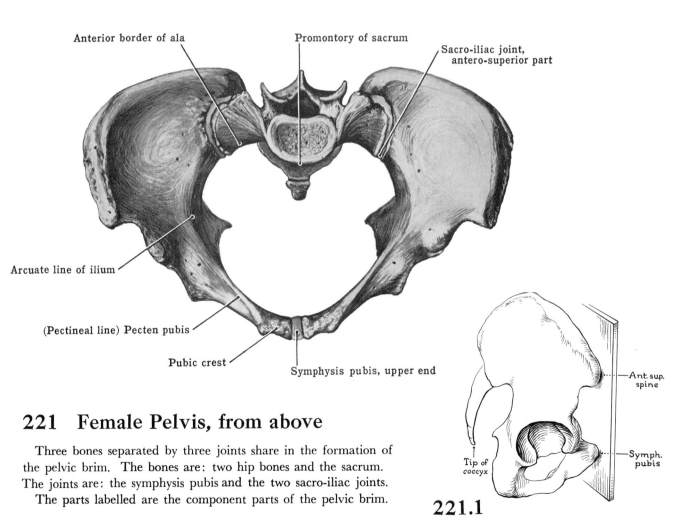

Anterior border of ala

Promontory of sacrum

Sacro-iliac joint,
antero-superior part

Arcuate line of ilium

(Pectineal line) Pecten pubis

Pubic crest

Symphysis pubis, upper end

221   Female Pelvis, from above

Three bones separated by three joints share in the formation of
the pelvic brim. The bones are: two hip bones and the sacrum.
The joints are: the symphysis pubis and the two sacro-iliac joints.
The parts labelled are the component parts of the pelvic brim.

Ant. sup.
spine

Symph.
pubis

Tip of
coccyx

221.1

Diagram. Orientation of pelvis. The ant.
sup. spines and the upper end of the
symphysis pubis lie in a vertical plane,
as though against a window or wall. The
tip of the coccyx is on a level with the
upper half of the body of the pubis.

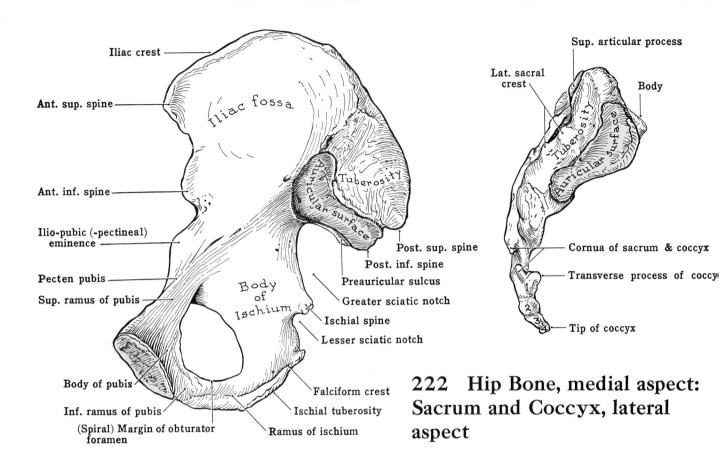

Iliac crest

Ant. sup. spine

Iliac fossa

Ant. inf. spine

Ilio-pubic (-pectineal) eminence

Pecten pubis

Sup. ramus of pubis

Tuberosity

Auricular surface

Post. sup. spine

Post. inf. spine

Preauricular sulcus

Greater sciatic notch

Ischial spine

Lesser sciatic notch

Body of Ischium

Body of pubis

Inf. ramus of pubis

(Spiral) Margin of obturator foramen

Falciform crest

Ischial tuberosity

Ramus of ischium

Sup. articular process

Lat. sacral crest

Body

Tuberosity

Auricular surface

Cornua of sacrum & coccyx

Transverse process of coccyx

Tip of coccyx

222   Hip Bone, medial aspect: Sacrum and Coccyx, lateral aspect

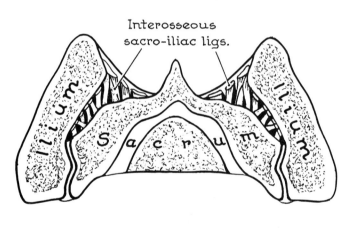

Interosseous sacro-iliac ligs.

Ilium

Ilium

Sacrum

223   Sacro-iliac Joint, transverse section

(*For dorsal sacro-iliac ligs. see fig. 273, sacro-tuberous and sacro-spinous ligs. figs. 217 & 273, and ilio-lumbar lig. fig. 190.*)

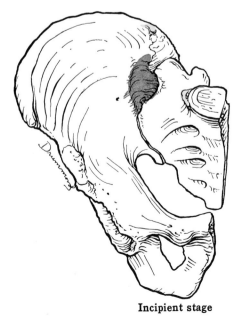

Incipient stage

223.1   Synostosis of the Sacro-iliac Joint

Synostosis of this joint was found in 14 of 182 half pelves (91 dissecting room subjects); 5 times on the right side only, 3 times on the left side only, and 3 times on both sides. One subject was a female (aged 64 years); the others were males, (aged 30 to 84 years). The ossification commonly begins, as here, (red) in the ventral sacro-iliac ligament and is associated with bony overgrowth elsewhere, e.g., acetabular margin, lumbo-sacral joint, and iliac crest (yellow). (*J.C.B.G.*)

224 Clitoris

This miniature penis comprises two corpora cavernosa which are bent, suspended by a suspensory ligament, and capped by a glans as in the male (fig. 198).

The male bulb and body of the corpus spongiosum (corpus cavernosum urethrae) are represented in the female by the bulbs of the vestibule and the commissure of the bulbs (pars intermedia). These, however, are not regarded as part of the clitoris and are not traversed by the urethra.

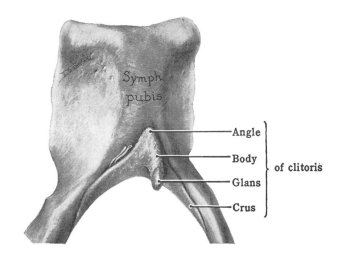

Symph pubis

Angle
Body
Glans
Crus

of clitoris

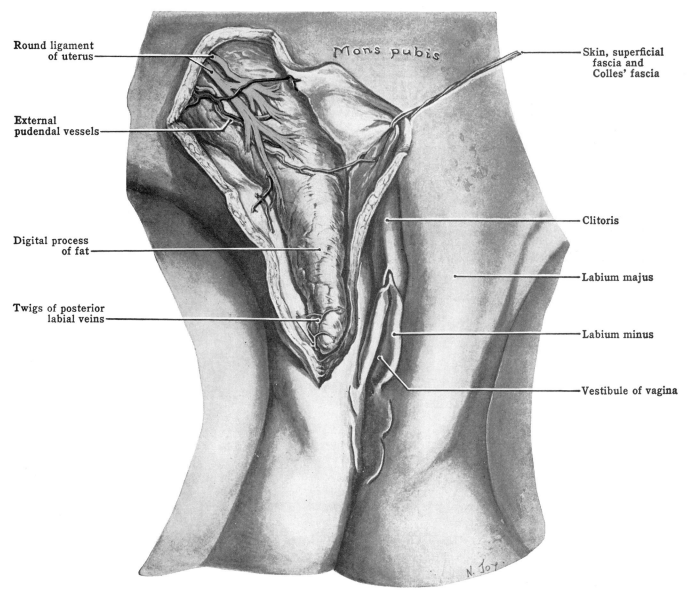

Round ligament of uterus

External pudendal vessels

Digital process of fat

Twigs of posterior labial veins

Mons pubis

Skin, superficial fascia and Colles' fascia

Clitoris

Labium majus

Labium minus

Vestibule of vagina

N. Joy.

225 Female Perineum—I

Observe:

1. A long digital, or finger-like, process of fat lying deep to the subcutaneous fatty tissue and descending far into the labium majus.

2. The thin transparent veil of areolar tissue that encloses the process and through which its lobulated nature is apparent.

3. The round ligament of the uterus (lig. teres uteri) ending as a branching band of fascia which spreads out in front of the digital process; and the (superficial) external pudendal vessels crossing the process.

4. The vestibule of the vagina, as the region between the labia minora and external to the hymen.

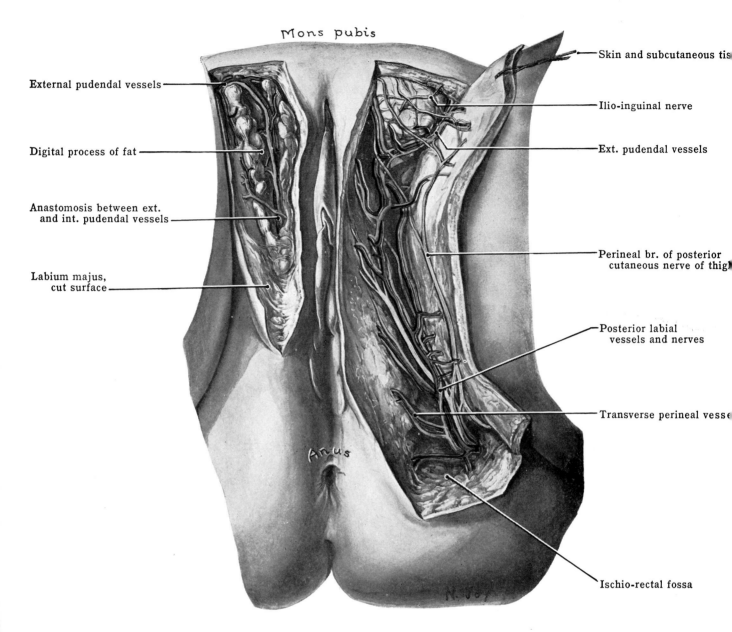

Mons pubis

External pudendal vessels

Digital process of fat

Anastomosis between ext.
and int. pudendal vessels

Labium majus,
cut surface

Anus

Skin and subcutaneous tis

Ilio-inguinal nerve

Ext. pudendal vessels

Perineal br. of posterior
cutaneous nerve of thigh

Posterior labial
vessels and nerves

Transverse perineal vesse

Ischio-rectal fossa

226   Female Perineum—II

Observe:

1. On left of page, the lobulated digital process of fat opened up, and anastomotic vessels, which unite the external to the internal pudendal vessels, running through its long axis like a core.

2. On right of page, the digital process of fat is largely removed. The posterior labial vessels and nerves (S.2, 3), joined by the perineal branch of the posterior cutaneous nerve of the thigh (S.1, 2, 3) running forwards almost to the mons pubis, the vessels there anastomosing with the external pudendal vessels, and the nerves meeting the ilio-inguinal nerve (L.1).

3. Note that there is here a hiatus in the numerical sequence of the nerve segments, accounted for by the fact that L.2, 3, 4, 5 and S.1 are drawn down into the lower limb with the result that L.1 is succeeded by S.2 (cf. the similar hiatus in the pectoral region between C.3 and 4 and T.2. See figs. 13 and 663).

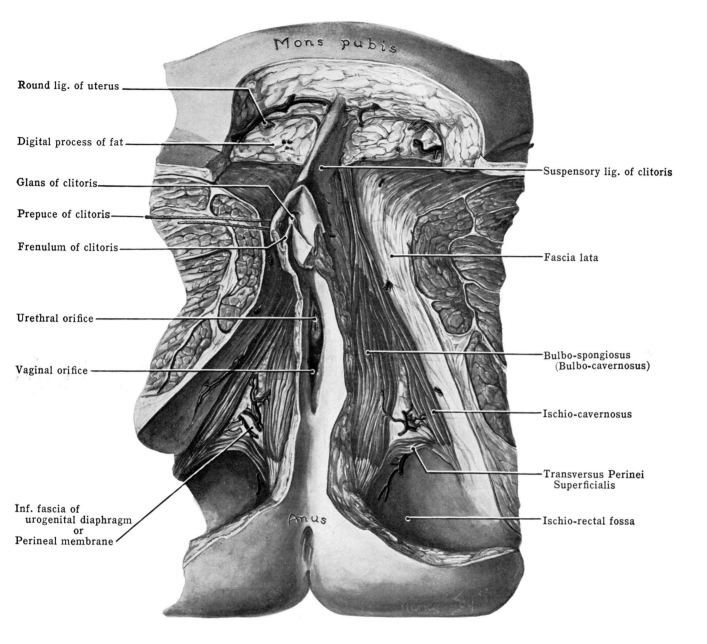

Round lig. of uterus

Digital process of fat

Glans of clitoris

Prepuce of clitoris

Frenulum of clitoris

Urethral orifice

Vaginal orifice

Inf. fascia of
urogenital diaphragm
or
Perineal membrane

Mons pubis

Suspensory lig. of clitoris

Fascia lata

Bulbo-spongiosus
(Bulbo-cavernosus)

Ischio-cavernosus

Transversus Perinei
Superficialis

Ischio-rectal fossa

Anus

227 Female Perineum—III

Observe:

1. The thickness of the superficial fatty tissue at the mons and the encapsuled digital process of fat deep to this. The suspensory ligament of the clitoris descending from the linea alba and symphysis pubis.

2. The prepuce of the clitoris, thrown like a hood over the clitoris, and the anterior ends of the labia minora uniting to form the frenulum of the clitoris.

3. The 3 muscles on each side: Bulbo-spongiosus, Ischio-cavernosus, and Transversus Perinei Superficialis, which when slightly separated reveal the perineal membrane. The Bulbo-spongiosus overlies the bulb of the vestibule. In the male, the muscles of the two sides are united by a median raphe (fig. 192); in the female, the orifice of the vagina separates the two.

4. The pin-point orifices of the right and the left paraurethral duct below the urethral orifice.

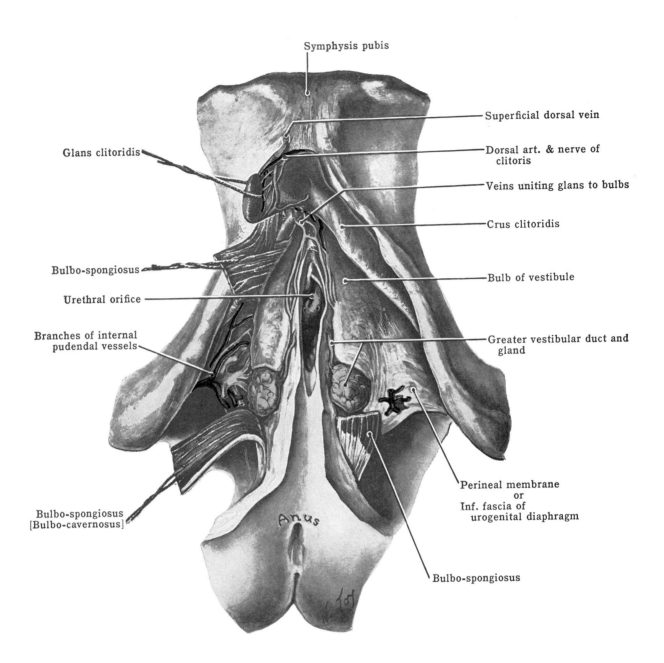

Symphysis pubis

Superficial dorsal vein

Dorsal art. & nerve of clitoris

Veins uniting glans to bulbs

Glans clitoridis

Crus clitoridis

Bulbo-spongiosus

Bulb of vestibule

Urethral orifice

Branches of internal pudendal vessels

Greater vestibular duct and gland

Perineal membrane
or
Inf. fascia of
urogenital diaphragm

Bulbo-spongiosus
[Bulbo-cavernosus]

Anus

Bulbo-spongiosus

228 Female Perineum—IV

On the right side the perineal membrane is removed.

Observe:

1. The paired Bulbo-spongiosus, divided and reflected on the right side, and largely excised on the left side.
2. The glans clitoridis, pulled over to the right side and the dorsal vessels and nerve of the clitoris running to it, as in the male (fig. 199).
3. The bulb of the vestibule (paired, right and left) one on each side of the vestibule of the vagina and therein differing from the bulb of the penis, which is unpaired (fig. 200).
4. Veins (pars intermedia) connecting the bulbs of the vestibule

to the glans of the clitoris.

5. The greater vestibular gland situated at the posterior blunt end of the bulb and like it covered with Bulbo-spongiosus, and having a long duct (about $\frac{3}{4}$") which opens into the vestibule (cf., the bulbo-urethral glands and ducts).
6. The perineal membrane to which the bulb is seen to be fastened, on the left side. On the right side the membrane is cut away thereby revealing the vessels of the bulb and the dorsal nerve and vessels of the clitoris within the deep perineal space.

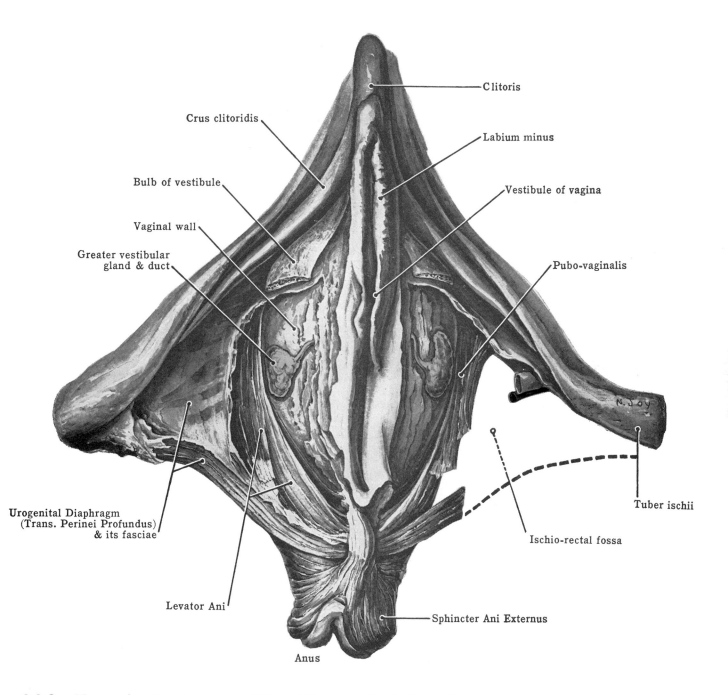

Clitoris

Crus clitoridis

Labium minus

Bulb of vestibule

Vestibule of vagina

Vaginal wall

Greater vestibular
gland & duct

Pubo-vaginalis

Urogenital Diaphragm
(Trans. Perinei Profundus)
& its fasciae

Tuber ischii

Ischio-rectal fossa

Levator Ani

Sphincter Ani Externus

Anus

229 Female Perineum: The Urogenital Diaphragm—V

Observe:

1. The bulbs of the vestibule cut short. The urogenital diaphragm and its fasciae partly cut away on the right side and extensively cut away on the left.

2. The urogenital diaphragm—a sheet of striated muscle, mainly Deep Transversus Perinei, placed between a superior and an inferior sheet of fascia, and having 2 parts: (a) a posterior which is a strong fleshy band that meets its fellow in the perineal body [central tendon of perineum] and (b) an anterior which is more areolar than fleshy.

3. Medially, the diaphragm and its fasciae have been raised from the sloping inferior surface of Levator Ani and detached from the sloping outer wall of vagina with which it fuses.

4. The anterior parts of the Levatores Ani (Pubo-vaginales) meeting behind the vaginal orifice. The greater vestibular glands and the bulbs of the vestibule applied to the sides of the vagina, medial to the anterior borders of the Levatores Ani.

5. The laminated nature of this part of the wall of the vagina. It is laminated because several layers of fascia fuse with it and lose their identity in it, namely the superficial perineal fascia, the diaphragm and its fasciae, and the fasciae of the Levatores Ani.

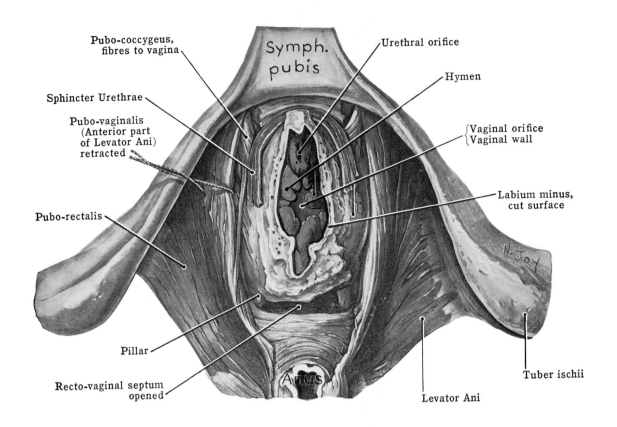

Pubo-coccygeus, fibres to vagina

Symph. pubis

Urethral orifice

Hymen

Sphincter Urethrae

Pubo-vaginalis (Anterior part of Levator Ani) retracted

{ Vaginal orifice
{ Vaginal wall

Pubo-rectalis

Labium minus, cut surface

N. Joy

Pillar

Recto-vaginal septum opened

Anus

Levator Ani

Tuber ischii

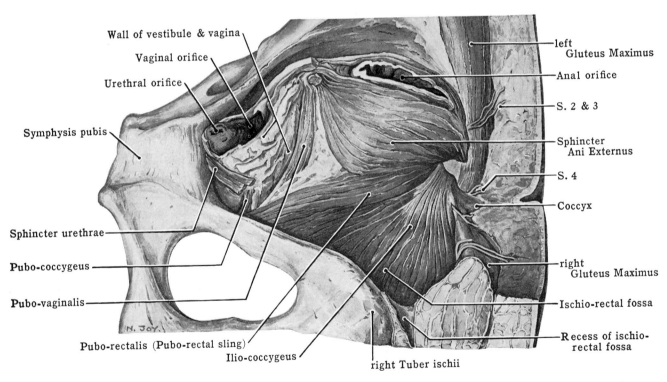

Wall of vestibule & vagina

Vaginal orifice

Urethral orifice

left Gluteus Maximus

Anal orifice

S. 2 & 3

Symphysis pubis

Sphincter Ani Externus

S. 4

Coccyx

Sphincter urethrae

Pubo-coccygeus

Pubo-vaginalis

right Gluteus Maximus

Ischio-rectal fossa

N. Joy

Recess of ischio-rectal fossa

Pubo-rectalis (Pubo-rectal sling)

Ilio-coccygeus

right Tuber ischii

230, 230.1   Female Perineum: The Levator Ani—VI

(The front view (above) and the obliquely tilted side view (below) are of different specimens.)

Observe:

1. The Sphincter Urethrae, of striated muscle, like a saddle, resting on the urethra and straddling the vagina.
2. The labia minora, cut short, bounding the vestibule of the vagina, and the hymen, separating the vestibule from the cavity of the vagina.

Continued on facing page

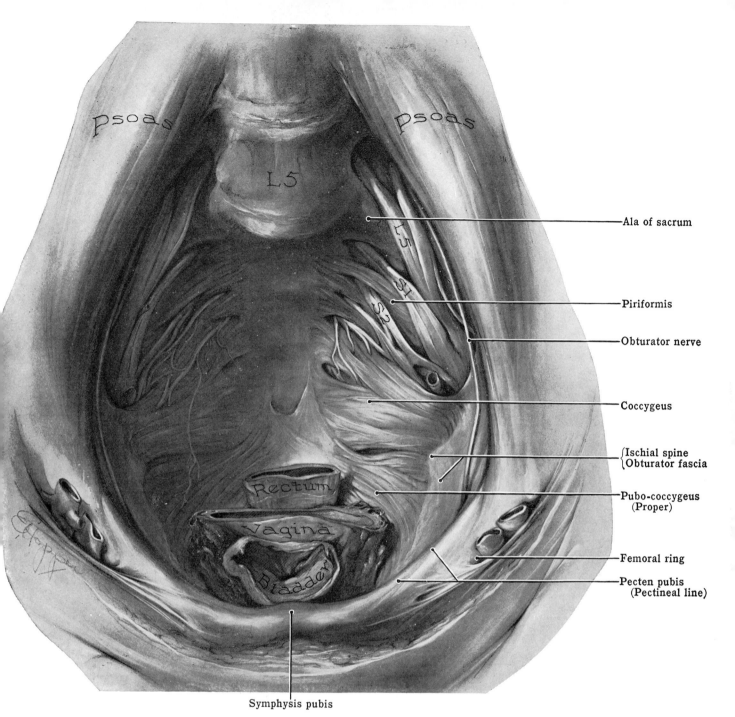

Psoas   Psoas

L5

L5

S1

S2

Ala of sacrum

Piriformis

Obturator nerve

Coccygeus

{ Ischial spine
{ Obturator fascia

Pubo-coccygeus
(Proper)

Femoral ring

Pecten pubis
(Pectineal line)

Rectum

Vagina

Bladder

Symphysis pubis

231   Floor of the Female Pelvis: Levator Ani

Note relative positions of bladder, vagina, and rectum.

Continued from facing page

3. The subdivisions of Levator Ani:

     A. { Pubo-coccygeus { Pubo-coccygeus Proper
                                  Pubo-vaginalis
                                  Pubo-rectalis
     B. { Ilio-coccygeus

4. The recto-vaginal (areolar) septum easily converted into a space, and limited on each side by a "fascial pillar" between rectal and vaginal fasciae.

5. The thick anterior pillar of Pubo-coccygeus Proper extending backwards to the vagina. Pubo-vaginal fibres of opposite sides meeting behind the vaginal orifice. Pubo-rectal fibres of opposite sides meeting in the ano-rectal junction to form the "pubo-rectal sling". Ilio-coccygeus meeting its fellow in an aponeurosis between rectum and coccyx.

6. The vaginal wall laminated, as in figure 229.

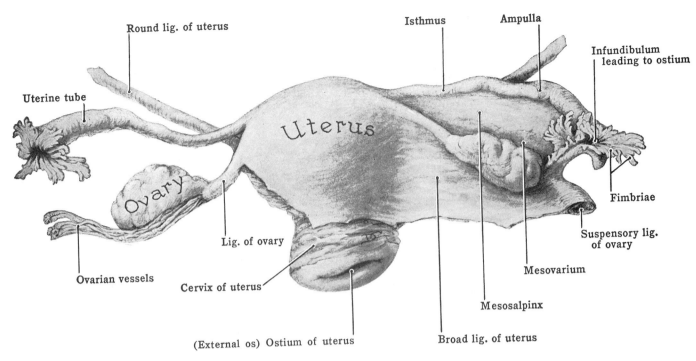

Round lig. of uterus

Isthmus

Ampulla

Infundibulum leading to ostium

Uterine tube

Uterus

Ovary

Fimbriae

Suspensory lig. of ovary

Lig. of ovary

Ovarian vessels

Cervix of uterus

Mesovarium

Mesosalpinx

(External os) Ostium of uterus

Broad lig. of uterus

232 Uterus and its Appurtenances, from behind

On the left side. The broad ligament of the uterus is removed, thereby setting free:—uterine tube, round ligament of uterus, and ligament of ovary. These three are attached to the side of the uterus close together, at the junction of its fundus and body.

On the right side. The "mesentery" of the uterus and tube is called the broad ligament. The ovary is attached

(a) to the broad ligament by a "mesentery" of its own, called the mesovarium; (b) to the uterus by the ligament of the ovary; and (c) near the pelvic brim, by the suspensory ligament of the ovary, which transmits the ovarian vessels. The part of the broad ligament above the level of the mesovarium is called the mesosalpinx.

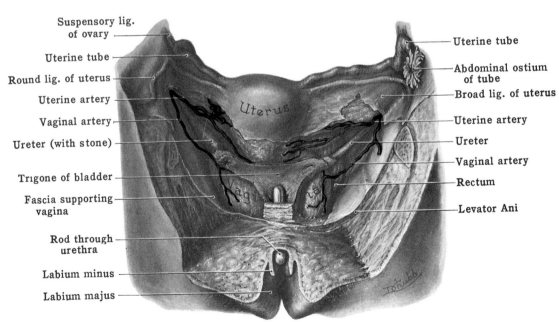

Suspensory lig. of ovary

Uterine tube

Round lig. of uterus

Uterine artery

Vaginal artery

Ureter (with stone)

Trigone of bladder

Fascia supporting vagina

Rod through urethra

Labium minus

Labium majus

Uterus

Uterine tube

Abdominal ostium of tube

Broad lig. of uterus

Uterine artery

Ureter

Vaginal artery

Rectum

Levator Ani

232.1 Uterus in its Setting, viewed from the front

The pubic bones and the bladder, trigone excepted, are removed.

Note: (a) Ureters, trigone of bladder, and urethra in relation to the asymmetrically placed uterus and vagina. (b) Ostium of left uterine tube here happens to face forwards, and (c) right ureter to contain a calculus (stone).

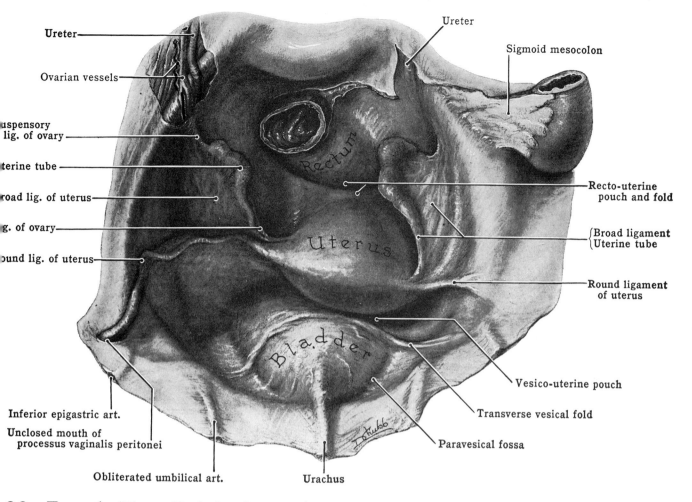

Ureter

Ovarian vessels

uspensory
lig. of ovary

terine tube

road lig. of uterus

g. of ovary

ound lig. of uterus

Inferior epigastric art.

Unclosed mouth of
processus vaginalis peritonei

Obliterated umbilical art.

Ureter

Sigmoid mesocolon

Rectum

Uterus

Bladder

Recto-uterine
pouch and **fold**

Broad ligament
Uterine tube

Round ligament
of uterus

Vesico-uterine pouch

Transverse vesical fold

Paravesical fossa

Urachus

33 Female True Pelvis, from above

bserve:

The pear-shaped uterus asymmetrically placed, as usual;
here leaning to the left.

The right round ligament [lig. teres uteri]; here longer
than the left and having an acquired "mesentery." The
round ligament of the female takes the same subperitoneal
course as the deferent duct of the male (fig. 210).

3. The free edge of the medial ⁴⁄₅ of the broad ligament [lig.
latum uteri] occupied by the uterine tube (Fallopian tube).
The lateral ⅕, occupied by the ovarian vessels, is the suspensory lig. of the ovary.

4. The ovarian vessels crossing the external iliac vessels very
close to the ureter; the left ureter crossing at the apex of
the inverted V-shaped root of the sigmoid mesocolon.

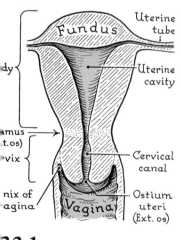

33.1

agram. The parts of the uterus.

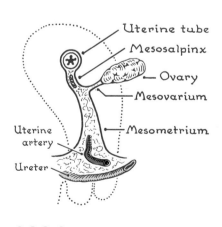

233.2

Diagram. Broad ligament in
paramedian section. (Metra is
Greek for uterus, and salpinx
for trumpet or tube.)

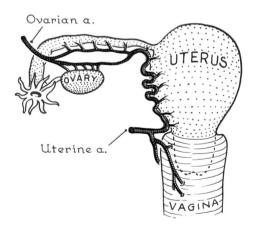

233.3

Diagram. The ovarian and uterine arteries
anastomose in the broad ligament.

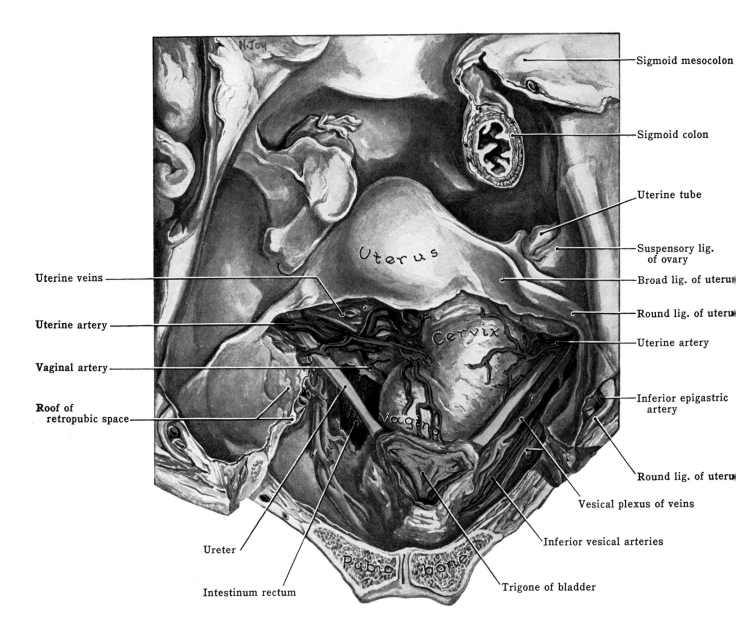

Labels on image:
- Sigmoid mesocolon
- Sigmoid colon
- Uterine tube
- Suspensory lig. of ovary
- Broad lig. of uterus
- Round lig. of uterus
- Uterine artery
- Inferior epigastric artery
- Round lig. of uterus
- Vesical plexus of veins
- Inferior vesical arteries
- Trigone of bladder
- Intestinum rectum
- Ureter
- Roof of retropubic space
- Vaginal artery
- Uterine artery
- Uterine veins
- Uterus
- Cervix
- Vagina
- Pubic bone

234 Female Genital Organs, from above—I

Part of the pubic bones and the whole of the bladder, excepting the trigone, are removed, and with them parts of the broad ligaments.

Observe:

1. The uterus asymmetrically placed, here leaning to the right, and also the vagina.

2. As a result, one ureter—in this instance the left—crosses the lateral fornix of the vagina and is close to the cervix of the uterus, the other being correspondingly farther away.

3. The uterine artery, lying with its veins in the base of the broad ligament and running up the side of the uterus.

4. A large vaginal artery, a branch of the uterine artery, supplying the cervix and the anterior surface of the vagina. The vaginal artery arising from the internal iliac artery and supplying the posterior surface of the vagina.

5. The rectal fascia (not labelled) intervening between the foregoing arteries and the rectum.

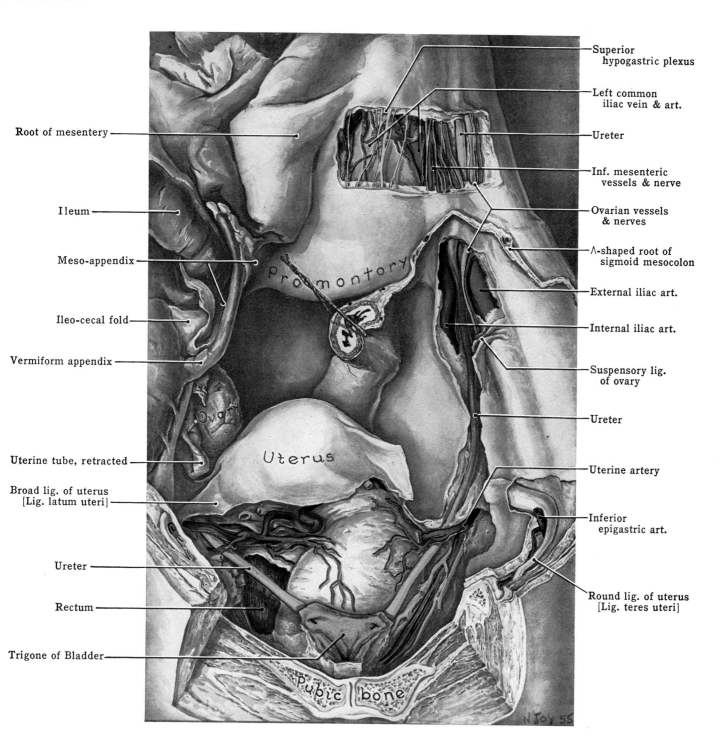

Root of mesentery

Ileum

Meso-appendix

Ileo-cecal fold

Vermiform appendix

Uterine tube, retracted

Broad lig. of uterus
[Lig. latum uteri]

Ureter

Rectum

Trigone of Bladder

Superior
hypogastric plexus

Left common
iliac vein & art.

Ureter

Inf. mesenteric
vessels & nerve

Ovarian vessels
& nerves

Λ-shaped root of
sigmoid mesocolon

External iliac art.

Internal iliac art.

Suspensory lig.
of ovary

Ureter

Uterine artery

Inferior
epigastric art.

Round lig. of uterus
[Lig. teres uteri]

promontory

Ovary

Uterus

Pubic bone

N Joy 55

235   Female Ureter in its Pelvic Course—II

Observe:

1. The superior hypogastric plexus and some lymph vessels anterior to the left common iliac vein.

2. The left ureter, which has just been crossed by the ovarian vessels and nerves, and which is about to be crossed by sigmoid branches of the inferior mesenteric vessels.

   The apex of the Λ-shaped root of the sigmoid mesocolon situated in front of the left ureter, and acting as a guide to it.

The ureter, crossing the external iliac artery—at the bifurcation of the common iliac artery and close behind the ovarian vessels—and descending in front of the internal iliac artery. Its subperitoneal course from where it enters the pelvis to where it passes deep to the broad ligament and is there crossed by the uterine artery.

3. The vermiform appendix in one of its rarer positions—post-ileal. The ileocecal fold extending from the end of the ileum to the meso-appendix.

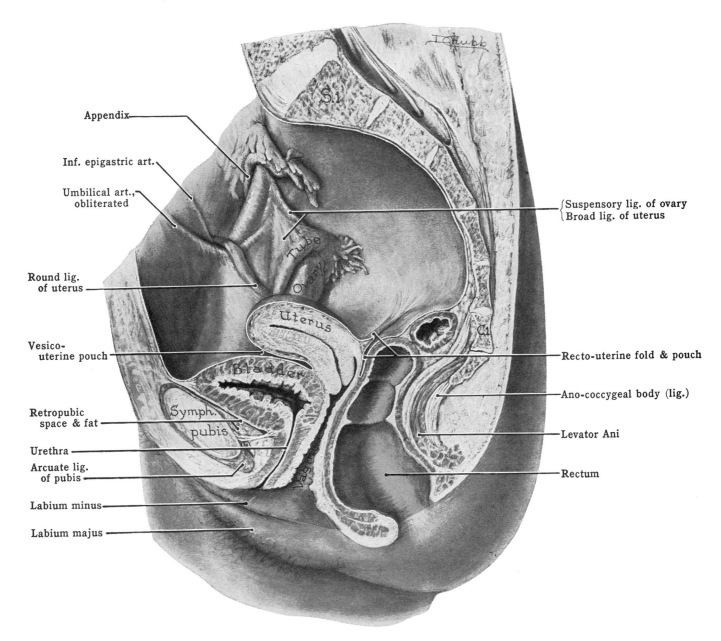

Appendix

Inf. epigastric art.

Umbilical art.,
obliterated

Round lig.
of uterus

Vesico-
uterine pouch

Retropubic
space & fat

Urethra

Arcuate lig.
of pubis

Labium minus

Labium majus

Suspensory lig. of ovary
Broad lig. of uterus

Recto-uterine fold & pouch

Ano-coccygeal body (lig.)

Levator Ani

Rectum

Tube

Ovary

Uterus

Bladder

Symph.
pubis

Vagina

S.1

Cx

236 Female True Pelvis, in median section

Plugs of cotton wool in the lower parts of the rectum and vagina had slightly distorted these parts. The uterus was sectioned in its own median plane and depicted as though this coincided with the median plane of the body—which is seldom the case.

Observe

1. The uterine tube and the ovary, in their virginal positions on the side wall of the pelvis, i.e., in the angle between:—ureter and the umbilical artery, and medial to the obturator nerve and vessels (fig. 210).

2. The uterus, bent on itself at the junction of body and cervix. The cervix, opening on the anterior wall of the vagina, and having a short, round, anterior lip and a long, thinner, posterior lip.

3. The ostium (external os) of the uterus, at the level of the upper end of the symphysis pubis.

4. The anterior fornix of the vagina, $\frac{1}{2}''$ or more from the vesico-uterine pouch. The posterior fornix covered with $\frac{1}{2}''$ or more of the recto-uterine pouch, which is the lowest part of the peritoneal cavity, when the subject is erect.

5. The urethra ($11\frac{1}{4}''$ long), the vagina, and the rectum parallel to one another and to the pelvic brim. The uterus, nearly at right angles to them, when the bladder is empty.

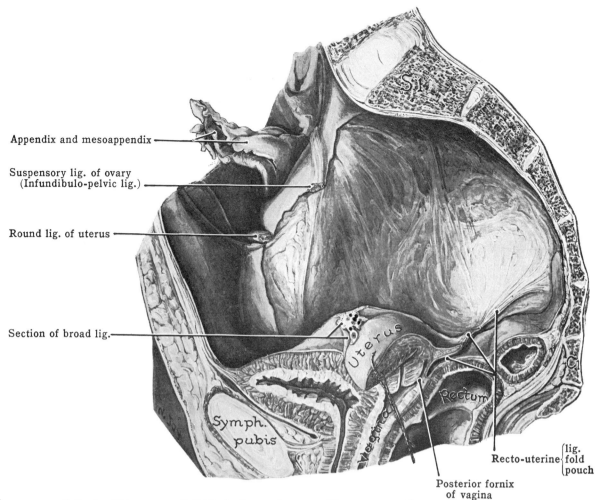

Appendix and mesoappendix

Suspensory lig. of ovary
(Infundibulo-pelvic lig.)

Round lig. of uterus

Section of broad lig.

Uterus

Symph. pubis

Rectum

Posterior fornix
of vagina

Recto-uterine {lig.
fold
pouch

37 Bed from which Figure 237.1 has been Removed

serve:

Divided at the pelvic brim are:–the round lig. and the suspensory lig. with the contained
ovarian vessels and nerves.

Divided at the side of the uterus are:–the broad lig. with the uterine tube in its free margin
the round lig. anteriorly, the lig. of the ovary posteriorly, and several branches of the uterine
vessels.

The structures shown in figure 237.1, thus set free, peeled off the side wall of the pelvis
leaving the subperitoneal fatty-areolar tissue (tela subserosa) exposed.

37.1 Broad Ligament and
s Related Structures,
moved from figure 237

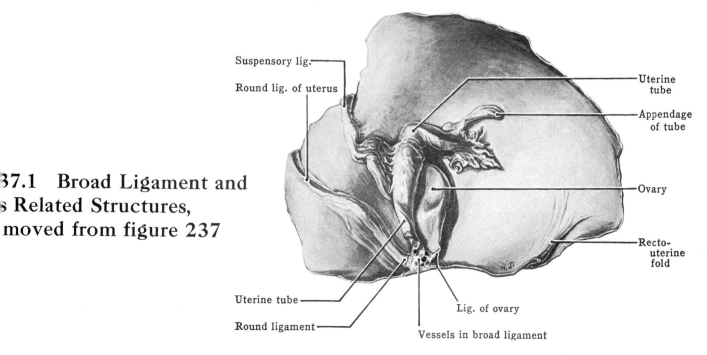

Suspensory lig.

Round lig. of uterus

Uterine tube

Appendage
of tube

Ovary

Recto-
uterine
fold

Uterine tube

Round ligament

Lig. of ovary

Vessels in broad ligament

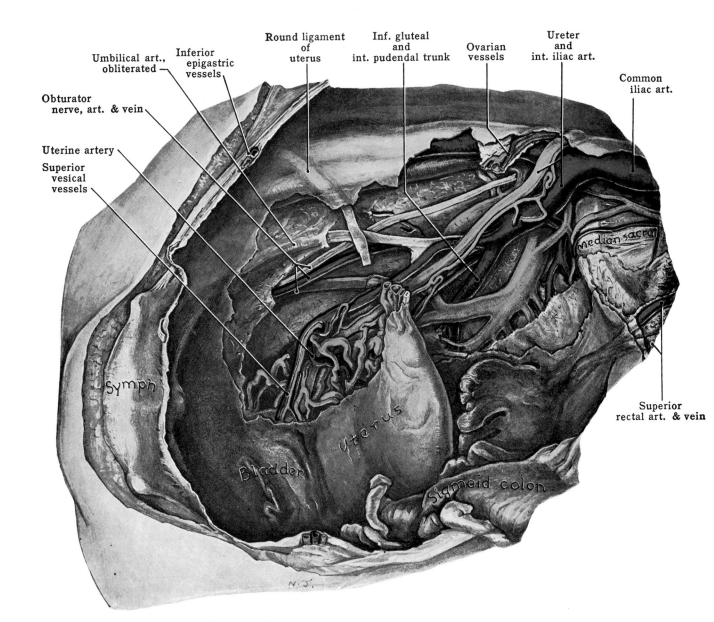

Umbilical art.,
obliterated

Inferior
epigastric
vessels

Round ligament
of
uterus

Inf. gluteal
and
int. pudendal trunk

Ovarian
vessels

Ureter
and
int. iliac art.

Common
iliac art.

Obturator
nerve, art. & vein

Uterine artery

Superior
vesical
vessels

Symph

median sacral

Bladder

Uterus

Sigmoid colon

Superior
rectal art. & vein

N. J.

238 Blood Vessels on the side wall of the Female Pelvis, viewed from the left side of a supine cadaver

In this older subject the uterus is retroverted. The inferior gluteal and internal pudendal arteries here spring from a common trunk, not separately as in figure 210.

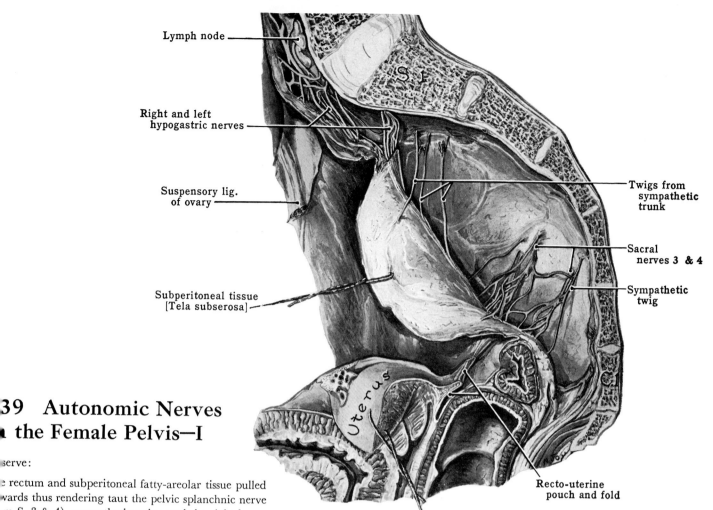

Lymph node

Right and left
hypogastric nerves

Suspensory lig.
of ovary

Subperitoneal tissue
[Tela subserosa]

Twigs from
sympathetic
trunk

Sacral
nerves **3** & **4**

Sympathetic
twig

Uterus

Recto-uterine
pouch and fold

39 Autonomic Nerves
the Female Pelvis—I

serve:

e rectum and subperitoneal fatty-areolar tissue pulled
wards thus rendering taut the pelvic splanchnic nerve
m S. 3 & 4), sympathetic twigs, and the right hypo-
tric nerve.

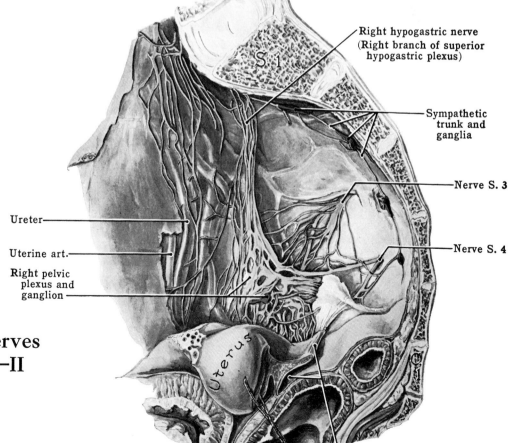

Right hypogastric nerve
(Right branch of superior
hypogastric plexus)

Sympathetic
trunk and
ganglia

Nerve S. **3**

Ureter

Uterine art.

Right pelvic
plexus and
ganglion

Nerve S. **4**

Uterus

40 Autonomic Nerves
the Female Pelvis—II

is is a later stage of figure 239.

Recto-uterine pouch and fold

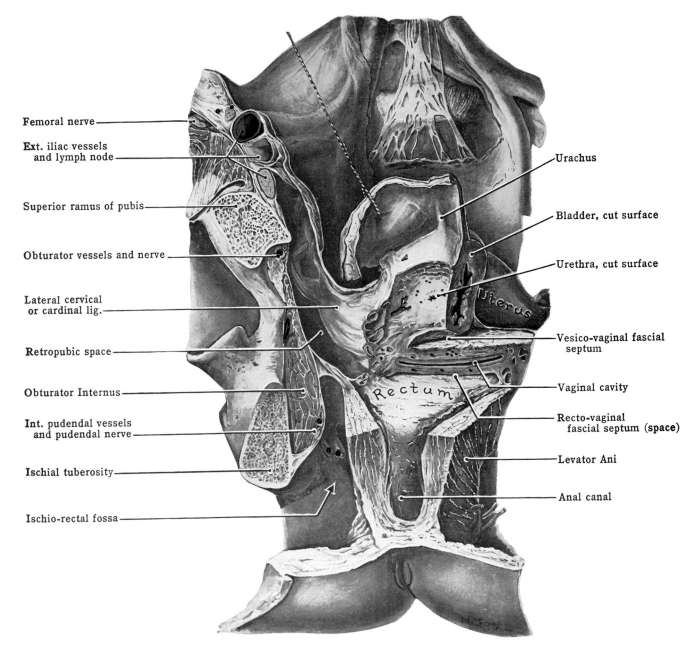

Femoral nerve

Ext. iliac vessels and lymph node

Superior ramus of pubis

Obturator vessels and nerve

Lateral cervical or cardinal lig.

Retropubic space

Obturator Internus

Int. pudendal vessels and pudendal nerve

Ischial tuberosity

Ischio-rectal fossa

Urachus

Bladder, cut surface

Urethra, cut surface

Vesico-vaginal fascial septum

Vaginal cavity

Recto-vaginal fascial septum (space)

Levator Ani

Anal canal

Uterus

Rectum

241 Suspensory and the Supporting Mechanism of the Vagina

This is approximately a coronal section of the pelvis. The neck of the bladder and the vagina are cut across transversely; the bladder is divided sagittally and is rotated backwards.

Observe:

1. The partition that separates the retropubic space from the ischiorectal fossa to be formed merely by the thin origin of Levator Ani from the Obturator Internus fascia, and its areolar coverings.

2. The rectum supporting the posterior wall of the vagina; the posterior wall supporting the anterior wall; and the anterior wall supporting the bladder.

3. The dense areolar tissue within which the vesico-vaginal plexus of veins passes postero-superiorly to join the internal iliac veins. This acts as a suspensory ligament for the cervix and vagina. It is called the cardinal ligament.

4. The cardinal ligament blending with the fascia that encapsules the vagina and with adjacent fasciae.

5. Anteriorly, the fascia encapsuling the vagina blending with the vesical fascia and intimately adherent to the urethra; and posteriorly, loosely attached to the rectal fascia.

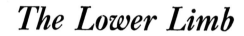

The Lower Limb

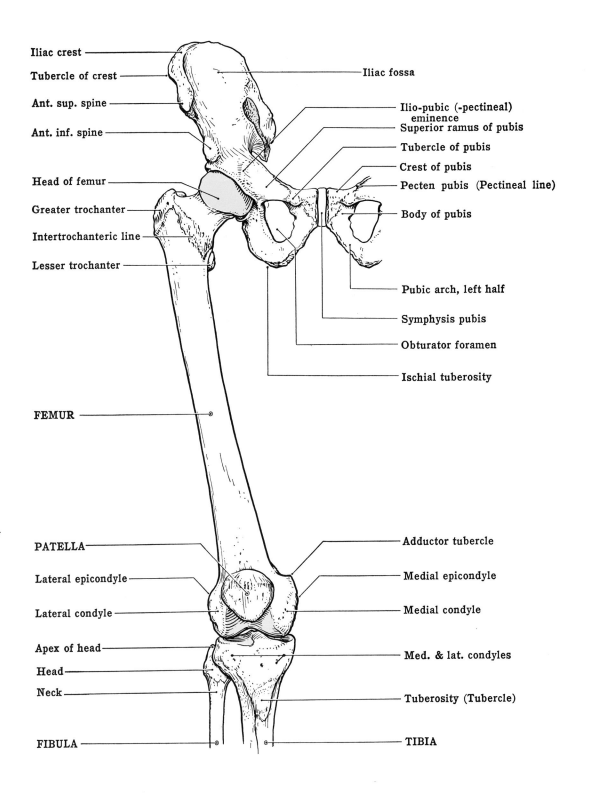

Iliac crest

Tubercle of crest

Ant. sup. spine

Ant. inf. spine

Head of femur

Greater trochanter

Intertrochanteric line

Lesser trochanter

FEMUR

PATELLA

Lateral epicondyle

Lateral condyle

Apex of head

Head

Neck

FIBULA

Iliac fossa

Ilio-pubic (-pectineal) eminence

Superior ramus of pubis

Tubercle of pubis

Crest of pubis

Pecten pubis (Pectineal line)

Body of pubis

Pubic arch, left half

Symphysis pubis

Obturator foramen

Ischial tuberosity

Adductor tubercle

Medial epicondyle

Medial condyle

Med. & lat. condyles

Tuberosity (Tubercle)

TIBIA

242   Bones of the Lower Limb, front view

(For Bones of Leg, see fig. 303. For Bones of Foot, dorsal aspect, see figs. 311–313 and 343.)

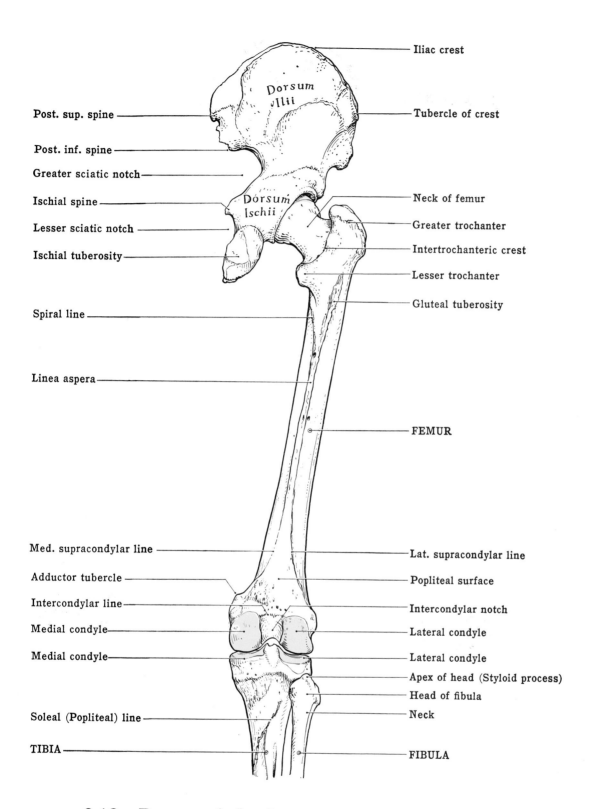

Iliac crest

Dorsum Ilii

Post. sup. spine

Tubercle of crest

Post. inf. spine

Greater sciatic notch

Ischial spine

Dorsum Ischii

Neck of femur

Greater trochanter

Intertrochanteric crest

Lesser sciatic notch

Ischial tuberosity

Lesser trochanter

Gluteal tuberosity

Spiral line

Linea aspera

FEMUR

Med. supracondylar line

Lat. supracondylar line

Adductor tubercle

Popliteal surface

Intercondylar line

Intercondylar notch

Medial condyle

Lateral condyle

Medial condyle

Lateral condyle

Apex of head (Styloid process)

Head of fibula

Soleal (Popliteal) line

Neck

TIBIA

FIBULA

243 Bones of the Lower Limb, posterior view

(For Bones of Leg, posterior view, see fig. 315. For Bones of Foot, plantar aspect, see fig. 314.)

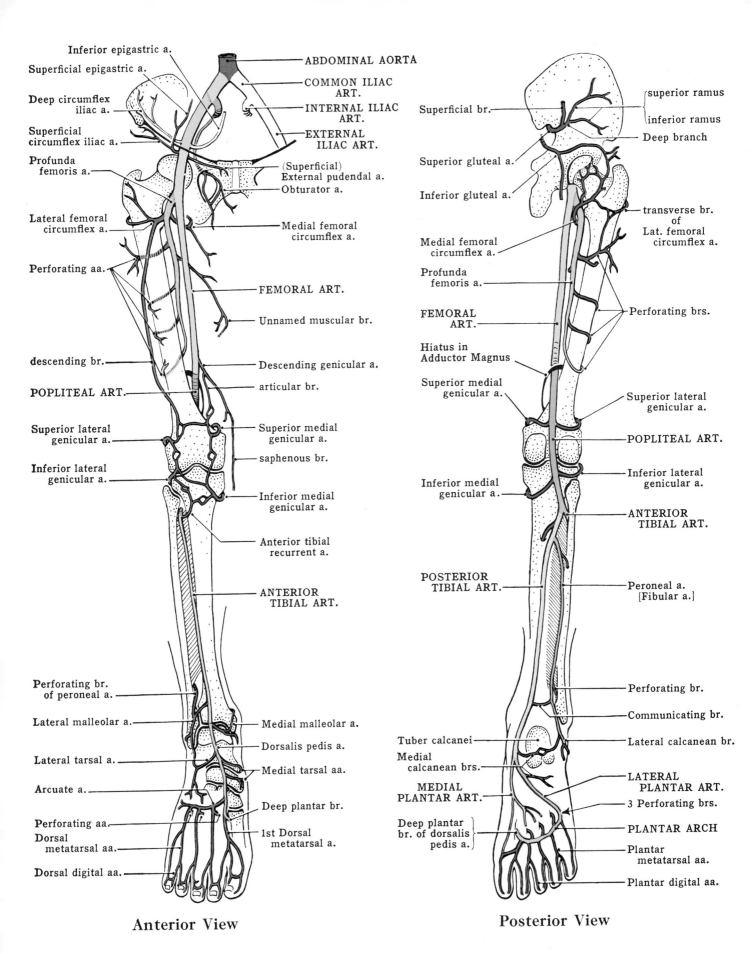

Anterior View

Inferior epigastric a.
Superficial epigastric a.
Deep circumflex iliac a.
Superficial circumflex iliac a.
Profunda femoris a.
Lateral femoral circumflex a.
Perforating aa.
descending br.
POPLITEAL ART.
Superior lateral genicular a.
Inferior lateral genicular a.
Perforating br. of peroneal a.
Lateral malleolar a.
Lateral tarsal a.
Arcuate a.
Perforating aa.
Dorsal metatarsal aa.
Dorsal digital aa.

ABDOMINAL AORTA
COMMON ILIAC ART.
INTERNAL ILIAC ART.
EXTERNAL ILIAC ART.
(Superficial) External pudendal a.
Obturator a.
Medial femoral circumflex a.
FEMORAL ART.
Unnamed muscular br.
Descending genicular a.
articular br.
Superior medial genicular a.
saphenous br.
Inferior medial genicular a.
Anterior tibial recurrent a.
ANTERIOR TIBIAL ART.
Medial malleolar a.
Dorsalis pedis a.
Medial tarsal aa.
Deep plantar br.
1st Dorsal metatarsal a.

Posterior View

Superficial br.
superior ramus
inferior ramus
Deep branch
Superior gluteal a.
Inferior gluteal a.
transverse br. of Lat. femoral circumflex a.
Medial femoral circumflex a.
Profunda femoris a.
FEMORAL ART.
Perforating brs.
Hiatus in Adductor Magnus
Superior medial genicular a.
Superior lateral genicular a.
POPLITEAL ART.
Inferior medial genicular a.
Inferior lateral genicular a.
ANTERIOR TIBIAL ART.
POSTERIOR TIBIAL ART.
Peroneal a. [Fibular a.]
Perforating br.
Communicating br.
Tuber calcanei
Medial calcanean brs.
Lateral calcanean br.
MEDIAL PLANTAR ART.
LATERAL PLANTAR ART.
3 Perforating brs.
Deep plantar br. of dorsalis pedis a.
PLANTAR ARCH
Plantar metatarsal aa.
Plantar digital aa.

244   A Diagram of the Arteries of the Lower Limb

A List of the Named Arteries of the Lower Limb

Internal iliac artery
  Obturator a.
    acetabular br.
    anterior br.
    posterior br.
  Superior gluteal a.
    Superficial br.
    Deep br.
      superior br.
      inferior br.
  Inferior gluteal a.
    branch to sciatic nerve

External iliac artery

Femoral artery
  Superficial epigastric a.
  Superficial circumflex iliac a.
  (Superficial) external pudendal a.
    Anterior scrotal [or labial] brs.
    Inguinal brs.
  Profunda femoris a.
    Medial femoral circumflex a.
      acetabular br.
      ascending br.
      transverse br.
    Lateral femoral circumflex a.
      ascending br.
      transverse br.
      descending br.
    Perforating branches
  Descending genicular a.
    (A. genu suprema)
      articular br.
      saphenous br.

Popliteal artery
  Superior lateral genicular a.
  Superior medial genicular a.
  Middle genicular a.
  Sural aa.
  Inferior lateral genicular a.
  Inferior medial genicular a.

Anterior tibial artery
  Anterior tibial recurrent a.
  Lateral malleolar a.
  Medial malleolar a.

Dorsalis pedis artery
  Lateral tarsal a.
  Medial tarsal aa.
  Arcuate a.
    Dorsal metatarsal aa.
      Dorsal digital aa.
  Deep plantar br.
  1st dorsal metatarsal a.

Posterior tibial artery
  Circumflex fibular br.
  Peroneal [Fibular] art.
    Perforating br.
    Communicating br.
    Lateral malleolar a.
    Lateral calcanean a.
  Medial malleolar a.
  Medial calcanean brs.

Medial plantar artery

Lateral plantar artery
  Plantar arch
    Plantar metatarsal aa.
    Perforating branches
      Plantar digital aa.

245 Superficial Veins of Lower Limb, antero-medial view

The arrows indicate where anastomotic veins perforate the deep fascia and bring the superficial and deep veins into communication with each other.

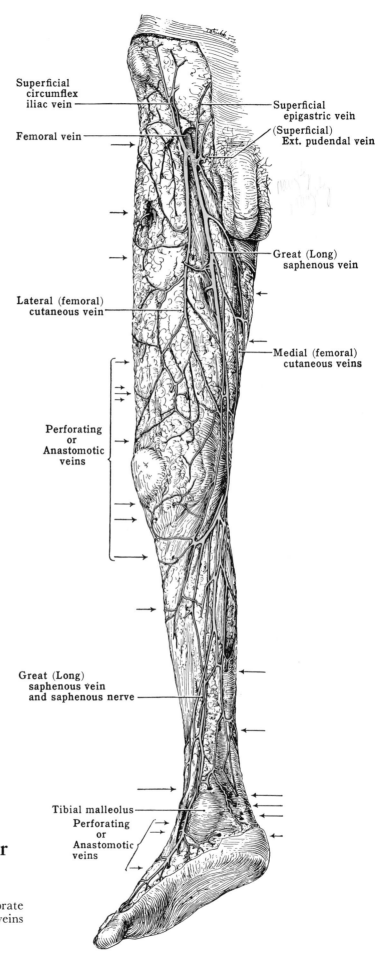

Superficial circumflex iliac vein

Femoral vein

Lateral (femoral) cutaneous vein

Perforating or Anastomotic veins

Great (Long) saphenous vein and saphenous nerve

Tibial malleolus

Perforating or Anastomotic veins

Superficial epigastric veih

(Superficial) Ext. pudendal vein

Great (Long) saphenous vein

Medial (femoral) cutaneous veins

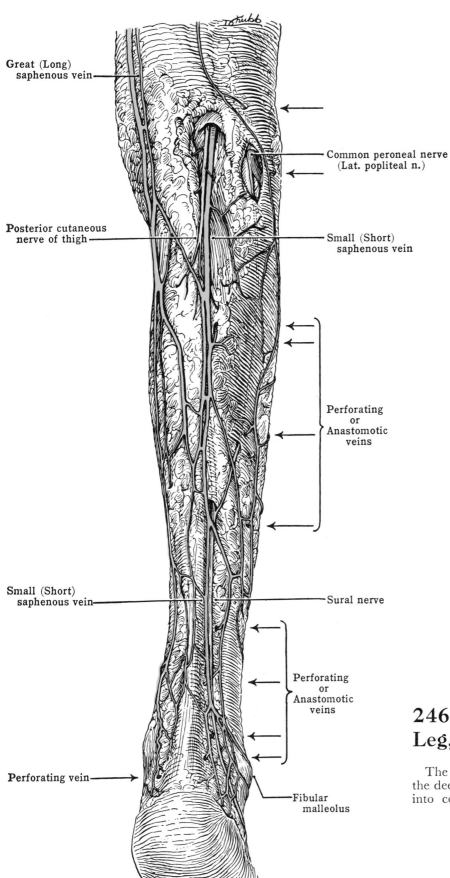

Great (Long) saphenous vein

Common peroneal nerve (Lat. popliteal n.)

Posterior cutaneous nerve of thigh

Small (Short) saphenous vein

Perforating or Anastomotic veins

Small (Short) saphenous vein

Sural nerve

Perforating or Anastomotic veins

Perforating vein

Fibular malleolus

246 Superficial Veins of the Leg, posterior view

The arrows indicate where anastomotic veins perf the deep fascia and bring the superficial and deep into communication with each other.

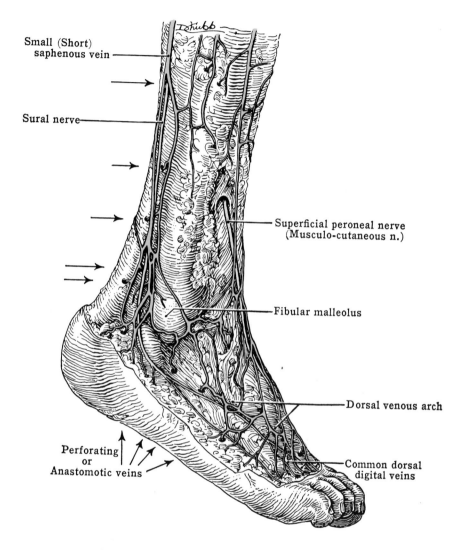

Small (Short) saphenous vein

Sural nerve

Superficial peroneal nerve
(Musculo-cutaneous n.)

Fibular malleolus

Dorsal venous arch

Perforating
or
Anastomotic veins

Common dorsal
digital veins

247 Superficial Veins of the Ankle and
Dorsum of the Foot, antero-lateral view

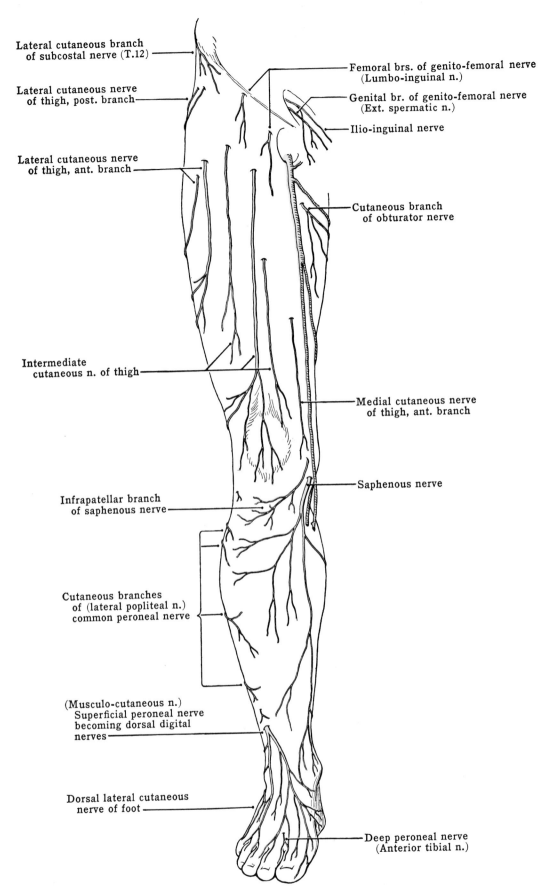

Lateral cutaneous branch
of subcostal nerve (T.12)

Lateral cutaneous nerve
of thigh, post. branch

Lateral cutaneous nerve
of thigh, ant. branch

Intermediate
cutaneous n. of thigh

Infrapatellar branch
of saphenous nerve

Cutaneous branches
of (lateral popliteal n.)
common peroneal nerve

(Musculo-cutaneous n.)
Superficial peroneal nerve
becoming dorsal digital
nerves

Dorsal lateral cutaneous
nerve of foot

Femoral brs. of genito-femoral nerve
(Lumbo-inguinal n.)

Genital br. of genito-femoral nerve
(Ext. spermatic n.)

Ilio-inguinal nerve

Cutaneous branch
of obturator nerve

Medial cutaneous nerve
of thigh, ant. branch

Saphenous nerve

Deep peroneal nerve
(Anterior tibial n.)

248 Cutaneous Nerves of the Lower Limb, front view

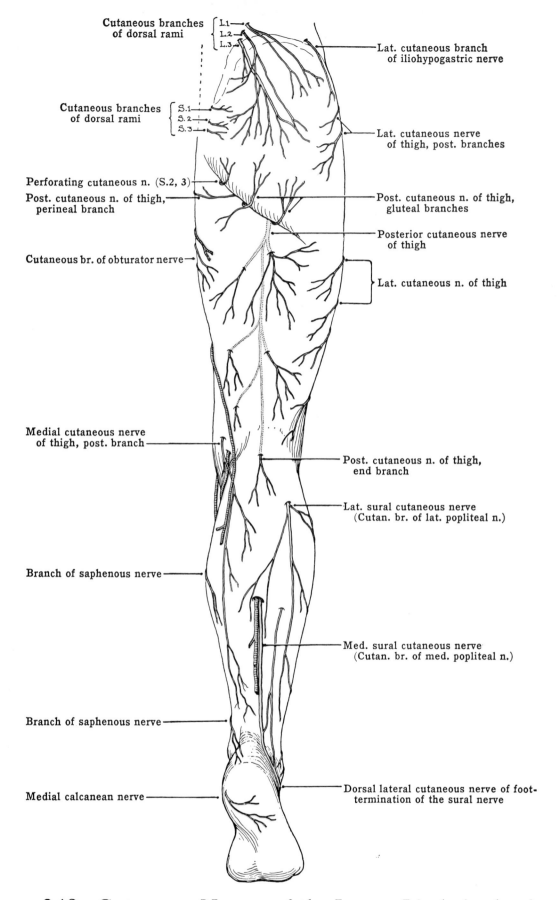

Cutaneous branches of dorsal rami
L.1
L.2
L.3

Lat. cutaneous branch of iliohypogastric nerve

Cutaneous branches of dorsal rami
S.1
S.2
S.3

Lat. cutaneous nerve of thigh, post. branches

Perforating cutaneous n. (S.2, 3)

Post. cutaneous n. of thigh, perineal branch

Post. cutaneous n. of thigh, gluteal branches

Posterior cutaneous nerve of thigh

Cutaneous br. of obturator nerve

Lat. cutaneous n. of thigh

Medial cutaneous nerve of thigh, post. branch

Post. cutaneous n. of thigh, end branch

Lat. sural cutaneous nerve (Cutan. br. of lat. popliteal n.)

Branch of saphenous nerve

Med. sural cutaneous nerve (Cutan. br. of med. popliteal n.)

Branch of saphenous nerve

Medial calcanean nerve

Dorsal lateral cutaneous nerve of foot- termination of the sural nerve

249   Cutaneous Nerves of the Lower Limb, back view

Note:

Sura is Latin for the calf. The medial sural cutaneous nerve is here joined close above the ankle by a communicating branch (not labelled) of the lateral sural cutaneous nerve to form the sural nerve. The level of the junction is variable, being here very low, in figure 286 very high, and in figure 246 in between.

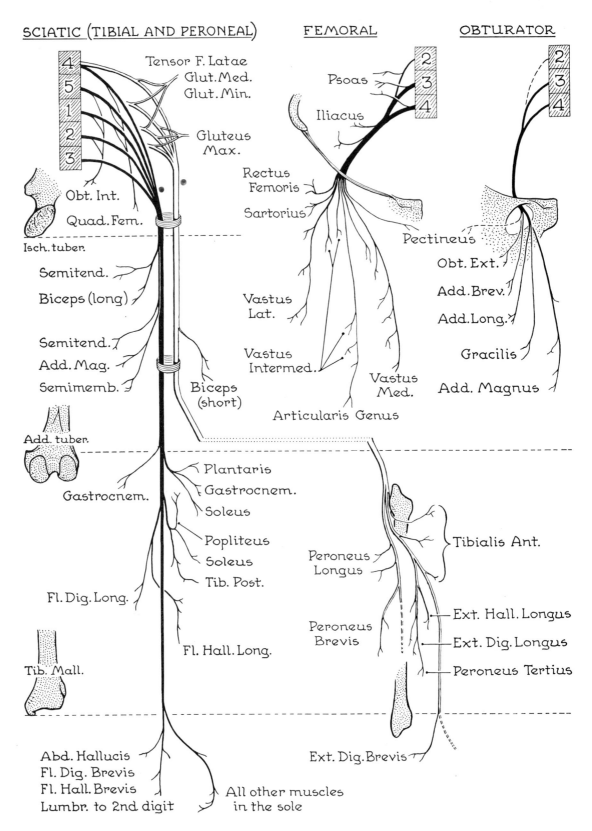

SCIATIC (TIBIAL AND PERONEAL)   **FEMORAL**   **OBTURATOR**

Tensor F. Latae
Glut. Med.
Glut. Min.

Gluteus Max.

Obt. Int.
Quad. Fem.

Isch. tuber.

Semitend.
Biceps (long)

Semitend.
Add. Mag.
Semimemb.

Biceps (short)

Add. tuber.

Gastrocnem.

Fl. Dig. Long.

Tib. Mall.

Abd. Hallucis
Fl. Dig. Brevis
Fl. Hall. Brevis
Lumbr. to 2nd digit

Plantaris
Gastrocnem.
Soleus
Popliteus
Soleus
Tib. Post.

Fl. Hall. Long.

All other muscles in the sole

Psoas
Iliacus

Rectus Femoris
Sartorius

Vastus Lat.

Vastus Intermed.

Vastus Med.

Articularis Genus

Pectineus
Obt. Ext.
Add. Brev.
Add. Long.

Gracilis

Add. Magnus

Peroneus Longus

Peroneus Brevis

Tibialis Ant.

Ext. Hall. Longus
Ext. Dig. Longus
Peroneus Tertius

Ext. Dig. Brevis

250 Scheme of the Motor Distribution of the Nerves of the Lower Limb

Levels at which the motor branches leave the stems of the main nerves are shown with reference to:—ischial tuberosity, adductor tubercle, and tibial malleolus.

Ilio-psoas
  Iliacus
  Psoas Major
Psoas Minor
Gluteus Maximus
Gluteus Medius
Gluteus Minimus
Tensor Fasciae Latae
Piriformis
Obturator Internus
Gemellus Superior
Gemellus Inferior
Quadratus Femoris
Sartorius
Quadriceps Femoris
  Rectus Femoris
  Vastus Lateralis
  Vastus Intermedius
  Vastus Medialis
Articularis Genus
Pectineus
Gracilis
Adductor Longus
Adductor Brevis
Adductor Magnus
Obturator Externus
Biceps Femoris
  long head
  short head
Semitendinosus
Semimembranosus
Tibialis Anterior
Extensor Digitorum Longus
Peroneus Tertius
Extensor Hallucis Longus
Peroneus Brevis
Peroneus Longus
Gastrocnemius
  lateral head
  medial head
Soleus
Plantaris
Popliteus
Tibialis Posterior
Flexor Digitorum Longus
Flexor Hallucis Longus
Extensor Hallucis Brevis
Extensor Digitorum Brevis
Abductor Hallucis
Flexor Hallucis Brevis
Adductor Hallucis
  oblique head
  transverse head
Abductor Digiti Minimi (V)
(Abductor Ossis Metatarsi Quinti)
Flexor Digiti Minimi Brevis
Flexor Digitorum Brevis
Flexor Digitorum Accessorius
Lumbricales
Interossei
  Dorsal
  Plantar

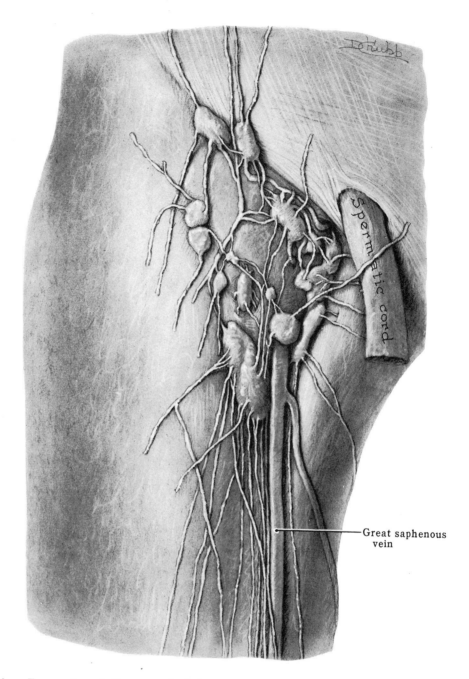

Great saphenous vein

251 Inguinal Lymph Nodes

Observe:

1. The arrangement of the nodes: (a) a proximal chain parallel to the inguinal ligament (superficial inguinal nodes); (b) a distal chain on the sides of the great saphenous vein (superficial subinguinal nodes); and above this, a chain of two or three nodes on the medial side of the femoral vein (deep inguinal nodes), one being below the femoral canal and one or two within it.

    These nodes receive the superficial and deep lymph vessels of the lower limb; the superficial vessels of the lower part of the abdominal wall; the vessels of the penis, including the glans penis and spongy urethra, and of the scrotum (but not of the testis or ovary); the vessels of the vulva, lower part of the vagina, and some vessels from the uterus that run with the round ligament; and vessels of the lower part of the anal canal.

2. The free anastomosis between the lymph vessels.

    About two dozen efferent vessels leave these nodes and, passing deep to the inguinal ligament, enter the external iliac nodes. Of these, less than half traverse the femoral canal; the others ascend along side the femoral artery and vein, some being inside the femoral sheath and some outside it. (fig. 110).

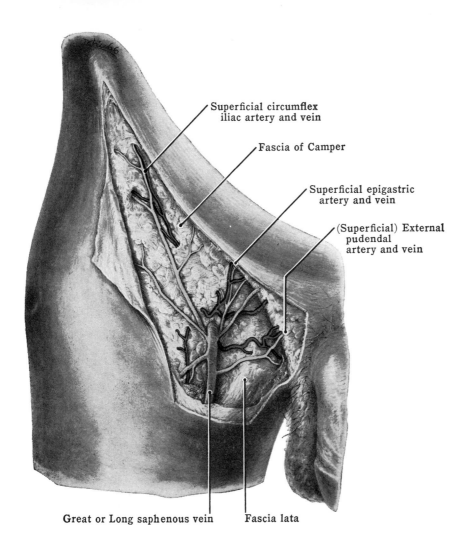

Superficial circumflex
iliac artery and vein

Fascia of Camper

Superficial epigastric
artery and vein

(Superficial) External
pudendal
artery and vein

Great or Long saphenous vein

Fascia lata

252 Superficial Inguina[l]
Arteries and Veins—I

The arteries are branches of the femor[al]
artery but the veins are tributaries of th[e]
great saphenous vein.

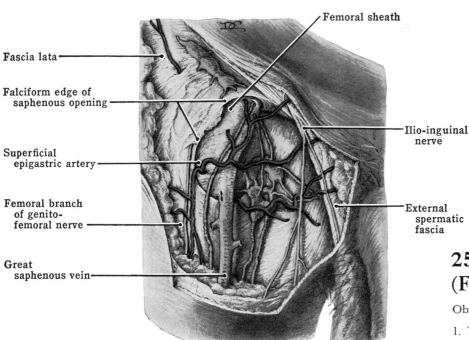

Femoral sheath

Fascia lata

Falciform edge of
saphenous opening

Superficial
epigastric artery

Femoral branch
of genito-
femoral nerve

Great
saphenous vein

Ilio-inguinal
nerve

External
spermatic
fascia

253 Saphenous Openin[g]
(Fossa Ovalis)—II

Observe:

1. The oval shape of this hiatus in the fascia lat[a]
   through which the great saphenous vei[n]
   passes to join the femoral vein, which lie[s]
   within the femoral sheath.
2. The sharp superior and inferior free margin[s]
   or cornua, of the opening and the less sharp[ly]
   definable lateral margin or falciform edge.
3. The great saphenous vein hooking over th[e]
   inferior cornu. Occasionally it joins the fem[-]
   oral vein 1 or even 2 cm. above this cornu[.]

serve:

The falciform edge of the saphenous opening or hiatus cut away.

The superior cornu of the opening passing towards the pubic tubercle and blending with the inguinal ligament and, in this specimen, with the lacunar ligament also.

The medial border of the opening formed by the fascia covering Pectineus and as such passing laterally behind the femoral sheath.

The 3 compartments of the sheath, each incised longitudinally:— (a) the lateral one for the artery, (b) the middle one for vein, and (c) the medial one, called the femoral canal, for lymph vessels.

The proximal end of the femoral canal, called the femoral ring, bounded:— medially by the lacunar ligament, anteriorly by the inguinal ligament, posteriorly by Pectineus & its fascia (fig. 274), and laterally by femoral vein.

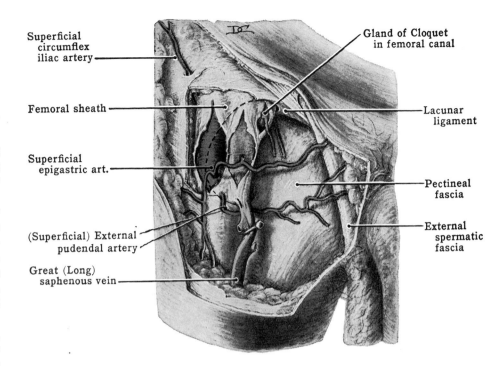

Superficial circumflex iliac artery

Femoral sheath

Superficial epigastric art.

(Superficial) External pudendal artery

Great (Long) saphenous vein

Gland of Cloquet in femoral canal

Lacunar ligament

Pectineal fascia

External spermatic fascia

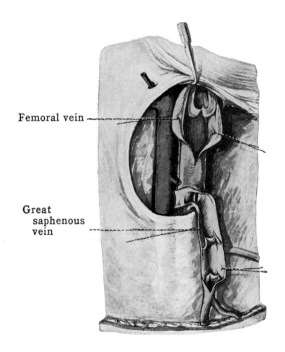

Femoral vein

Great saphenous vein

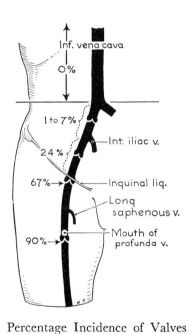

Inf. vena cava

0%

1 to 7%

Int. iliac v.

24%

67%

Inquinal liq.

Long saphenous v.

90%

Mouth of profunda v.

Percentage Incidence of Valves

255

Valves at Proximal Ends of the Femoral and Great Saphenous Veins—IV

Between the mouth of the great saphenous vein and the heart there were no valves in 21% of 506 limbs, 1 valve in 71%, 2 in 7%, and 3 in 1%.

Valves in the common iliac vein are rarely competent, but $\frac{2}{3}$ of those in the external iliac vein are competent.

(Data collected and summarized by Dr. J. V. Basmajian.)

(For most proximal valve, see fig. 281.)

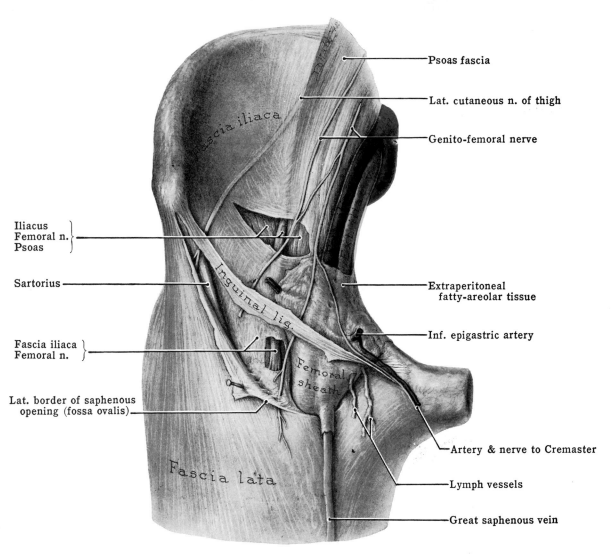

Psoas fascia

Lat. cutaneous n. of thigh

Genito-femoral nerve

Iliacus
Femoral n.
Psoas

Sartorius

Extraperitoneal
fatty-areolar tissue

Inf. epigastric artery

Fascia iliaca
Femoral n.

Lat. border of saphenous
opening (fossa ovalis)

Artery & nerve to Cremaster

Lymph vessels

Great saphenous vein

fascia iliaca

Inguinal lig.

Femoral sheath

Fascia lata

256 Femoral Sheath

The three flat muscles of the abdominal wall are cut away fr●
the upper border of the inguinal ligament, and the fascia lata fr●
the lower border. The falciform margin of the saphenous openi●
or hiatus in the fascia lata is cut and reflected.

Observe:

1. The fascia iliaca, continuous medially with the Psoas fascia and carri●
   downwards in front of Iliacus into the thigh. As it passes behind t●
   inguinal ligament it adheres to it.

2. The extraperitoneal fatty-areolar tissue, which lines the abdomi●
   cavity and in which the external iliac vessels run, carried downwa●
   around these vessels into the thigh as a delicate funnel-shaped s●
   called the femoral sheath. This is loosely adherent to the inguinal li●
   ment in front and to the pecten pubis behind.

3. The femoral sheath containing the femoral artery, vein, and lym●
   vessels; the femoral nerve, being behind the fascia iliaca, is *outside* t●
   sheath.

4. The falciform margin of the saphenous opening (part of the fascia la●
   lying in front of the femoral sheath. Medially the fascia passses beh●
   the sheath as the pectineal fascia.

5. The genito-femoral nerve pierces the Psoas fascia high up in one or t●
   branches; the lateral cutaneous nerve of the thigh pierces the fas●
   iliaca at a variable point, commonly, as here, low down near the a●
   terior superior iliac spine.

Note: The inferior epigastric artery is pulled medially; the deep c●
cumflex iliac artery is not labelled.

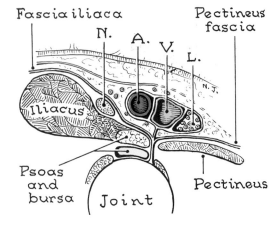

Fascia iliaca   Pectineus fascia

N.   A. V. L.

N. J.

Iliacus

Psoas
and
bursa   Joint

Pectineus

256.1

Diagram. Relationship of femoral vessels and
nerve to each other and to hip joint. Tough
Psoas tendon separates artery from joint.

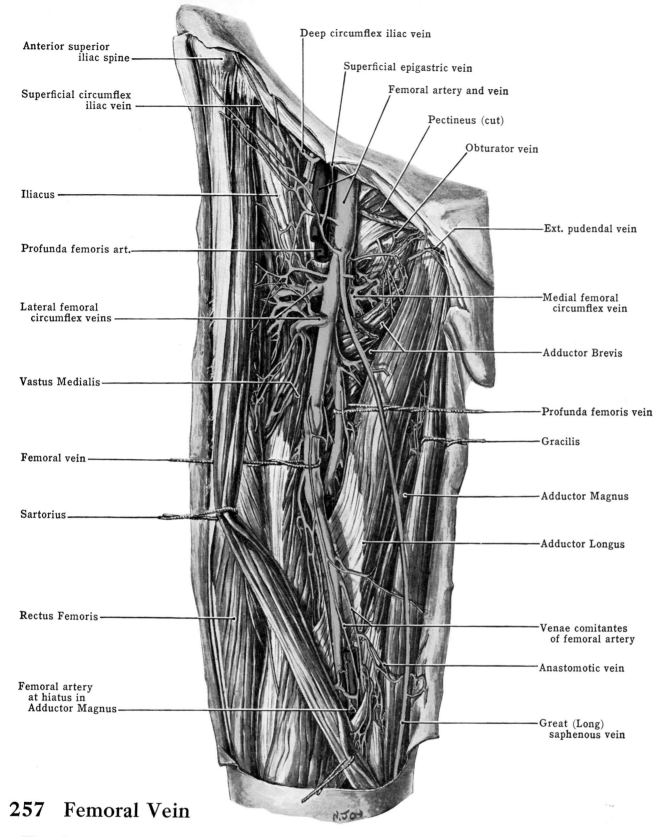

Anterior superior iliac spine

Superficial circumflex iliac vein

Iliacus

Profunda femoris art.

Lateral femoral circumflex veins

Vastus Medialis

Femoral vein

Sartorius

Rectus Femoris

Femoral artery at hiatus in Adductor Magnus

Deep circumflex iliac vein

Superficial epigastric vein

Femoral artery and vein

Pectineus (cut)

Obturator vein

Ext. pudendal vein

Medial femoral circumflex vein

Adductor Brevis

Profunda femoris vein

Gracilis

Adductor Magnus

Adductor Longus

Venae comitantes of femoral artery

Anastomotic vein

Great (Long) saphenous vein

N.Joy

257 Femoral Vein

The veins are injected with latex. Only the stumps of the arteries remain. (The limb is rotated laterally at the hip joint through the force of gravity.)

Observe:

1. The profunda femoris artery arising from the femoral artery about 1½″ below the inguinal ligament. The profunda femoris vein joining the femoral vein twice that distance below the ligament; indeed, in 90 limbs the average distance below the inguinal ligament (actually, below a straight line joining the anterior superior spine to the pubic tubercle) at which the profunda artery sprang from the femoral artery was 5.2 cm. (ranging from 1.0 cm. to 8.5 cm.); whereas the average distance below this line at which the profunda vein joined the femoral vein was 8.4 cm. (ranging from 4.6 cm. to 12.2 cm.). (J. F. R. Fleming and L. F. Levy.)

2. The large size of the lateral femoral circumflex vein, here double and, like the medial femoral circumflex, ending in the femoral vein.

3. The many long, slender, paired venae comitantes that accompany the various arteries.

4. The superficial circumflex iliac vein, in this specimen receiving the superficial epigastric vein, communicating with the veins proximal and distal to it, and ending both in the great saphenous and in the femoral vein.

5. The great saphenous vein communicating with a vena comitans of the femoral artery. The medial femoral circumflex vein communicating with the obturator vein.

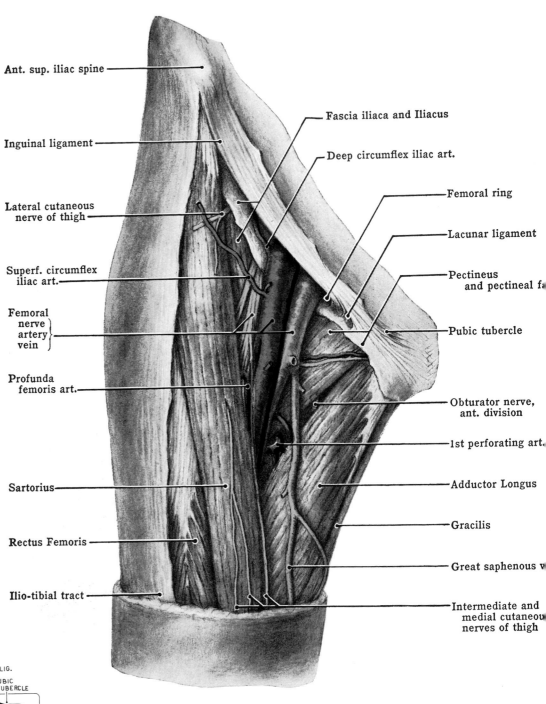

Ant. sup. iliac spine

Inguinal ligament

Lateral cutaneous
nerve of thigh

Superf. circumflex
iliac art.

Femoral
nerve
artery
vein

Profunda
femoris art.

Sartorius

Rectus Femoris

Ilio-tibial tract

Fascia iliaca and Iliacus

Deep circumflex iliac art.

Femoral ring

Lacunar ligament

Pectineus
and pectineal fa

Pubic tubercle

Obturator nerve,
ant. division

1st perforating art.

Adductor Longus

Gracilis

Great saphenous v

Intermediate and
medial cutaneou
nerves of thigh

258.1

A. S. SPINE
INGUINAL LIG.
PUBIC
TUBERCLE
SARTORIUS
ADD. LONGUS
3½"
APEX
OF
TRIANGLE
ADDUCTOR
TUBERCLE

Diagram. Boundaries of triangle;
relationship of artery to femur.

258 Femoral Triangle

Observe:

1. The boundaries of the triangle: The inguinal ligament, which curves gently from
   sup. spine to pubic tubercle, being the base; the medial border of Sartorius bein
   lateral side; the lateral border of Adductor Longus being the medial side; an
   point where the two converging sides meet distally being the apex. (Some au
   regard the medial border of Add. Longus as the medial side of the triangle.)

2. The femoral artery and vein lying in front of the fascia covering Ilio-psoas
   Pectineus, and the femoral nerve lying behind.

3. The artery appearing midway between the anterior superior spine and the
   tubercle, and disappearing where the medial border of Sartorius crosses the l
   border of Adductor Longus—in short, from the midpoint of the base of the tri
   to the apex.

4. That when the adjacent borders of Pectineus and Adductor Longus are not
   tiguous, as here, a glimpse is had of the anterior branch of the obturator nerve
   in front of Adductor Brevis.

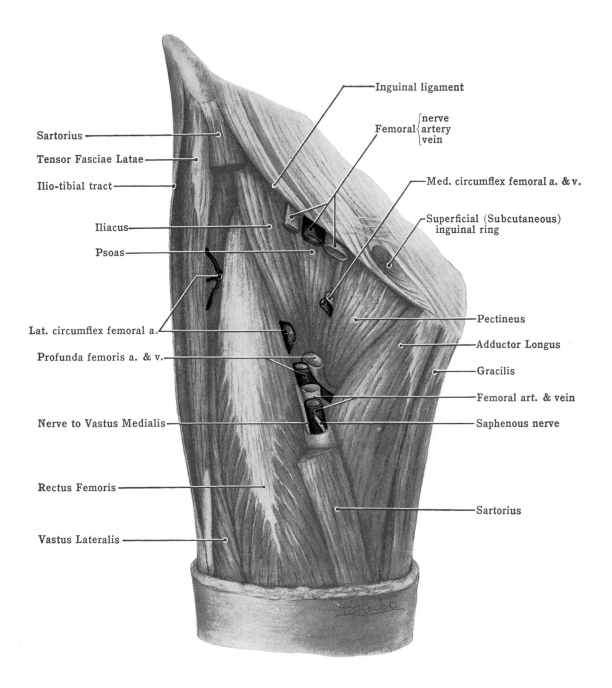

Sartorius

Tensor Fasciae Latae

Ilio-tibial tract

Iliacus

Psoas

Lat. circumflex femoral a.

Profunda femoris a. & v.

Nerve to Vastus Medialis

Rectus Femoris

Vastus Lateralis

Inguinal ligament

Femoral { nerve / artery / vein }

Med. circumflex femoral a. & v.

Superficial (Subcutaneous) inguinal ring

Pectineus

Adductor Longus

Gracilis

Femoral art. & vein

Saphenous nerve

Sartorius

259 Floor of the Femoral Triangle

Sections are removed from Sartorius and from the femoral vessels and nerve.

Observe:

1. The floor of the triangle to be a trough with sloping lateral and medial walls. This is notably so, if Adductor Longus is included with Pectineus in the medial wall: Ilio-psoas, (medial border of Rectus Femoris) and Sartorius form the lateral wall.

2. The trough to be shallow at the base and deep at the apex.

3. At the apex four vessels, one in front of the other, and two nerves pass into the adductor canal of Hunter (subsartorial canal).

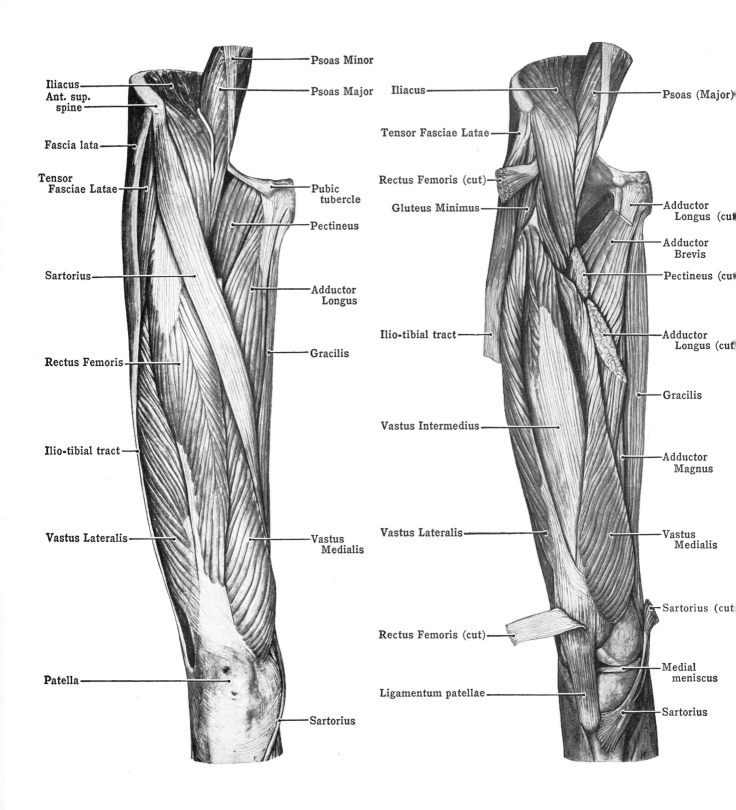

Iliacus
Ant. sup. spine
Fascia lata
Tensor Fasciae Latae
Sartorius
Rectus Femoris
Ilio-tibial tract
Vastus Lateralis
Patella

Psoas Minor
Psoas Major
Pubic tubercle
Pectineus
Adductor Longus
Gracilis
Vastus Medialis
Sartorius

Iliacus
Tensor Fasciae Latae
Rectus Femoris (cut)
Gluteus Minimus
Ilio-tibial tract
Vastus Intermedius
Vastus Lateralis
Rectus Femoris (cut)
Ligamentum patellae

Psoas (Major)
Adductor Longus (cut
Adductor Brevis
Pectineus (cut
Adductor Longus (cut
Gracilis
Adductor Magnus
Vastus Medialis
Sartorius (cut
Medial meniscus
Sartorius

260 Muscles of the Front of the Thigh—I

261 Muscles of the Front of the Thigh—II

Sections of Sartorius, Rectus Femoris, Pectineus and Adductor Longus are excised.

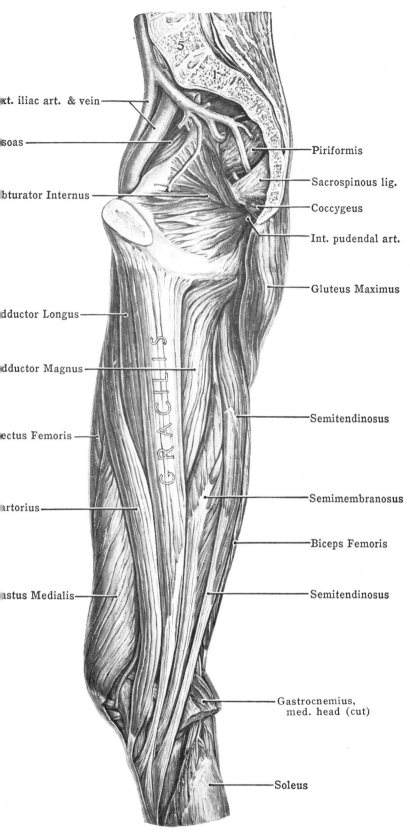

Ext. iliac art. & vein

Psoas

Obturator Internus

Adductor Longus

Adductor Magnus

Rectus Femoris

Sartorius

Vastus Medialis

GRACILIS

Piriformis

Sacrospinous lig.

Coccygeus

Int. pudendal art.

Gluteus Maximus

Semitendinosus

Semimembranosus

Biceps Femoris

Semitendinosus

Gastrocnemius, med. head (cut)

Soleus

262 Muscles of the Medial Side of the Thigh—III

(*For posterior views, see figs. 267–269.*)

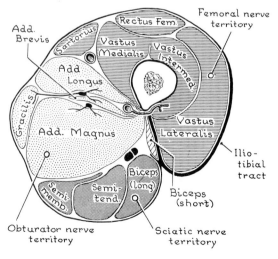

Add. Brevis

Sartorius

Rectus Fem.

Femoral nerve territory

Vastus Medialis

Vastus Intermed.

Add. Longus

Gracilis

Add. Magnus

Vastus Lateralis

Ilio-tibial tract

Biceps (short)

Biceps (Long)

Semi-tend.

Semi-memb.

Obturator nerve territory

Sciatic nerve territory

262

Diagram. Cross section of thigh showing muscles divided into 3 territories—anterior, medial and posterior—according to the nerve supply.

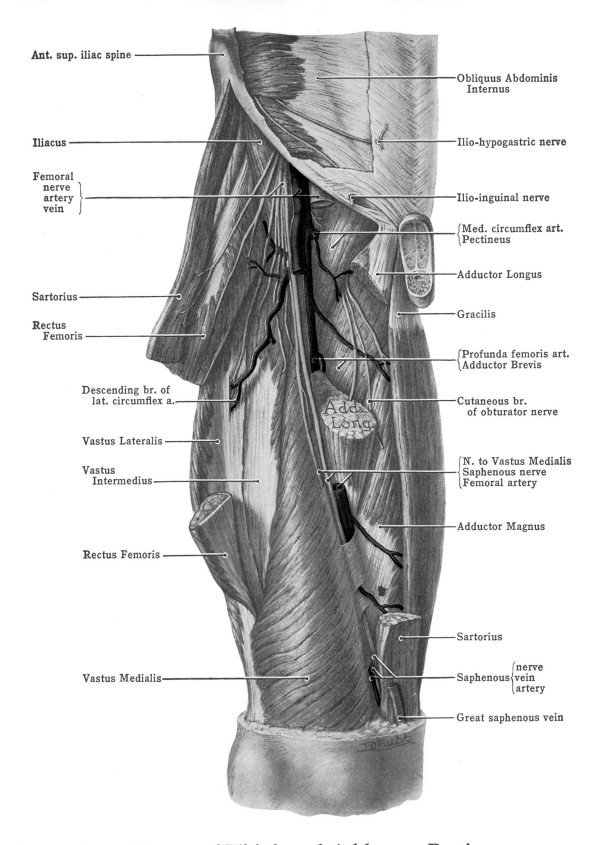

Ant. sup. iliac spine

Iliacus

Femoral
nerve
artery
vein

Sartorius

Rectus
Femoris

Descending br. of
lat. circumflex a.

Vastus Lateralis

Vastus
Intermedius

Rectus Femoris

Vastus Medialis

Obliquus Abdominis
Internus

Ilio-hypogastric nerve

Ilio-inguinal nerve

{ Med. circumflex art.
Pectineus

Adductor Longus

Gracilis

{ Profunda femoris art.
Adductor Brevis

Cutaneous br.
of obturator nerve

{ N. to Vastus Medialis
Saphenous nerve
Femoral artery

Adductor Magnus

Sartorius

Saphenous { nerve
vein
artery

Great saphenous vein

Add.
Long.

263 Dissection of Front of Thigh and Adductor Region

(The limb is rotated laterally)

Observe:

1. The femoral nerve breaking up into a leash of nerves on entering the thigh.

2. The femoral artery lying between two motor territories, namely that of the obturator nerve which is medial, and that of the femoral nerve which is lateral. No motor nerve crosses in front of the femoral artery, but the twig to Pectineus is seen crossing behind it.

3. The nerve to Vastus Medialis and the saphenous nerve accompanying the femoral artery into the adductor canal. The saphenous nerve and artery and their companion anastomotic vein emerging from the lower end of the canal. They become superficial between Sartorius and Gracilis.

4. The profunda femoris artery arising $1\frac{1}{2}''$ below the inguinal ligament, lying behind the femoral artery, and disappearing behind Adductor Longus.

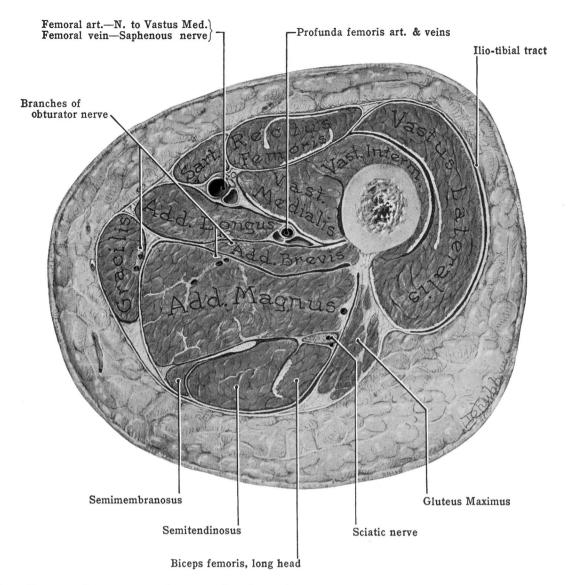

Femoral art.—N. to Vastus Med.
Femoral vein—Saphenous nerve

Profunda femoris art. & veins

Ilio-tibial tract

Branches of
obturator nerve

Sart. Rectus Femoris
Vast. Interm.
Vast. Medialis
Add. Longus
Add. Brevis
Gracilis
Add. Magnus
Vastus Lateralis

Semimembranosus

Semitendinosus

Biceps femoris, long head

Gluteus Maximus

Sciatic nerve

4   Cross Section through the thigh, female

erve:

evel of section—(a) through the insertion of Gluteus Maximus,
herefore above the origin of short head of Biceps; (b) below in-
rtion of Pectineus, above that of Adductor Longus and therefore,
hrough that of Adductor Brevis; (c) through the adductor canal
nd therefore below the apex of the femoral triangle—say 4″–6″
own the femur.

Gracilis abutting against the free, medial borders of the Adductor
uscles.

dductor Longus intervening between the femoral and the
rofunda femoris vessels.

dductor Brevis intervening between the anterior and the pos-
erior division of the obturator nerve.

Aponeurosis of semimembranosus not dissimilar from the sciatic
erve and mistakable for it.

Vastus Intermedius arising from the anterior and lateral surfaces
f the shaft of the femur; Vastus Medialis covering the medial
urface but not arising from it. That is to say, Vastus Intermedius
lone arises from the surfaces, the other muscles are relegated to
he linea aspera or to its upward and downward extensions.
roximally, Lateralis is large.

he considerable amount of subcutaneous fat present in the
male.

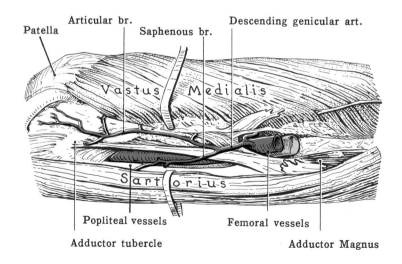

Patella
Articular br.
Saphenous br.
Descending genicular art.

Vastus   Medialis

Sartorius

Popliteal vessels
Femoral vessels

Adductor tubercle
Adductor Magnus

264.1

Femoral artery becomes popliteal artery at the (tendinous)
opening in Adductor Magnus (Adductor hiatus).

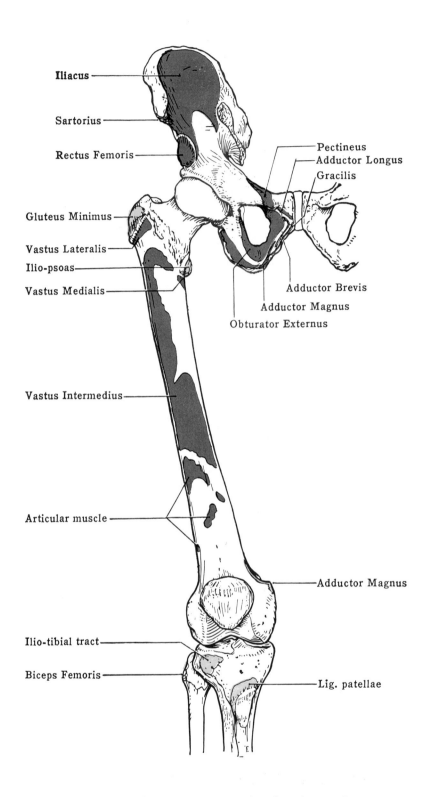

Iliacus

Sartorius

Rectus Femoris

Pectineus
Adductor Longus
Gracilis

Gluteus Minimus

Vastus Lateralis

Ilio-psoas

Vastus Medialis

Adductor Brevis

Adductor Magnus

Obturator Externus

Vastus Intermedius

Articular muscle

Adductor Magnus

Ilio-tibial tract

Biceps Femoris

Lig. patellae

**265   Bones of the Lower Limb showing
Attachments of Muscles, anterior view**

(For Tibia and Fibula, see fig. 303; Bones of Foot, dorsal aspect, see figs. 311, 312 & 313.)

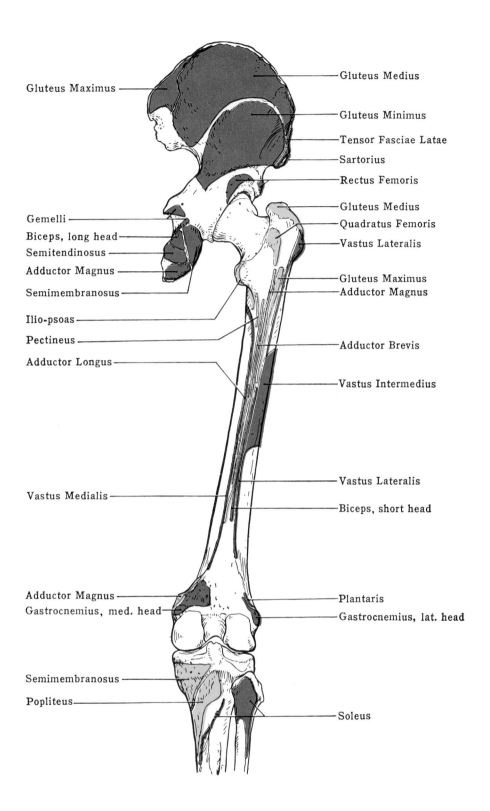

Gluteus Maximus

Gluteus Medius

Gluteus Minimus

Tensor Fasciae Latae

Sartorius

Rectus Femoris

Gemelli

Gluteus Medius

Biceps, long head

Quadratus Femoris

Semitendinosus

Vastus Lateralis

Adductor Magnus

Semimembranosus

Gluteus Maximus

Adductor Magnus

Ilio-psoas

Pectineus

Adductor Brevis

Adductor Longus

Vastus Intermedius

Vastus Medialis

Vastus Lateralis

Biceps, short head

Adductor Magnus

Gastrocnemius, med. head

Plantaris

Gastrocnemius, lat. head

Semimembranosus

Popliteus

Soleus

266 Bones of the Lower Limb showing Attachments of Muscles, posterior view

(For Tibia and Fibula, posterior aspect, see fig. 316; Bones of Foot, plantar aspect, see fig. 314.)

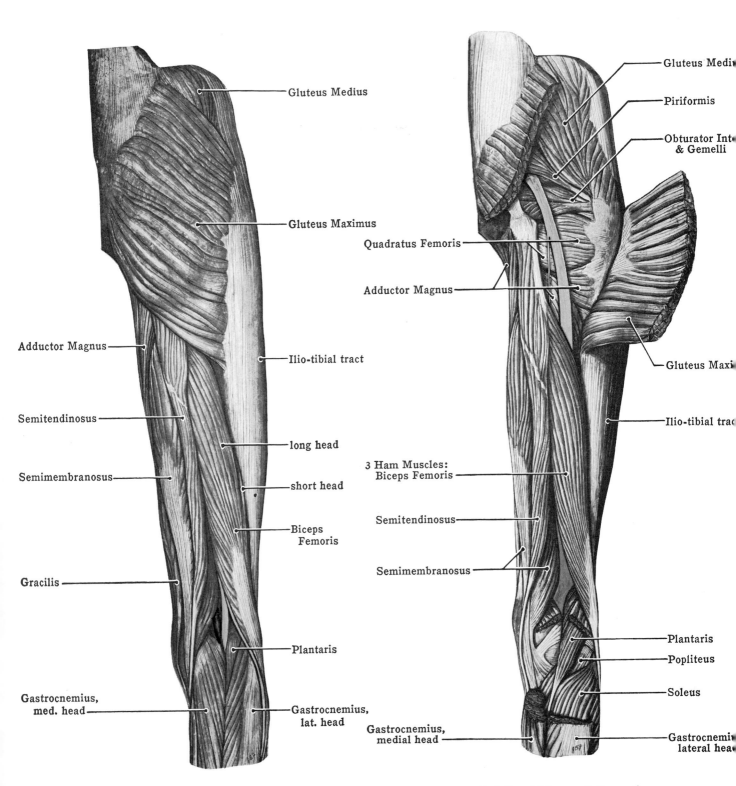

Gluteus Medius

Gluteus Maximus

Ilio-tibial tract

long head

short head

Biceps
Femoris

Plantaris

Gastrocnemius,
lat. head

Adductor Magnus

Semitendinosus

Semimembranosus

Gracilis

Gastrocnemius,
med. head

Gluteus Medi

Piriformis

Obturator Inte
& Gemelli

Quadratus Femoris

Adductor Magnus

Gluteus Maxi

Ilio-tibial trac

3 Ham Muscles:
Biceps Femoris

Semitendinosus

Semimembranosus

Plantaris

Popliteus

Soleus

Gastrocnemi
lateral hea

Gastrocnemius,
medial head

**267 Muscles of the Gluteal
Region and Back of the Thigh**

268 Ham Muscles

(Gluteus Maximus, reflected; Gastrocnemiu
partly excised.)

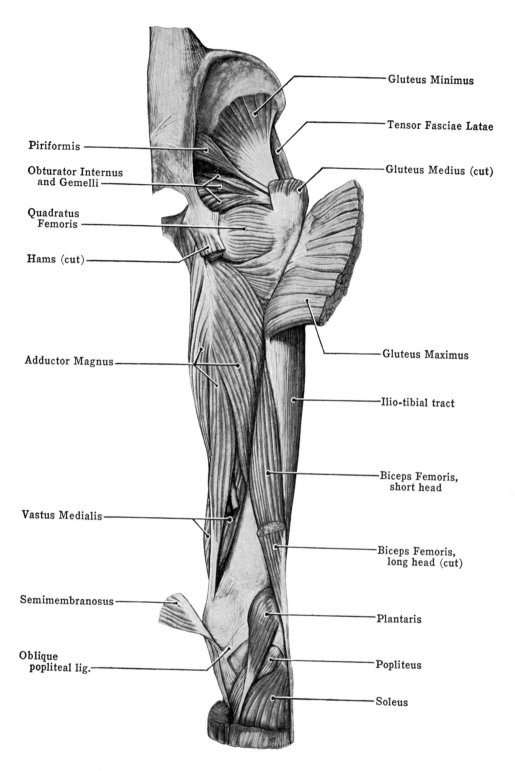

Gluteus Minimus

Tensor Fasciae Latae

Piriformis

Gluteus Medius (cut)

Obturator Internus
and Gemelli

Quadratus
Femoris

Hams (cut)

Gluteus Maximus

Adductor Magnus

Ilio-tibial tract

Biceps Femoris,
short head

Vastus Medialis

Biceps Femoris,
long head (cut)

Semimembranosus

Plantaris

Oblique
popliteal lig.

Popliteus

Soleus

269 Adductor Magnus, from behind

(Gluteus Medius and Ham muscles, excised.)
(For anterior and medial views, see figs. 260-262.)

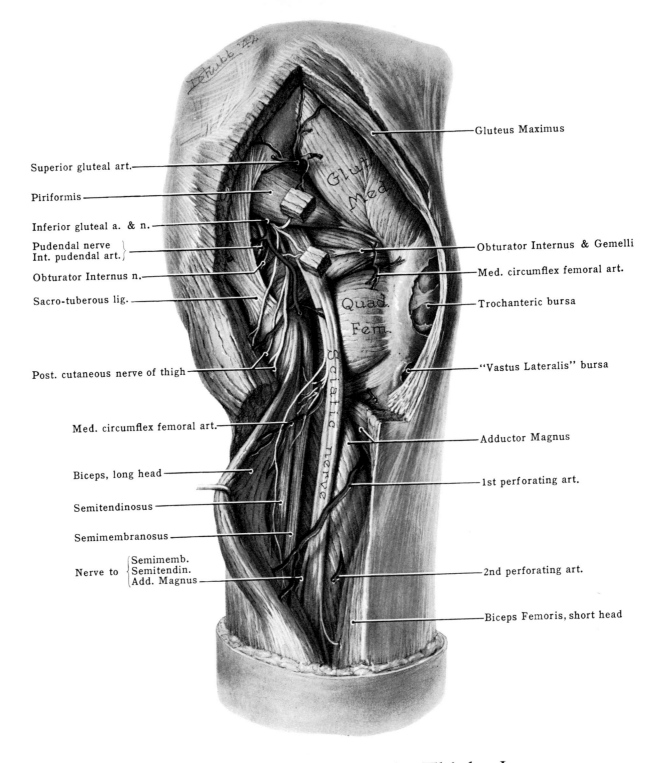

Superior gluteal art.

Piriformis

Inferior gluteal a. & n.

Pudendal nerve
Int. pudendal art.

Obturator Internus n.

Sacro-tuberous lig.

Post. cutaneous nerve of thigh

Med. circumflex femoral art.

Biceps, long head

Semitendinosus

Semimembranosus

Nerve to { Semimemb.
Semitendin.
Add. Magnus

Gluteus Maximus

Glut Med

Quad. Fem.

Sciatic nerve

Obturator Internus & Gemelli

Med. circumflex femoral art.

Trochanteric bursa

"Vastus Lateralis" bursa

Adductor Magnus

1st perforating art.

2nd perforating art.

Biceps Femoris, short head

270 Gluteal Region and the Back of the Thigh—I

Gluteus Maximus is split, both above and below, in the direction of its fibres, and the middle part excised, but two cubes remain to identify its nerve.

Observe:

1. Gluteus Maximus is the only muscle to cover the greater trochanter. It is aponeurotic where it plays on the trochanter and the aponeurosis of Vastus Lateralis, and has underlying bursae.

2. The nerve (inf. gluteal n.) enters Gluteus Maximus in two chief branches near its centre.

3. Above Piriformis is Gluteus Medius, which covers Gluteus Minimus (fig. 271).

4. The sciatic nerve appears below Piriformis and crosses in turn:—dorsum ischii, Obturator Internus and Gemelli, Quadratus Femoris, and Adductor Magnus. Its branches spring from its medial side at variable levels to supply the hams and part of Adductor Magnus. Only the branch to Biceps (short head) springs (usually low down) from its lateral side, which, therefore, is the safer side to dissect on.

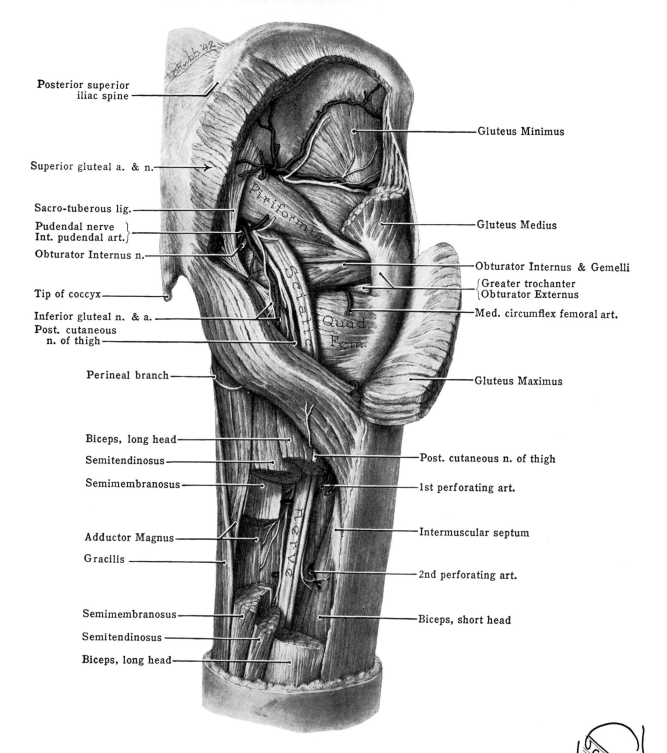

Posterior superior iliac spine

Superior gluteal a. & n.

Sacro-tuberous lig.

Pudendal nerve
Int. pudendal art.

Obturator Internus n.

Tip of coccyx

Inferior gluteal n. & a.
Post. cutaneous n. of thigh

Perineal branch

Biceps, long head

Semitendinosus

Semimembranosus

Adductor Magnus

Gracilis

Semimembranosus

Semitendinosus

Biceps, long head

Gluteus Minimus

Piriformis

Sciatic

Quad. Fem.

nerve

Gluteus Medius

Obturator Internus & Gemelli

Greater trochanter
Obturator Externus

Med. circumflex femoral art.

Gluteus Maximus

Post. cutaneous n. of thigh

1st perforating art.

Intermuscular septum

2nd perforating art.

Biceps, short head

271   Gluteal Region and the Back of the Thigh—II

The upper three quarters of Gluteus Maximus is reflected, and parts of Gluteus
Medius and the three ham muscles are excised.

Observe:

1. The superior gluteal vessels and nerve appearing above Piriformis; all other vessels and
nerves appearing below it.

2. There are no nerves and no vessels of importance lateral to the sciatic nerve.

3. The horizontal groove (the natal fold) crossing the lower border of Gluteus Maximus
indicates the upper limit of the sleeve-like deep fascia of the thigh.

4. Gluteus Maximus consisting of bundles of parallel fibres. It is rhomboidal and the deep
fascia covering it is thin. Gluteus Medius arising in part from the covering deep fascia
which, therefore, is strong and thick. It is fan-shaped.

5. The sciatic nerve is accessible deep in the angle between the lower border of Gluteus Maximus and the lateral border of the long head of Biceps.

Sciatic nerve

271.1

Diagram. Exaggerated to show
that the sciatic nerve is most
readily accessible in the angle deep
to Gluteus Maximus and Long
head of Biceps. Check with fig. 271.

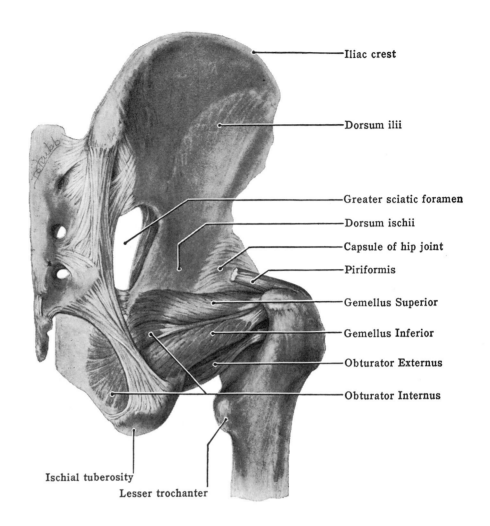

- Iliac crest
- Dorsum ilii
- Greater sciatic foramen
- Dorsum ischii
- Capsule of hip joint
- Piriformis
- Gemellus Superior
- Gemellus Inferior
- Obturator Externus
- Obturator Internus
- Ischial tuberosity
- Lesser trochanter

272 Obturator Muscles, from behind

Observe:

1. Obturator Internus and Gemelli fill the gap between Piriformis above and Quadratus Femoris below. (Origin, within pelvis (fig. 216.)
2. Obturator Externus passing obliquely, below neck of femur, to its insertion. (Origin, see figs. 274 & 276.)

   Note:—The lower end of the ischial tuberosity is on the level of the lesser trochanter.

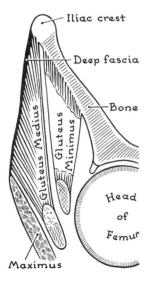

- Iliac crest
- Deep fascia
- Bone
- Gluteus Medius
- Gluteus Minimus
- Head of Femur
- Maximus

272.1

Tracing. The most anterior part of Gluteus Medius has but little bone available to it (fig. 284), so it uses extensively, as an aponeurosis, the deep fascia covering it.

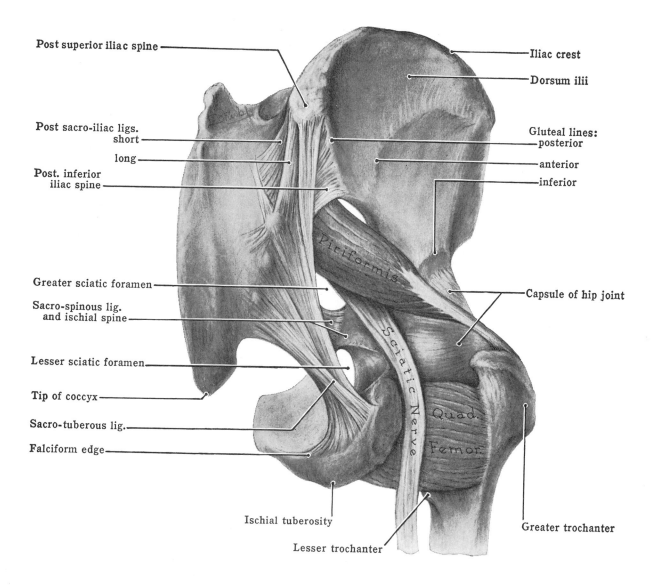

Post superior iliac spine

Iliac crest

Dorsum ilii

Post sacro-iliac ligs.
short

long

Post. inferior
iliac spine

Gluteal lines:
posterior

anterior

inferior

Piriformis

Greater sciatic foramen

Sacro-spinous lig.
and ischial spine

Lesser sciatic foramen

Capsule of hip joint

Sciatic Nerve

Tip of coccyx

Sacro-tuberous lig.

Falciform edge

Quad.

Femor.

Ischial tuberosity

Greater trochanter

Lesser trochanter

273 Bony and Ligamentous Parts of Gluteal Region: Certain Landmarks

Observe:

1. The tip of the coccyx lies above the level of the ischial tuberosity and below that of the ischial spine.

2. The lower border of Piriformis is defined by joining the midpoint between the tip of the coccyx and the posterior superior iliac spine to the top of the greater trochanter.

3. The lower border of Quadratus Femoris is level with the lower end of the ischial tuberosity and it crosses the lesser trochanter.

4. The lateral border of the sciatic nerve lies midway between the lateral surface of the greater trochanter and the medial surface of the ischial tuberosity, provided the body is in the ana-tomical posture—toes pointing forward.

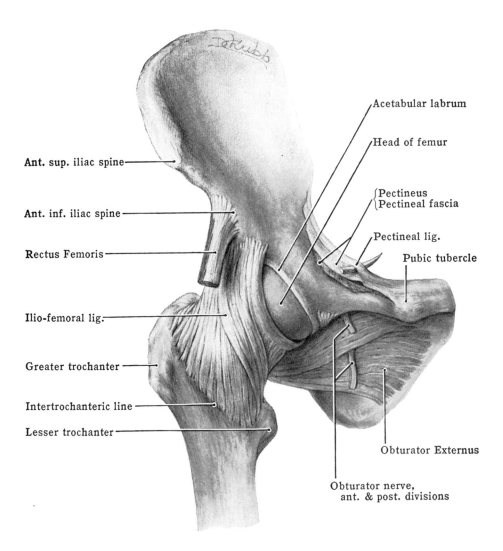

Acetabular labrum

Head of femur

Ant. sup. iliac spine

{ Pectineus
{ Pectineal fascia

Ant. inf. iliac spine

Pectineal lig.

Rectus Femoris

Pubic tubercle

Ilio-femoral lig.

Greater trochanter

Intertrochanteric line

Lesser trochanter

Obturator Externus

Obturator nerve,
ant. & post. divisions

274 Hip Joint, from the front

Observe:

1. The head of the femur exposed just medial to the ilio-femoral lig. and facing not only upwards and medially, but also forwards. Here, at the site of the Psoas bursa, the capsule is weak or, as in this specimen, partially deficient, but it is guarded by the Psoas tendon.

2. The ilio-femoral lig., shaped like an inverted Y, attached above deep to Rectus Femoris, and so directed as to become taut on medial rotation of the femur (figs. 276 and 276.I).

3. Obturator Externus crossing obliquely below the neck of the femur (see fig. 272).

4. The thinness of Pectineus; and its fascia blending with the pectineal ligament (Cooper's lig.) along the pecten pubis (pectineal line).

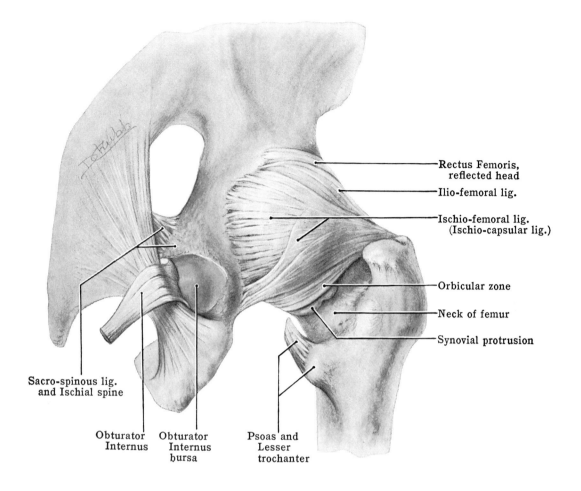

Rectus Femoris,
reflected head

Ilio-femoral lig.

Ischio-femoral lig.
(Ischio-capsular lig.)

Orbicular zone

Neck of femur

Synovial protrusion

Sacro-spinous lig.
and Ischial spine

Obturator
Internus

Obturator
Internus
bursa

Psoas and
Lesser
trochanter

275 Hip Joint, from behind

Observe:

1. The fibres of the capsule so directed spirally as to become taut during extension and medial rotation of the femur.

2. The fibres crossing the neck posteriorly, but not attached to it; indeed, the synovial membrane protrudes below the fibrous capsule and there forms a bursa for the tendon of Obturator Externus.

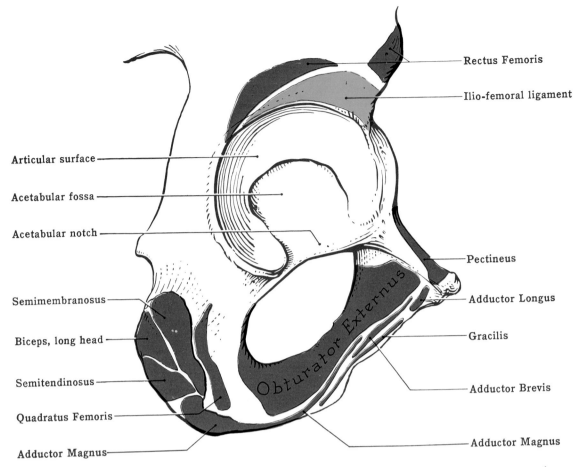

Rectus Femoris

Ilio-femoral ligament

Articular surface

Acetabular fossa

Acetabular notch

Pectineus

Semimembranosus

Adductor Longus

Biceps, long head

Gracilis

Obturator Externus

Semitendinosus

Adductor Brevis

Quadratus Femoris

Adductor Magnus

Adductor Magnus

276   Acetabular Region: Origins of Neighbouring Muscles

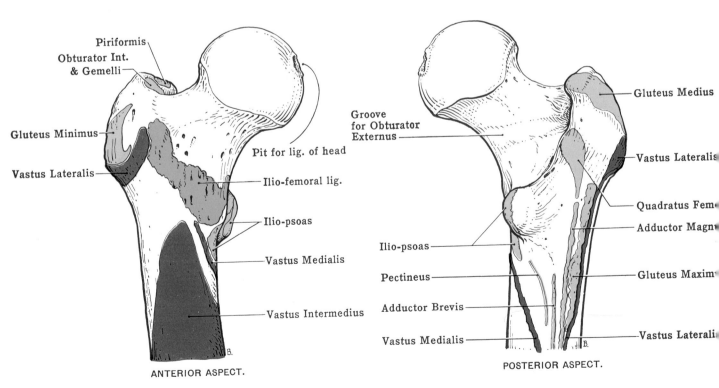

Piriformis
Obturator Int.
& Gemelli

Gluteus Medius

Gluteus Minimus

Vastus Lateralis

Pit for lig. of head

Vastus Lateralis

Ilio-femoral lig.

Groove
for Obturator
Externus

Ilio-psoas

Quadratus Fem

Vastus Medialis

Adductor Magn

Ilio-psoas

Vastus Intermedius

Gluteus Maxim

Pectineus

Adductor Brevis

Vastus Medialis

Vastus Laterali

ANTERIOR ASPECT.

POSTERIOR ASPECT.

276.1   Upper End of Femur showing Attachments of Muscles

277 Hip Bone in Youth, external aspect

The three elements of the hip bone meet in the acetabulum at a tri-radiate synchondrosis. Of these, the pubis contributes least to the acetabulum, the ilium next least, and the ischium most, including the non-articular part.

Secondary centres of ossification appear:— (a) along the whole length of the iliac crest (attachment of the 3 flat abdominal muscles); (b) at the anterior inferior spine (origin of Rectus Femoris); (c) at the ischial tuberosity (origin of the ham muscles); and also (d) at the symphysis pubis, hence the wavy surfaces.

These appear about puberty. Fusion may start as early as the 17th or 18th year; complete fusion is never delayed beyond the 23rd year (McK. & S.).

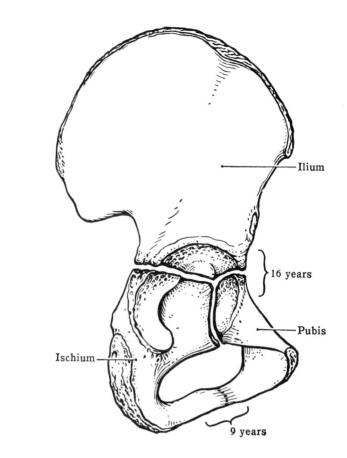

278 Consolidation of the Acetabulum: The Os Acetabuli

One or more centres of ossification appear in the triradiate cartilage of the acetabulum about the 12th year. One of these, the os acetabuli, extends widely over the acetabular surface of the pubic bone.

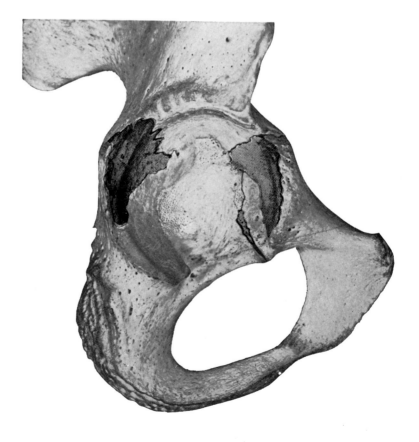

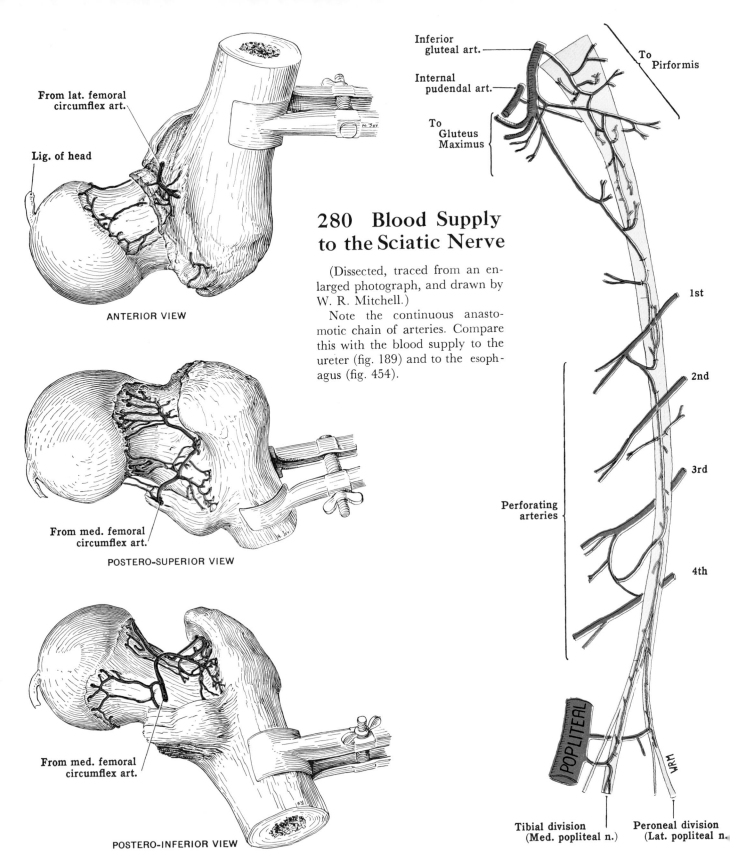

From lat. femoral circumflex art.

Lig. of head

ANTERIOR VIEW

From med. femoral circumflex art.

POSTERO-SUPERIOR VIEW

From med. femoral circumflex art.

POSTERO-INFERIOR VIEW

Inferior gluteal art.

Internal pudendal art.

To Pirformis

To Gluteus Maximus

1st

2nd

3rd

4th

Perforating arteries

POPLITEAL

WRM

Tibial division (Med. popliteal n.)

Peroneal division (Lat. popliteal n.)

280 Blood Supply to the Sciatic Nerve

(Dissected, traced from an enlarged photograph, and drawn by W. R. Mitchell.)

Note the continuous anastomotic chain of arteries. Compare this with the blood supply to the ureter (fig. 189) and to the esophagus (fig. 454).

279 Blood Supply to the Head of the Femur

Note:—

The head receives 3 sets of arteries:—(a) the never-failing and main set of 3 or 4 ascends in the synovial retinacula on the postero-superior and postero-inferior parts of the neck, to perforate just distal to the head, bend at 45° towards its centre, and anastomose freely with (b) terminal branches of the medullary artery of the shaft, and in 80% of cases with (c) the artery of the lig. of the head. This last artery enters the head only when the centre of ossification has extended to the pit for the lig. of the head (12th to 14th year). This anastomosis persists even in advanced age; but in 20% it is never established. (Wolcott.)

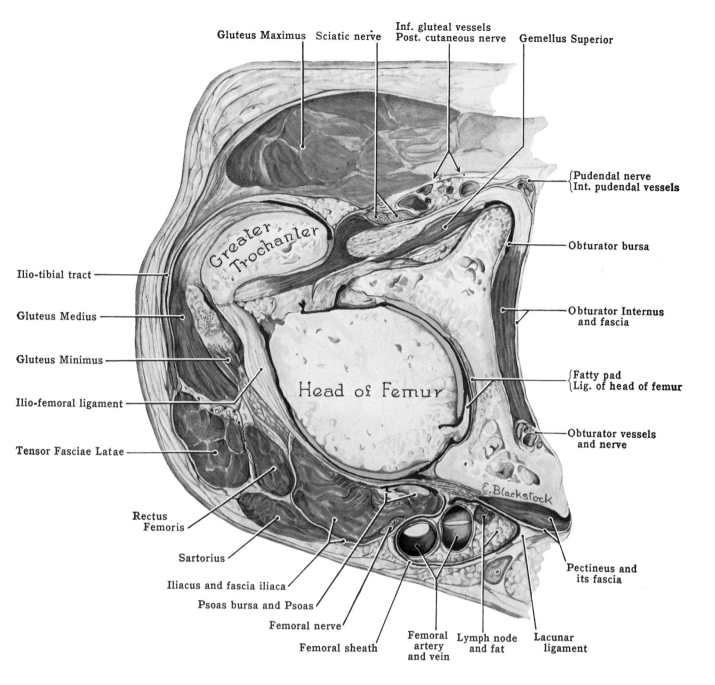

Gluteus Maximus Sciatic nerve

Inf. gluteal vessels
Post. cutaneous nerve Gemellus Superior

Pudendal nerve
Int. pudendal vessels

Obturator bursa

Obturator Internus
and fascia

Fatty pad
Lig. of head of femur

Obturator vessels
and nerve

Pectineus and
its fascia

Ilio-tibial tract

Gluteus Medius

Gluteus Minimus

Ilio-femoral ligament

Tensor Fasciae Latae

Greater Trochanter

Head of Femur

E. Blackstock

Rectus
Femoris

Sartorius

Iliacus and fascia iliaca

Psoas bursa and Psoas

Femoral nerve

Femoral sheath

Femoral
artery
and vein

Lymph node
and fat

Lacunar
ligament

281 Transverse Section through the Thigh at the Level of the Hip Joint

Observe:

1. The articular cartilage spread unevenly over the head of the femur.
2. The fibrous capsule of the joint to be very thick where forming the ilio-femoral ligament, and thin dorsal to the Psoas tendon, the Psoas bursa here intervening.
3. The femoral sheath, which encloses the femoral artery, vein, lymph node, lymph vessels and fat, to be free except posteriorly where, between Psoas and Pectineus, it is attached to the capsule of the hip joint.
4. The femoral artery separated from the joint by the tough Psoas tendon; the vein at the interval between Psoas and Pectineus; the lymph node anterior to Pectineus. The femoral nerve lying between Iliacus and fascia Iliaca.
5. The two cusps of the valve in the femoral vein so placed that pressure on the skin surface closes the valve. (For data on valves, see fig. 255.)
6. The sciatic nerve descending between Gluteus Maximus and the short lateral rotators of the femur.

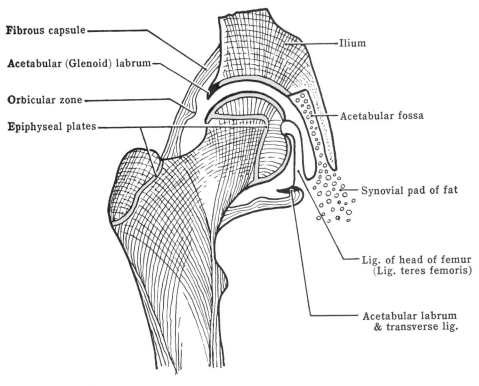

Fibrous capsule

Acetabular (Glenoid) labrum

Orbicular zone

Epiphyseal plates

Ilium

Acetabular fossa

Synovial pad of fat

Lig. of head of femur
(Lig. teres femoris)

Acetabular labrum
& transverse lig.

282 Hip Joint on Coronal Section, partly schematic

Observe:

1. The bony trabeculae of the ilium projecte⊙ into the head of the femur as lines of pres⊙ sure and the trabeculae that cross these a⊙ lines of tension.

2. The epiphysis of the head of the femur, en⊙ tirely within the capsule of the joint.

3. The lig. of the head of the femur, as ⊙ synovial tube that is fixed above at the pi⊙ (fovea) on the head of the femur and ope⊙ below at the acetabular foramen where it i⊙ continuous with the synovial membran⊙ covering the fat in the acetabular fossa an⊙ also with the synovial membrane coverin⊙ the transverse ligament (fig. 284).

4. The ligament of the head, obviously be⊙ comes taut during adduction of the hi⊙ joint, as when crossing the legs.

5. The fluid fat below the joint can be sucke⊙ into the acetabular fossa during flexion⊙

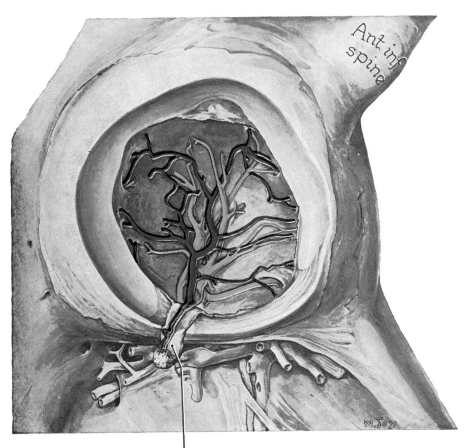

Ant. inf.
spine

Lig. of head
of femur

283 Blood Vessels of the Acetabular Fossa

Prepared by Dr. K. O. McCuaig.

The acetabular branches (an artery a⊙ a vein) of the posterior division of t⊙ obturator vessels pass through the ac⊙ tabular foramen and enter the acetabul⊙ fossa where they ramify in the fatty-areol⊙ tissue. The branches, mostly in pairs (⊙ artery and a vein) radiate to the marg⊙ of the fossa where they enter nutrie⊙ foramina. One pair runs through t⊙ ligament of the head of the femur to t⊙ head. Twigs supply the fat.

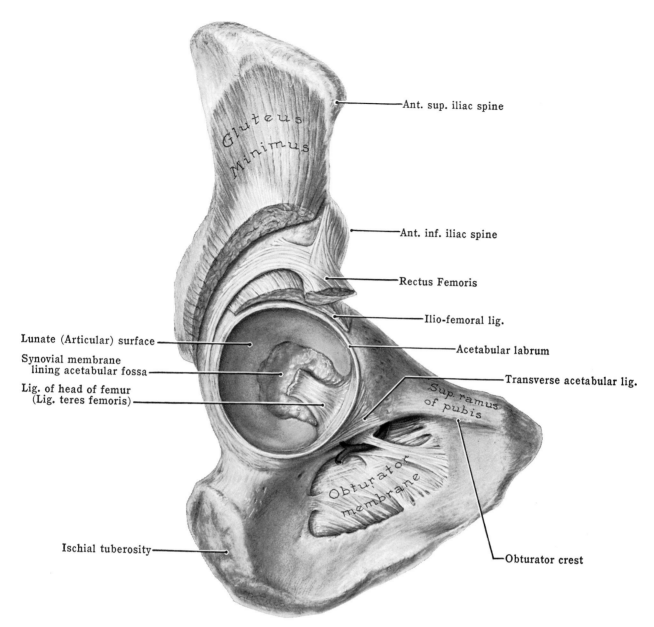

Ant. sup. iliac spine

Ant. inf. iliac spine

Rectus Femoris

Ilio-femoral lig.

Lunate (Articular) surface

Acetabular labrum

Synovial membrane
lining acetabular fossa

Transverse acetabular lig.

Lig. of head of femur
(Lig. teres femoris)

Sup. ramus of pubis

Obturator membrane

Ischial tuberosity

Obturator crest

284   Socket for the Head of the Femur

Observe:

1. The transverse acetabular ligament (whose fibres decussate like the limbs of a St. Andrew's cross) converting the acetabular notch into the acetabular foramen.

2. The acetabular labrum, attached to the acetabular rim and to the transverse ligament. It forms a complete ring around the head of the femur beyond its equator.

3. The articular or lunate surface.

4. The synovial membrane attached to the margin of the articular cartilage and covering the pad of fat and the vessels in the acetabular fossa.

5. The ligament of the head of the femur, which is a hollow cone of synovial membrane compressed between the head of the femur and its socket. It resembles a collapsed bell tent. It envelops ligamentous fibres; these are attached above to the pit on the head of the femur, and below to the transverse ligament and the margins of the acetabular notch. Through it passes the artery to the head of the femur (fig. 283).

6. Gluteus Minimus which, being a medial rotator as well as an abductor of the hip joint, is thickest in front. It covers the two heads of Rectus femoris which in turn cover, and are nearly co-extensive with, the attachment of the ilio-femoral ligament. (fig. 276).

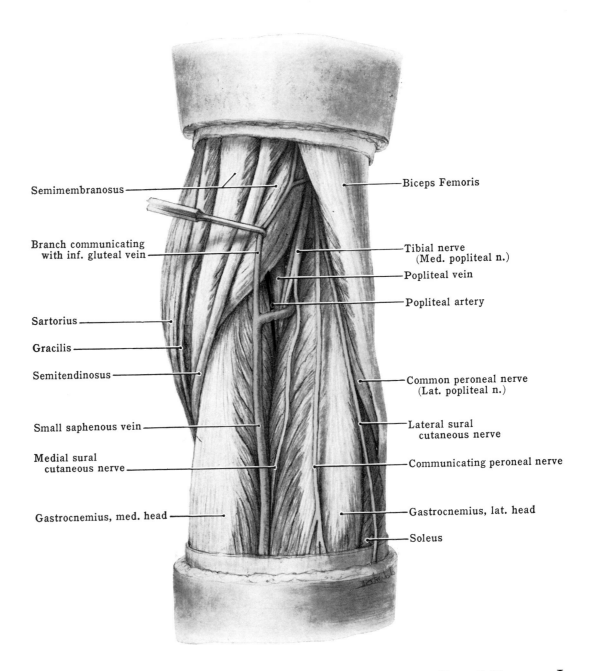

Semimembranosus

Branch communicating with inf. gluteal vein

Sartorius

Gracilis

Semitendinosus

Small saphenous vein

Medial sural cutaneous nerve

Gastrocnemius, med. head

Biceps Femoris

Tibial nerve (Med. popliteal n.)

Popliteal vein

Popliteal artery

Common peroneal nerve (Lat. popliteal n.)

Lateral sural cutaneous nerve

Communicating peroneal nerve

Gastrocnemius, lat. head

Soleus

285 Superficial Dissection of the Popliteal Fossa—I

Observe:

1. The two heads of Gastrocnemius, embraced on the medial side by Semimembranosus, which is overlaid by Semitendinosus, and on the lateral side by Biceps. The result is the lozenge-shaped popliteal fossa.

2. The small saphenous vein running between the two heads of Gastrocnemius. Deep to this vein is the medial sural cutaneous nerve which, followed proximally, leads to the tibial nerve. The tibial nerve is superficial to the popliteal vein, which in turn is superficial to the popliteal artery.

3. The common peroneal nerve following the posterior border of Biceps, and here giving off two cutaneous branches. (See cutaneous nerves, fig. 249).

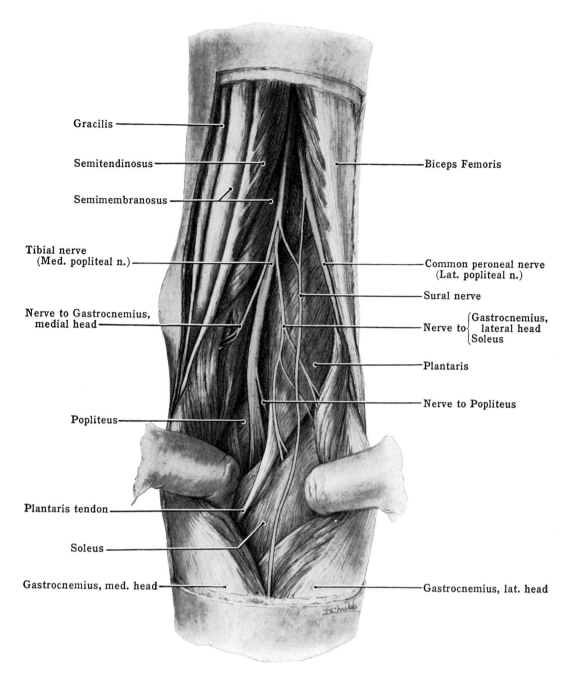

Gracilis

Semitendinosus

Semimembranosus

Tibial nerve
(Med. popliteal n.)

Nerve to Gastrocnemius,
medial head

Popliteus

Plantaris tendon

Soleus

Gastrocnemius, med. head

Biceps Femoris

Common peroneal nerve
(Lat. popliteal n.)

Sural nerve

Nerve to {Gastrocnemius,
          lateral head
          Soleus

Plantaris

Nerve to Popliteus

Gastrocnemius, lat. head

286 Nerves of the Popliteal Fossa—II

The two heads of Gastrocnemius are pulled forcibly apart.

Observe:

1. A cutaneous branch of the tibial nerve joining a cutaneous branch of the common peroneal nerve to form the sural nerve. Here the junction is very high—usually it is two or three inches above the ankle.

2. All motor branches in this region springing from the tibial nerve, one branch coming from its medial side, the others from its lateral side. Hence, it is safer to dissect on the medial side.

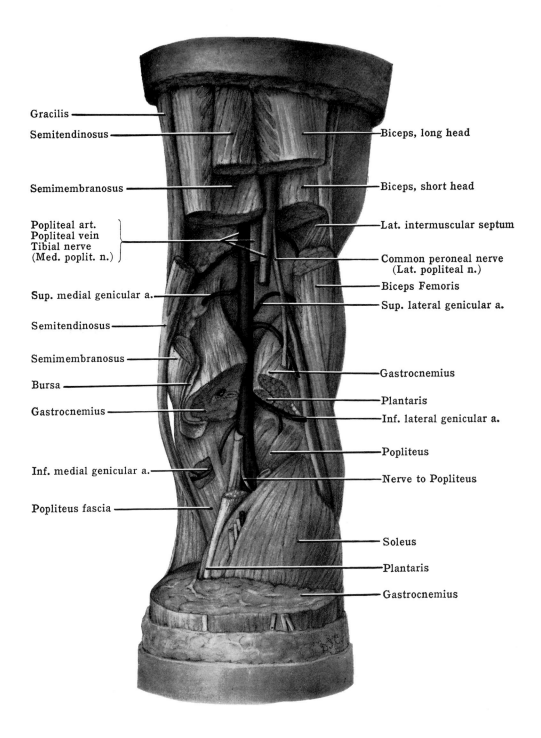

Gracilis

Semitendinosus

Semimembranosus

Popliteal art.
Popliteal vein
Tibial nerve
(Med. poplit. n.)

Sup. medial genicular a.

Semitendinosus

Semimembranosus

Bursa

Gastrocnemius

Inf. medial genicular a.

Popliteus fascia

Biceps, long head

Biceps, short head

Lat. intermuscular septum

Common peroneal nerve
(Lat. popliteal n.)

Biceps Femoris

Sup. lateral genicular a.

Gastrocnemius

Plantaris

Inf. lateral genicular a.

Popliteus

Nerve to Popliteus

Soleus

Plantaris

Gastrocnemius

287 Step Dissection of the Popliteal Fossa—III

Observe:

1. The thickness of the various muscles.

2. The popliteal artery lying on the floor of the fossa (i.e. femur, capsule of joint, Popliteus fascia), much fat intervening, and giving off genicular branches which also lie on the floor, and ending by bifurcating into the anterior and the posterior tibial artery at the upper border of Soleus.

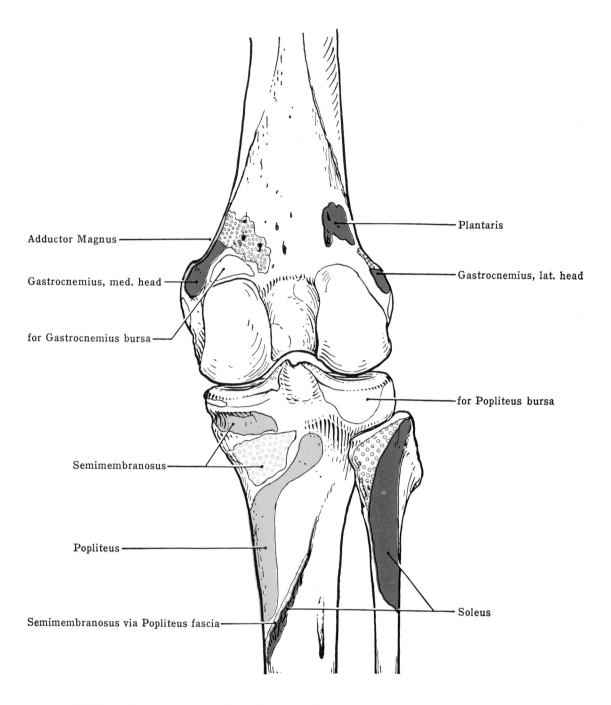

Adductor Magnus

Gastrocnemius, med. head

for Gastrocnemius bursa

Semimembranosus

Popliteus

Semimembranosus via Popliteus fascia

Plantaris

Gastrocnemius, lat. head

for Popliteus bursa

Soleus

**288   Bones of the Knee Joint showing
Attachments of Muscles, from behind—IV**

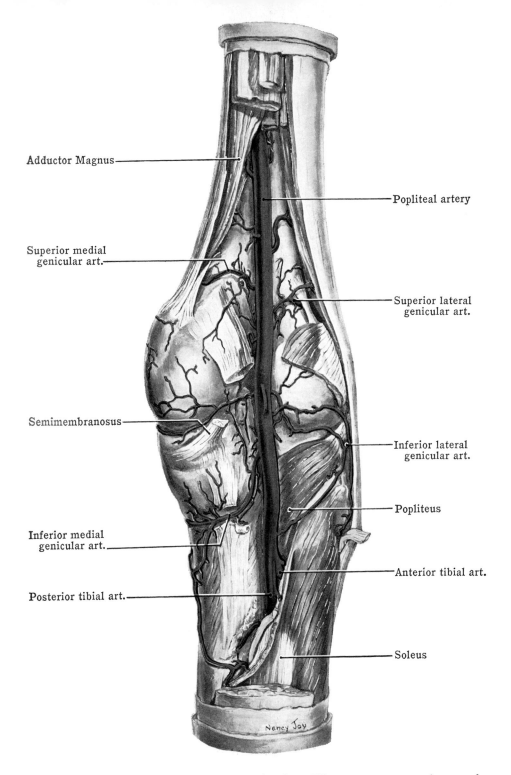

Adductor Magnus

Popliteal artery

Superior medial
genicular art.

Superior lateral
genicular art.

Semimembranosus

Inferior lateral
genicular art.

Popliteus

Inferior medial
genicular art.

Anterior tibial art.

Posterior tibial art.

Soleus

Nancy Joy

289 Anastomoses around the Knee, posterior view

Latex injection. *Dissection by Dr. J. S. Simpson.*

Observe:

1. The popliteal artery throughout its course, from the hiatus in Adductor Magnus proximally to the lower border of Popliteus distally (or, if you prefer, to the upper border of Soleus), where it bifurcates into the anterior and posterior tibial arteries.

2. The 3 ventral relations of the artery:—(a) femur (fat intervening), (b) capsule of the joint, and (c) Popliteus (covered with popliteus fascia).

3. The 4 named genicular branches that hug the skeletal plane, nothing intervening except the popliteus tendon which the inferior lateral genicular artery must cross. (The median genicular art. is not in view.)

4. An unnamed genicular artery arising on each side.

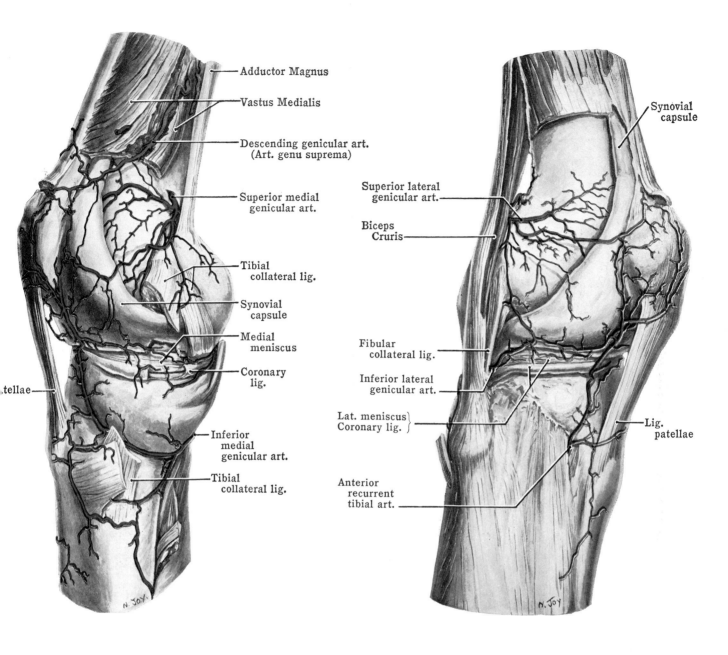

Adductor Magnus

Vastus Medialis

Descending genicular art.
(Art. genu suprema)

Superior medial
genicular art.

Tibial
collateral lig.

Synovial
capsule

Medial
meniscus

Coronary
lig.

tellae

Inferior
medial
genicular art.

Tibial
collateral lig.

Synovial
capsule

Superior lateral
genicular art.

Biceps
Cruris

Fibular
collateral lig.

Inferior lateral
genicular art.

Lat. meniscus
Coronary lig.

Lig.
patellae

Anterior
recurrent
tibial art.

290 Antero-medial view   **291 Antero-lateral view**

Anastomoses around the Knee

Observe:

1. Two named genicular branches of the popliteal artery, on each side—a superior and an inferior.

2. Three supplementary arteries:—(a) descending genicular branch of the femoral artery, supero-medially; (b) descending branch of lateral femoral circumflex artery, supero-laterally (fig. 244); and (c) anterior recurrent branch of anterior tibial artery, infero-laterally (fig. 306).

3. The inferior lateral genicular artery running along the lateral meniscus; an unnamed artery running similarly along the medial meniscus.

292 Cruciate Ligaments

In each illustration one half of the femur is removed with the proximal part of the corresponding cruciate ligament.

Observe:

1. The posterior cruciate ligament, which prevents forward sliding of the femur, particularly when the knee is flexed.
2. The anterior cruciate ligament, which prevents backward sliding of the femur and hyperextension of the knee, and limits medial rotation of the femur when the foot is on the ground—i.e., when the leg is fixed.

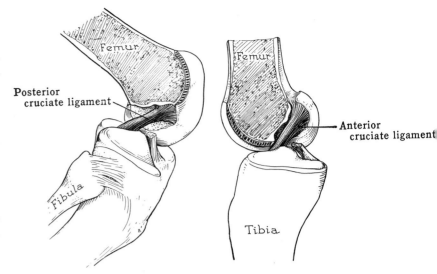

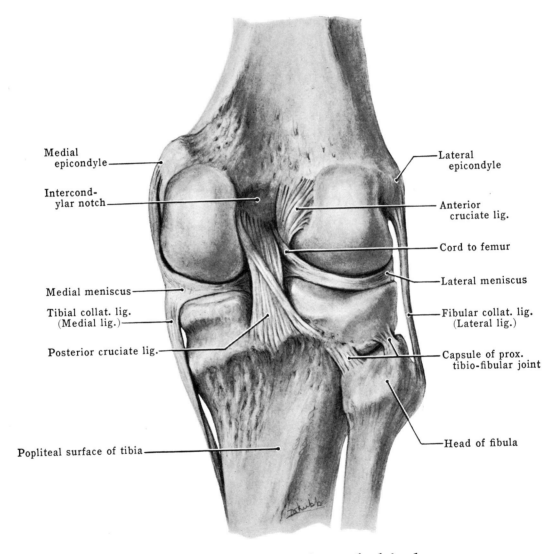

293 Ligaments of the Knee Joint, from behind

Observe:

1. The bandlike medial ligament attached to the medial meniscus (semilunar cartilage). The cordlike lateral ligament separated from the lateral meniscus by the width of the Popliteus tendon (removed).

2. The posterior cruciate ligament joined by a cord from the lateral meniscus and passing to the fore part of the medial condyle of the femur. The anterior cruciate ligament attached to the hinder part of the lateral condyle.

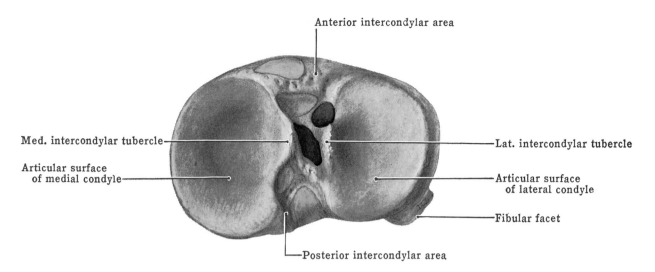

Anterior intercondylar area

Med. intercondylar tubercle

Articular surface
of medial condyle

Lat. intercondylar tubercle

Articular surface
of lateral condyle

Fibular facet

Posterior intercondylar area

Superior Aspect of the Proximal End of the Tibia

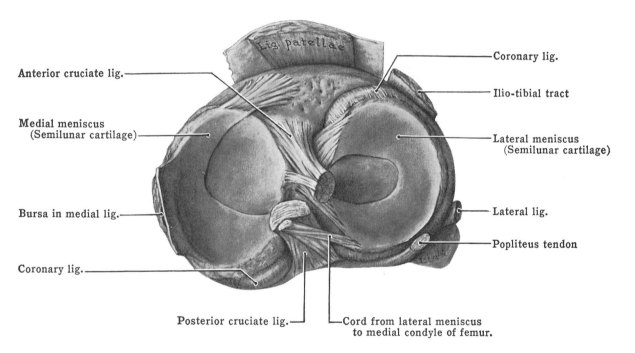

Lig. patellae

Anterior cruciate lig.

Coronary lig.

Ilio-tibial tract

Medial meniscus
(Semilunar cartilage)

Lateral meniscus
(Semilunar cartilage)

Bursa in medial lig.

Lateral lig.

Popliteus tendon

Coronary lig.

Posterior cruciate lig.

Cord from lateral meniscus
to medial condyle of femur.

294 Cruciate Ligaments and the Menisci (Semilunar Cartilages)

The sites of attachment of the cruciate ligaments are coloured yellow; those of the medial meniscus, blue; and those of the lateral meniscus, red.

Of the tibial condyles, the lateral is flatter, shorter from front to back, and more circular; the medial is concave, longer from front to back, and more oval.

The menisci are cartilaginous and tough where compressed between femur and tibia, but ligamentous and pliable at their attachments—as is the case with other intra-articular fibro-cartilages.

The menisci conform to the shapes of the surfaces on which they rest. Since the horns of the lateral meniscus are attached close together and its coronary ligament is slack, this meniscus can slide forwards and backwards on the (flat) condyle; since the horns of the medial meniscus are attached far apart, its movements on the (concave) condyle are restricted.

Note the bursa between the long and short parts of the medial ligament of the knee.

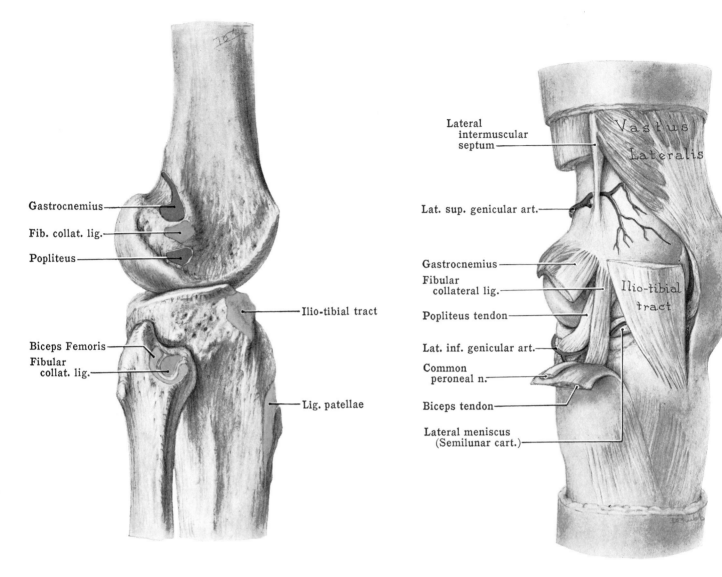

Gastrocnemius

Fib. collat. lig.

Popliteus

Biceps Femoris

Fibular collat. lig.

Ilio-tibial tract

Lig. patellae

Lateral intermuscular septum

Vastus Lateralis

Lat. sup. genicular art.

Gastrocnemius

Fibular collateral lig.

Popliteus tendon

Ilio-tibial tract

Lat. inf. genicular art.

Common peroneal n.

Biceps tendon

Lateral meniscus (Semilunar cart.)

295   Bones of the Knee Joint: Attachments of Muscles and Ligaments, lateral view

296   Dissection of the Knee, lateral aspect

Observe:

1. The ilio-tibial tract intervening between the skin and the synovial membrane and which, by virtue of its toughness, protects this exposed aspect of the joint.
2. The 3 structures that arise from the lateral epicondyle and that are uncovered by reflecting Biceps. Of these, Gastrocnemius is postero-superior; Popliteus is antero-inferior; the fibular collateral lig. is in between, and it crosses superficial to Popliteus.
3. The lateral inferior genicular artery coursing along the lateral meniscus.

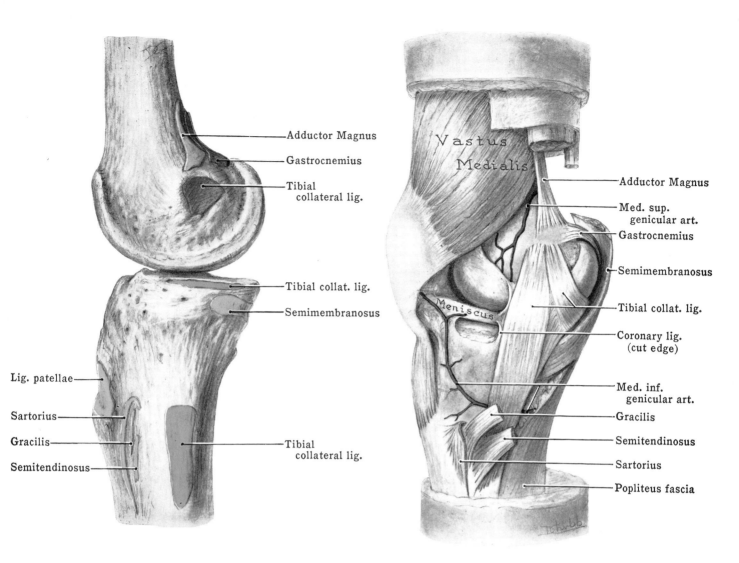

Adductor Magnus

Gastrocnemius

Tibial
collateral lig.

Tibial collat. lig.

Semimembranosus

Lig. patellae

Sartorius

Gracilis

Semitendinosus

Tibial
collateral lig.

*Vastus
Medialis*

Adductor Magnus

Med. sup.
genicular art.

Gastrocnemius

Semimembranosus

Tibial collat. lig.

Coronary lig.
(cut edge)

Meniscus

Med. inf.
genicular art.

Gracilis

Semitendinosus

Sartorius

Popliteus fascia

297   Bones of the Knee Joint
Attachments of Muscles and
Ligaments, medial view

298   Dissection of the Knee,
medial aspect

Note: The band-like part of the tibial collateral ligament of the knee: attached to the medial
epicondyle; almost in line with Adductor Magnus tendon; crossing the insertion of Semimembranosus; crossing the medial inferior genicular artery; and crossed by the tendons of 3 medial
rotators (Sartorius, Gracilis, Semitendinosus), each of which is supplied by a different nerve
(femoral, obturator, sciatic) (fig. 262).

298.1

Articularis Genus, (or deepest muscular
bands of Vastus Intermedius), is inserted
into the synovial capsule, which it retracts during extension of the knee joint.

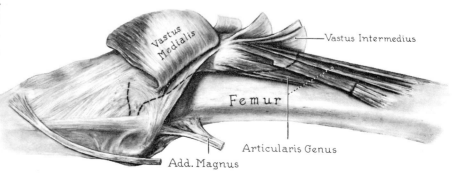

*Vastus
Medialis*

Vastus Intermedius

Femur

Add. Magnus

Articularis Genus

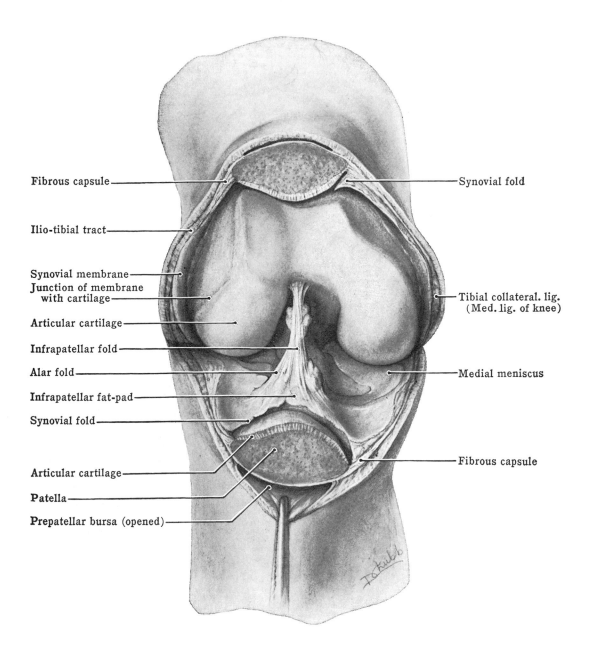

Fibrous capsule

Ilio-tibial tract

Synovial membrane
Junction of membrane
 with cartilage

Articular cartilage

Infrapatellar fold

Alar fold

Infrapatellar fat-pad

Synovial fold

Articular cartilage

Patella

Prepatellar bursa (opened)

Synovial fold

Tibial collateral. lig.
 (Med. lig. of knee)

Medial meniscus

Fibrous capsule

299 Knee Joint, opened from the front

The patella is sawn through; the skin and joint capsule are cut through; and the joint is flexed.

Observe:

1. The articular cartilage of the patella, not of uniform thickness but spread unevenly, as on other bones.
2. The infrapatellar synovial fold resembling a partially collapsed bell-tent whose apex is attached to the intercondylar notch and whose base is below the patella (cf. lig. of the head of femur, fig. 282). The infrapatellar pad of fat is continued into the tent.
3. A fracture of the patella would bring the prepatellar bursa into communication with the joint cavity.
4. Articular cartilage and synovial membrane continuous with each other on the side of the condyle, as in other joints.

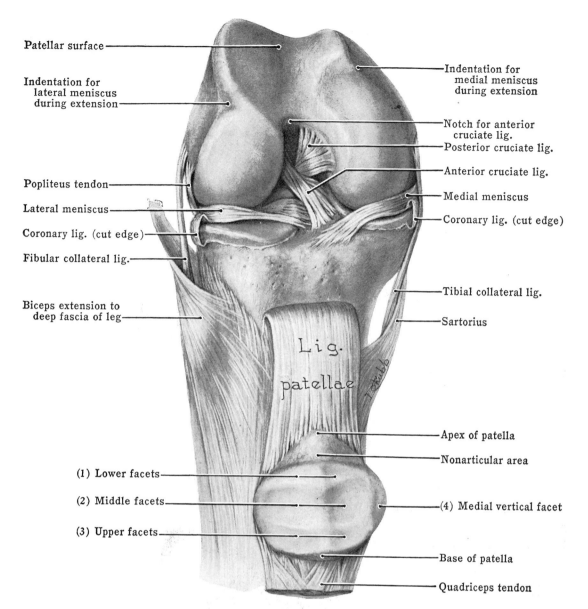

Patellar surface

Indentation for
lateral meniscus
during extension

Popliteus tendon

Lateral meniscus

Coronary lig. (cut edge)

Fibular collateral lig.

Biceps extension to
deep fascia of leg

(1) Lower facets

(2) Middle facets

(3) Upper facets

Indentation for
medial meniscus
during extension

Notch for anterior
cruciate lig.

Posterior cruciate lig.

Anterior cruciate lig.

Medial meniscus

Coronary lig. (cut edge)

Tibial collateral lig.

Sartorius

Apex of patella

Nonarticular area

(4) Medial vertical facet

Base of patella

Quadriceps tendon

Lig. patellae

300 Ligaments of the Knee Joint, front view

The patella is thrown down and the joint is flexed.

Observe:

The indentations on the sides of the femoral condyles at the junction of
the patellar and tibial articular areas. The lateral tibial articular area, shorter
than the medial one.

The subsidiary notch, at the antero-lateral part of the intercondylar notch,
for the reception of the anterior cruciate ligament on full extension.

The three paired facets on the posterior surface of the patella for articulation
with the patellar surface of the femur successively during (1) extension,
(2) slight flexion, (3) flexion; and the most medial facet on the patella
(4) for articulation during full flexion with the crescentic facet that skirts
the medial margin of the intercondylar notch of the femur.

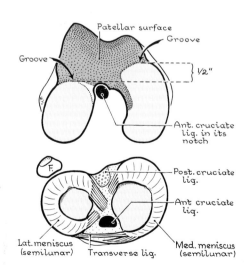

Patellar surface

Groove

Groove

½"

Ant. cruciate
lig. in its
notch

Post. cruciate
lig.

Ant. cruciate
lig.

Lat. meniscus
(semilunar)

Transverse lig.

Med. meniscus
(semilunar)

300.1

Diagram. Articular surfaces of knee joint,
and the menisci. (See text.)

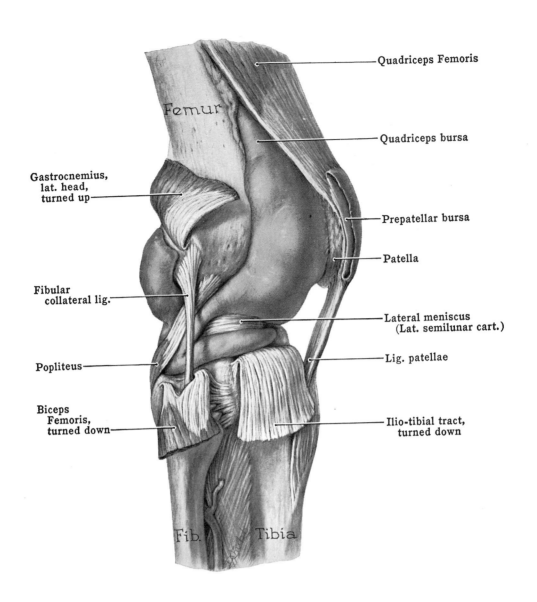

Quadriceps Femoris

Quadriceps bursa

Prepatellar bursa

Patella

Gastrocnemius,
lat. head,
turned up

Lateral meniscus
(Lat. semilunar cart.)

Fibular
collateral lig.

Lig. patellae

Popliteus

Biceps
Femoris,
turned down

Ilio-tibial tract,
turned down

Femur

Fib.   Tibia

301   Distended Knee Joint, lateral view

Latex is injected into the joint cavity and fixed with acetic acid; the distended synovial capsule is exposed and cleaned. Gastrocnemius is thrown up; Biceps and the ilio-tibial tract are thrown down. The latex, in this specimen, has flowed into the proximal tibio-fibular joint cavity.

Observe:

1. The extent of the synovial capsule:—
   (a) Superiorly, it rises about two fingers' breadth above the patella and here rests on a layer of fat which allows it to glide freely in movements of the joint. This upper part, called the suprapatellar (Quadriceps Femoris) bursa, is obviously not a frictional bursa.
   (b) Posteriorly, it rises as high as the origin of Gastrocnemius.
   (c) Laterally, it curves below the lateral femoral epicondyle where popliteus tendon and the fibular collateral ligament are attached.
   (d) Inferiorly, it bulges below the lateral meniscus, overlapping about $\frac{1}{3}''$ of the tibia. The coronary ligament is removed to show this.
2. Biceps and ilio-tibial tract protecting the joint laterally.
3. The prepatellar bursa, here more extensive than usual, more than covering the patella.

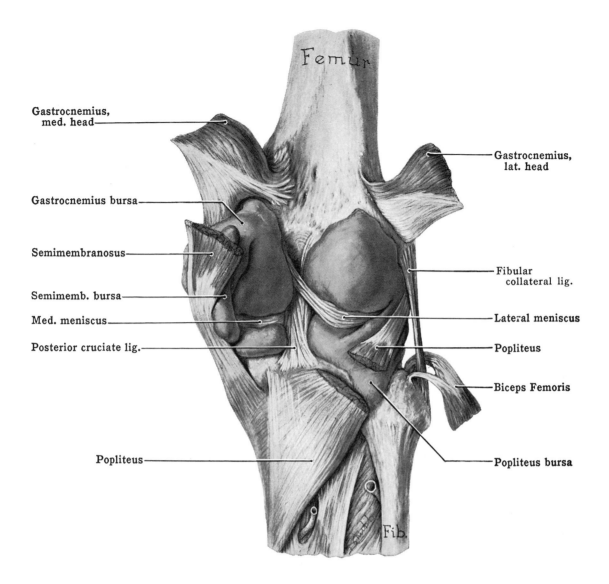

Gastrocnemius, med. head

Gastrocnemius, lat. head

Gastrocnemius bursa

Semimembranosus

Fibular collateral lig.

Semimemb. bursa

Med. meniscus

Lateral meniscus

Posterior cruciate lig.

Popliteus

Biceps Femoris

Popliteus

Popliteus bursa

Femur

Fib.

302   Distended Knee Joint, posterior view

Both heads of Gastrocnemius are thrown up; Biceps is thrown down; and a section is removed from Popliteus.

Observe:

1. The posterior cruciate ligament exposed from behind without opening the synovial capsule [articular cavity].
2. The origins of Gastrocnemius limiting the extent to which the synovial capsule can rise.
3. Semimembranosus bursa here communicating with Gastrocnemius bursa, which in turn communicates with the synovial cavity (as in fig. 287).
4. The Popliteus tendon separated from the lateral meniscus, the upper end of the tibia, and the proximal tibio-fibular joint by an elongated bursa.

    This Popliteus bursa communicates with the synovial cavity of the knee joint both above and below the meniscus, and in this specimen it also communicates with the proximal tibio-fibular synovial cavity, as revealed by figure 301.

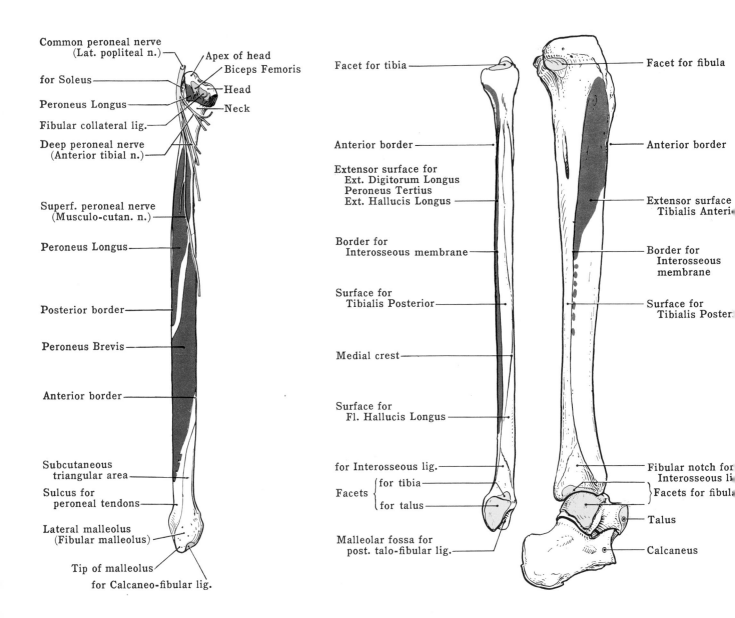

Common peroneal nerve
(Lat. popliteal n.)
Apex of head
Biceps Femoris
for Soleus
Head
Peroneus Longus
Neck
Fibular collateral lig.
Deep peroneal nerve
(Anterior tibial n.)
Superf. peroneal nerve
(Musculo-cutan. n.)
Peroneus Longus
Posterior border
Peroneus Brevis
Anterior border
Subcutaneous
triangular area
Sulcus for
peroneal tendons
Lateral malleolus
(Fibular malleolus)
Tip of malleolus
for Calcaneo-fibular lig.

Facet for tibia
Facet for fibula
Anterior border
Anterior border
Extensor surface for
Ext. Digitorum Longus
Peroneus Tertius
Ext. Hallucis Longus
Extensor surface
Tibialis Anteri●
Border for
Interosseous membrane
Border for
Interosseous
membrane
Surface for
Tibialis Posterior
Surface for
Tibialis Poster●
Medial crest
Surface for
Fl. Hallucis Longus
for Interosseous lig.
Fibular notch for
Interosseous li●
Facets {
for tibia
Facets for fibul●
for talus
Talus
Malleolar fossa for
post. talo-fibular lig.
Calcaneus

303 Lateral Surface of Fibula

Tibia and Fibula, opposed aspec●

Observe:

1. The lateral (or peroneal) surface of the fibula describing a quarter of a spiral, its distal end being grooved and facing posteriorly. This allows the lateral malleolus to act as a pulley for the long and short peroneal tendons.

2. The common peroneal nerve and its terminal branches having long contact with the fibula.

3. On the fibula, 2 small articular facets for the tibia; one proximally and one distally. Below the latter a large tri-

angular facet for articulation with almost the entire depth of the lateral surface of the body of the talus.

4. Interosseous borders of the tibia and fibula, for the attachment of the interosseous membrane, separating the anterior or extensor surface from the posterior or flexor surface. Each of these borders widening below into a triangular area for the interosseous ligament.

5. The extensor surface of the fibula narrow below and almost linear above.

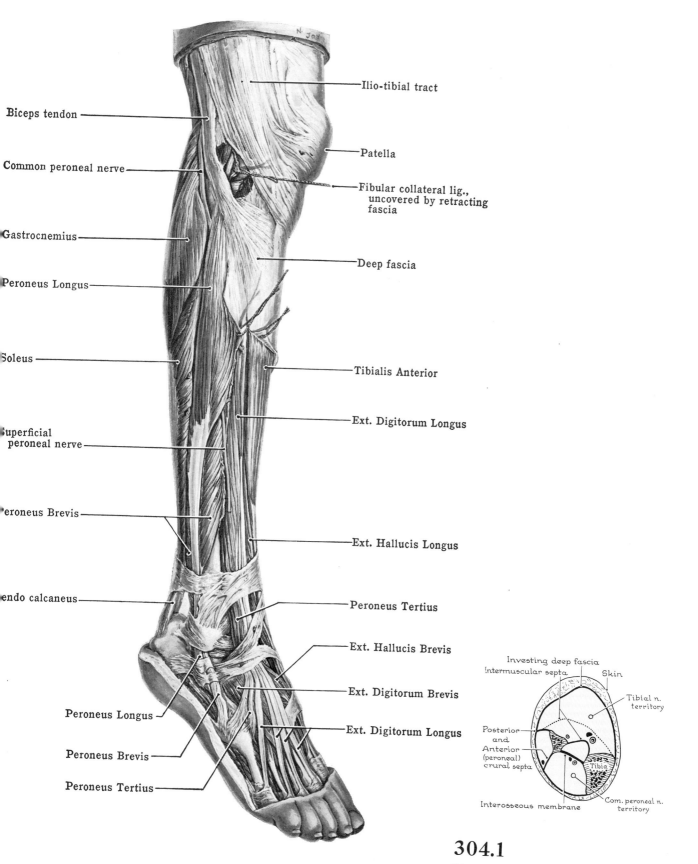

Biceps tendon

Common peroneal nerve

Gastrocnemius

Peroneus Longus

Soleus

Superficial peroneal nerve

Peroneus Brevis

endo calcaneus

Peroneus Longus

Peroneus Brevis

Peroneus Tertius

Ilio-tibial tract

Patella

Fibular collateral lig., uncovered by retracting fascia

Deep fascia

Tibialis Anterior

Ext. Digitorum Longus

Ext. Hallucis Longus

Peroneus Tertius

Ext. Hallucis Brevis

Ext. Digitorum Brevis

Ext. Digitorum Longus

Investing deep fascia
Intermuscular septa
Skin
Tibial n. territory
Posterior and Anterior (peroneal) crural septa
Tibia
Interosseous membrane
Com. peroneal n. territory

304 Muscles of the Leg and Foot, antero-lateral view

304.1

Diagram. Cross section of leg, showing muscles divided into a large dorsal tibial nerve territory and an anterior and lateral common peroneal nerve territory. (For detail, see fig. 310.)

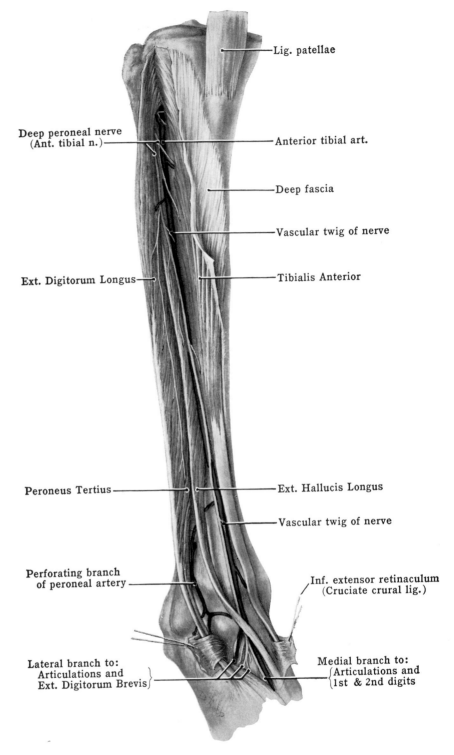

Lig. patellae

Deep peroneal nerve
(Ant. tibial n.)

Anterior tibial art.

Deep fascia

Vascular twig of nerve

Ext. Digitorum Longus

Tibialis Anterior

Peroneus Tertius

Ext. Hallucis Longus

Vascular twig of nerve

Perforating branch
of peroneal artery

Inf. extensor retinaculum
(Cruciate crural lig.)

Lateral branch to:
Articulations and
Ext. Digitorum Brevis

Medial branch to:
Articulations and
1st & 2nd digits

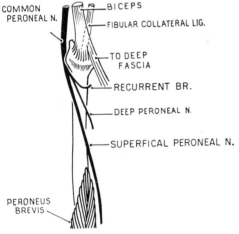

COMMON
PERONEAL N.

BICEPS

FIBULAR COLLATERAL LIG.

TO DEEP
FASCIA

RECURRENT BR.

DEEP PERONEAL N.

SUPERFICAL PERONEAL N.

PERONEUS
BREVIS

305.1

Diagram. The exposed position of the
common peroneal nerve. It is applied
to the back of the head of the fibula (a
film of Soleus intervening); its branches
are applied directly to the neck and
body of the fibula for 3 or 4 inches deep
to Peroneus Longus, as shown in fig.
306.

305 Front of the Leg

The muscles are separated in order to display the artery and nerve.

Observe:

1. Tibialis Anterior, arising in part from the deep fascia which, therefore, is stron[
   longitudinal fibres, and makes sharp the upper part of the anterior border of the[

2. Peroneus Tertius being merely the lower part of Ext. Digitorum Longus.   H[
   Longus extending farther proximally than usual. These three muscles are unipe[
   and arise from the fibula.

3. The vascular and articular branches of the deep peroneal nerve.

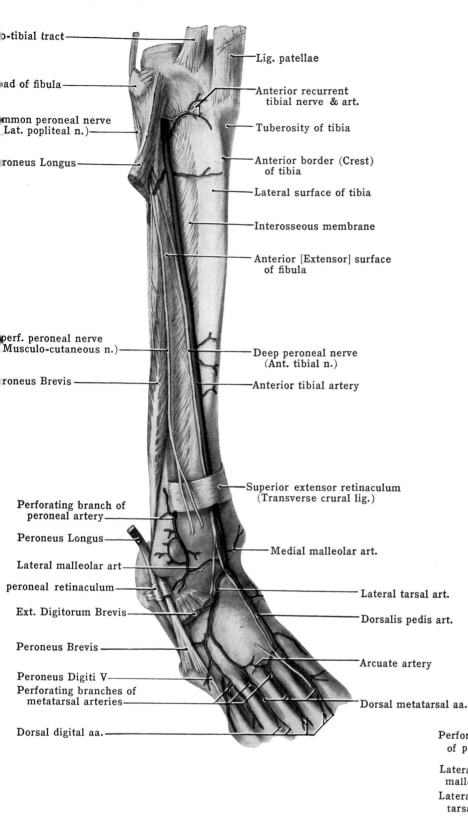

Ilio-tibial tract

Head of fibula

Common peroneal nerve
(Lat. popliteal n.)

Peroneus Longus

Superf. peroneal nerve
(Musculo-cutaneous n.)

Peroneus Brevis

Lig. patellae

Anterior recurrent
tibial nerve & art.

Tuberosity of tibia

Anterior border (Crest)
of tibia

Lateral surface of tibia

Interosseous membrane

Anterior [Extensor] surface
of fibula

Deep peroneal nerve
(Ant. tibial n.)

Anterior tibial artery

Superior extensor retinaculum
(Transverse crural lig.)

Perforating branch of
peroneal artery

Peroneus Longus

Lateral malleolar art.

peroneal retinaculum

Ext. Digitorum Brevis

Peroneus Brevis

Peroneus Digiti V
Perforating branches of
metatarsal arteries

Dorsal digital aa.

Medial malleolar art.

Lateral tarsal art.

Dorsalis pedis art.

Arcuate artery

Dorsal metatarsal aa.

306 Arteries and Nerves of the Front and Dorsum of Foot

The anterior crural muscles are removed and Peroneus Longus is excised.

Observe:

1. The anterior tibial artery entering the region in contact with the medial side of the neck of the fibula; the deep peroneal nerve in contact with the lateral side. Hence, the nerve approaches the artery from the lateral side (fig. 303).

2. The artery and nerve and their named branches lying strictly on the skeletal plane and undisturbed by the removal of the muscles.

3. The superficial peroneal nerve following the anterior border of Peroneus Brevis which guides it to the surface a variable distance above the triangular subcutaneous area of the fibula.

4. The fibres of the interosseous membrane, so directed as to allow the fibula to be forced upwards but not pulled downwards.

306.1

Diagram Arteries of dorsum of foot. Compare with those of hand, figure 78.

(For plantar arteries, fig. 326; for variations, fig. 324.)

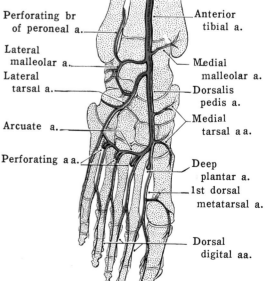

Perforating br
of peroneal a.

Lateral
malleolar a.

Lateral
tarsal a.

Arcuate a.

Perforating aa.

Anterior
tibial a.

Medial
malleolar a.

Dorsalis
pedis a.

Medial
tarsal aa.

Deep
plantar a.

1st dorsal
metatarsal a.

Dorsal
digital aa.

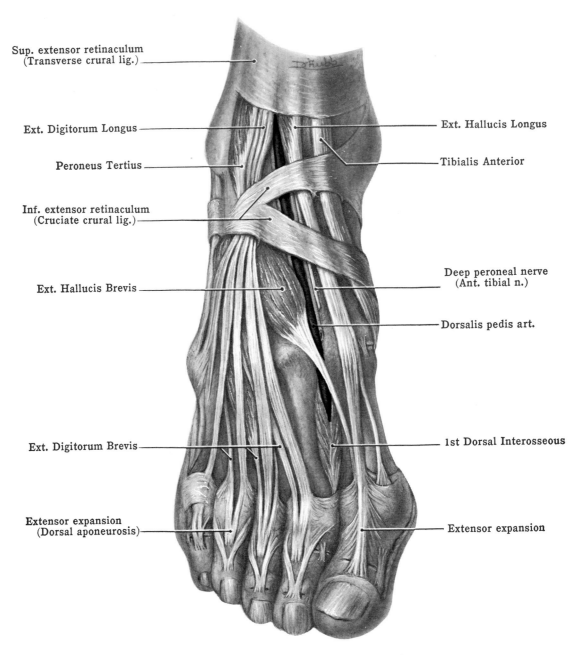

Sup. extensor retinaculum
(Transverse crural lig.)

Ext. Digitorum Longus

Peroneus Tertius

Inf. extensor retinaculum
(Cruciate crural lig.)

Ext. Hallucis Brevis

Ext. Digitorum Brevis

Extensor expansion
(Dorsal aponeurosis)

Ext. Hallucis Longus

Tibialis Anterior

Deep peroneal nerve
(Ant. tibial n.)

Dorsalis pedis art.

1st Dorsal Interosseous

Extensor expansion

307 Dorsum of the Foot, front view

The vessels and nerves are cut short.

Observe:

1. At the ankle, the vessels and nerve lying midway between the malleoli and having two tendons on each side.

2. On the dorsum of the foot, the artery crossed by Ext. Hallucis Brevis and disappearing between the two heads of the 1st Dorsal Interosseous (cf. the radial artery on the dorsum of the hand, figs. 78 and 79).

3. The inferior extensor retinaculum restraining the tendons from bowstringing forwards and also from bowstringing medially; i.e., it restrains them in two planes.

308 Dorsum of the Foot, lateral view

The ankle, subtalar, and calcaneo-cuboid joints are exposed in order to reveal their positions.

Observe:

1. The calcaneo-fibular ligament attached to the fibular malleolus in front of its tip, thereby allowing that tip to overlap the Peronei tendons and so prevent them from slipping forwards.

2. The inferior peroneal retinaculum attached to the lateral surface of the calcaneus, and in line with the inferior extensor retinaculum which is attached to the superior surface.

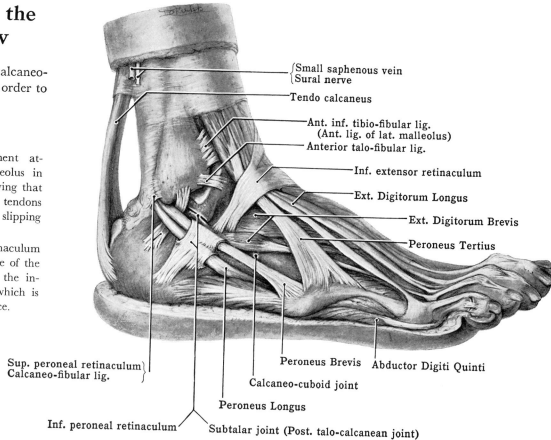

Small saphenous vein
Sural nerve
Tendo calcaneus
Ant. inf. tibio-fibular lig. (Ant. lig. of lat. malleolus)
Anterior talo-fibular lig.
Inf. extensor retinaculum
Ext. Digitorum Longus
Ext. Digitorum Brevis
Peroneus Tertius

Sup. peroneal retinaculum
Calcaneo-fibular lig.
Inf. peroneal retinaculum
Peroneus Brevis
Abductor Digiti Quinti
Calcaneo-cuboid joint
Peroneus Longus
Subtalar joint (Post. talo-calcanean joint)

309 Synovial Sheaths of the Tendons at the Ankle, antero-lateral view

The tendons of Peroneus Longus and Peroneus Brevis are enclosed in a common synovial sheath behind the fibular malleolus and this sheath splits into two, one for each tendon, behind the peroneal trochlea.

The tendon of Peroneus Longus has a second sheath (not in view) which accompanies it across the sole of the foot.

In 46.6 per cent of 131 feet, the two sheaths of the Longus were demonstrated by injection to be in continuity on their deep, or frictional, surface—though not on their superficial surface (*R. K. G.*).

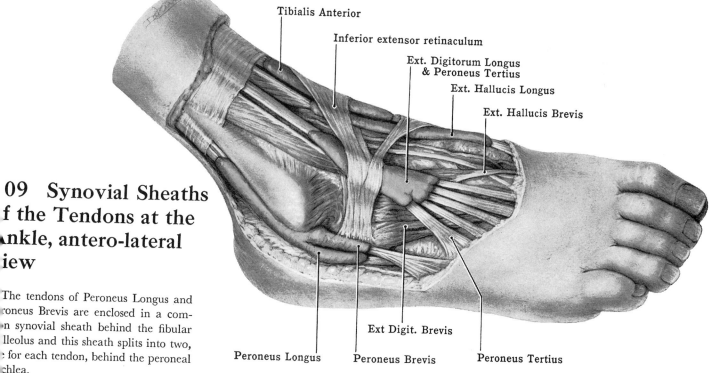

Tibialis Anterior
Inferior extensor retinaculum
Ext. Digitorum Longus & Peroneus Tertius
Ext. Hallucis Longus
Ext. Hallucis Brevis
Peroneus Longus
Ext Digit. Brevis
Peroneus Brevis
Peroneus Tertius

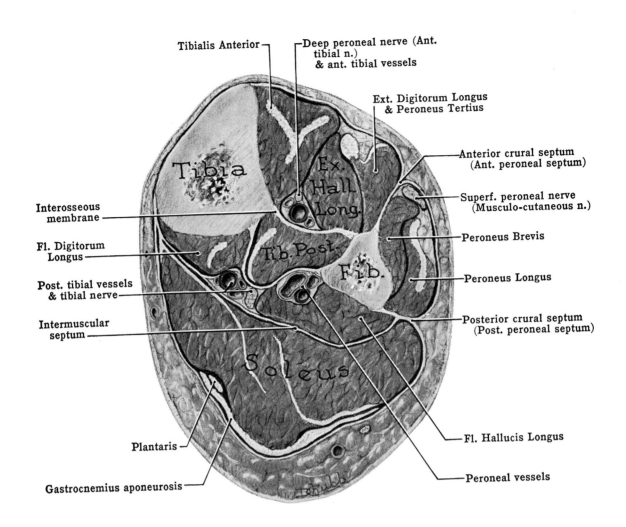

Tibialis Anterior

Deep peroneal nerve (Ant. tibial n.) & ant. tibial vessels

Ext. Digitorum Longus & Peroneus Tertius

Anterior crural septum (Ant. peroneal septum)

Superf. peroneal nerve (Musculo-cutaneous n.)

Peroneus Brevis

Peroneus Longus

Posterior crural septum (Post. peroneal septum)

Fl. Hallucis Longus

Peroneal vessels

Interosseous membrane

Fl. Digitorum Longus

Post. tibial vessels & tibial nerve

Intermuscular septum

Plantaris

Gastrocnemius aponeurosis

310 Cross Section through the Leg, male

Observe:

1. *The Level of the Section*—(a) Extensor and Flexor Hallucis Longus are both present and Tibialis Anterior has ceased to arise from the deep fascia, therefore the section is below the upper ⅓rd of the leg; (b) the anterior tibial artery has not yet moved on to the front of the tibia, therefore it is above the lower ⅓rd; (c) Peronei Longus et Brevis are both arising from the fibula, therefore it is in the middle ⅓rd. (d) Gastrocnemius is aponeurotic, therefore, it is in the lower ½—say through the lower part of the middle ⅓rd.

2. *The Anterior Tibio-fibular Compartment*, bounded by tibia, interosseous membrane, fibula, anterior intermuscular crural septum and deep fascia, and containing the anterior tibial vessels and deep peroneal nerve. (*Peroneal* is Greek for *fibular*, which is Latin.)

3. *The Peroneal or Fibular Compartment* bounded by fibula, anterior and posterior intermuscular crural septa and the deep fascia, and containing the superficial peroneal nerve.

4. *The Posterior Tibio-fibular Compartment* bounded by tibia, interosseous membrane, fibula, posterior intermuscular crural septum and deep fascia. This compartment is subdivided by two coronal septa into three subcompartments:—1st, or deepest, contains Tibialis Posterior; the 2nd, or intermediate, contains Flexor Hallucis Longus, Flexor Digitorum Longus and posterior tibial vessels and tibial nerve; and the 3rd, or most superficial, contains Soleus, Gastrocnemius and Plantaris.

311 Bones of the Foot, medial aspect

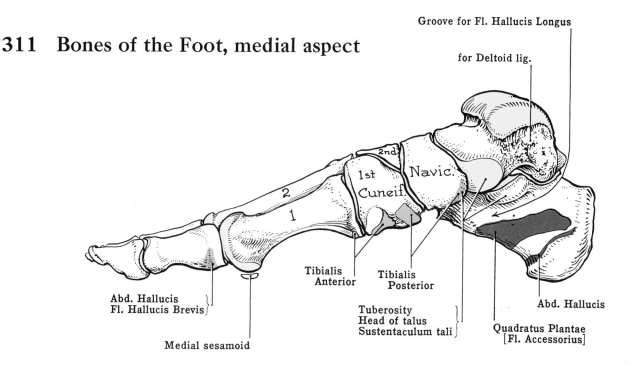

Groove for Fl. Hallucis Longus

for Deltoid lig.

2nd

1st Cuneif.

Navic.

2

1

Tibialis Anterior

Tibialis Posterior

Abd. Hallucis
Fl. Hallucis Brevis

Medial sesamoid

Tuberosity
Head of talus
Sustentaculum tali

Abd. Hallucis

Quadratus Plantae
[Fl. Accessorius]

312 Bones of the Foot, lateral aspect

Terminology: The trochlea of the talus is the part of the body of the talus that articulates with the ankle socket. It has an upper, a medial malleolar, and a lateral malleolar part.

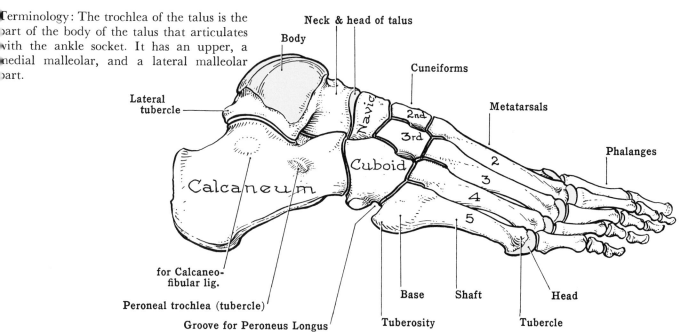

Neck & head of talus

Body

Cuneiforms

Metatarsals

Lateral tubercle

2nd

3rd

Navic

Cuboid

2

Phalanges

3

Calcaneum

4

5

for Calcaneofibular lig.

Peroneal trochlea (tubercle)

Groove for Peroneus Longus

Base

Tuberosity

Shaft

Head

Tubercle

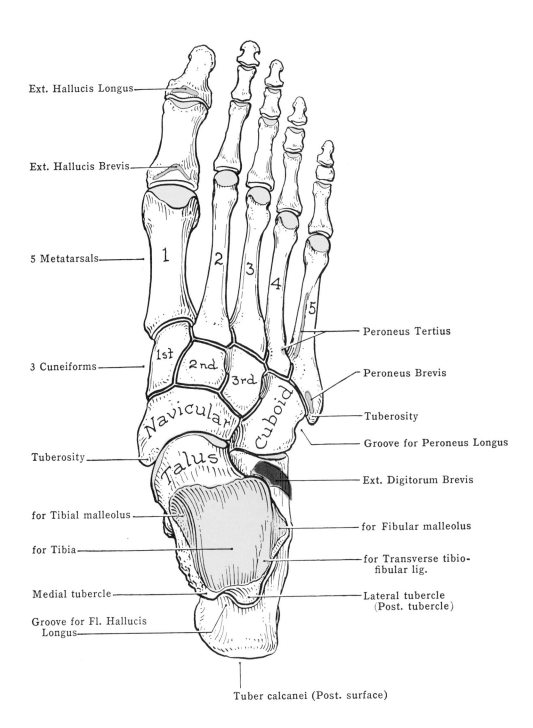

Ext. Hallucis Longus

Ext. Hallucis Brevis

5 Metatarsals

3 Cuneiforms

Tuberosity

for Tibial malleolus

for Tibia

Medial tubercle

Groove for Fl. Hallucis Longus

1

2

3

4

5

1st

2nd

3rd

Navicular

Cuboid

Talus

Peroneus Tertius

Peroneus Brevis

Tuberosity

Groove for Peroneus Longus

Ext. Digitorum Brevis

for Fibular malleolus

for Transverse tibio-fibular lig.

Lateral tubercle (Post. tubercle)

Tuber calcanei (Post. surface)

313 Bones of the Foot, dorsal aspect

(For upper surface of calcaneus, see fig. 344.)

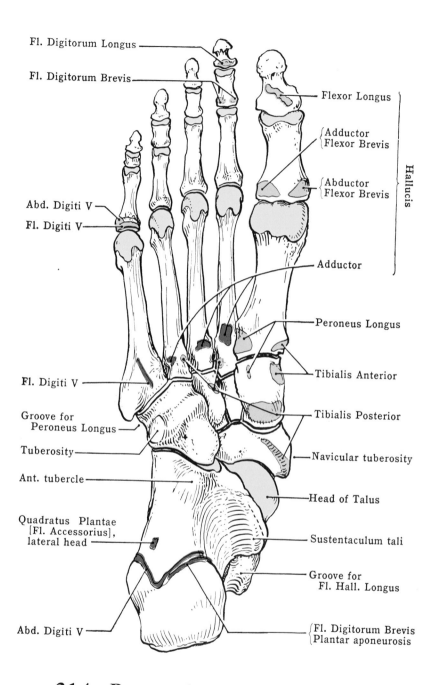

Fl. Digitorum Longus

Fl. Digitorum Brevis

Flexor Longus

Adductor
Flexor Brevis

Abductor
Flexor Brevis

Hallucis

Abd. Digiti V

Fl. Digiti V

Adductor

Peroneus Longus

Fl. Digiti V

Tibialis Anterior

Groove for
Peroneus Longus

Tibialis Posterior

Tuberosity

Navicular tuberosity

Ant. tubercle

Head of Talus

Quadratus Plantae
[Fl. Accessorius],
lateral head

Sustentaculum tali

Groove for
Fl. Hall. Longus

Abd. Digiti V

Fl. Digitorum Brevis
Plantar aponeurosis

314   Bones of the Foot, plantar aspect

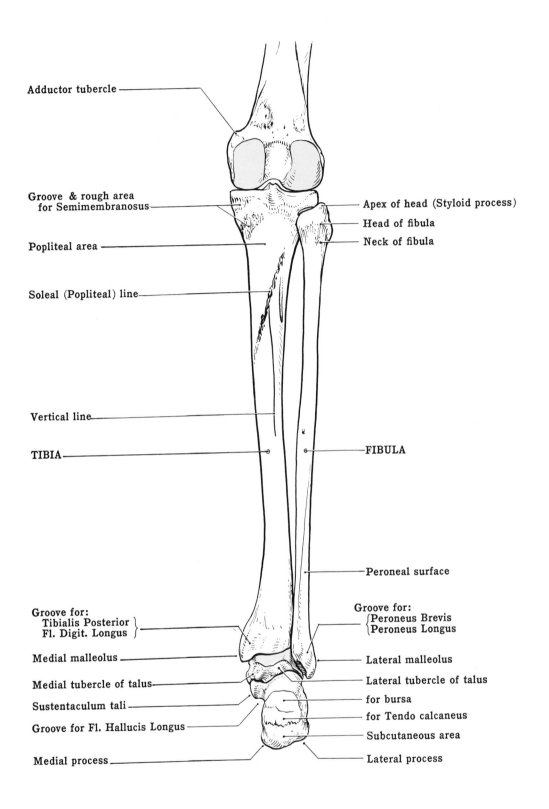

Adductor tubercle

Groove & rough area
for Semimembranosus

Popliteal area

Soleal (Popliteal) line

Vertical line

TIBIA

Groove for:
  Tibialis Posterior
  Fl. Digit. Longus

Medial malleolus

Medial tubercle of talus

Sustentaculum tali

Groove for Fl. Hallucis Longus

Medial process

Apex of head (Styloid process)
Head of fibula
Neck of fibula

FIBULA

Peroneal surface

Groove for:
  Peroneus Brevis
  Peroneus Longus

Lateral malleolus

Lateral tubercle of talus

for bursa

for Tendo calcaneus

Subcutaneous area

Lateral process

315 Bones of the Leg, posterior view

(For anterior view, see fig. 303; for os coxae and femur, see figs. 242 & 243.)

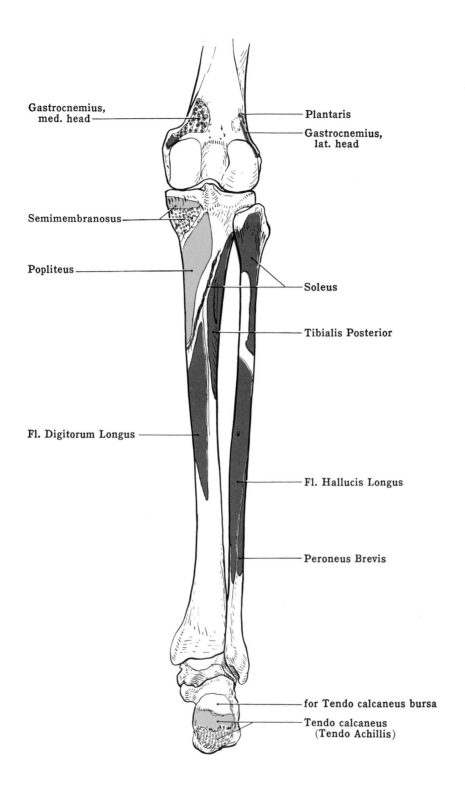

Gastrocnemius, med. head

Plantaris

Gastrocnemius, lat. head

Semimembranosus

Popliteus

Soleus

Tibialis Posterior

Fl. Digitorum Longus

Fl. Hallucis Longus

Peroneus Brevis

for Tendo calcaneus bursa

Tendo calcaneus (Tendo Achillis)

316 Bones of the Leg showing Attachments of Muscles, posterior view

(For Os coxae and Femur, posterior aspect, see fig. 266; Bones of Foot, plantar aspect, see fig. 314.)

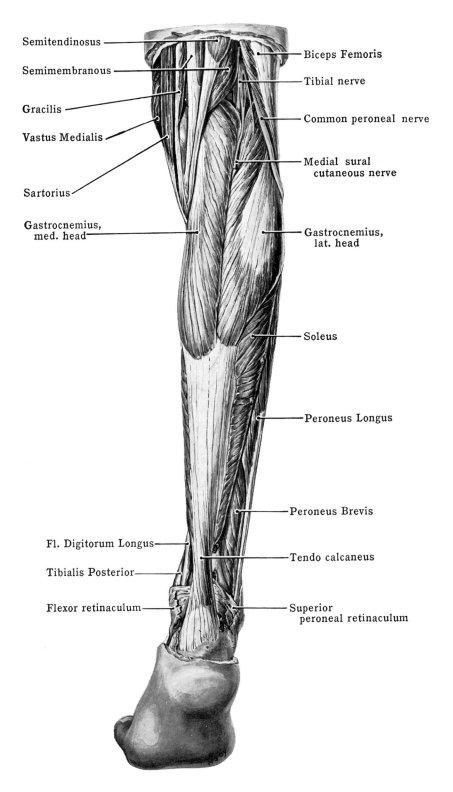

Semitendinosus

Semimembranous

Gracilis

Vastus Medialis

Sartorius

Gastrocnemius,
med. head

Biceps Femoris

Tibial nerve

Common peroneal nerve

Medial sural
cutaneous nerve

Gastrocnemius,
lat. head

Soleus

Peroneus Longus

Peroneus Brevis

Fl. Digitorum Longus

Tibialis Posterior

Flexor retinaculum

Tendo calcaneus

Superior
peroneal retinaculum

317 Muscles of the Leg, posterior view—I

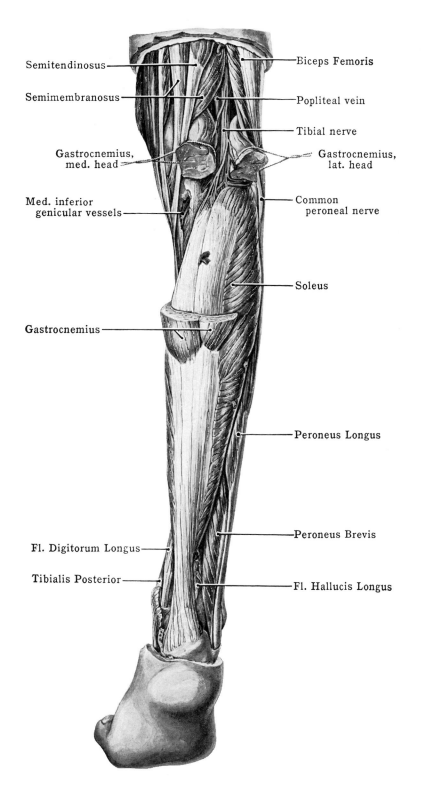

Semitendinosus

Semimembranosus

Gastrocnemius,
med. head

Med. inferior
genicular vessels

Gastrocnemius

Fl. Digitorum Longus

Tibialis Posterior

Biceps Femoris

Popliteal vein

Tibial nerve

Gastrocnemius,
lat. head

Common
peroneal nerve

Soleus

Peroneus Longus

Peroneus Brevis

Fl. Hallucis Longus

318 Muscles of the Leg, posterior view—II

The fleshy bellies of Gastrocnemius are largely excised, and the origin of
Soleus is thereby exposed. Plantaris is absent from this specimen.

319 Back of the Leg, deep structures undisturbed

Tendo calcaneus is divided; Gastrocnemius and a horseshoe-shaped section of Soleus are removed.

Observe:

1. The bipennate structure of the large Flexor Hallucis Longus and of the smaller Flexor Digitorum Longus.

2. The posterior tibial artery and the tibial nerve descending between these two muscles, on a layer of fascia that covers Tibialis Posterior (For cross section, see fig. 310.)

3. The tough, intermuscular fascial septum deep to Soleus and tendo calcaneus that acts as a restraining anklet at the ankle and there blends medially with the weaker investing deep fascia to form the flexor retinaculum.

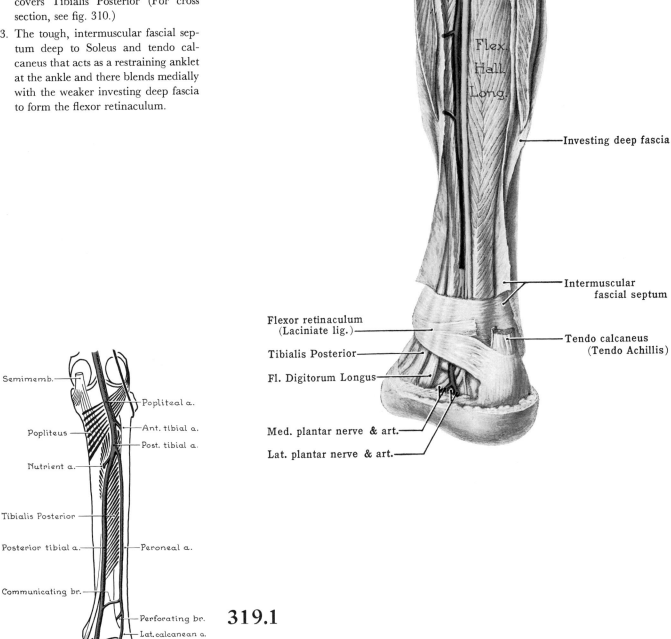

Semimembranosus

Popliteus fascia

Fl. Digitorum Longus
Post. tibial artery
(Post.) Tibial nerve

Flex. Hall. Long.

Tibial nerve (Med. popliteal n.)
Popliteus
Common peroneal nerve (Lat. popliteal n.)

Soleus

Fibula
Tibialis Posterior
Peroneal artery

Investing deep fascia

Intermuscular fascial septum

Flexor retinaculum (Laciniate lig.)

Tibialis Posterior

Fl. Digitorum Longus

Med. plantar nerve & art.

Lat. plantar nerve & art.

Tendo calcaneus (Tendo Achillis)

Semimemb.

Popliteus

Nutrient a.

Tibialis Posterior

Posterior tibial a.

Communicating br.

Plantar aa.

Popliteal a.

Ant. tibial a.

Post. tibial a.

Peroneal a.

Perforating br.

Lat. calcanean a.

319.1

Diagram. Arteries of back of leg. (For variations, see fig. 324.)

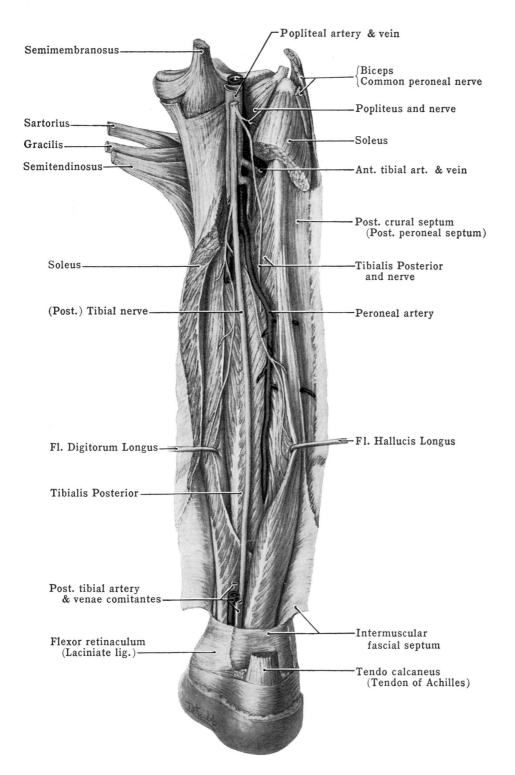

Semimembranosus

Popliteal artery & vein

Biceps
Common peroneal nerve

Popliteus and nerve

Sartorius

Gracilis

Soleus

Semitendinosus

Ant. tibial art. & vein

Post. crural septum
(Post. peroneal septum)

Soleus

Tibialis Posterior
and nerve

(Post.) Tibial nerve

Peroneal artery

Fl. Digitorum Longus

Fl. Hallucis Longus

Tibialis Posterior

Post. tibial artery
& venae comitantes

Intermuscular
fascial septum

Flexor retinaculum
(Laciniate lig.)

Tendo calcaneus
(Tendon of Achilles)

320 Back of the Leg, deep structures displayed

Soleus is largely cut away; the two long digitial flexors are pulled apart; the posterior tibial artery is partly excised.

Observe:

1. Tibialis Posterior, bipennate and powerful, lying deep to the two long digital flexors.
2. The peroneal artery overlapped by Fl. Hallucis Longus.
3. The nerve to Tibialis Posterior arising in conjunction with the nerve to Popliteus, and the nerve to Fl. Digitorum Longus arising in conjunction with the nerve to Fl. Hallucis Longus.
4. In the popliteal fossa the nerve is superficial to the artery: at the ankle the artery is superficial to the nerve.

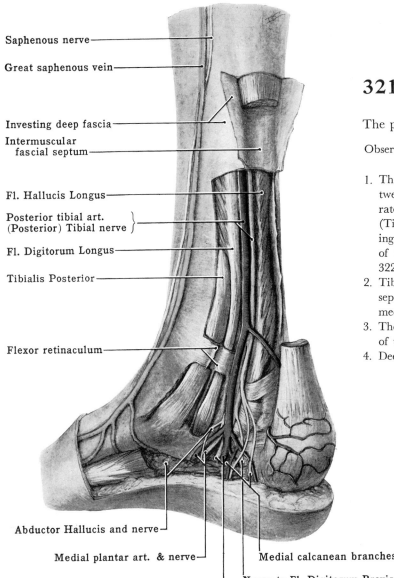

Saphenous nerve

Great saphenous vein

Investing deep fascia

Intermuscular
  fascial septum

Fl. Hallucis Longus

Posterior tibial art.
(Posterior) Tibial nerve

Fl. Digitorum Longus

Tibialis Posterior

Flexor retinaculum

Abductor Hallucis and nerve

Medial plantar art. & nerve

Lateral plantar nerve & art.

Medial calcanean branches

Nerve to Fl. Digitorum Brevis

321 Ankle and Heel, medial view—

The posterior part of Abductor Hallucis is excised.

Observe:

1. The posterior tibial artery and the tibial nerve lying between Fl. Digitorum Longus and Fl. Hallucis Longus; separated from the tibial malleolus by the width of two tendons (Tibialis Posterior and Fl. Digitorum Longus); and dividing into medial and lateral plantar branches on the surface of the osseo-fibrous tunnel of Fl. Hallucis Longus (figs. 322 and 333).
2. Tibialis Posterior and Fl. Digitorum Longus occupying separate and individual occeofibrous tunnels behind the medial malleolus, which is their pulley.
3. The medial and lateral plantar nerves lying within the fork of the medial and lateral plantar arteries.
4. Deep veins of foot emerging to join the great saphenous vein.

321.1 Structures on Medial Side of the Ankle, lateral view

The talus has been removed from its socket to show the structures medial to the ankle.

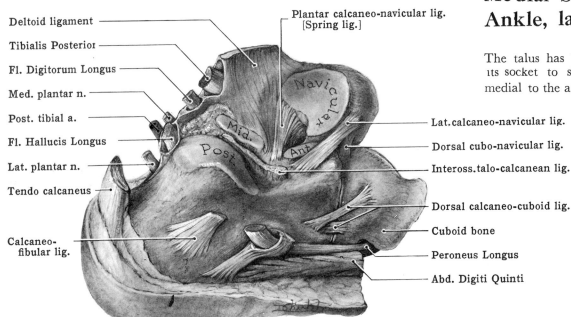

Deltoid ligament

Tibialis Posterior

Fl. Digitorum Longus

Med. plantar n.

Post. tibial a.

Fl. Hallucis Longus

Lat. plantar n.

Tendo calcaneus

Calcaneo-
  fibular lig.

Plantar calcaneo-navicular lig.
[Spring lig.]

Navicular

Mid.

Post.

Ant.

Lat. calcaneo-navicular lig.

Dorsal cubo-navicular lig.

Inteross. talo-calcanean lig.

Dorsal calcaneo-cuboid lig.

Cuboid bone

Peroneus Longus

Abd. Digiti Quinti

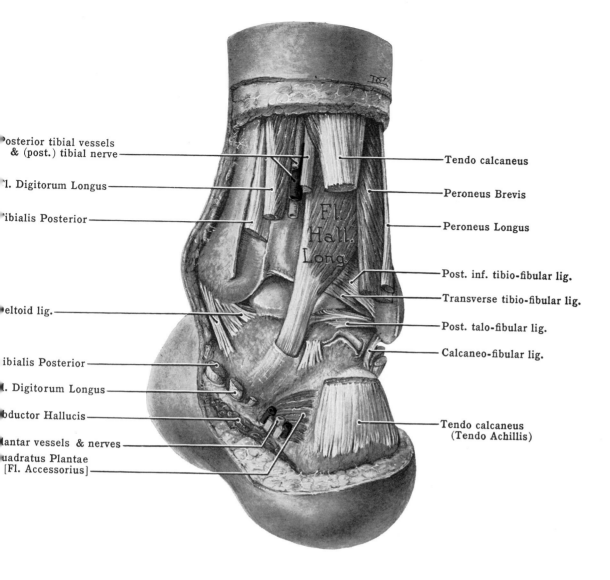

Posterior tibial vessels & (post.) tibial nerve

Fl. Digitorum Longus

Tibialis Posterior

Fl. Hall. Long.

Deltoid lig.

Tibialis Posterior

Fl. Digitorum Longus

Abductor Hallucis

Plantar vessels & nerves

Quadratus Plantae [Fl. Accessorius]

Tendo calcaneus

Peroneus Brevis

Peroneus Longus

Post. inf. tibio-fibular lig.

Transverse tibio-fibular lig.

Post. talo-fibular lig.

Calcaneo-fibular lig.

Tendo calcaneus (Tendo Achillis)

322   Ankle and Heel, posterior view—II

Observe:

1. Fl. Hallucis Longus placed midway between the two malleoli; and having the two tendons (Fl. Digitorum Longus and Tibialis Posterior) that groove the tibial malleolus medial to it and the two tendons (Peronei Longus et Brevis) that groove the fibular malleolus lateral to it.

2. The entrance to the sole "porta pedis" lying deep to Abd. Hallucis. The plantar vessels and nerves, the two long digital flexors, and part of Tibialis Posterior enter here. Quadratus Plantae serves as a soft pad for the vessels and nerves.

3. The posterior tibial artery and the tibial nerve lying medial to Fl. Hallucis Longus above and, after bifurcating, postero-lateral to it below. The crossing takes place where the long flexor is within its osseo-fibrous tunnel.

4. The strongest parts of the ligaments of the ankle are those that prevent forward displacement of the leg bones, viz. posterior part of the deltoid (posterior tibio-talar), posterior talo-fibular, tibio-calcanean, and calcaneo-fibular.

321.2

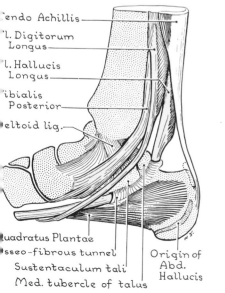

Tendo Achillis

Fl. Digitorum Longus

Fl. Hallucis Longus

Tibialis Posterior

Deltoid lig.

Quadratus Plantae

Osseo-fibrous tunnel

Sustentaculum tali

Med. tubercle of talus

Origin of Abd. Hallucis

Diagram. Only Fl. Hallucis Longus uses the sustentaculum as a pulley (trochlea).

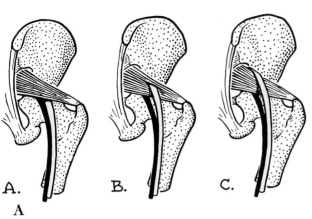

A

The Relationship of the Sciatic Nerve to Piri-formis. (a) In 87.3% of 640 limbs both the tibial and the peroneal division of the sciatic nerve passed below Piriformis; (b) in 12.2% the peroneal division passed through Piriformis; and (c) in 0.5% it passed above. (*J. C. B. G.*)

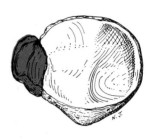

C

Bipartite Patella, posterior view. Occasionally the supero-lateral angle of the patella ossifies independently and remains discrete.

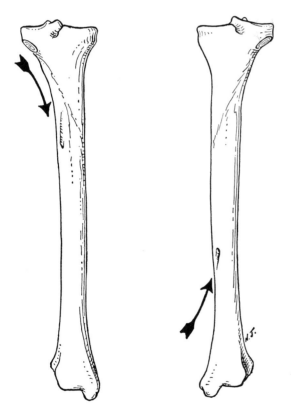

B

The Nutrient Canals of Long Bones are directed away from the more actively growing ends of the bones, but in this pair of tibiae (taken from the same subject) they take opposite directions.

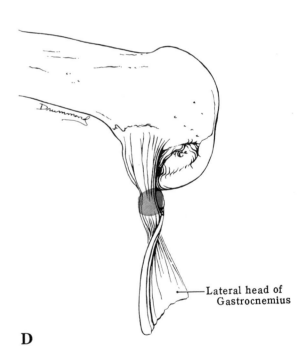

D

A Sesamoid Bone (Fabella) in the Lateral Head of Gastrocnemius was present in 21.6% of 116 limbs. (*J. C. B. G.*)

323 Variations and Anomalies

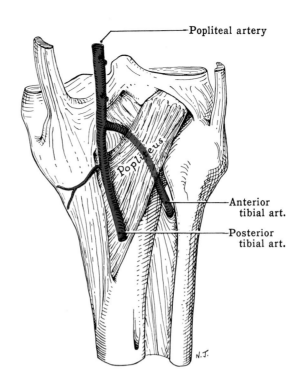

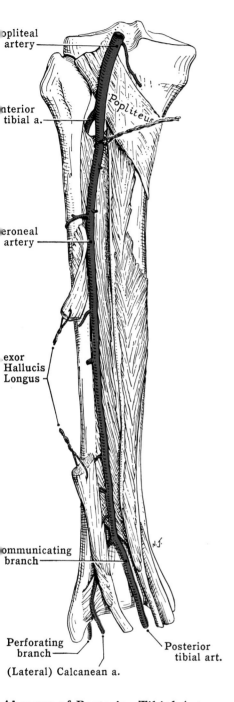

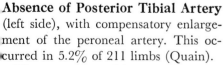

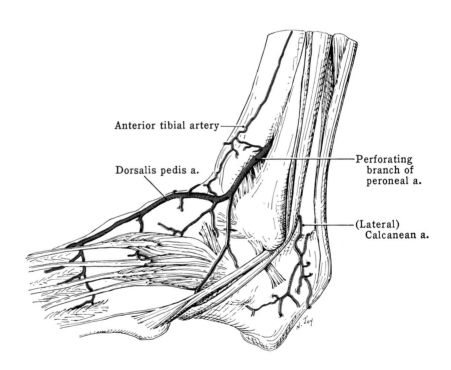

High Division of Popliteal Artery with the anterior tibial artery descending anterior to Popliteus occurred in 1.8% of 218 limbs (Quain).

Absence of Posterior Tibial Artery (left side), with compensatory enlargement of the peroneal artery. This occurred in 5.2% of 211 limbs (Quain).

The reverse condition, i.e., absence of peroneal artery with enlargement of the posterior tibial artery probably never occurs (Senior)

The Dorsalis Pedis Artery (left side) as a continuation of the perforating branch of the peroneal artery. When this occurs (3.7% of 592 limbs) the anterior tibial artery either fails to reach the ankle or is a very slender vessel. (J. C. B. G.)

324   Variations and Anomalies

(Anomalies of tarsal bones, see fig. 356.)

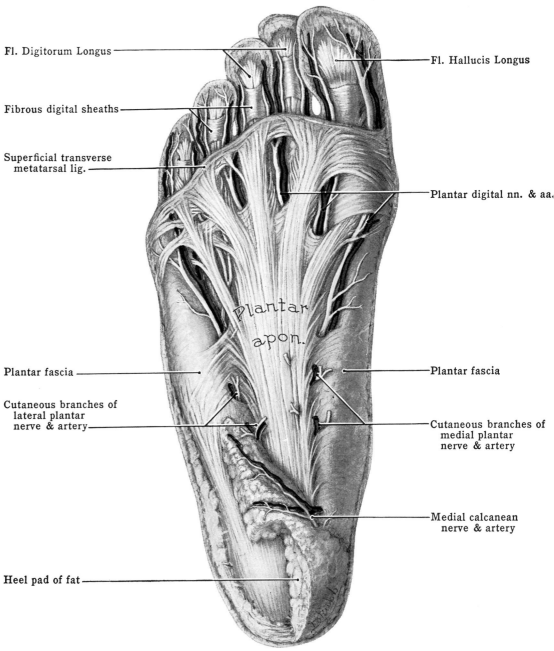

Fl. Digitorum Longus

Fibrous digital sheaths

Superficial transverse
metatarsal lig.

Fl. Hallucis Longus

Plantar digital nn. & aa.

plantar
apon.

Plantar fascia

Plantar fascia

Cutaneous branches of
lateral plantar
nerve & artery

Cutaneous branches of
medial plantar
nerve & artery

Medial calcanean
nerve & artery

Heel pad of fat

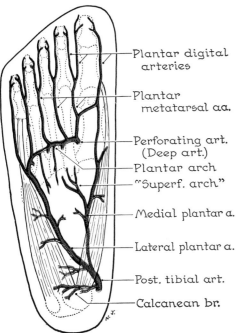

Plantar digital
arteries

Plantar
metatarsal aa.

Perforating art.
(Deep art.)
Plantar arch
"Superf. arch"

Medial plantar a.

Lateral plantar a.

Post. tibial art.

Calcanean br.

325   Superficial Dissection of Plantar Aspect, or Sole, of the Foot

The plantar aponeurosis, the medial and lateral parts of the plantar fascia, and the digital vessels and nerves should be compared and contrasted with the corresponding structures in the palm (figs. 59, 67, & 68).

326   Diagram of plantar arteries.

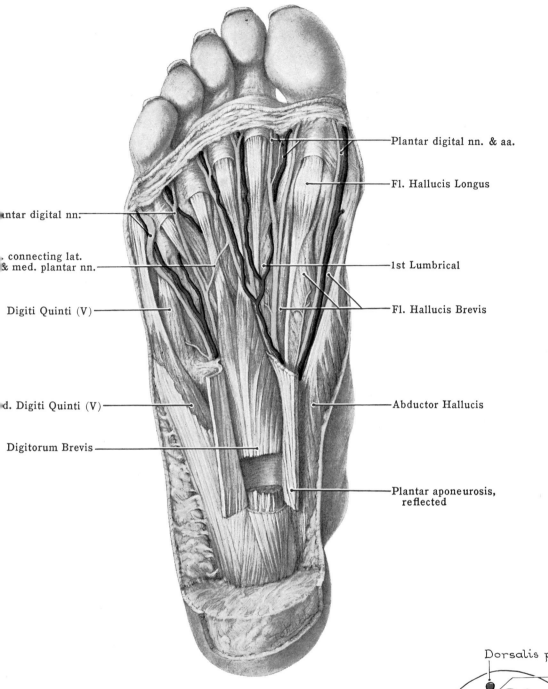

Plantar digital nn. & aa.

Fl. Hallucis Longus

ntar digital nn.

1st Lumbrical

connecting lat.
& med. plantar nn.

Fl. Hallucis Brevis

Digiti Quinti (V)

d. Digiti Quinti (V)

Abductor Hallucis

Digitorum Brevis

Plantar aponeurosis,
reflected

27   The First Layer of Plantar
Iuscles, Digital Nerves and Arteries

The muscles are:—Abd. Digiti Quinti, Fl. Digitorum Brevis, Abd.
allucis.

The plantar aponeurosis and fascia are reflected or removed, and a
ction is taken from Fl. Digitorum Brevis in order to show the fibrous
ox encasing it.

The lateral and medial plantar digital nerves, like the corresponding
lmar digital branches of the ulnar and median nerves, supply $1\frac{1}{2}$ and
  digits respectively and are united by a connecting (communicating)
anch (cf. fig. 68).

The lateral nerve to the little toe is here thickened. Fl. Digitorum
evis here, as commonly, fails to send a tendon to the little toe.

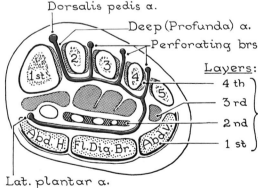

Dorsalis pedis a.

Deep (Profunda) a.

Perforating brs

Layers:

4 th

3 rd

2 nd

1 st

Lat. plantar a.

327.1

Diagram. Cross section of foot, near bases of
metatarsals.

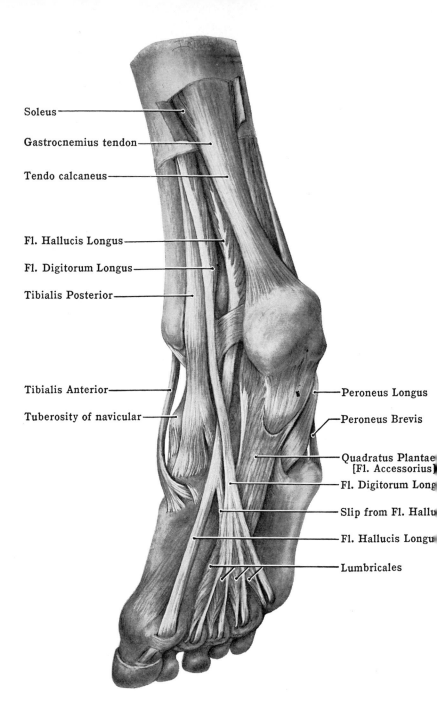

Soleus

Gastrocnemius tendon

Tendo calcaneus

Fl. Hallucis Longus

Fl. Digitorum Longus

Tibialis Posterior

Tibialis Anterior

Tuberosity of navicular

Peroneus Longus

Peroneus Brevis

Quadratus Plantae
[Fl. Accessorius]

Fl. Digitorum Long

Slip from Fl. Hallu

Fl. Hallucis Longu

Lumbricales

328   Second Layer of Plantar Muscles

Fl. Hallucis Longus, Fl. Digitorum Longus $\left\{\begin{array}{l}\text{Four Lumbricals}\\\text{Quadratus Plantae}\end{array}\right.$

Observe:

1. Fl. Digitorum Longus crossing superficial to Tibialis Posterior behind the medial malleol
   and superficial to Fl. Hallucis Longus abreast of the tuberosity of the navicular bone.
2. The four Lumbricals passing to the hallux side of the toes just as, in the hand, they pass
   the pollex side of the fingers (fig. 61).
3. Fl. Hallucis Longus sending a strong tendinous slip to Fl. Digitorum Longus.

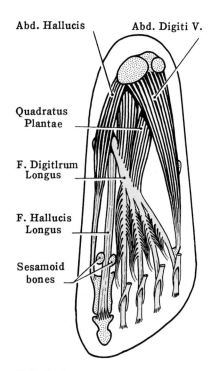

Abd. Hallucis

Abd. Digiti V.

Quadratus
Plantae

F. Digitlrum
Longus

F. Hallucis
Longus

Sesamoid
bones

328.1

Diagram. 2nd layer of muscles,
framed by abductors of 1st layer.

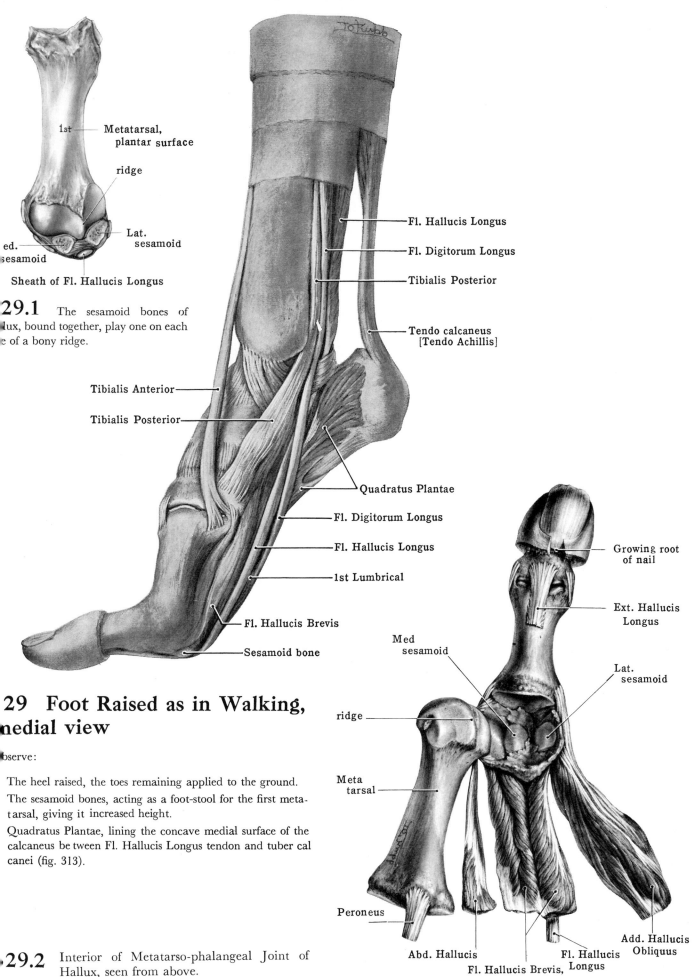

1st —— Metatarsal,
plantar surface

ridge

Lat.
sesamoid

ed.
sesamoid

Sheath of Fl. Hallucis Longus

29.1 The sesamoid bones of
lux, bound together, play one on each
e of a bony ridge.

Fl. Hallucis Longus

Fl. Digitorum Longus

Tibialis Posterior

Tendo calcaneus
[Tendo Achillis]

Tibialis Anterior ——

Tibialis Posterior ——

Quadratus Plantae

Fl. Digitorum Longus

Fl. Hallucis Longus

1st Lumbrical

Fl. Hallucis Brevis

Sesamoid bone

Growing root
of nail

Ext. Hallucis
Longus

Lat.
sesamoid

Med
sesamoid

ridge

Meta
tarsal

Peroneus

Abd. Hallucis

Fl. Hallucis Brevis,

Fl. Hallucis
Longus

Add. Hallucis
Obliquus

29 Foot Raised as in Walking,
medial view

bserve:

The heel raised, the toes remaining applied to the ground.

The sesamoid bones, acting as a foot-stool for the first metatarsal, giving it increased height.

Quadratus Plantae, lining the concave medial surface of the
calcaneus between Fl. Hallucis Longus tendon and tuber cal
canei (fig. 313).

29.2 Interior of Metatarso-phalangeal Joint of
Hallux, seen from above.

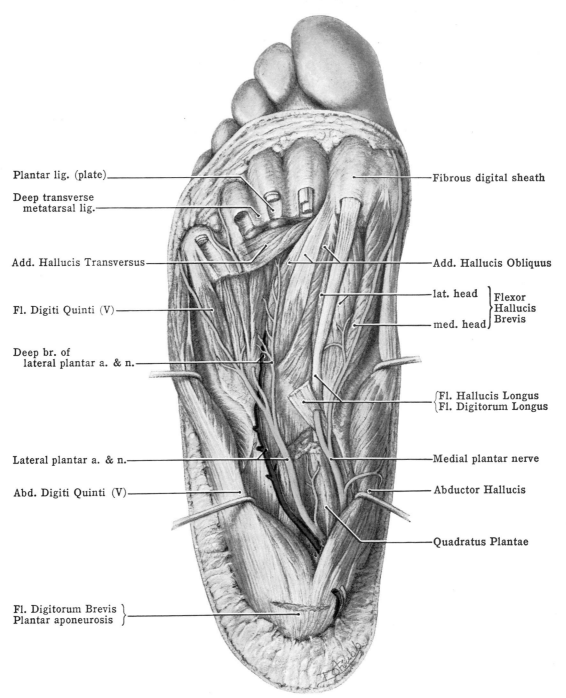

Plantar lig. (plate)

Deep transverse metatarsal lig.

Add. Hallucis Transversus

Fl. Digiti Quinti (V)

Deep br. of lateral plantar a. & n.

Lateral plantar a. & n.

Abd. Digiti Quinti (V)

Fl. Digitorum Brevis }
Plantar aponeurosis }

Fibrous digital sheath

Add. Hallucis Obliquus

lat. head } Flexor
} Hallucis
med. head } Brevis

{ Fl. Hallucis Longus
{ Fl. Digitorum Longus

Medial plantar nerve

Abductor Hallucis

Quadratus Plantae

330   Third Layer of Plantar Muscles

These are:—Fl. Digiti V,   Add. Hallucis Transversus,   and Fl. Hallucis Brevis, which form three sides of a square in the anterior half of the sole, largely filled by Add. Hallucis Obliquus.

Of the 1st layer, Abd. Digiti V and Abd. Hallucis are pulled aside and Fl. Digitorum Brevis is cut short. Of the 2nd layer, Fl. Digitorum Longus and Lumbricales are excised and Quadratus Plantae is cut long.

The lateral Interossei are seen in the floor of the square.

The lateral plantar nerve and artery course laterally between muscles of the 1st and 2nd layers; their deep branches then course medially between muscles of the 3rd and 4th layers.

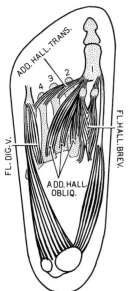

ADD. HALL. TRANS.

4 3 2

FL. DIG. V.

FL. HALL. BREV.

ADD. HALL. OBLIQ.

330.1

Diagram. The 3rd layer of muscles.

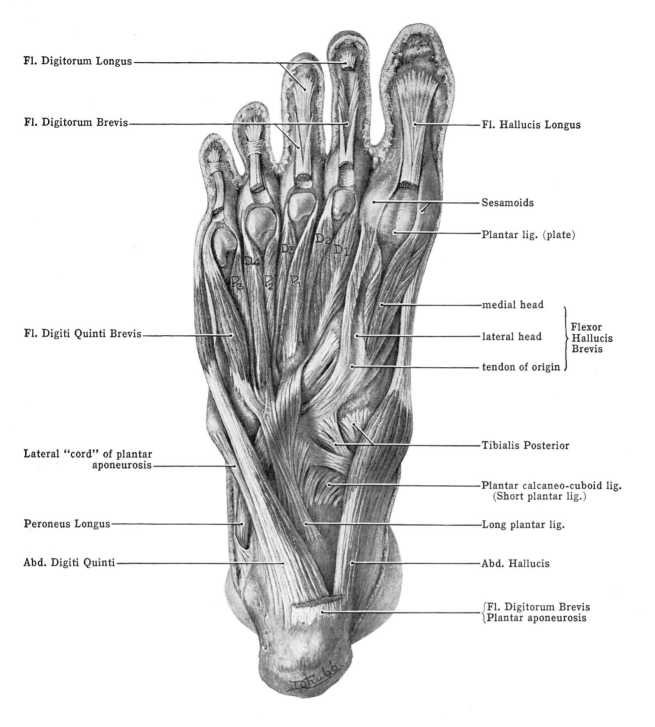

Fl. Digitorum Longus

Fl. Digitorum Brevis

Fl. Hallucis Longus

Sesamoids

Plantar lig. (plate)

D2
D3
D1
D4
P3
P2
P1

medial head

Fl. Digiti Quinti Brevis

lateral head

Flexor
Hallucis
Brevis

tendon of origin

Tibialis Posterior

Lateral "cord" of plantar
aponeurosis

Plantar calcaneo-cuboid lig.
(Short plantar lig.)

Long plantar lig.

Peroneus Longus

Abd. Digiti Quinti

Abd. Hallucis

Fl. Digitorum Brevis
Plantar aponeurosis

331　Fourth Layer of Plantar Muscles

These are:—(a) three Plantar and four Dorsal Interossei in the anterior half of the foot and (b) the tendon of Peroneus Longus and of Tibialis Posterior in the posterior half.

Of the first three layers, Abductor and Flexor Brevis of the fifth toe and Abductor and Flexor Brevis of the big toe remain for purposes of orientation.

Note: Plantar Interossei adduct the three lateral toes towards an axial line that passes through the 2nd metatarsal bone and second toe; whereas Dorsal Interossei abduct from this line.

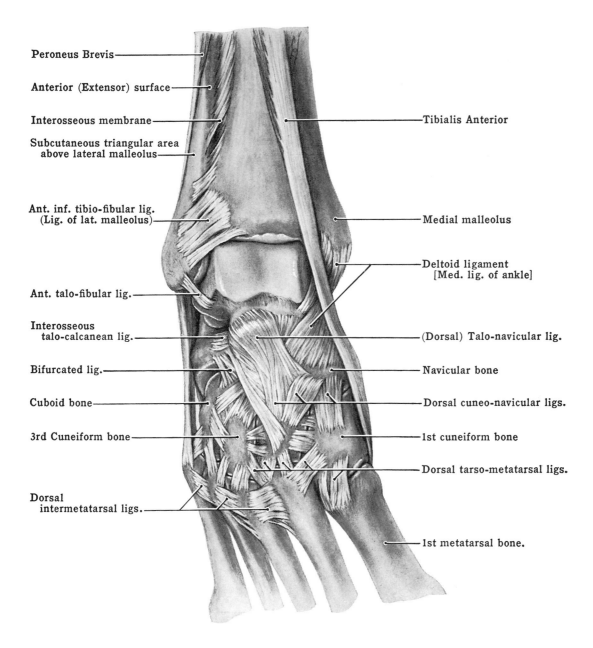

Peroneus Brevis

Anterior (Extensor) surface

Interosseous membrane

Subcutaneous triangular area above lateral malleolus

Ant. inf. tibio-fibular lig. (Lig. of lat. malleolus)

Ant. talo-fibular lig.

Interosseous talo-calcanean lig.

Bifurcated lig.

Cuboid bone

3rd Cuneiform bone

Dorsal intermetatarsal ligs.

Tibialis Anterior

Medial malleolus

Deltoid ligament [Med. lig. of ankle]

(Dorsal) Talo-navicular lig.

Navicular bone

Dorsal cuneo-navicular ligs.

1st cuneiform bone

Dorsal tarso-metatarsal ligs.

1st metatarsal bone.

332   Ankle Joint and the Joints of the Foot, dorsal view

The ankle joint is extended (plantar-flexed), its anterior capsular fibers are removed.

Observe:

1. The fibers of the membrane and ligaments uniting the fibula to the tibia are so directed as to resist the downward pull of (eight) muscles, but allowing the fibula to be forced upwards.

2. The anterior talo-fibular ligament is but a weak band, easily torn (fig. 338).

3. The dorsal ligaments of the foot resist the same thrusts as the plantar ligaments, and, therefore, are identically disposed, as reference to figure 342 shows. The plantar ligaments, however, act also as tie-beams for the arches of the foot and, therefore, are stronger.

4. Tibialis Anterior clinging to the skeleton throughout its entire course, as does Tibialis Posterior (figs. 320 & 341).

333 Horizontal Section through the Ankle Joint

Observe:

1. The body of the talus on section, wedge-shaped and grasped by the malleoli, which are bound to it by the deltoid and the posterior talo-fibular ligament and are thereby prevented from sliding forward.

2. Several synovial folds projecting into the joint.

3. Flexor Hallucis Longus, within its fibro-osseous sheath, lying between medial and lateral tubercles of talus.

   2 tendons each within a separate sheath (fibrous and synovial) behind the medial malleolus, and 2 within a common sheath behind the lateral malleolus.

4. Because of the intervening fibrous sheath, the posterior tibial vessels and the tibial nerve are not disturbed by the excursions of Fl. Hallucis Longus.

5. The small inconstant bursa superficial to tendo Achillis and the large constant bursa deep to it and containing a long synovial fold.

6. The anterior tibial artery and its companion nerve at the mid-point of the front of the ankle, with 2 tendons medial to it and 2 lateral to it (fig. 307).

7. The intermuscular fascial septum, shown and described in fig. 319.

334 Vertical Section through Ankle Region

Observe:

1. Tibia resting on the talus, and talus resting on the calcaneus, and between the calcaneus and the skin several large and many small encapsuled cushions of fat.

2. Fibular malleolus descending much farther than tibial malleolus. The weak interosseous tibio-fibular ligament.

3. The interosseous band between talus and calcaneus separating the subtalar or posterior talo-calcanean joint from the talo-calcaneo-navicular joint. (For clarification see fig. 337.)

4. Sustentaculum tali acting as a pulley for Fl. Hallucis Longus and giving attachment to the calcaneo-tibial band of the deltoid ligament. Tibialis Posterior rubbing on the band and Flexor Digitorum Longus on the sustentaculum.

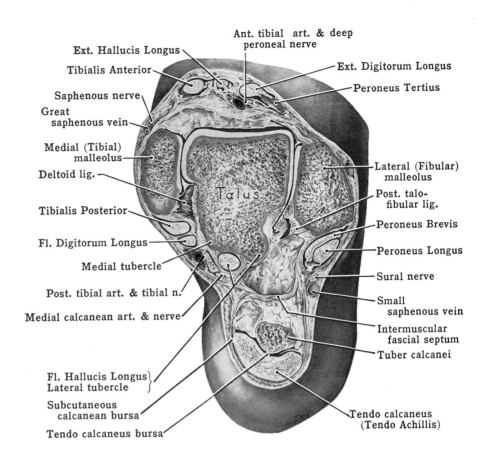

Ext. Hallucis Longus — Tibialis Anterior — Ant. tibial art. & deep peroneal nerve — Ext. Digitorum Longus — Peroneus Tertius — Saphenous nerve — Great saphenous vein — Medial (Tibial) malleolus — Deltoid lig. — Tibialis Posterior — Lateral (Fibular) malleolus — Post. talo-fibular lig. — Peroneus Brevis — Peroneus Longus — Fl. Digitorum Longus — Medial tubercle — Sural nerve — Post. tibial art. & tibial n. — Medial calcanean art. & nerve — Small saphenous vein — Intermuscular fascial septum — Tuber calcanei — Fl. Hallucis Longus Lateral tubercle — Subcutaneous calcanean bursa — Tendo calcaneus bursa — Tendo calcaneus (Tendo Achillis)

Talus

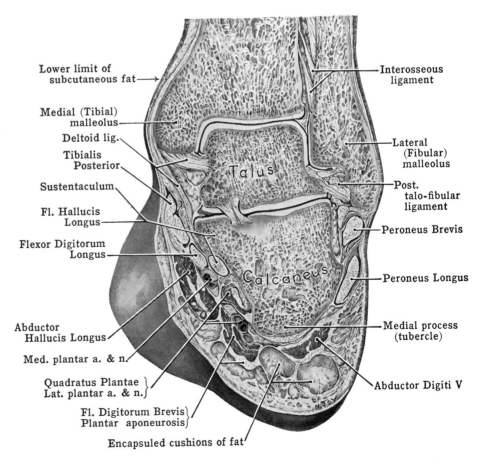

Lower limit of subcutaneous fat → — Interosseous ligament — Medial (Tibial) malleolus — Deltoid lig. — Tibialis Posterior — Sustentaculum — Fl. Hallucis Longus — Flexor Digitorum Longus — Lateral (Fibular) malleolus — Post. talo-fibular ligament — Peroneus Brevis — Peroneus Longus — Medial process (tubercle) — Abductor Hallucis Longus — Med. plantar a. & n. — Quadratus Plantae Lat. plantar a. & n. — Fl. Digitorum Brevis Plantar aponeurosis — Encapsuled cushions of fat — Abductor Digiti V

Talus

Calcaneus

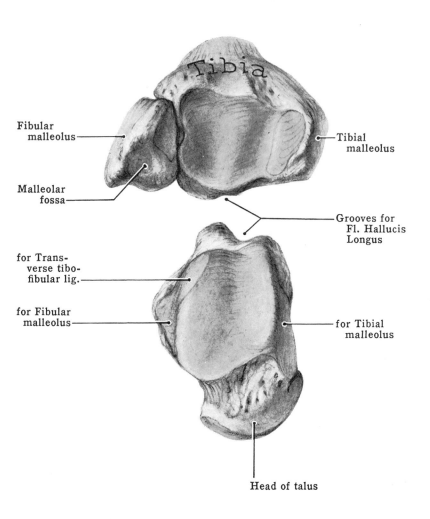

Fibular malleolus

Tibia

Tibial malleolus

Malleolar fossa

Grooves for Fl. Hallucis Longus

for Transverse tibo-fibular lig.

for Fibular malleolus

for Tibial malleolus

Head of talus

Note:

The superior articular surface of [the] talus is broader in front than beh[ind,] hence the tibial and fibular mal[leoli,] which grasp the sides of the talus t[end,] in dorsiflexion, to be forced apart. [By] virtue of the inferior tibio-fibular j[oint] on which the brunt of the strain [then] falls, is in the resilience it gives to [the] ankle joint.

336 Joints of Inversi[on] and Eversion

The ankle joint has been [im-] mobilized by nailing together t[ibia,] fibula and talus, thereby makin[g a] single rigid unit of these 3 bones. [The] remaining bones of the foot—all [but] talus—have been wired together [as] another unit. Movements betw[een] these 2 units constitute inversion [and] eversion of the foot.

The talus takes part in 3 jo[ints:]
1. "*Supratalar joint*", i.e., the a[nkle] joint.
2. "*Infratalar joints*"
   - posterior talo-calcanean or subtalar joint
   - anterior talo-calcanean joint
3. "*Pretalar joint*", i.e., the talo-navicular joint

talo-calca[nean] navicula[r] joint.

At the supratalar joint only m[ove-] ments of flexion and extension [are] normally permitted—they are [here] eliminated by a nail.

At the infratalar and pret[alar] joints movements of inversion [and] eversion take place.

The 2 parts of the infratalar j[oint] are separated from each other by [the] sulcus tali and the sulcus calca[nei] which, when the talus and calca[neus] are in articulation, become [the] tarsal sinus or tunnel.

The convex posterior talar f[acet] of the calcaneus, the concave mi[ddle] and anterior talar facets, and [the] concave talar facet of the navic[ular] all have their counterparts on [the] talus. The star (*) is at the site of [the] spring ligament. The middle t[alar] facet is the cartilage-covered up[per] surface of the sustentaculum tali.

The calcaneo-cuboid joint is [ac-] cessory to the foregoing joints.

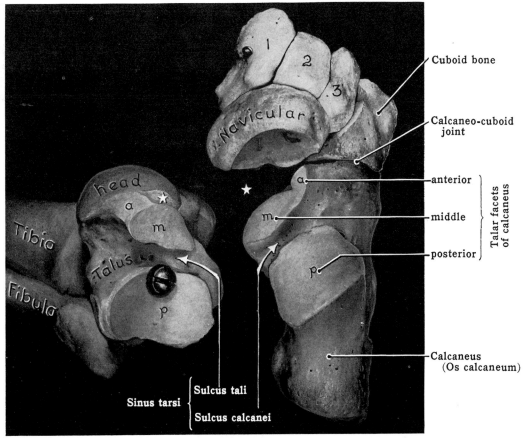

Cuboid bone

Calcaneo-cuboid joint

anterior

middle

posterior

Talar facets of calcaneus

Calcaneus (Os calcaneum)

Tibia

Fibula

Talus

head

Navicular

Sinus tarsi

Sulcus tali

Sulcus calcanei

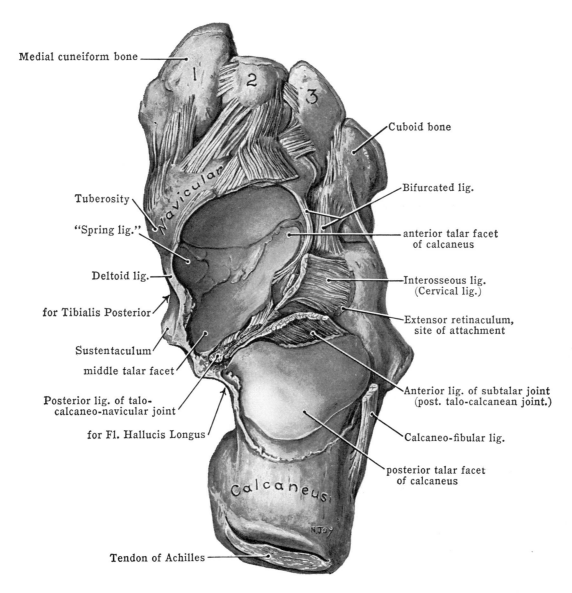

Medial cuneiform bone

Cuboid bone

Bifurcated lig.

anterior talar facet of calcaneus

Tuberosity

"Spring lig."

Interosseous lig. (Cervical lig.)

Deltoid lig.

Extensor retinaculum, site of attachment

for Tibialis Posterior

Sustentaculum

middle talar facet

Anterior lig. of subtalar joint (post. talo-calcanean joint.)

Posterior lig. of talo-calcaneo-navicular joint

Calcaneo-fibular lig.

for Fl. Hallucis Longus

posterior talar facet of calcaneus

Tendon of Achilles

337 Joints of Inversion (Supination) and Eversion (Pronation)

This specimen was prepared by sawing through the body of the talus and, after discarding it, by nibbling away the neck and head of the talus, thereby fully exposing the structures in the tarsal sinus. (Prepared by Dr. J. E. Anderson.)

Observe:

1. The convex, posterior talar facet separated from the concave, middle and anterior facets by the ligamentous structures within the tarsal sinus.

2. At the wide lateral end of the sinus: (a) the strong interosseous talo-calcanean ligament; and (b) in blue, the attachments of the extensor retinaculum, which extends medially between the posterior lig. of the anterior talo-calcanean joint and the anterior lig. of the posterior talo-calcanean, or subtalar, joint.

3. The subtalar joint has a synovial cavity to itself; whereas the talo-navicular joint and the anterior talo-calcanean

joint share a common synovial cavity, hence the collective title—talo-calcaneo-navicular joint.

4. The angular space between the navicular bone and the middle talar facet, on the sustentaculum tali, to be bridged by the plantar calcaneo-navicular, or spring, lig., the central part of which is fibro-cartilaginous.

5. The socket for the head of the talus to be deepened medially by the part of the deltoid lig. that is attached to the spring lig., and laterally by the calcaneo-navicular part of the bifurcated lig.

6. Various synovial folds overlying the margins of the articular cartilage; some of these containing fat.

(For plantar aspect, see figs. 341 and 342.)

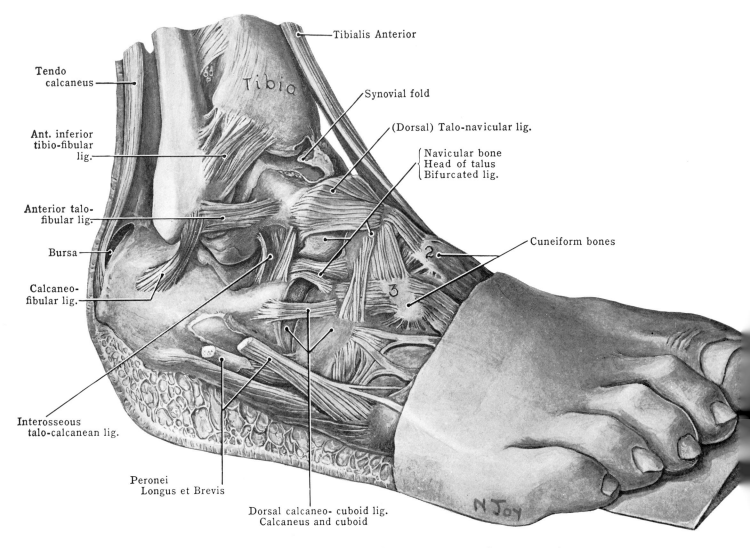

Tibialis Anterior

Tendo calcaneus

Ant. inferior tibio-fibular lig.

Anterior talo-fibular lig.

Bursa

Calcaneo-fibular lig.

Interosseous talo-calcanean lig.

Peronei Longus et Brevis

Synovial fold

(Dorsal) Talo-navicular lig.

Navicular bone
Head of talus
Bifurcated lig.

Cuneiform bones

Dorsal calcaneo- cuboid lig.
Calcaneus and cuboid

N Joy

338 Ankle Joint and the Joints of Inversion and Eversion, lateral view

The joints of inversion and eversion are:—(1) the subtalar (i.e., posterior talo-calcanean) joint, (2) the talo-calcaneo-navicular (i.e., combined anterior talocalcanean and talo-navicular) joint, and (3) the transverse tarsal (i.e., combined calcaneo-cuboid and talo-navicular) joint. Hence, the talo-navicular joint is twice involved.

The foot has been inverted in order to demonstrate:—(a) the areas of articular surface uncovered, and (b) the ligaments rendered taut, on inverting the foot.

Observe:

1. The uncovered articular parts are:—(a) posterior talar facet of calcaneus, (b) anterior surface of the calcaneus, and (c) head of the talus, all of which are palpable. Since inversion of the foot is commonly associated with plantar flexion of the ankle joint, (d) the upper and side parts of the trochlea of the talus are commonly uncovered too.

2. The ligaments that resist further inversion.

3. The anterior talo-fibular lig. and the dorsal calcaneo-cuboid lig. are weak and easily torn; the bifurcated and talo-navicular ligs. are under strain. The strong calcaneo-fibular lig., not attached to the tip of the malleolus but to a facet in front of the tip. Hence, the projecting tip, being free, helps to retain the peroneal tendons.

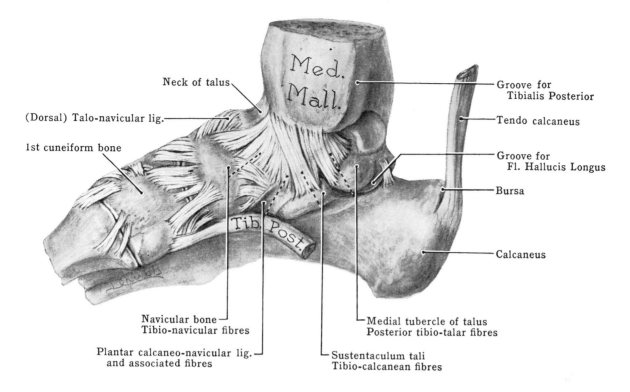

Neck of talus

(Dorsal) Talo-navicular lig.

1st cuneiform bone

Med. Mall.

Groove for Tibialis Posterior

Tendo calcaneus

Groove for Fl. Hallucis Longus

Bursa

Tib. Post.

Calcaneus

Navicular bone
Tibio-navicular fibres

Plantar calcaneo-navicular lig. and associated fibres

Medial tubercle of talus
Posterior tibio-talar fibres

Sustentaculum tali
Tibio-calcanean fibres

339   Ligaments of the Ankle Joint and Foot, medial view

Observe:

1. Tibialis Posterior displaced from its bed—malleolus, deltoid lig., and plantar calcaneo-navicular, or spring, lig.
2. The bed of Fl. Hallucis Longus—the groove between the two tubercles of the talus and the continuation of that groove beneath the sustentaculum tali.

3. The chief parts of the deltoid lig. passing downwards and backwards and thereby resisting forward displacement of the bones of the leg. The parts of the deltoid lig. are: tibio-navicular, tibio-(spring lig.), ant. tibio-talar, tibio-calcanean, and post. tibio-talar.

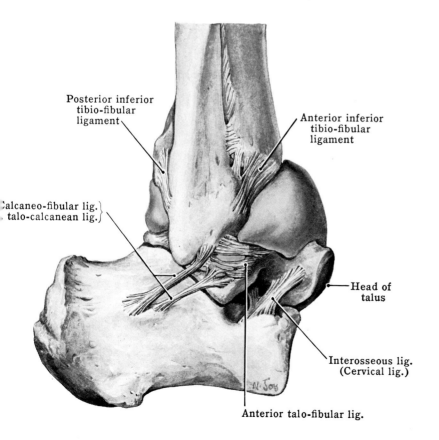

Posterior inferior tibio-fibular ligament

Anterior inferior tibio-fibular ligament

Calcaneo-fibular lig.
talo-calcanean lig.

Head of talus

Interosseous lig. (Cervical lig.)

Anterior talo-fibular lig.

340   A Distended Ankle Joint

Observe:

1. The far forward extension of the synovial cavity on the neck of the talus.
2. Posteriorly and laterally, the closeness of the synovial cavity of the ankle joint to that of the subtalar joint (posterior talo-calcanean joint).

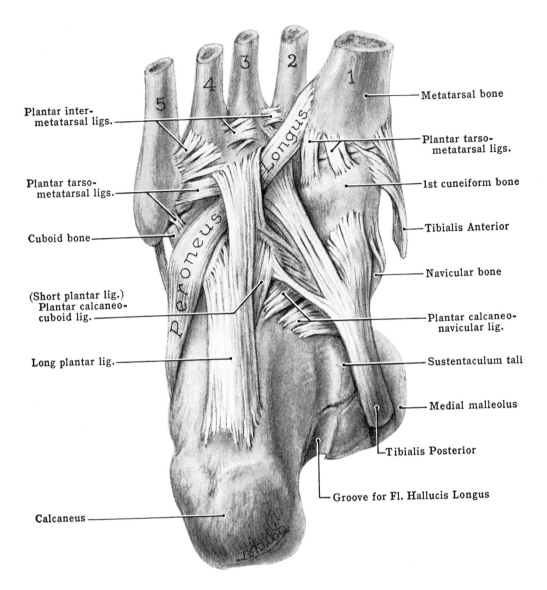

Plantar inter-metatarsal ligs.

Plantar tarso-metatarsal ligs.

Cuboid bone

(Short plantar lig.)
Plantar calcaneo-cuboid lig.

Long plantar lig.

Calcaneus

Metatarsal bone

Plantar tarso-metatarsal ligs.

1st cuneiform bone

Tibialis Anterior

Navicular bone

Plantar calcaneo-navicular lig.

Sustentaculum tali

Medial malleolus

Tibialis Posterior

Groove for Fl. Hallucis Longus

341 Plantar Ligaments. Insertions of Three Long Tendons—I

Observe:

1. The tendons are:—Peroneus Longus, Tibialis Anterior, Tibialis Posterior.

2. The tendon of Peroneus Longus crossing the sole in the groove in front of the ridge of the cuboid; bridged by some fibres of the long plantar ligament; and inserted into the base of the 1st metatarsal. Usually, like Tibialis Anterior, it is also inserted into the 1st cuneiform. It is an evertor (pronator) of the foot. (Fig. 314.)

3. Slips of the tendon of Tibialis Posterior extending like the fingers of an open hand to grasp the bones anterior to the transverse tarsal joint (i.e. the five small tarsal bones and several metatarsal bones, fig. 343). It is an invertor (supinator) of the foot.

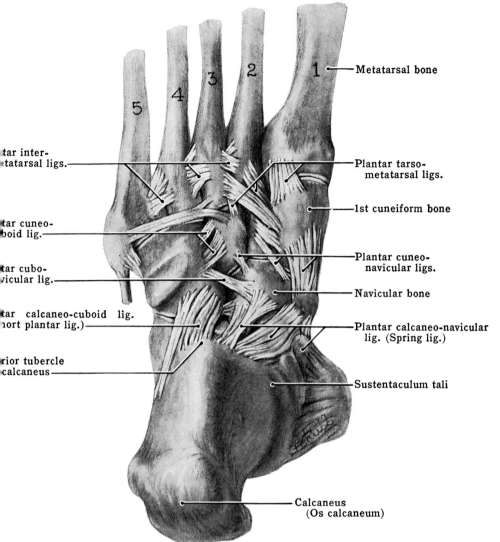

Metatarsal bone

Plantar tarso-
metatarsal ligs.

1st cuneiform bone

Plantar cuneo-
navicular ligs.

Navicular bone

Plantar calcaneo-navicular
lig. (Spring lig.)

Sustentaculum tali

Calcaneus
(Os calcaneum)

tar inter-
tatarsal ligs.

tar cuneo-
boid lig.

tar cubo-
vicular lig.

tar calcaneo-cuboid lig.
ort plantar lig.)

rior tubercle
calcaneus

342 Plantar Ligaments—II

Observe:

1. The plantar calcaneo-cuboid (or short plantar) lig. and the plantar calcaneo-navicular (or spring) lig. are the inferior ligaments of the transverse tarsal joint. Having a common purpose, they have a common direction.

2. The ligaments in the fore part of the foot diverge backwards from each side of the long axis of the 3rd metatarsal and 3rd cuneiform. Hence a backward thrust to the 1st metatarsal, as when rising on the big toe in walking, is transmitted directly to the navicular and talus by the 1st cuneiform, and indirectly by the 2nd metatarsal and 2nd cuneiform and also by the 3rd metatarsal and 3rd cuneiform.

3. A backward thrust to the 4th and 5th metatarsals is transmitted directly to the cuboid and calcaneus. That these four bones (i.e., the bones of the lateral longitudinal arch of the foot) are not displaced backwards is to the credit of the adjoining ligaments.

(For dorsal aspect, see fig. 337.)

342.1

Structures necessary for support of head of talus—plantar calcaneo-navicular lig. and tendon of Tibialis Posterior (fig. 341), seen from below.
(For upper & side views, see figs. 337 & 338.)

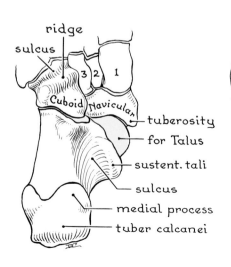
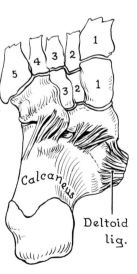

ridge

sulcus

Cuboid Navicular

tuberosity

for Talus

sustent. tali

sulcus

medial process

tuber calcanei

Calcaneus

Deltoid lig.

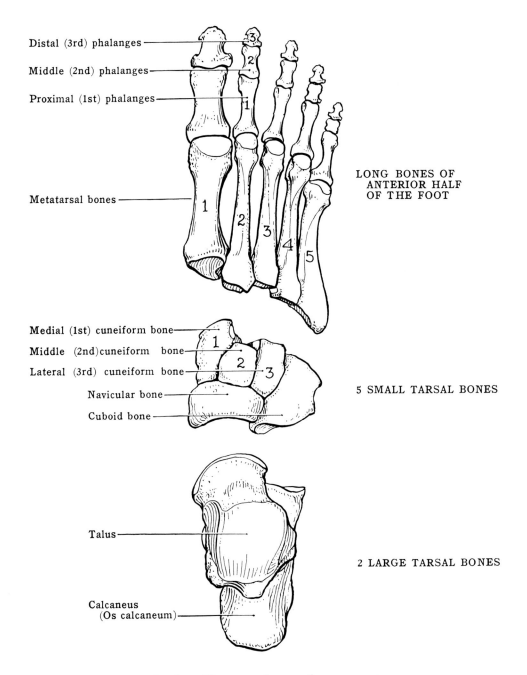

Distal (3rd) phalanges

Middle (2nd) phalanges

Proximal (1st) phalanges

Metatarsal bones

LONG BONES OF
ANTERIOR HALF
OF THE FOOT

Medial (1st) cuneiform bone

Middle (2nd) cuneiform bone

Lateral (3rd) cuneiform bone

Navicular bone

Cuboid bone

5 SMALL TARSAL BONES

Talus

2 LARGE TARSAL BONES

Calcaneus
(Os calcaneum)

343 Bones of the Foot, dorsal aspect

The bones are divisible, at the transverse tarsal and tarso-metatarsal joints, into three sections—anterior, middle, and posterior.

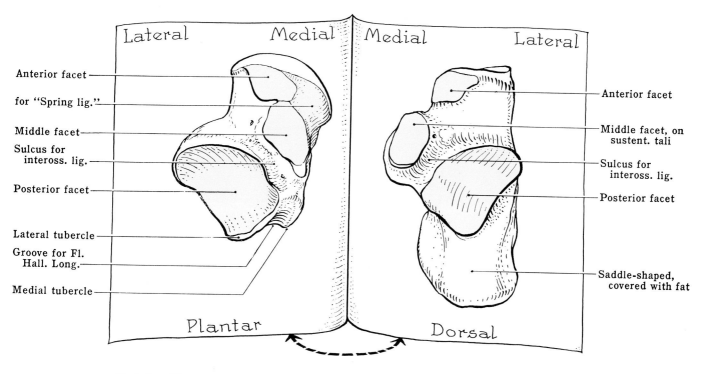

Lateral   Medial   Medial   Lateral

Anterior facet
for "Spring lig."
Middle facet
Sulcus for
inteross. lig.
Posterior facet

Lateral tubercle
Groove for Fl.
Hall. Long.
Medial tubercle

Plantar   Dorsal

Anterior facet
Middle facet, on
sustent. tali
Sulcus for
inteross. lig.
Posterior facet

Saddle-shaped,
covered with fat

344   Bony Surfaces of the Talo-calcanean Joints

The under or plantar surface of the talus and the upper or dorsal surface of the calcaneus are displayed.

The joints are gliding joints, hence apposed or corresponding facets are not exact counterparts of each other, one being more extensive than the other.

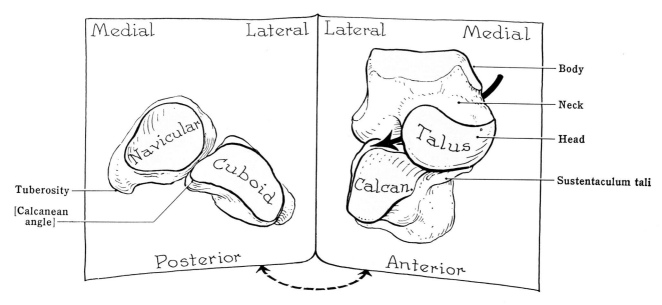

Medial   Lateral   Lateral   Medial

Navicular   Cuboid

Tuberosity
[Calcanean
angle]

Posterior   Anterior

Body
Neck
Head

Talus

Calcan.

Sustentaculum tali

345   Bony Surfaces of the Transverse Tarsal Joint (talo-navicular and calcaneo-cuboid)

The posterior surfaces of the navicular and cuboid bones, and the anterior surfaces of the talus and calcaneus are displayed. The black arrow traverses the tarsal sinus (tunnel), which lodges the interosseous talo-calcanean ligament (fig. 337).

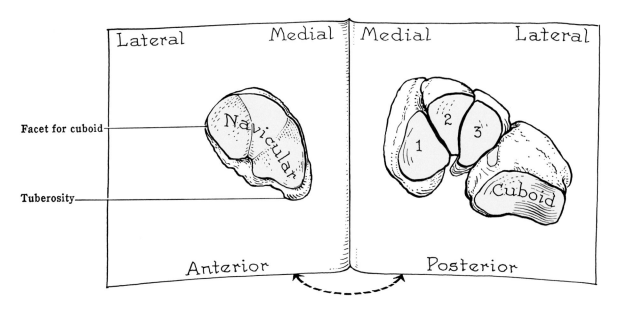

346 Bony Surfaces of the Cuneo-navicular and Cubo-navicular Joints

The anterior surface of the navicular bone, the posterior surfaces of the three cuneiform bones, and the medial and posterior surfaces of the cuboid bone are displayed.

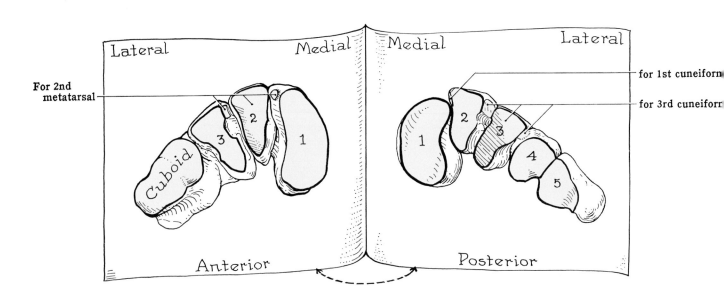

347 Bony Surfaces of the Tarso-metatarsal Joints

The anterior surfaces of the cuboid and 3 cuneiform bones, and the posterior surfaces of the bases of the 5 metatarsal bones are displayed.

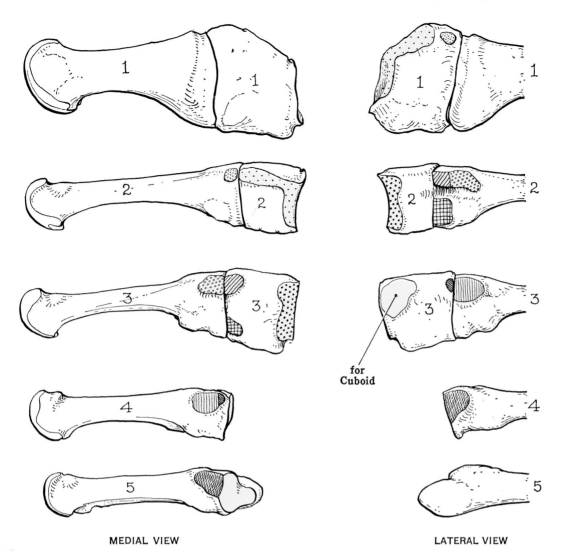

MEDIAL VIEW   LATERAL VIEW

348   Bony Surfaces of the Intercuneiform and Intermetatarsal Joints

The medial and lateral surfaces of the 3 cuneiform and 5 metatarsal bones are displayed.

The joints are gliding joints, hence apposed or corresponding facets are not exact counterparts of each other, one being more extensive than the other.

For purposes of identification, corresponding facets have been marked with corresponding designs.

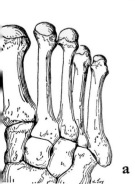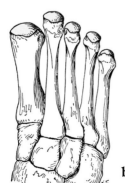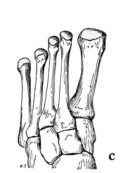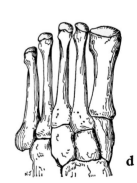

349   Long and Short 1st Metatarsal Bones

The extent of the forward projection of the 1st, 2nd, and 3rd metatarsal bones varies: In (a) the 1st and 2nd metatarsals project equally far; in (b) the 2nd projects much farther than either the 1st or 3rd; in (c) the 1st is the most projecting; and in (d) the 2nd and 3rd project equally far.

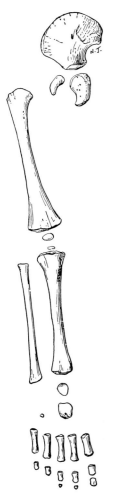

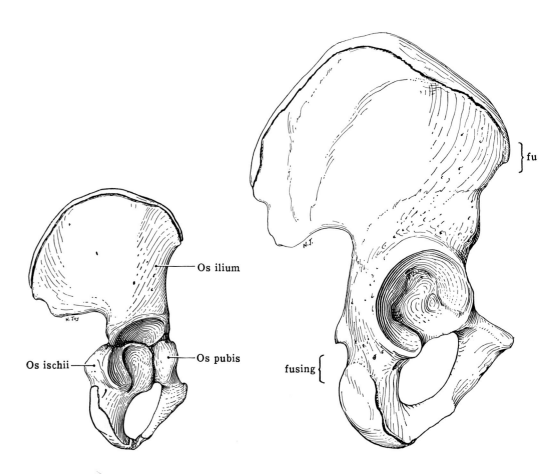

350 Bones of Lower Limb at Birth

The hip bone is in 3 primary parts—ilium, ischium, and pubis. The diaphyses of the long bones are well ossified. Certain epiphyses and certain tarsal bones have started to ossify, namely, the distal epiphysis of the femur and perhaps the proximal epiphysis of the tibia; the calcaneus, talus, and perhaps the cuboid.

351 Epiphyses of the Hip Bone

Hip Bone, aged about 5 years

The triradiate cartilage in the acetabulum is ossified and fused before the end of the 16th year. A bar of cartilage that unites the pubic and ischial rami ossifies about the 9th year. There is a cartilaginous epiphysis along the whole length of the iliac crest and one on the ischial tuberosity and ramus.

(*All ages given in figures 350—356 are for males.*)

Hip Bone, aged about 19 years

The acetabulum and the pubic arch now consolidated. The epiphysis along iliac crest and that on the ischial tuber are ossified and fusion is beginning—i one, anteriorly; in the other, superi Fusion starts in many cases before the year: most (80%) crests are partly fuse 18th year and most tuberosities by the Complete fusion is never delayed beyon 23rd year (*T. W. McKern & T. D. Ste* (*See also figures 277 & 278.*)

OSSIFICATION—EPIPHYSES

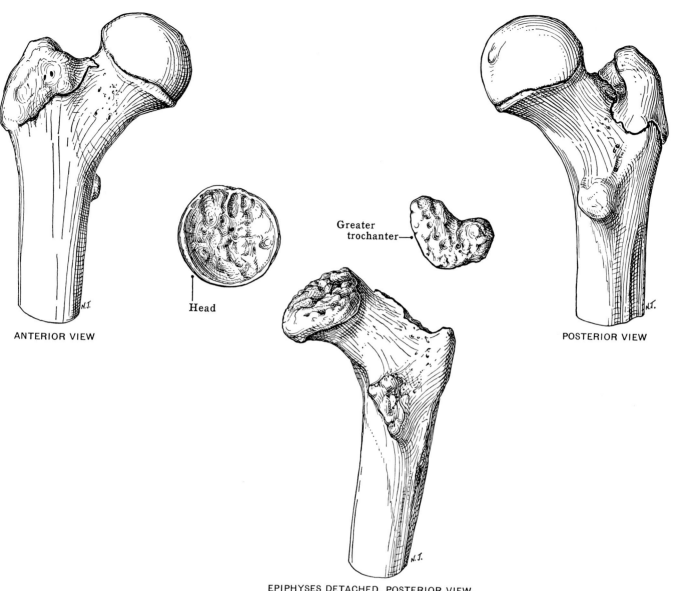

Head

Greater trochanter⟶

ANTERIOR VIEW

POSTERIOR VIEW

EPIPHYSES DETACHED, POSTERIOR VIEW.

352   Epiphyses at the Proximal End of the Femur

The epiphysis of the head fits like a cap on to the slightly conical end of the diaphysis. The apposed surfaces are billowy—pitted and ridged—as at other epiphyses. The articular cartilage of the head is carried for a few mm. on to the inferior aspect of the neck, compare the humerus (fig. 101). The epiphysis of the greater trochanter lies above the site of confluence of the shaft and neck. That of the lesser trochanter is a thick scale.

The epiphysis of the head begins to ossify during the 1st year; that of the greater trochanter before the 5th year; and that of the lesser trochanter before the 14th year. These have in most cases fused completely with the shaft before the end of the 18th year, and in all cases by the 20th (*McK. & S.*).

OSSIFICATION—EPIPHYSES

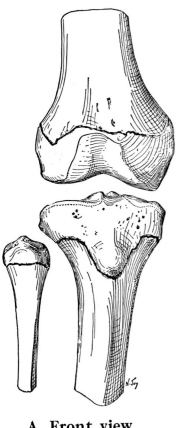

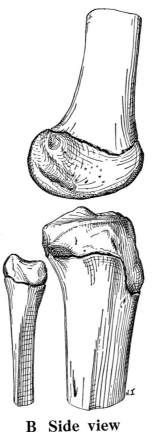

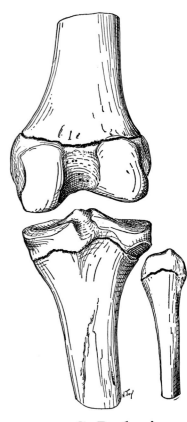

A Front view   **B Side view**   **C Back view**

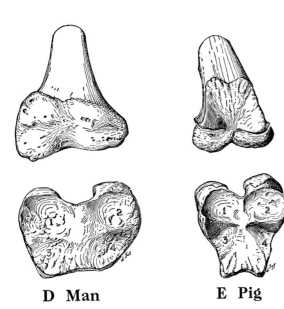

D Man   **E Pig**

353 Epiphyses at the Knee Joint

A, B, C.—The epiphyseal plate splits the adductor tubercle, skims above the patellar trochlea, shaves the cartilage of the lateral condyle, and follows along the intercondylar line.

The proximal epiphyseal plate of the tibia shaves the fibular facet and passes below the groove for the Semimembranosus tendon. Anteriorly, it dips down like a tongue to include the tuberosity. The epiphyseal plate of the fibula lies well above the neck.

The distal epiphysis of the femur begins to ossify before birth; that of the tibia soon follows it; that of the fibula begins to ossify before the 5th year. These 3 epiphyses at the knee have usually completely fused with their respective diaphyses before the end of the 19th year, and always by the 22nd—that of the tibia may be the 23rd (*McK. & S.*). A separate centre for the tibial tuberosity may appear before puberty.

D, E.—A quadruped walks with bent knees and the distal epiphysis of its femur has 4 deep pits into which 4 prongs project. In man, who walks erect, these are replaced by shallow impressions and slight bosses.

OSSIFICATION—EPIPHYSES

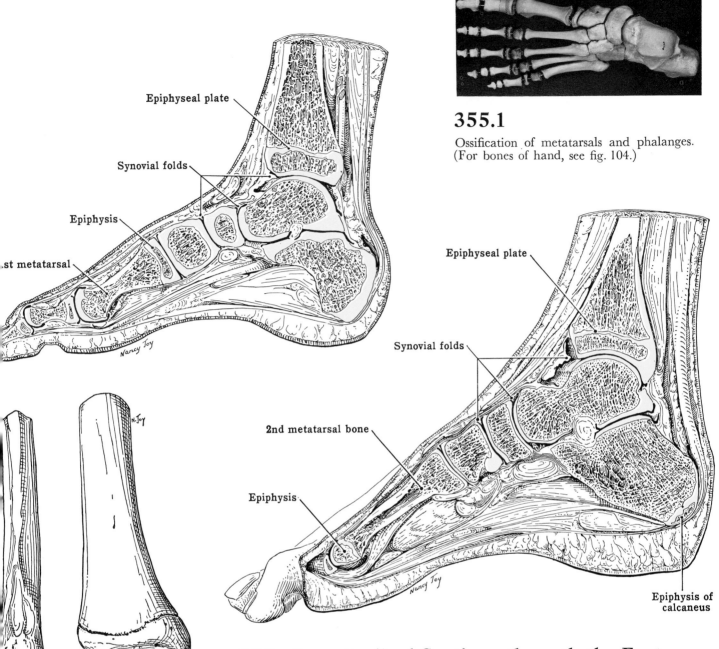

Epiphyseal plate

Synovial folds

Epiphysis

st metatarsal

Nancy Joy

355.1

Ossification of metatarsals and phalanges. (For bones of hand, see fig. 104.)

Epiphyseal plate

Synovial folds

2nd metatarsal bone

Epiphysis

Epiphysis of calcaneus

Nancy Joy

N-Joy

ANTERIOR VIEW

DIAL VIEW

4 Distal Epiphyses
the Tibia and Fibula

he epiphyseal plate of the fibula lies at
level of the ankle joint, and, therefore,
ssarily below the level of the epiphyseal
e of the tibia. The tibial epiphysis starts
ssify during the 1st year; the fibular
ng the 1st or 2nd year (*C. C. Francis*
.). Fusion is usually complete by the
or 18th year, and in all cases by the
(*McK. & S.*).

355 Longitudinal Sections through the Feet
of Children aged about 4 and 10 years

Observe:

1. From the younger foot, that epiphyses of long bones (e.g., tibia, metatarsals, and phalanges) ossify like short bones (i.e., carpal and tarsal bones)—the ossific centres being
   enveloped in cartilage; and that ossification has already extended to the surface of the
   larger tarsal bones.

2. From the older foot, that ossification has spread to the dorsal and plantar surfaces of all
   the tarsal bones in view; and that cartilage persists on the articular surfaces only.

3. The traction epiphysis of the calcaneus for the tendo Achillis and plantar aponeurosis.
   This starts to ossify between the ages of 6 and 10 years (C. C. Francis).

4. That the 1st metatarsal bone behaves as a phalanx in that its epiphysis is at its base and
   not at its head like the 2nd and other metatarsal bones (c.f. the hand, fig. 104).

5. The synovial folds projecting between the articular cartilages where they are liable to be
   pinched.

(For epiphyses of upper limb, see figs. 98—104.)

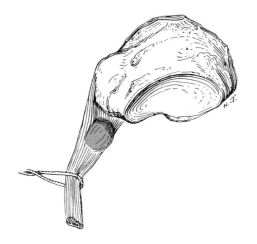

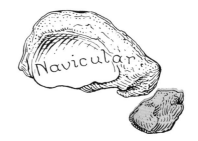

A Sesamoid Bone in Tibialis Posterior Tendon was found in 80 or 23 % of 348 adult feet; 42 were paired and 38 unpaired (C. E. Storton).

Accessory Navicular Bone (Tibiale Exter num). The tuberosity of the navicular bone, t which Tibialis Posterior is largely inserted, appeared as an independent bone in 4.1 % of 3619 men ex amined by X-ray (R. I. Harris and T. Beath).

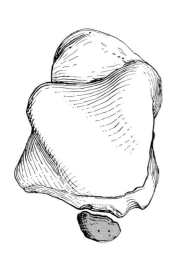
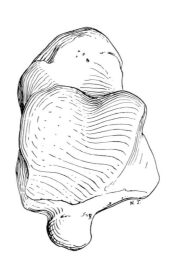

Os Trigonum. The lateral (posterior) tubercle of the talus has a separate centre of ossification, whic appears between the ages of 7 and 13 years. Ha (50 %) of these fuse at the age of 12 years. (C. C. F. When this fails to fuse with the body of the talus, a in the left bone of this pair, it is called an os tri gonum. It was found in 43 or 7.7 % of 558 adul feet; 22 were paired, 21 were unpaired. (C. E. S.

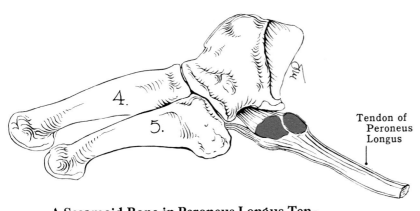

Tendon of
Peroneus
Longus

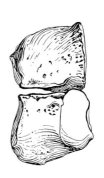
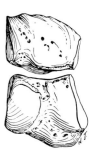

A Sesamoid Bone in Peroneus Longus Tendon was found in 26 % of 92 feet. In this specimen it is bipartite, and Peroneus Longus has an additional attachment to the 5th metatarsal bone. (*C.E.S.*)

A Bipartite Medial Cuneiform Bone, i dorsal and plantar halves, is not common.

356 Anomalies of the Tarsal Bones

(Anomalies of hip, knee and leg. figs. 323—324.)

The Vertebrae and
the Vertebral Column

FUNCTIONS: PARTS:

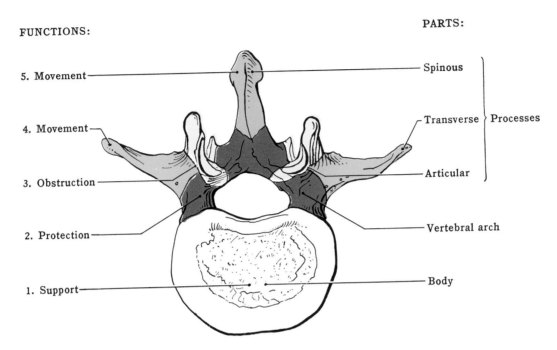

5. Movement ——————————————————— Spinous

4. Movement ——————————————— Transverse } Processes

3. Obstruction ———————————————— Articular

2. Protection ——————————————————— Vertebral arch

1. Support ——————————————————————— Body

357   Functions of Constituent Parts of a Vertebra

A typical vertebra comprises the following parts:

1. A columnar body, situated anteriorly or ventrally. Its function, like that of the femur and tibia, is to support weight. Like them and other long bones, it is narrow about its middle and expanded at both ends. These ends also are articular and during growth have epiphyses (fig. 361).

2. A vertebral arch, placed behind the body. With the body this arch encloses a foramen, called the vertebral foramen. Collectively, the vertebral foramina constitute the vertebral canal wherein lodges the spinal cord. The function of a vertebral arch is to afford protection to the cord much as the bones of the vault of the skull afford protection to the brain.

3. Three processes—2 transverse and 1 spinous. These project from the vertebral arch like spokes from a capstan. They afford attachment to muscles. Indeed, they are the levers that help to move the vertebrae.

4. Four articular processes—2 superior and 2 inferior. These project (cranially and caudally) respectively from the arch and come into apposition with the corresponding processes of the vertebrae above and below. Their function is to restrict movements to certain directions, or at least to decree in what directions movements may be permitted, and they prevent the vertebrae from slipping forwards. When one rises from the flexed position, they bear weight temporarily. The lower articular processes of the 5th lumbar vertebra bear weight even in the erect posture (fig. 383).

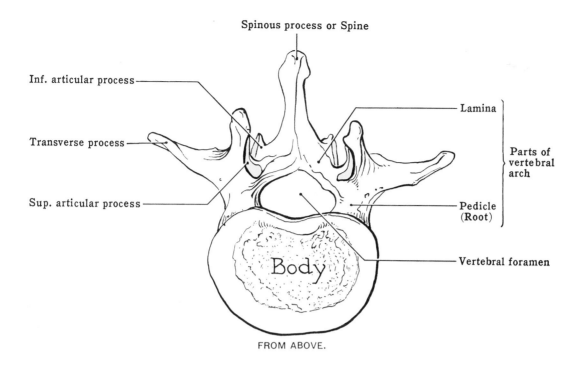

Spinous process or Spine

Inf. articular process

Lamina

Transverse process

Parts of vertebral arch

Sup. articular process

Pedicle (Root)

Body

Vertebral foramen

FROM ABOVE.

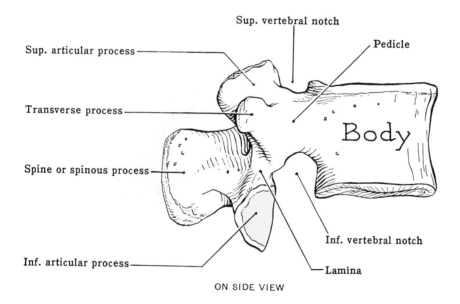

Sup. vertebral notch

Sup. articular process

Pedicle

Transverse process

Body

Spine or spinous process

Inf. vertebral notch

Inf. articular process

Lamina

ON SIDE VIEW

358 A Vertebra

(Second lumbar vertebra.)

Observe:

1. The vertebral arch. It consists of two stout, rounded pedicles, one on each side, which spring from the body and which are united posteriorly by two flat plates or laminae.
2. A small notch above the pedicle and a larger one below it, called the superior and the inferior vertebral notch. When two vertebrae are in articulation, the two adjacent vertebral notches become an intervertebral foramen for the transmission of a spinal nerve and its accompanying intervertebral vessels.
3. Obviously, each articular process has an articular facet—the two terms are not synonymous.

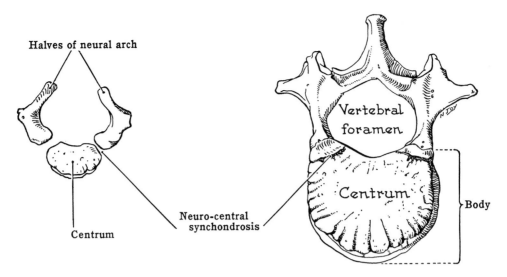

Halves of neural arch

Neuro-central
synchondrosis

Centrum

Vertebral
foramen

Centrum

Body

359 A Vertebra at Birth

360 A Vertebra in Childhood

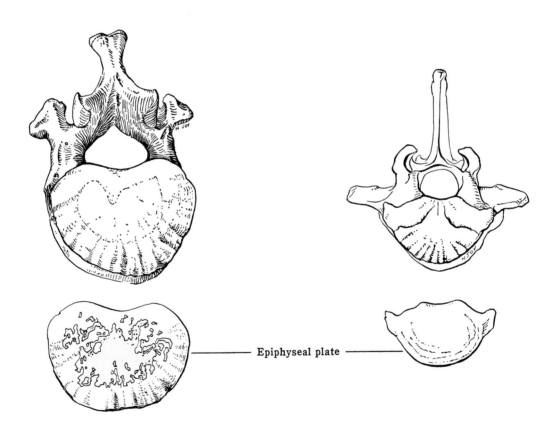

Epiphyseal plate

361 A Vertebra in Adolescence

362 A Vertebra of a sheep

Observe:

1. At birth each typical vertebra consists of three bony parts, united by hyaline cartilage (fig. 359).

2. The synchondrosis between the two halves of the neural arch undergoes synostosis before the neuro-central synchondroses (fig. 360).

3. The body of a vertebra, being the upper and lower epiphyseal plates and the part of the vertebra between them, includes the entire centrum and the anterior ends of the neural arch. The rest of the neural arch is the vertebral arch.

4. The epiphyseal plate is a plate of hyaline cartilage and a circumferential bony ring—that is, in man (fig. 361). In other mammals it is a complete bony plate (fig. 362).

5. The apposed surfaces of the plate and centrum are corrugated. Their interlocking acts as a nonslipping device.

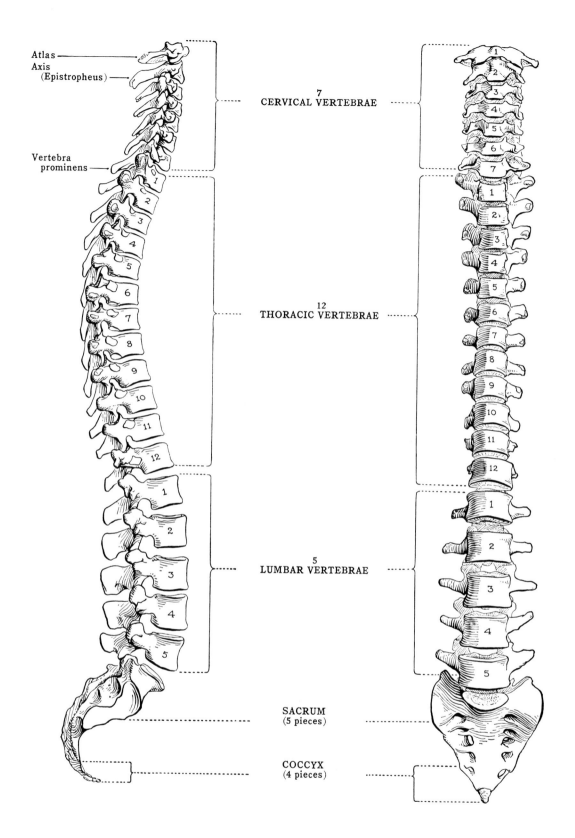

Atlas
Axis (Epistropheus)

Vertebra prominens

1
2
3
4
5
6
7
8
9
10
11
12

12 THORACIC VERTEBRAE

1
2
3
4
5

5 LUMBAR VERTEBRAE

SACRUM (5 pieces)

COCCYX (4 pieces)

63   Vertebral Column, side view

364   Vertebral Column, front view

bserve:

The vertebral column comprises 24 true or pre-sacral vertebrae and 2 composite vertebrae—the sacrum and the coccyx. Of the 24 pre-sacral vertebrae, 12 (50 percent) support ribs and therefore are thoracic; of the other 12, 7 are in the neck and 5 are in the lumbar region.

Vertebrae lying behind bony cavities (the thoracic vertebrae behind the thoracic cavity, and the sacrum and coccyx behind the pelvic cavity) are concave forwards; but elsewhere (in the cervical and lumbar regions), by way of compensation, they are convex forwards.

3. The transverse processes of the atlas spread widely; those of C. 7 spread almost as far; those of C. 2 to C. 6 much less. The spread diminishes progressively from T. 1 to T. 12. In the lumbar region it is greatest at L. 3.

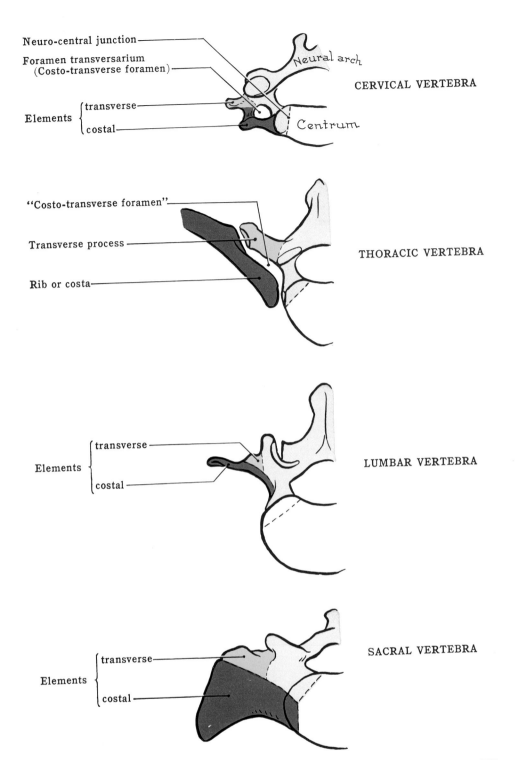

Neuro-central junction

Foramen transversarium
(Costo-transverse foramen)

Elements { transverse
            costal

Neural arch

CERVICAL VERTEBRA

Centrum

"Costo-transverse foramen"

Transverse process

Rib or costa

THORACIC VERTEBRA

Elements { transverse
            costal

LUMBAR VERTEBRA

Elements { transverse
            costal

SACRAL VERTEBRA

365 Diagram of the Homologous Parts of the Vertebrae

Red = rib or costal element; blue = neural arch
and its processes; uncoloured = centrum.

Note:

1. A rib or costa is a free element in the thoracic region. In the cervical region it is represented by the anterior part of a transverse process; in the lumbar region likewise by the anterior part of a transverse process; and in the sacrum by the anterior part of the pars lateralis (lateral mass, fig. 373).

2. The heads of the ribs (thoracic region) articulate with the sides of the bodies of the vertebrae posterior to the neuro-central junctions, i.e., not with the centra, but with the neural arches.

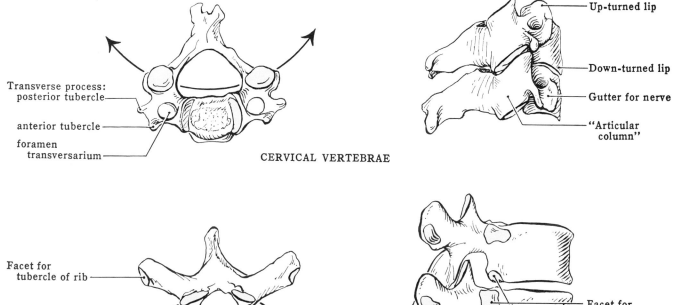

Transverse process:
posterior tubercle

anterior tubercle

foramen
transversarium

CERVICAL VERTEBRAE

Up-turned lip

Down-turned lip

Gutter for nerve

"Articular
column"

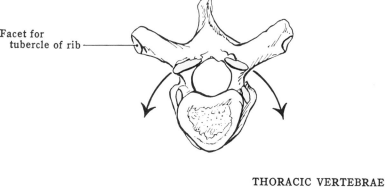

Facet for
tubercle of rib

THORACIC VERTEBRAE

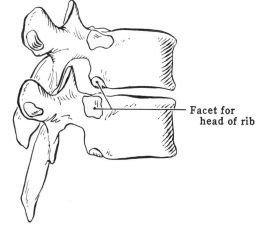

Facet for
head of rib

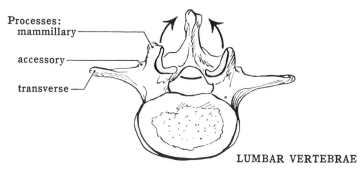

Processes:
mammillary

accessory

transverse

LUMBAR VERTEBRAE

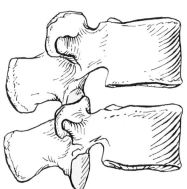

366 Distinguishing Features and the Movements of the Free Vertebrae

Distinctive Features:

Foramina transversaria are distinctive of all cervical vertebrae; facets for the heads of ribs are distinctive of all thoracic vertebrae; the absence of these proclaims a vertebra to be lumbar.

Typical Features:

1. The *Bodies* of cervical and lumbar vertebrae are greater in the transverse diameter than in the antero-posterior, and the vertebral foramina are triangular. In thoracic vertebrae the two diameters are about equal and the foramen is circular. Further, the superior surface of the body of a cervical vertebra ends at each side in an up-turned lip, hence it is concave from side to side. The inferior surface ends anteriorly in a down-turned lip. The superior and inferior surfaces of thoracic and lumbar bodies are flat.

2. A *Transverse Process* in the cervical region points laterally, downwards and forwards, and ends in two tubercles with a gutter between them. In the thoracic region it points laterally, backwards and upwards, has a facet for the tubercle of a rib, and is stout. In the lumbar region it points laterally, and is long and slender.

3. *Spinous Processes* are bifid if cervical, spine-like if thoracic, and oblong if lumbar.

4. *Articular Processes* in the cervical region collectively form a cylinder which is in part weight-bearing; it is cut obliquely into segments. In the thoracic and lumbar regions, the superior articular facets lie behind the pedicles, and the inferior facets are in front of the laminae.

Superior Articular Facets in the cervical region face mainly upwards; in the thoracic region mainly backwards; in the lumbar region mainly medially. The change in direction is gradual from cervical to thoracic, but from thoracic to lumbar it is abrupt.

Movements: In all three regions the articular processes permit flexion and extension and side to side movement. Cervical vertebrae allow one to look sideways up. Thoracic vertebrae allow of medial and lateral rotation, but lumbar vertebrae do not.

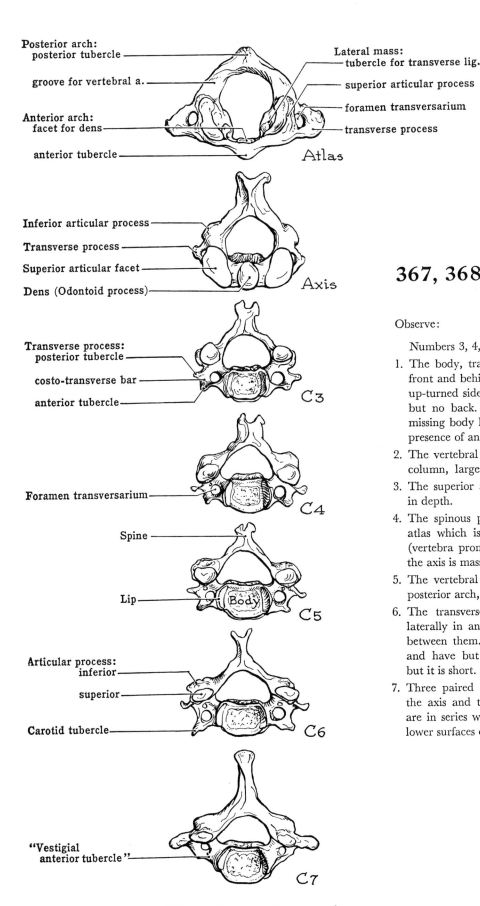

Posterior arch:
posterior tubercle

groove for vertebral a.

Anterior arch:
facet for dens

anterior tubercle

Lateral mass:
tubercle for transverse lig.

superior articular process

foramen transversarium

transverse process

Atlas

Inferior articular process

Transverse process

Superior articular facet

Dens (Odontoid process)

Axis

Transverse process:
posterior tubercle

costo-transverse bar

anterior tubercle

C3

Foramen transversarium

C4

Spine

Lip

Body

C5

Articular process:
inferior

superior

Carotid tubercle

C6

"Vestigial
anterior tubercle"

C7

367, 368   Cervical Vertebrae

Observe:

Numbers 3, 4, 5 and 6 are typical; 1, 2 and 7 are peculiar

1. The body, transversely elongated. It is of equal depth in front and behind. Its upper surface, resembling a seat with up-turned side arms, which bear facets, and rounded from but no back. The absence of a body for the atlas—the missing body having joined the axis as the dens,—and the presence of an anterior arch which lies in front of the dens

2. The vertebral foramen, in this most mobile section of the column, large and triangular. It is largest in the atlas

3. The superior and inferior vertebral notches, nearly equal in depth.

4. The spinous process, short and bifid, except that of the atlas which is reduced to a tubercle, and that of C. 7 (vertebra prominens) which is long and nonbifid. That of the axis is massive.

5. The vertebral arch, also massive in the axis but, as the posterior arch, slender in the atlas.

6. The transverse processes, short, perforated and ending laterally in anterior and posterior tubercles with a gutter between them. Those of the atlas and of C. 7 are longer and have but one (posterior) tubercle; so has the axis, but it is short.

7. Three paired articular facets, viz., the superior facets of the axis and the inferior and superior facets of the atlas are in series with the facets at the sides of the upper and lower surfaces of the bodies.

367   Cervical Vertebrae, from above

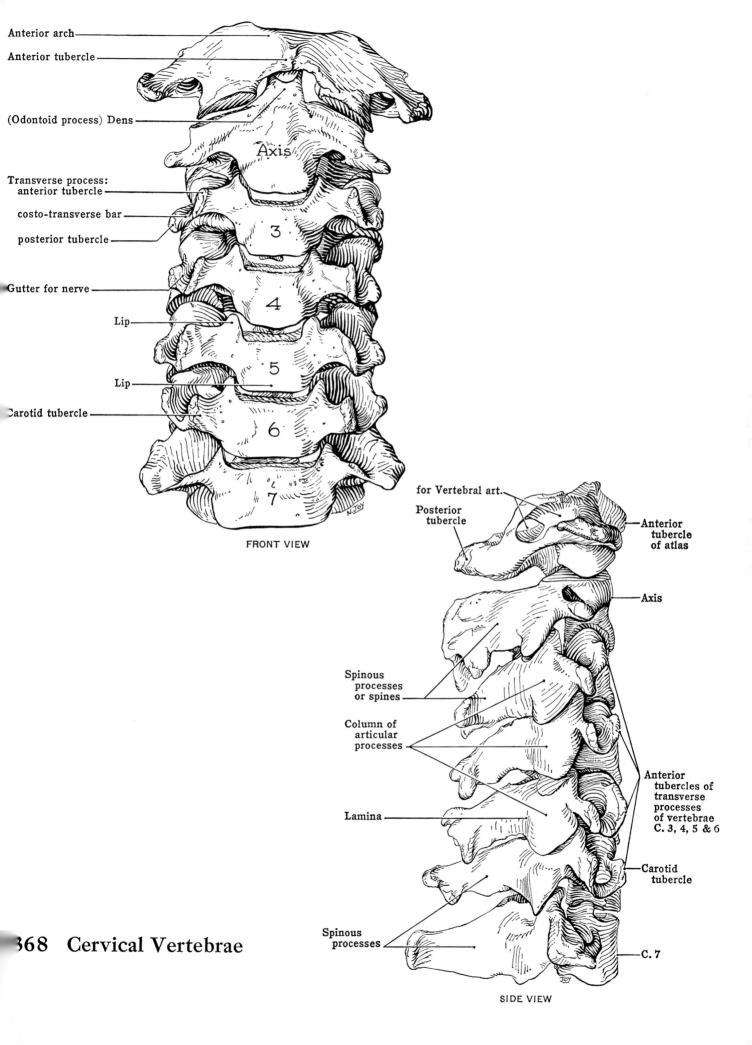

Anterior arch

Anterior tubercle

(Odontoid process) Dens

Axis

Transverse process:
anterior tubercle

costo-transverse bar

posterior tubercle

3

Gutter for nerve

4

Lip

5

Lip

Carotid tubercle

6

7

N.JOY

FRONT VIEW

for Vertebral art.

Posterior
tubercle

Anterior
tubercle
of atlas

Axis

Spinous
processes
or spines

Column of
articular
processes

Anterior
tubercles of
transverse
processes
of vertebrae
C. 3, 4, 5 & 6

Lamina

Carotid
tubercle

Spinous
processes

C. 7

JOY

368 Cervical Vertebrae

SIDE VIEW

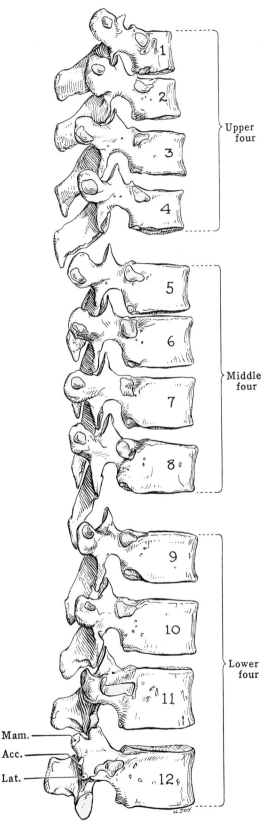

369 Thoracic Vertebrae, side view

369, 370 Thoracic Vertebrae

Observe:

1. The middle 4 are typical; those at the ends have cervical and lumbar features respectively.

2. The body, deeper dorsally than ventrally; with flat upper and lower surfaces; the surface area (weight-bearing surface) increasing from T.1 to T.12. (Indeed, from C.3 to L.5.) The triangular shape of the middle 4 (i.e., equal antero-posterior and transverse diameters), the transverse diameter increasing towards the cervical and lumbar ends of the series.

3. The rib facet at the upper postero-lateral angle of the body encroaching on the lower postero-lateral angle of the body above; except the facets of (T.10), 11 and 12 which are on the pedicles.

4. The superior vertebral notch, present on T.1 only.

5. The vertebral foramen, circular and smaller than a finger-ring, and becoming triangular towards the cervical and lumbar ends.

6. The spines of the middle 4, which are long, over-lapping and nearly vertical. Those of 1, 2 and 11, 12 which are nearly horizontal; and those of 3, 4 and 9, 10 which are oblique.

7. The stretch of the transverse processes diminishing progressively from T.1 to T.12. T.1 to T.10 having rib facets on the transverse processes. These are concave and placed anteriorly on T.1 to T.7; flat and superiorly placed on T.8 to T.10.

8. The cervical features of T.1—possession of superior vertebral notches, and upturned side lips on the body.

9. The lumbar features of T.12—the lateral direction of the inferior articular processes; possession of mamillary, accessory and lateral tubercles.

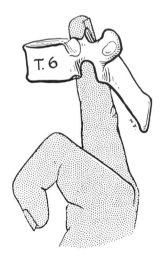

369.1
Demonstrating the small size of a vertebral foramen.

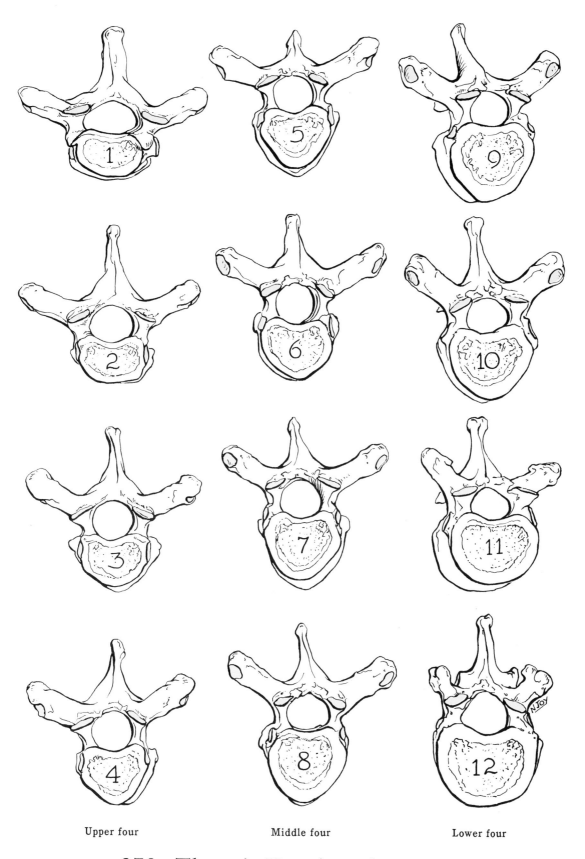

Upper four   Middle four   Lower four

370   Thoracic Vertebrae, from above

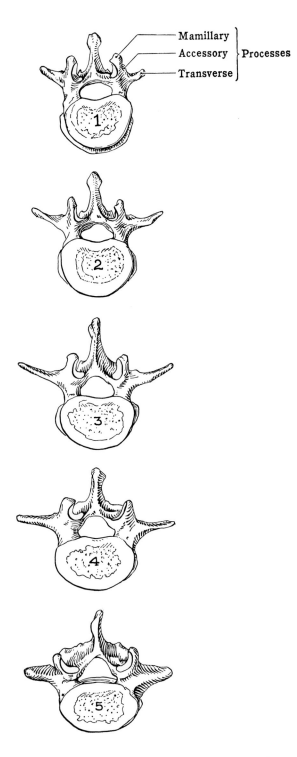

Mamillary ⎫
Accessory ⎬ Processes
Transverse ⎭

371, 372 Lumbar Vertebrae

Observe:

1. The kidney–shaped bodies, greater in transverse diameter than in antero–posterior. Bodies L.1 and L.2 deeper behind; L.4 and L.5 deeper in front; L.3 transitional, being sometimes deeper behind and sometimes deeper in front.

2. The vertebral foramina, small and triangular, and having pinched lateral angles in L.5.

3. The slight superior vertebral notches.

4. The large, oblong, and horizontal spinous processes.

5. The long, slender, horizontal transverse processes. That of L.3 projecting furthest; that of L.5 spreading forward on to the body, being conical and its apex having an upward tilt. The mamillary process (for origin of Multifidus) on the superior articular process. The accessory process (for insertion of Longissimus) on the transverse process.

6. The superior articular processes, facing each other and grasping the inferior processes of the vertebra above. The inferior articular processes, close together in L.1, but far apart in L.5 and facing more anteriorly.

371 Lumbar Vertebrae, from above

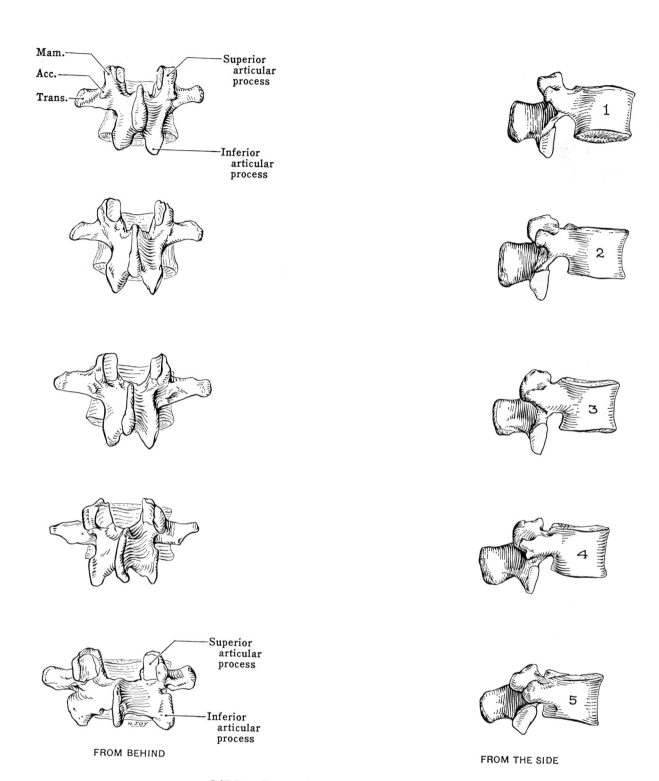

Mam.
Acc.
Trans.

Superior
articular
process

Inferior
articular
process

Superior
articular
process

Inferior
articular
process

FROM BEHIND

FROM THE SIDE

372   Lumbar Vertebrae

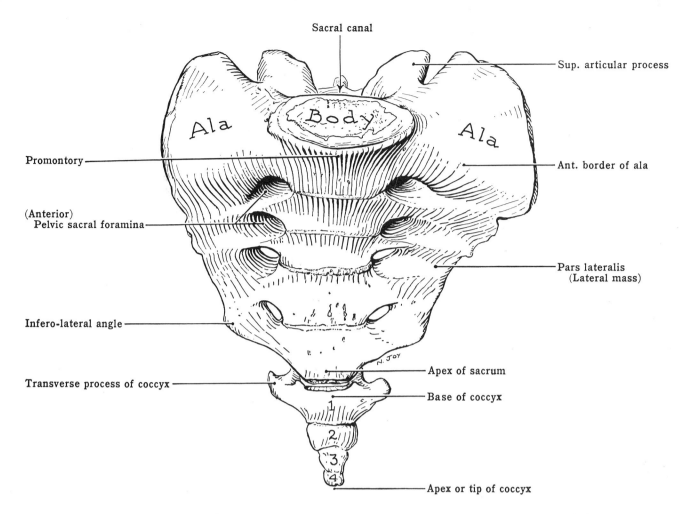

Sacral canal

Sup. articular process

Ala

Body

Ala

Promontory

Ant. border of ala

(Anterior)
Pelvic sacral foramina

Pars lateralis
(Lateral mass)

Infero-lateral angle

N. JOY

Apex of sacrum

Transverse process of coccyx

Base of coccyx

1

2

3

4

Apex or tip of coccyx

373   Sacrum and Coccyx, pelvic surface and base

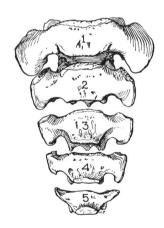

373.1   Sacrum in Youth

The costal elements (fig. 365) begin to fuse with each other about puberty. The bodies begin to fuse with each other from below upwards about the 17th–18th year, fusion being complete by the 23rd year. A gap, however, may persist between the 3rd and 2nd bodies until the 24th year, and between the 2nd and 1st until the 33rd year. (McKern & Stewart.)

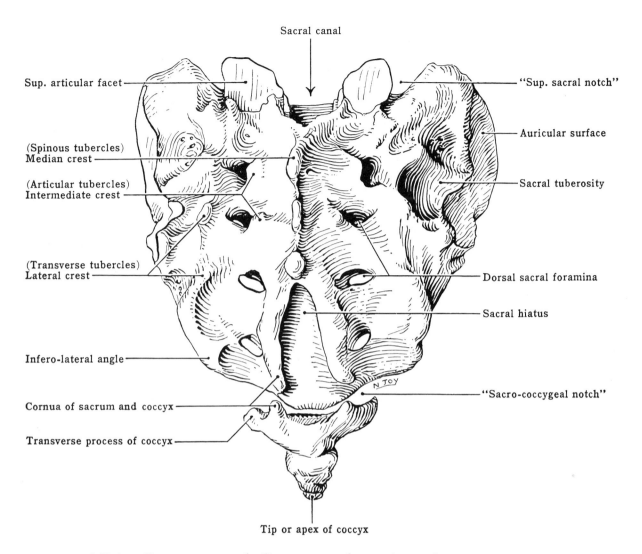

Sacral canal

Sup. articular facet

"Sup. sacral notch"

Auricular surface

(Spinous tubercles)
Median crest

(Articular tubercles)
Intermediate crest

Sacral tuberosity

(Transverse tubercles)
Lateral crest

Dorsal sacral foramina

Sacral hiatus

Infero-lateral angle

N TOY

"Sacro-coccygeal notch"

Cornua of sacrum and coccyx

Transverse process of coccyx

Tip or apex of coccyx

374 Sacrum and Coccyx, dorsal surface

Observe, on *Anterior View* (fig. 373):

1. The 5 sacral bodies, demarcated by 4 transverse lines which end laterally in 4 pairs of pelvic (anterior) sacral foramina.

2. The foramina of the two sides, approximately equidistant throughout. Their margins rounded laterally, but sharp elsewhere, indicating the courses of the emerging nerves.

3. The coccyx having 4 pieces. The 1st piece having a pair of transverse processes and a pair of cornua; the other 3 pieces being nodular.

Observe, on *Posterior View* (fig. 374):

4. The absence of the 4th and 5th sacral spines and laminae.

5. The superior articular processes, the intermediate crest, and the sacral and coccygeal cornua are serially homologous;

6. so, likewise, are the "superior sacral notch", the 4 dorsal sacral foramina, and the "sacro-coccygeal notch";

7. and, likewise, the postero-superior angle of the ala, the lateral crest, the inferolateral angle, and the transverse process of the coccyx.

8. A straight probe can be passed through a lower dorsal foramen, across the sacral canal, and through a pelvic foramen. Side view see figure 222.

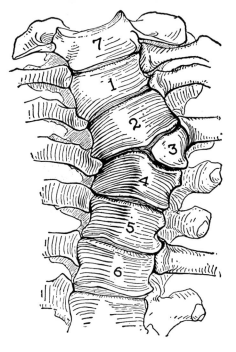

375   A Half Vertebra

The entire right half of the 3rd thoracic vertebra and the corresponding rib are absent. The left lamina and the spine are fused throughout with those of T.4, and the left intervertebral foramen is reduced in size. Observe the associated scoliosis (lateral curvature). (From the Anatomy Department, University of Manitoba, courtesy of Professor I. Maclaren Thompson.)

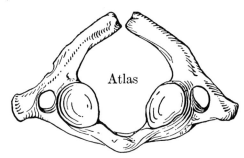

376   Instance of Failure of Two Halves of a Vertebral Arch to undergo Synostosis

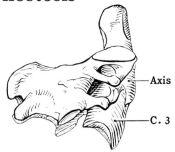

377   Congenital Synostosis of Axis and 3rd Cervical Vertebra

It is not very rare for the laminae and articular processes of these two bones to be fused together.

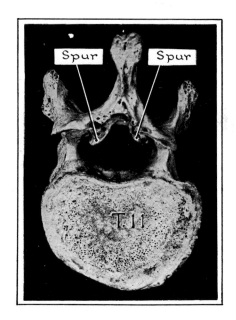

378   Ossifying Ligamenta Flava

Sharp, bony spurs commonly grow from the laminae caudally into the ligg. flava thereby reducing the lengths of these elastic bands. Hence, when the vertebral column is flexed, they are likely to be torn. Restricted to the thoracic and lumbar regions, commonest and largest on T. 11, they diminish in size and frequency cranially to T. 1 and caudally to L. 5 (*G. T. Ho*).

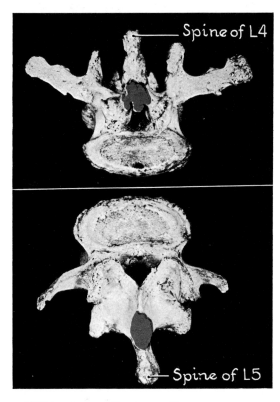

379   "Kissing Spines"

In macerated vertebral columns contact facets, either horizontal or obliquely overlapping, between lumbar spines (1 & 2), 2 & 3, 3 & 4, and 4 & 5 are commonly found (fig. 386). (*J.C.B.G.*)

ANOMALIES OF THE VERTEBRAE

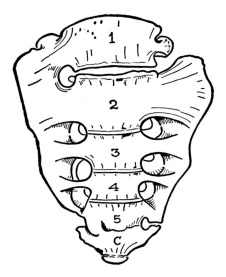

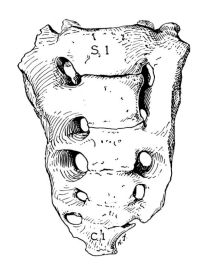

380 A Transitional Lumbo-sacral Vertebra

In this instance, the 1st sacral vertebra is partly free (lumbarized). Not uncommonly the 5th lumbar vertebra is partly fused to the sacrum (sacralized).

381 Maldevelopment of the Sacrum

The left side of the sacrum is imperfectly developed.

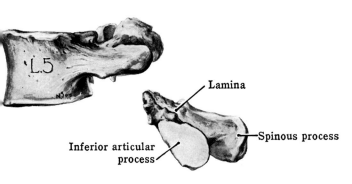

Lamina

Spinous process

Inferior articular process

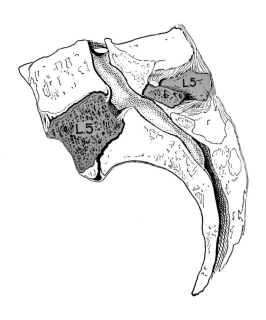

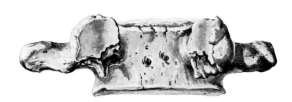

383 Spondylolisthesis

382, 383. Commonly (in 5% of vertebral columns) the 5th lumbar vertebra is in two pieces, the inferior articular processes, the laminae, and the spine forming a separate unit. Hence, the body and the superimposed vertebrae tend to slide forwards (spondylolisthesis). Less often the 4th lumbar vertebra is bipartite. (*See T. D. Stewart.*)

382 A Bipartite Fifth Lumbar Vertebra

ANOMALIES OF THE VERTEBRAE

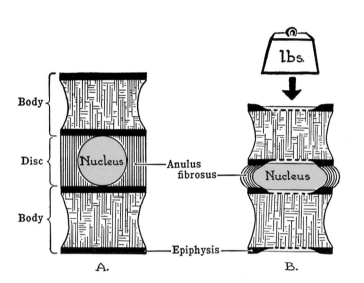

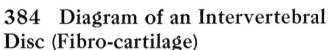

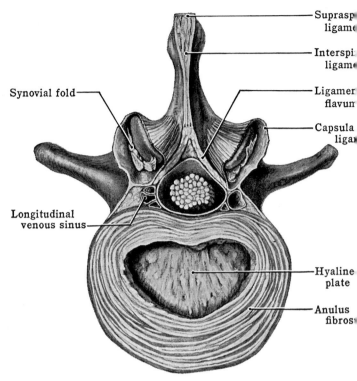

384 Diagram of an Intervertebral Disc (Fibro-cartilage)

To illustrate the cushioning value of the nucleus pulposus and the presence of a thin, hyaline epiphyseal plate.

385 An Intervertebral Disc and Ligaments, on cross section

The nucleus pulposus has been scooped out and the cartilaginous epiphyseal plate exposed.

Observe:

1. The rings of the anulus fibrosus, least numerous dorsally.
2. The continuity of the following ligaments—capsular, flavum, interspinous, and supraspinous.
3. The synovial fold, containing a pad of fat, such as is present in all synovial joints.
4. The longitudinal vertebral venous sinuses which extend extradurally throughout the length of the vertebral canal (fig. 390).
5. The cauda equina of the spinal cord (not labelled) lying free within the subarachnoid space.

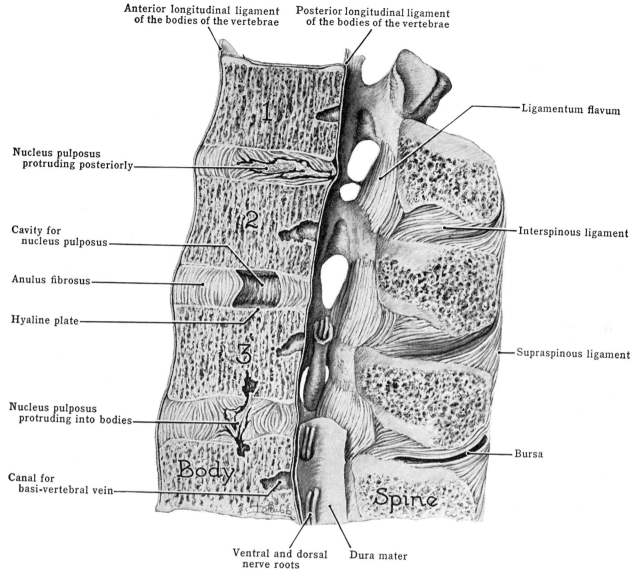

Anterior longitudinal ligament
of the bodies of the vertebrae

Posterior longitudinal ligament
of the bodies of the vertebrae

Ligamentum flavum

Nucleus pulposus
protruding posteriorly

Cavity for
nucleus pulposus

Interspinous ligament

Anulus fibrosus

Hyaline plate

Supraspinous ligament

Nucleus pulposus
protruding into bodies

Bursa

Canal for
basi-vertebral vein

Body

Spine

Ventral and dorsal
nerve roots

Dura mater

386 An Intervertebral Disc (Fibro-cartilage) and Ligaments, on median section

Observe:

1. The nucleus pulposus of the normal disc between the 2nd and 3rd vertebrae has been scooped out from the enclosing anulus fibrosus.

2. The ligamentum flavum, extending from the upper border and adjacent part of the posterior aspect of one lamina to the lower border and adjacent part of the anterior aspect of the lamina above, and extending laterally to the intervertebral foramen which it bounds posteriorly.

3. The interspinous ligament, uniting obliquely the upper and lower borders of two adjacent spines. Elastic fibers are sparce. The supraspinous lig. extended as far caudally as L.3 in 22% of 100 specimens, to L.4 in 73%, to L.5 in 5%, and to the sacrum never. Many of the fibers shown above are not ligamentous, but the fibrous attachments of thoracolumbar fascia, Longissimus, and Multifidus (figs. 479–481. (Rissanen.)

4. The adventitious bursa between the 3rd and 4th lumbar spines, acquired presumably as the result of habitual hyperextension which brings the lumbar spines into contact, as in fig. 379.

5. Two degenerative changes—(a) The pulp of the disc between the 1st and 2nd vertebrae has herniated backwards through the anulus, and (b) the pulp of the disc between the 3rd and 4th vertebrae has herniated through the cartilaginous epiphyseal plates into the bodies of the vertebrae above and below.

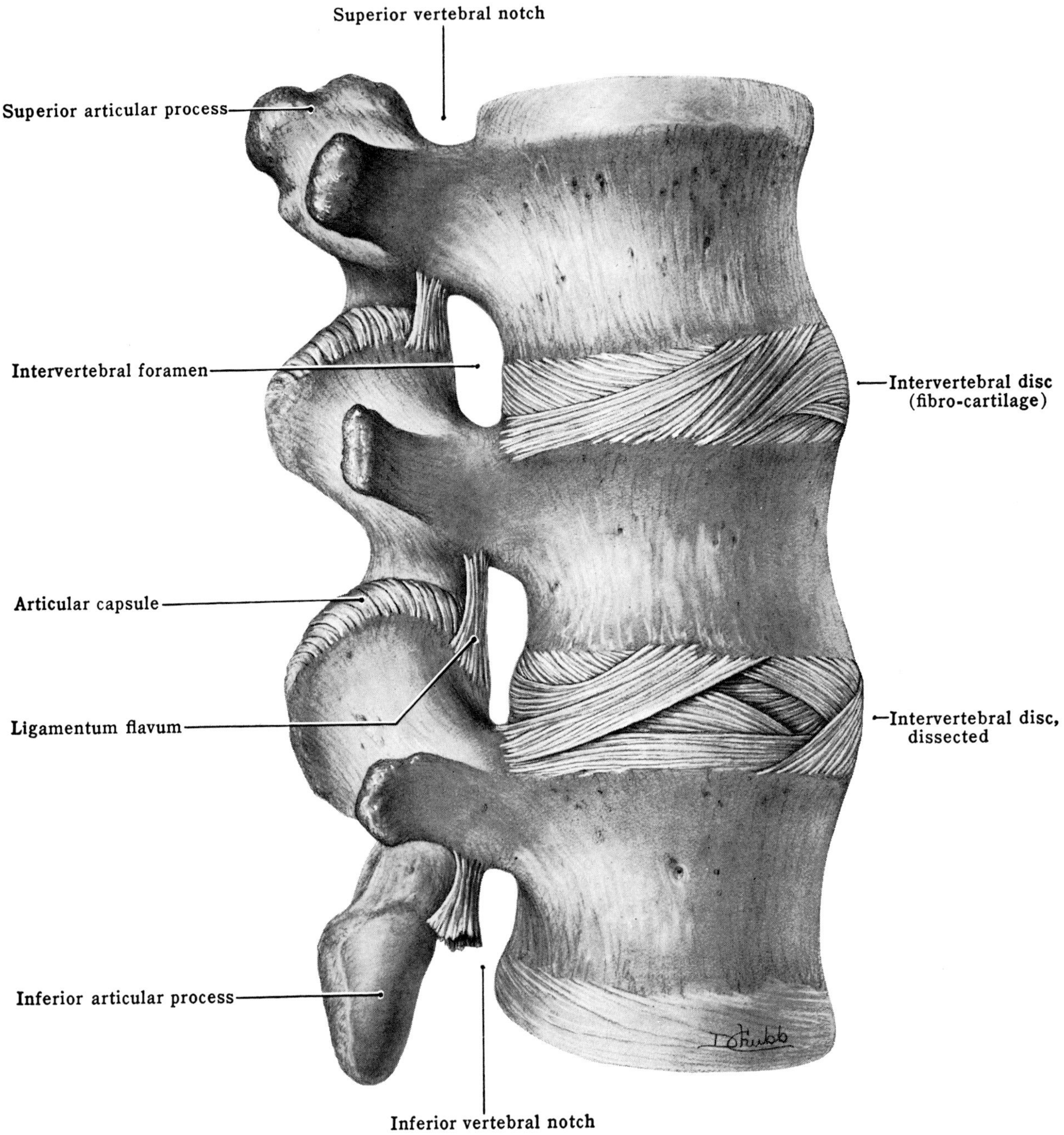

Superior vertebral notch

Superior articular process —

Intervertebral foramen —

Articular capsule —

Ligamentum flavum —

Inferior articular process —

— Intervertebral disc
(fibro-cartilage)

— Intervertebral disc,
dissected

Inferior vertebral notch

387 An Intervertebral Disc, side view

Sections have been removed from the superficial layers of the lower disc, in order to show the directions of the fibres.

Observe:

1. The anulus fibrosus, resembling the flat muscles of the abdominal wall in being arranged in layers of parallel fibres which criss-cross those of the next layer.

2. An intervertebral foramen, resulting from the apposition of a superior and an inferior vertebral notch, bounded above and below by pedicles, in front by an intervertebral disc and parts of the two bodies united by that disc, and behind by a capsular ligament and parts of the two articular processes united by that capsular ligament. Further, the anterior part of the capsule is strengthened by the lateral border of the ligamentum flavum.

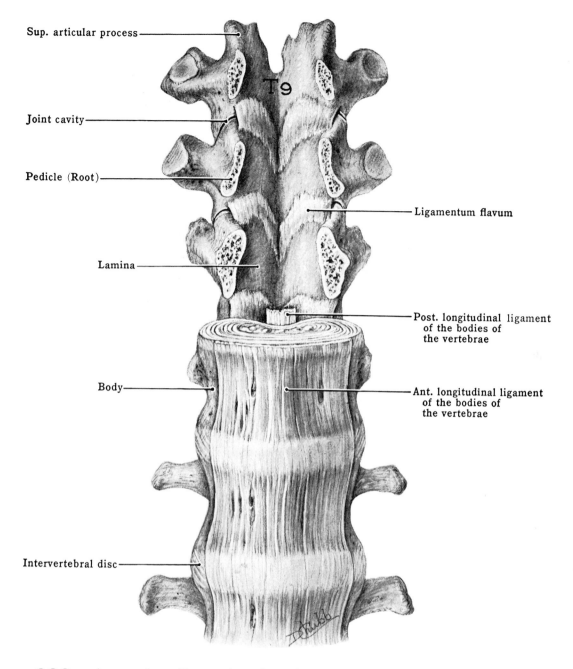

Sup. articular process

Joint cavity

Pedicle (Root)

Lamina

Body

Intervertebral disc

T9

Ligamentum flavum

Post. longitudinal ligament of the bodies of the vertebrae

Ant. longitudinal ligament of the bodies of the vertebrae

388 Anterior Longitudinal Ligament and the Ligamenta Flava, anterior view

The pedicles of the 9th, 10th, and 11th thoracic vertebrae have been sawn through and their bodies discarded.

Note:

1. The anterior and posterior longitudinal ligaments are ligaments of the bodies; the ligamenta flava are ligaments of the vertebral arches.

2. The anterior longitudinal ligaments are broad, strong, fibrous bands. They are attached to the intervertebral discs and to the adjacent parts of the fronts of the bodies. They have foramina for veins and arteries passing from and to the bodies.

3. The ligamenta flava, composed of yellow or elastic fibres, extend between adjacent laminae. Those of opposite sides meet and blend in the median plane. They extend laterally to the articular processes where they blend with the anterior fibres of the capsule of the joint. Being elastic, they tend, at all times, to restore the vertebral column to the extended or erect position. Above, they are in series with the posterior atlanto-axial and posterior atlanto-occipital membranes.

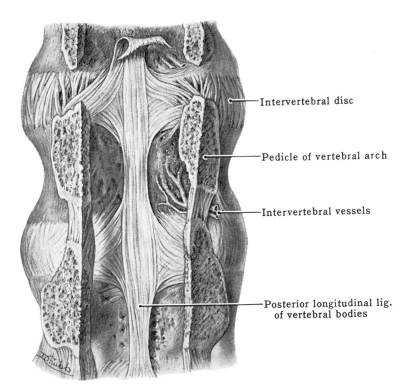

Intervertebral disc

Pedicle of vertebral arch

Intervertebral vessels

Posterior longitudinal lig.
of vertebral bodies

389 Posterior Longitudinal Ligament, posterior view

The vertebral arches have been sawn through
and largely removed.

Observe:

1. This taut but somewhat flimsy band passing from
   disc to disc, spanning the posterior surfaces of the
   bodies of the vertebrae, and rendering smooth the
   anterior wall of the vertebral canal.
2. The diamond shape taken by the ligament behind
   each disc, where it both gives and receives fibers.
3. Between the ligament and a vertebral body, a
   plexus of veins which receives the basivertebral
   vein from the body (fig. 386), communicates with
   the longitudinal vertebral venous sinus on each
   side, and drains by way of the intervertebral veins.

   The ligament extends to the sacrum below, it
becomes the strong membrana tectoria above (fig.
565).

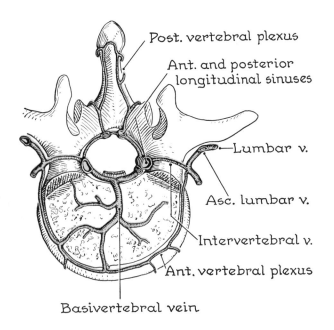

Post. vertebral plexus

Ant. and posterior
longitudinal sinuses

Lumbar v.

Asc. lumbar v.

Intervertebral v.

Ant. vertebral plexus

Basivertebral vein

390 Diagram of the Vertebral Venous Plexuses

The Internal Plexus: The vertebral canal contains a plexus of thin
walled, valveless veins which surround like a basket-work the dura
mater of the spinal cord and also the posterior longitudinal ligament.
Anterior and posterior longitudinal channels (ant. and post. longitudinal venous sinuses) can be discerned in this plexus. Above, the
plexus communicates through the foramen magnum with the occipital and basilar sinuses. At each spinal segment the plexus receives
veins from the spinal cord and a basivertebral vein from the body
of a vertebra. The plexus in turn is drained by intervertebral veins
which pass through the intervertebral and sacral foramina to the
vertebral, intercostal, lumbar, and lateral sacral veins.

The External Plexus: Through the body of each vertebra come
veins which form a meagre anterior vertebral plexus, and through
the ligamenta flava pass veins which form a well marked posterior
vertebral plexus.

In the cervical region, these plexuses communicate freely with
the occipital and profunda cervicis veins which receive from the
sigmoid sinus the mastoid and condyloid emissary veins. In the
thoracic, lumbar, and pelvic regions the azygos (or hemiazygos),
the ascending lumbar, and the lateral sacral veins respectively
further link segment to segment. (*See Batson, O. V.*)

The Thorax

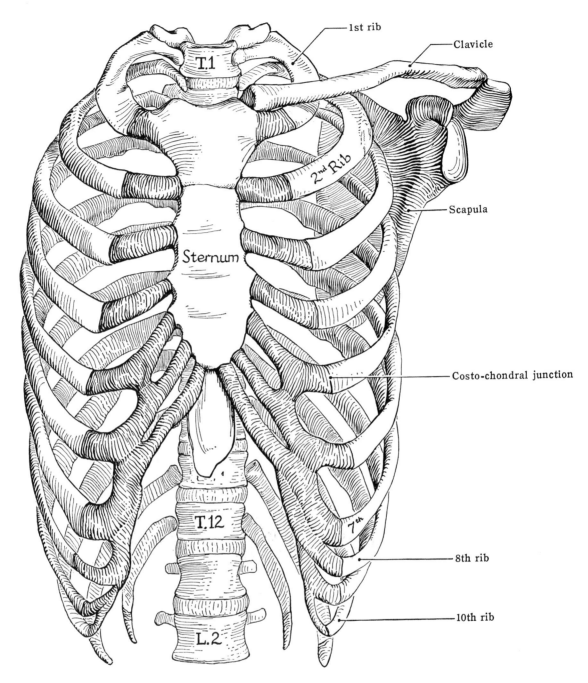

- 1st rib
- Clavicle
- T.1
- 2nd Rib
- Scapula
- Sternum
- Costo-chondral junction
- T.12
- 7th
- 8th rib
- 10th rib
- L.2

391 Bony Thorax, anterior aspect

Observe from figures 391 and 392:

1. The component parts of the bony thorax —12 vertebrae, 12 pairs of ribs and cartilages, and the sternum.

2. Each rib articulating posteriorly with the vertebral column.

3. The cartilages of the upper seven pairs of ribs articulating directly with the sternum. (The eighth pair may do so, as in fig. 406.) The 8th, 9th and (10th) cartilages articulating with the cartilages next above; the 11th and 12th cartilages being free or floating anteriorly.

4. The downward inclination of all ribs. The cartilages of the upper two and of the lower two pairs of ribs, continuing this downward inclination (the 2nd cartilages, however, may be horizontal); the cartilages of the 3rd to 10th ribs inclining upwards.

5. The side to which a detached rib belongs may be told at a glance by the fact that the front of its neck faces *upwards* and forwards. (This does not apply to the uppermost two or three ribs.)

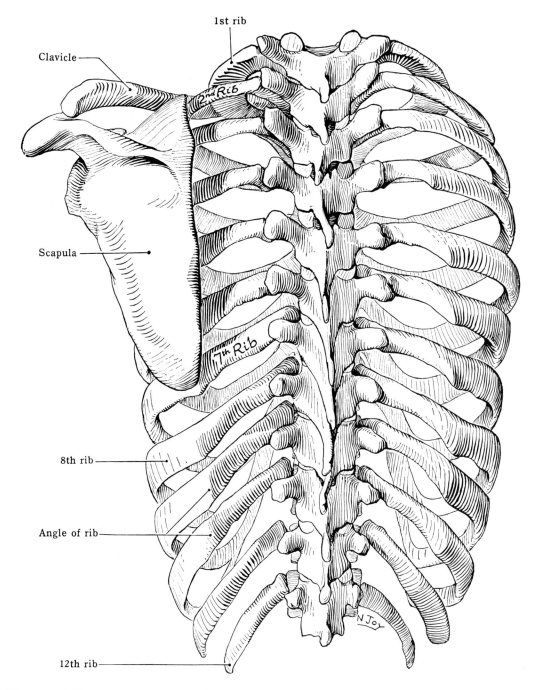

Clavicle

1st rib

2nd Rib

Scapula

7th Rib

8th rib

Angle of rib

12th rib

392 Bony Thorax, posterior aspect

6. The progressive increase in length of the first seven ribs and of the first seven cartilages. The seventh rib is the longest rib, but the eighth and ninth are more oblique.

7. The sternal end of the first costal cartilage, being about $1\frac{1}{2}$ inches below the level of the head of its rib. The tip of the twelfth costal cartilage, being at the level of the second lumbar vertebra.

8. The tenth ribs and cartilages, being the lowest ribs and cartilages visible from the front.

9. The clavicle, thrusting the scapula laterally and backwards. The scapula crossing 50 per cent of the twelve ribs, namely, 2nd–7th inclusive.

10. The distance between the spines of the vertebrae and the angles of the ribs diminishing from the eighth rib upwards.

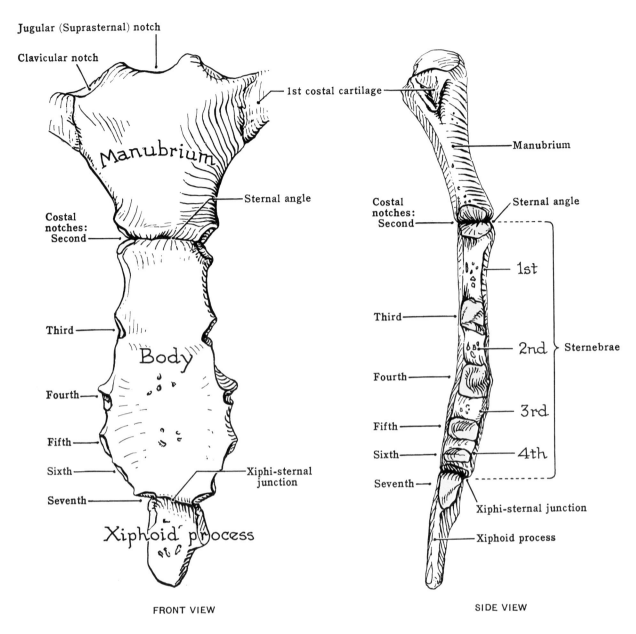

Jugular (Suprasternal) notch

Clavicular notch

1st costal cartilage

Manubrium

Sternal angle

Costal notches: Second

Third

Body

Fourth

Fifth

Sixth

Seventh

Xiphi-sternal junction

Xiphoid process

FRONT VIEW

Costal notches: Second

Sternal angle

Manubrium

1st

Third

2nd ⎫ Sternebrae

Fourth

3rd

Fifth

Sixth

4th

Seventh

Xiphi-sternal junction

Xiphoid process

SIDE VIEW

393 Sternum

Observe:

1. The great thickness of the upper third of the manubrium, between the clavicular notches.

2. The thin and tapering tip and sides of the xiphoid process, which give attachment to the linea alba and to the Transversus Abdominis aponeurosis.

3. Two landmarks—(a) The sternal angle at the junction of the manubrium and body, at the level of the 2nd costal cartilages; and (b) the sharp lower edge of the body, at the xiphi-sternal junction.

4. Seven pairs of costal cartilages articulating with the sternum; the 1st by synchondrosis; the 6th at the sides of the 4th sternebra; the other 5, at the angles between two pieces of the sternum. Of these, the 7th lies in front of the xiphoid process. The 8th costal cartilages sometimes articulates with the sternum, as in figure 406.

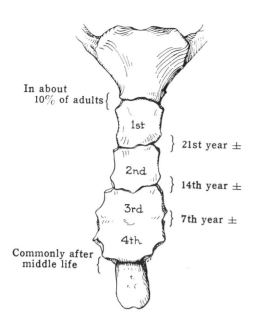

394 Young Sterum

Times of synostosis are shown. The four sternebrae fuse together from below upwards. Numbers, 4, 3 and 2 are usually fused together not later than the 17th or 18th year, and 2 to 1 not later than the 23rd year. They may, however, be delayed. (McK. & Stewart.) Synostosis of manubrium and body was found in about 10% of adults, aged 30 to 80 years. It is apparently unrelated to age. (Trotter, M.)

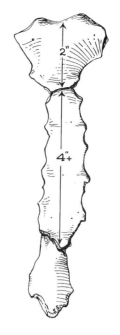

395 Common Form of Sternum

The manubrium is 2″ long and the body 4″ +. It is a variant of figure 393.

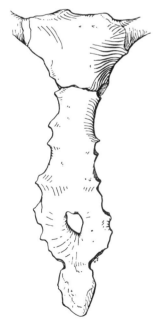

396 Sternal Foramen

This defect of ossification, suggestive of a bullet wound is common. Note synostosis of xiphisternal joint.

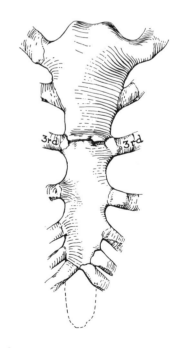

397 Low Sternal Angle

This, at the level of the 3rd costal cartilages, is usual in the gibbon; rare in man.

[From the Anatomy Department, University of Manitoba, courtesy of Professor I. Maclaren Thompson.]

OSSIFICATION—VARIATIONS

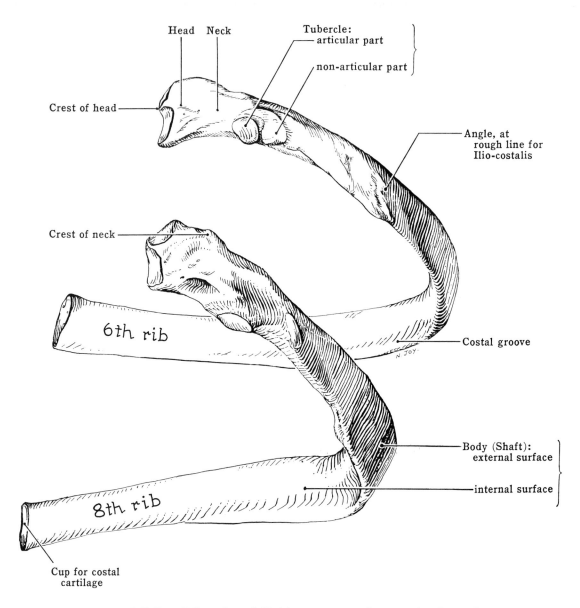

Head   Neck

Crest of head

Tubercle:
  articular part
  non-articular part

Angle, at
rough line for
Ilio-costalis

Crest of neck

6th rib

Costal groove

Body (Shaft):
external surface

internal surface

8th rib

Cup for costal
cartilage

398   Typical Ribs, seen from behind

Observe:

1. The wedge-shaped head, with a larger lower facet for its own vertebra (6th or 8th) an smaller facet for the vertebra above.

2. The crest of the head, which is joined to the intervertebral disc by an intra-articular li ment.

3. The posterior surface of the neck, rough for the costo-transverse ligament (lig. of the ne

4. The crest of the neck, sharp for the superior costo-transverse ligament.

5. The non-articular part of the tubercle, for the lateral costo-transverse ligament (lig. of tubercle) (fig. 411).

6. The articular part of the tubercle, convex and on the posterior aspect of the upper se (vertebro-sternal) ribs, but flat and on the inferior aspect of the 8th, 9th and 10th (verteb chondral) ribs. Indeed, on the 7th it is transitional, being either convex or flat.

7. The posterior part of the shaft is round on cross-section; the anterior part is flattened. anterior end, being articular, is slightly enlarged.

8. The rough line for the attachment of Ilio-costalis where the rib takes not only a bend also a twist, on which account it will not lie flat on a table.

9. The costal groove, which lodges the intercostal vein, artery and nerve.

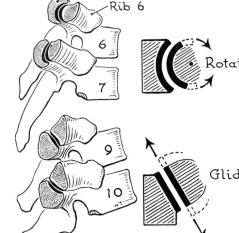

Transverse
process

Rib 6

6

7

Rotates

9

10

Glides   **398.1**

Diagram of costo-transverse joints. At the upper joints the ribs rotate; at 8th, 9th & 10th they glide, increasing the transverse diameter of upper abdomen.

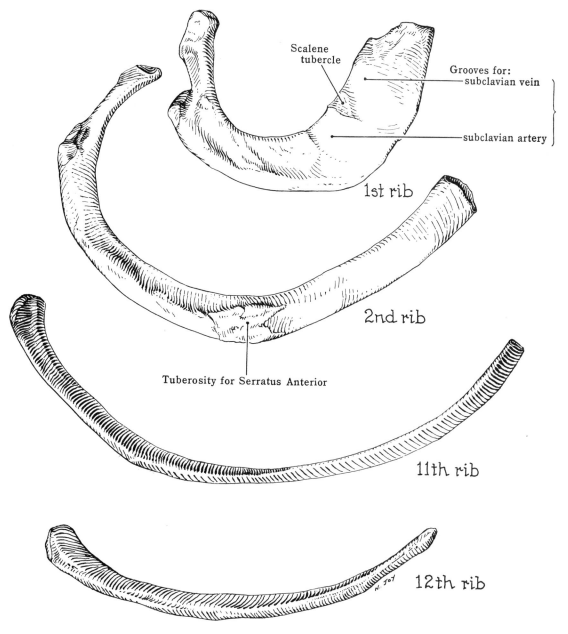

Scalene tubercle

Grooves for:
— subclavian vein

— subclavian artery

1st rib

2nd rib

Tuberosity for Serratus Anterior

11th rib

12th rib

399 Peculiar or Atypical Ribs—1st, 2nd, 11th and 12th—viewed from above

Observe:

These 4 ribs have but faint angles (i.e., twists), if any, and can lie flat on the table.

The 1st is superlative in being the highest, shortest, broadest, strongest, and most curved. Its head and neck are directed medially and downwards—not medially and upwards—and the head has a single facet. Its tubercle is the most prominent of all, for here tubercle and angle coincide. The tubercle for Scalenus Anterior on the upper (external) surface of the shaft separates the groove for the subclavian vein in front from the groove for the subclavian artery and lowest trunk of the brachial plexus behind.

The 2nd rib is marked by the tuberosity for Serratus Anterior. The 11th and 12th ribs, or floating ribs, have each a single facet on the head, no tubercle, and a tapering end.

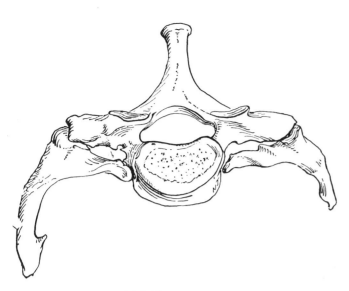

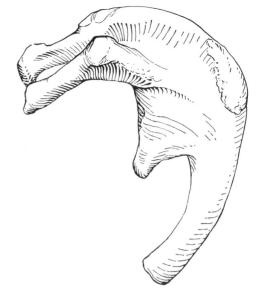

400   Cervical Ribs

A cervical rib is an enlarged costal element (fig. 365) of the 7th cervical vertebra. The subclavian artery and the lowest root of the brachial plexus arch over such ribs. Radiologically, they occur in 5.6 patients per 1000; twice as often in females as in males; and 50% occur bilaterally (Adson). [From the Anatomy Department, University of Manitoba, by the courtesy of Professor I. Maclaren Thompson.]

401   Bicipital Rib

This was occasioned by the partial fusion of th[e] 1st and 2nd thoracic ribs. A similar condition resul[ts] from the partial fusion of a cervical rib and the 1st thoracic rib. [Courtesy of Dr. H. A. Cates.]

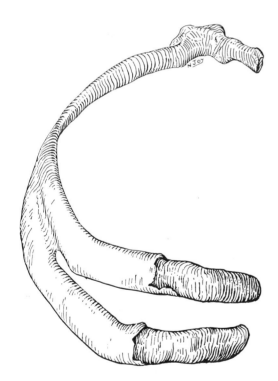

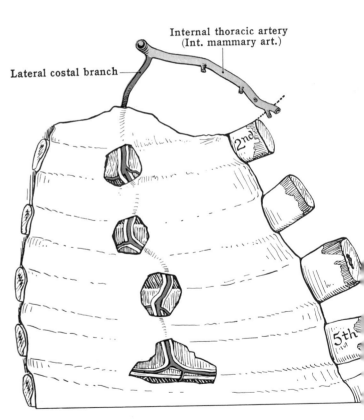

402   Bifid Rib

The upper limb of this 3rd rib is supernumerary. It articulated with the side of the 1st sternebra of the body of the sternum; the lower limb articulated in the normal situation for a 3rd rib, i.e., at the junction of the 1st and 2nd sternebrae. The condition is not uncommon.

403   Lateral Costal Artery

This branch of the int. thoracic artery, which desce[nds] near the midlateral line, was found in 31 (about 25[%]) of 112 cadavera. It was bilateral in six. Of these [29] arteries, 14 reached the 1st or 2nd intercostal spac[e;] the 3rd space; 10 the 4th; and 5 the 5th or 6th. (Kro[ll] B. N.)

VARIATIONS—ANOMALIES

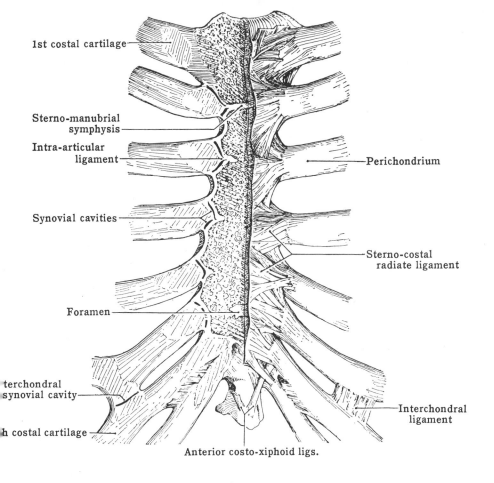

1st costal cartilage

Sterno-manubrial symphysis

Intra-articular ligament

Perichondrium

Synovial cavities

Sterno-costal radiate ligament

Foramen

terchondral synovial cavity

h costal cartilage

Interchondral ligament

Anterior costo-xiphoid ligs.

The cortex of the right half of the sternum and of the right costal cartilages has been shaved away.

Observe:

1. The fibres of the perichondrium, parallel to the long axes of the costal cartilages and therefore acting as ligaments which end as radiate ligaments.

2. The joint between the 1st costal cartilage and the manubrium is a synchondrosis, so, in this instance is the joint between the 7th costal cartilage and the sternum.
The sterno-manubrial joint is a symphysis.
The other sterno-costal joints and the interchondral joints are synovial joints with or without intra-articular ligaments.

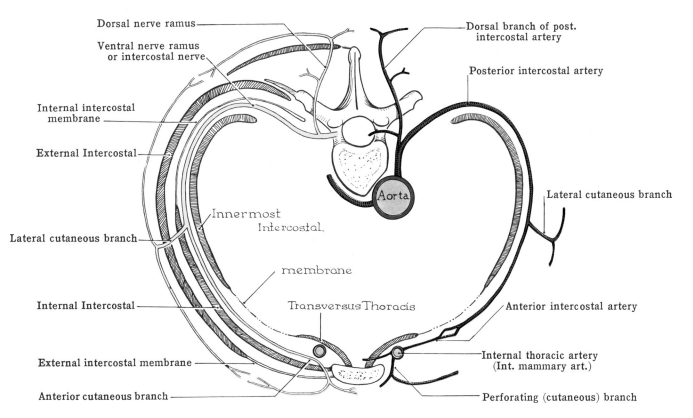

Dorsal nerve ramus

Ventral nerve ramus or intercostal nerve

Internal intercostal membrane

External Intercostal

Lateral cutaneous branch

Internal Intercostal

External intercostal membrane

Anterior cutaneous branch

Dorsal branch of post. intercostal artery

Posterior intercostal artery

Aorta

Innermost Intercostal.

membrane

Transversus Thoracis

Lateral cutaneous branch

Anterior intercostal artery

Internal thoracic artery (Int. mammary art.)

Perforating (cutaneous) branch

405   Diagram of an Intercostal Space

Observe:

1. Three layers: (a) External Intercostal muscle and membrane, (b) Internal Intercostal muscle and membrane, and (c) Innermost Intercostal and Transversus Thoracis muscles and the membrane connecting them.

2. The intercostal vessels and nerves running in the plane between the middle and innermost layers of muscles. Subsequently, the lower intercostal vessels and nerves occupy the corresponding morphological plane in the abdominal wall (figs. 106 and 408).

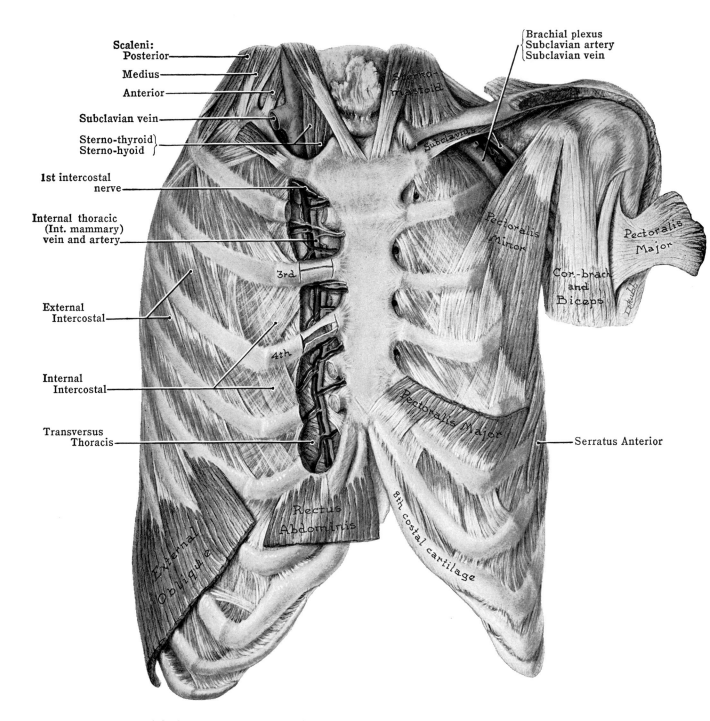

Scaleni:
Posterior
Medius
Anterior
Subclavian vein
Sterno-thyroid
Sterno-hyoid
1st intercostal nerve
Internal thoracic (Int. mammary) vein and artery
External Intercostal
Internal Intercostal
Transversus Thoracis

Brachial plexus
Subclavian artery
Subclavian vein

Sterno-mastoid
Subclavius
Pectoralis Minor
Cor.-brach. and Biceps
Pectoralis Major
3rd
4th
Pectoralis Major
Serratus Anterior
8th costal cartilage
Rectus Abdominis
External Oblique

406   Anterior Thoracic Wall, front view—I

Observe:

1. Preparatory. Muscles to be removed before dissection begins:—External Oblique, Rectus Abdominis, Pectoralis Major, Pectoralis Minor, Subclavius, sternal head of Sternomastoid, and Scalenus Posterior at the front; Serratus Anterior and Latissimus Dorsi at the sides (figs. 23 & 24); Serrati Posteriores, Longissimus, and Ilio-costalis at the back (fig. 409).

2. Pulling the arm backwards and downwards forces the clavicle, padded with Subclavius, to compress the subclavian vessels against the 1st rib and thus arrest the blood flow.

3. The 11th and 12th ribs are too short to be seen from the front.

4. The 7th costal cartilages are usually the last to reach the sternum, although not uncommonly, as here, the 8th also do so.

5. The H-shaped cut made through the perichondrium of the 3rd and 4th cartilages prior to shelling out segments of cartilage.

6. The internal thoracic vessels, crossed anteriorly by the intercostal nerves, and associated with parasternal lymph nodes.

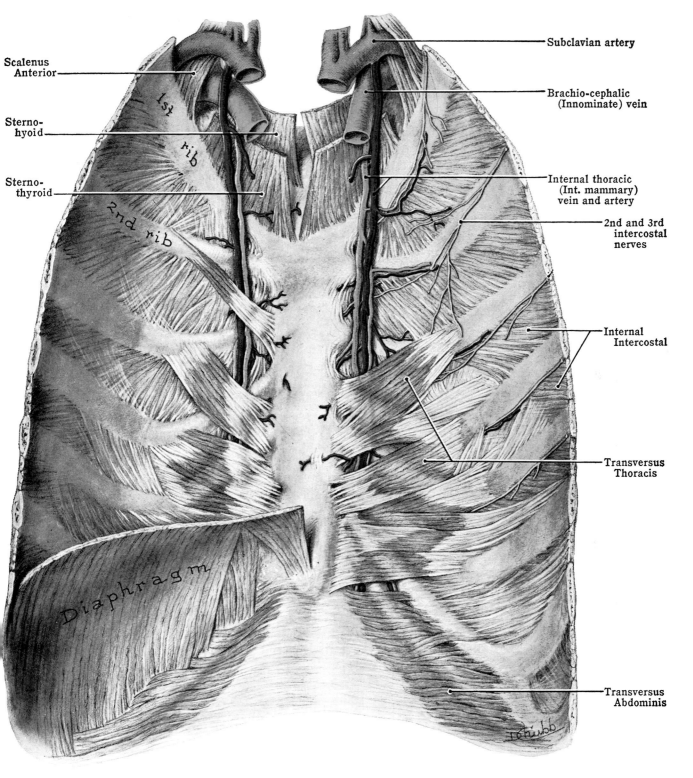

Scalenus Anterior

Sterno-hyoid

Sterno-thyroid

1st rib

2nd rib

Diaphragm

Subclavian artery

Brachio-cephalic (Innominate) vein

Internal thoracic (Int. mammary) vein and artery

2nd and 3rd intercostal nerves

Internal Intercostal

Transversus Thoracis

Transversus Abdominis

407 Anterior Thoracic Wall, from behind—II

(*Dissection by Dr. S. A. Crooks*)

Observe:

1. The continuity of Transversus Thoracis with Transversus Abdominis, these being the inner-most layer of the three flat muscles of the thoraco-abdominal wall (fig. 405).

2. The internal thoracic artery, arising from the first part of the subclavian artery, accom-panied by two veins (venae comitantes) up to the 3rd or 2nd intercostal space and above this by a single vein (internal thoracic vein), which proceeds to the brachio-cephalic vein.

3. The lower portions of the internal thoracic vessels, covered posteriorly with Transversus Thoracis; the upper portions in contact with parietal pleura (removed).

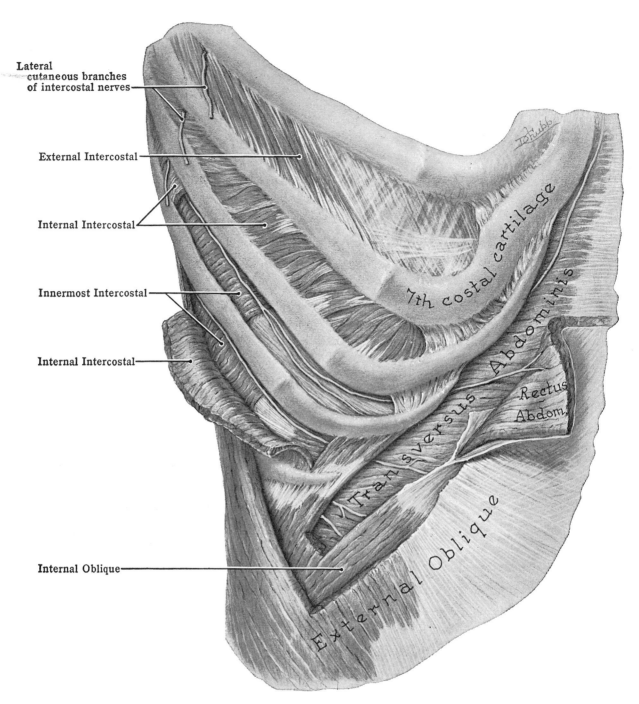

Lateral cutaneous branches of intercostal nerves

External Intercostal

Internal Intercostal

Innermost Intercostal

Internal Intercostal

Internal Oblique

7th costal cartilage

Transversus-Abdominis

Rectus Abdom.

External Oblique

408 Anterior Ends of Lower Intercostal Spaces, front view—I

Observe:

1. The common direction of the fibres of the External Intercostal and External Oblique.

2. The continuity of the Internal Intercostal with the Internal Oblique, at the anterior ends of the 9th, 10th, and 11th intercostal spaces.

3. The morphological plane in which an intercostal nerve lies—deep to an Internal Intercostal but superficial to an Innermost Intercostal and either the Transversus Thoracis or the Transversus Abdominis, according to the level (as fig. 405 explains).

4. The direction in which an intercostal nerve runs—first, parallel to the ribs immediately above and below, and then, parallel to the costal cartilages. Thus, on gaining the abdominal walls nerves T.7 and T.8 continue upwards, T.9 continues nearly horizontally, and T.10 continue, downwards towards the umbilicus.

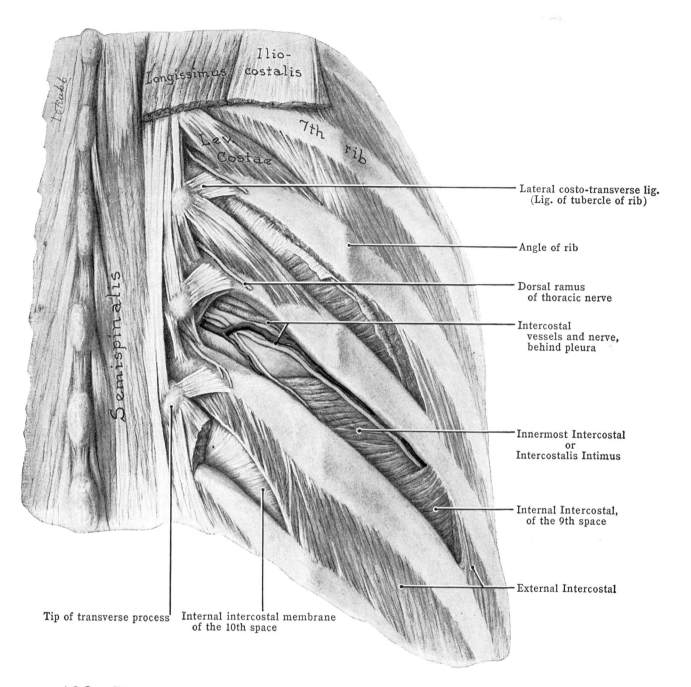

Longissimus Ilio-costalis

7th rib

Lev. Costae

Semispinalis

Lateral costo-transverse lig.
(Lig. of tubercle of rib)

Angle of rib

Dorsal ramus
of thoracic nerve

Intercostal
vessels and nerve,
behind pleura

Innermost Intercostal
or
Intercostalis Intimus

Internal Intercostal,
of the 9th space

External Intercostal

Tip of transverse process   Internal intercostal membrane
of the 10th space

409   Posterior End of an Intercostal Space, from behind—II

Note:

1. Medial to the angles of ribs—Ilio-costalis and Longissimus have been removed and Levatores Costarum thereby uncovered.

2. Of the five intercostal spaces depicted:—(a) the upper two (viz., the 6th & 7th spaces) are intact; (b) from the lowest or 10th space Levator Costae and the underlying part of the External Intercostal have been removed thereby revealing the internal intercostal membrane;   (c) from the 8th space more of the External Intercostal has been removed and the Internal intercostal membrane is seen extending laterally as an areolar sheet; (d) finally, in the 9th space this sheet has been removed in order to show the intercostal vessels and nerve (a) appearing medially between the superior costo-transverse ligament and the pleura and (b) disappearing laterally between the Internal Intercostal and the Innermost Intercostal.

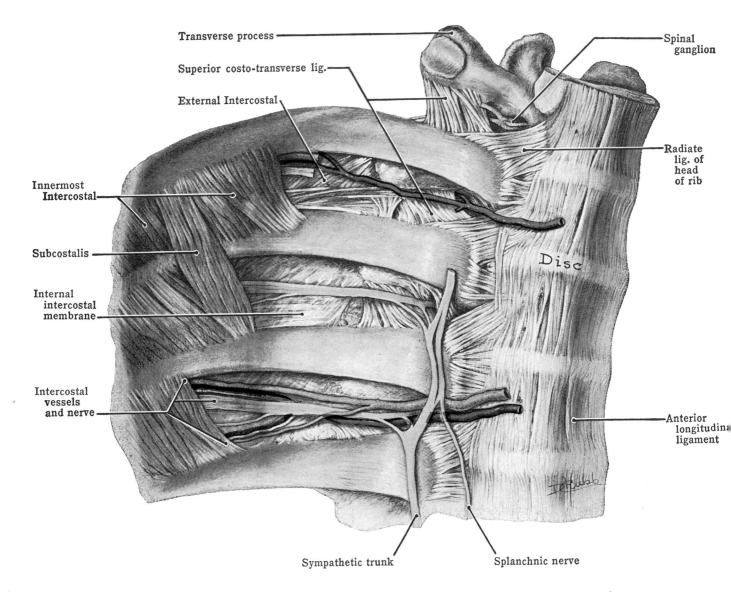

Transverse process

Superior costo-transverse lig.

External Intercostal

Spinal ganglion

Radiate lig. of head of rib

Innermost Intercostal

Subcostalis

Internal intercostal membrane

Disc

Intercostal vessels and nerve

Anterior longitudinal ligament

Sympathetic trunk

Splanchnic nerve

410 Vertebral End of an Intercostal Space and the Costo-vertebral Ligaments, anterior view—III

Observe:

1. Portions of the Innermost Intercostal muscle that bridge two intercostal spaces are called Subcostal muscles.
2. An External Intercostal muscle in the uppermost space.
3. An internal intercostal membrane in the middle space, continuous medially with a superior costo-transverse ligament.
4. In the lowest space, the order of the structures—intercostal vein, artery, and nerve. Note their collateral branches.
5. The ventral ramus of a thoracic nerve, crossing in front of a superior costo-transverse ligament and a dorsal ramus crossing behind.

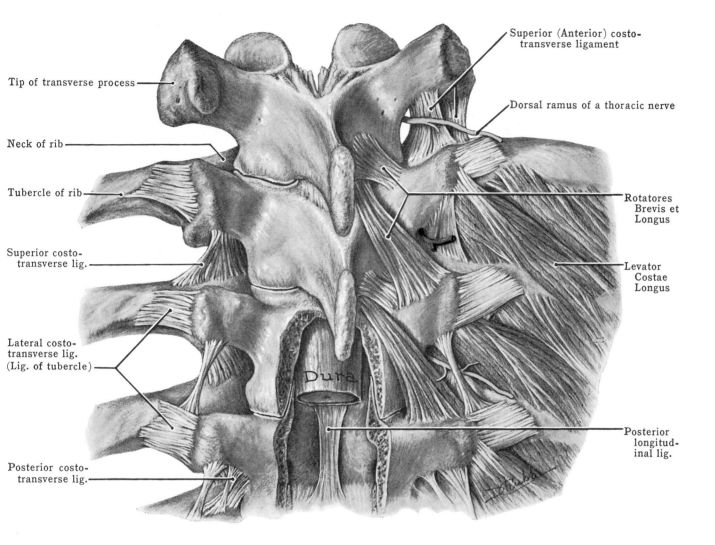

Tip of transverse process

Neck of rib

Tubercle of rib

Superior costo-
transverse lig.

Lateral costo-
transverse lig.
(Lig. of tubercle)

Posterior costo-
transverse lig.

Superior (Anterior) costo-
transverse ligament

Dorsal ramus of a thoracic nerve

Rotatores
Brevis et
Longus

Levator
Costae
Longus

Posterior
longitud-
inal lig.

Dura

411 Rotatores and the Costo-transverse Ligaments—IV

Note:

1. Of the 3 layers of Transverso-spinalis or oblique muscles of the back: —Semispinales, Multifidus, Rotatores —the Rotatores are the deepest and shortest. They pass from the root of one
transverse process to the junction of the transverse process and lamina of the vertebra next
above; but some (Rotatores Longi) pass to the vertebra two above.

2. Similarly, the Levatores Costarum pass from the tip of one transverse process to the rib
next below; but some (Levatores Longi) pass to the rib two below.

3. Of the 3 sets of costo-transverse ligaments—superior, lateral, and medial—

   (a) The superior ligament splits laterally into two sheets between which the medial border
of a Levator Costae and of an External Intercostal are received. The dorsal ramus of a thoracic
nerve passes behind this ligament and the ventral ramus, (intercostal nerve) passes in front.

   (b) The lateral ligament is strong and, if there were no joint cavity between transverse
process and rib, it would be continuous with the medial ligament (lig. of the neck, fig. 431).

   (c) The medial ligament passes between the front of a transverse process and the back of
the neck of its own rib. It is called "the" costo-transverse ligament. (A few fibers of little
account, lying postero-medial to the superior lig. constitute a posterior costo-transverse lig.)

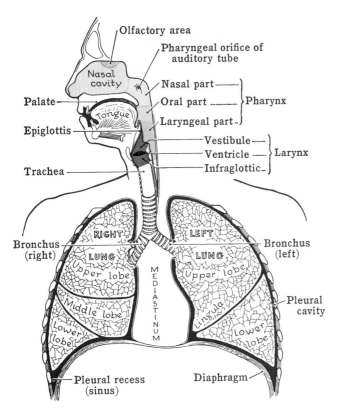

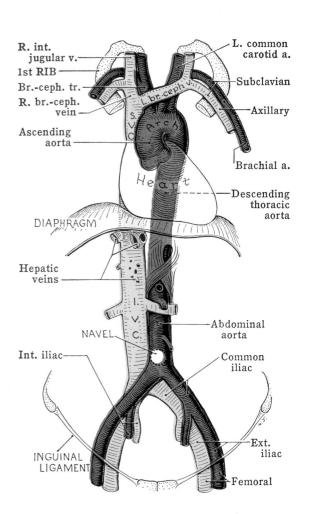

412   Diagram of Respiratory System

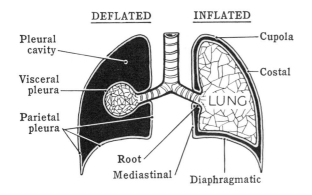

412.1   Scheme of Pleural Cavity and Pleura

The parts of the parietal pleura are labelled on the right side.
(Visceral pleura = pulmonary pleura.)

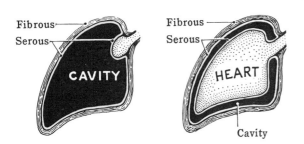

412.2   Scheme of Fibrous and Serous Pericardia

Parietal pericardium is fibrous pericardium lined with serous.
Visceral pericardium, called epicardium, is serous only.

413   Diagram of Great Arteries and Veins

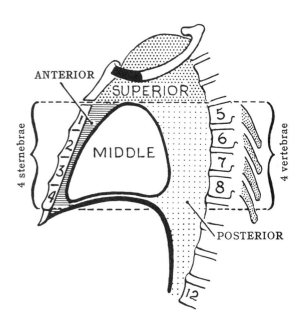

413.1   Subdivisions of Mediastinum

These are 4—middle, superior, posterior, and
anterior.

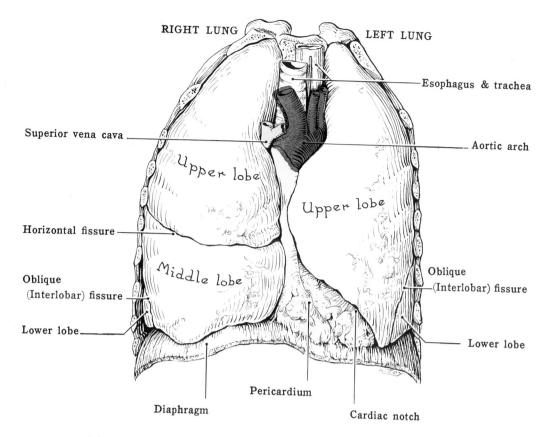

Esophagus & trachea

RIGHT LUNG LEFT LUNG

Superior vena cava

Aortic arch

Upper lobe

Upper lobe

Horizontal fissure

Oblique
(Interlobar) fissure

Middle lobe

Oblique
(Interlobar) fissure

Lower lobe

Lower lobe

Diaphragm

Pericardium

Cardiac notch

414   Lungs and Pericardium, front view

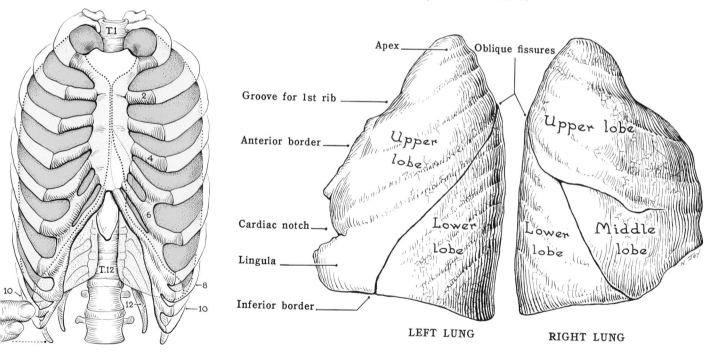

Apex

Oblique fissures

Groove for 1st rib

Upper
lobe

Upper lobe

Anterior border

Cardiac notch

Lower
lobe

Lingula

Lower
lobe

Middle
lobe

Inferior border

LEFT LUNG

RIGHT LUNG

414.1   Lungs, lateral views

Observe:

1. The three lobes of the right lung and the two lobes of the left.

2. The middle lobe (of the right lung) lying at the front of the thorax; i.e., it is entirely anterior to the midlateral line.

3. The deficiency of the upper lobe of the left lung, called the cardiac notch, allowing the pericardium to appear.

4. A horizontal fissure (of the right lung), complete in figure 414 and incomplete in figure 414.1.

3.2

Pleura rises to, but not above, neck of 1st rib.
ht & left **Sternocostal Reflexions** meet behind
num above level of 2nd ribs, descend together to
ribs where left pleura deviates variably to 6th or
rib (fig. 431), is in midclavicular line at 8th rib, in
lateral line at 10th rib (2 fingers's breadth above
gin of bony thorax, fig. 126); thence, as **Vertebral
flexion** it ascends on vertebral bodies Th. 12th to
(fig. 455). (Partly after Cunningham, and Wood-
ne.)

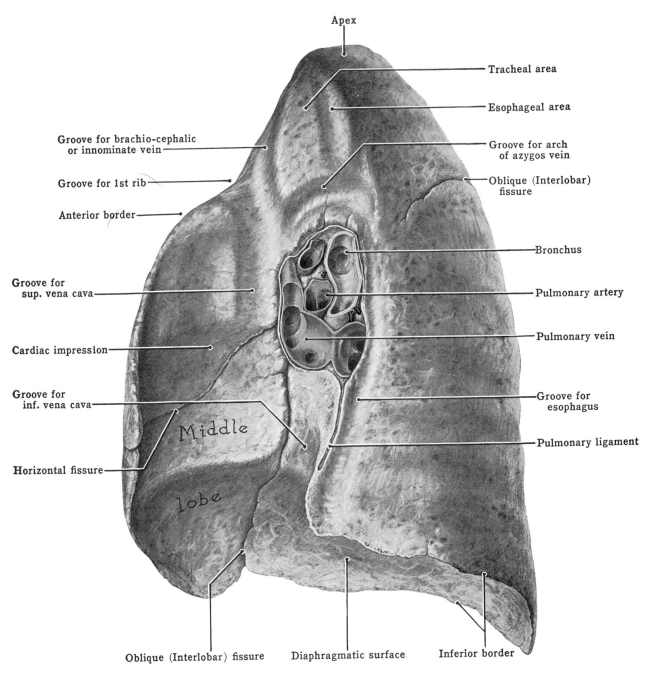

Apex

Tracheal area

Esophageal area

Groove for brachio-cephalic or innominate vein

Groove for arch of azygos vein

Groove for 1st rib

Oblique (Interlobar) fissure

Anterior border

Bronchus

Groove for sup. vena cava

Pulmonary artery

Pulmonary vein

Cardiac impression

Groove for inf. vena cava

Groove for esophagus

Pulmonary ligament

Middle

Horizontal fissure

lobe

Oblique (Interlobar) fissure   Diaphragmatic surface   Inferior border

415 Mediastinal Surface of the Right Lung

Observe:

1. The lungs, resembling inflated balloons in that they take the impressions of the structures with which they come into contact. Thus, the base is fashioned by the cupola of the diaphragm; the costal surface bears the impressions of the ribs; distended vessels leave their mark; empty vessels and nerves do not.

2. The somewhat pear-shaped root of the lung near the centre of the mediastinal surface, and the pulmonary ligament descending like a stalk from the root.

3. The groove for (or line of contact with) the esophagus throughout the length of the lung, except where the arch of the azygos vein intervenes. This groove passes behind the root and therefore behind the pulmonary ligament, which separates it from the groove for the l.v. cava.

4. The oblique (interlobar) fissure, here incomplete, but complete in figure 416.

5. The two pulmonary veins, here uniting unusually close to the lung.

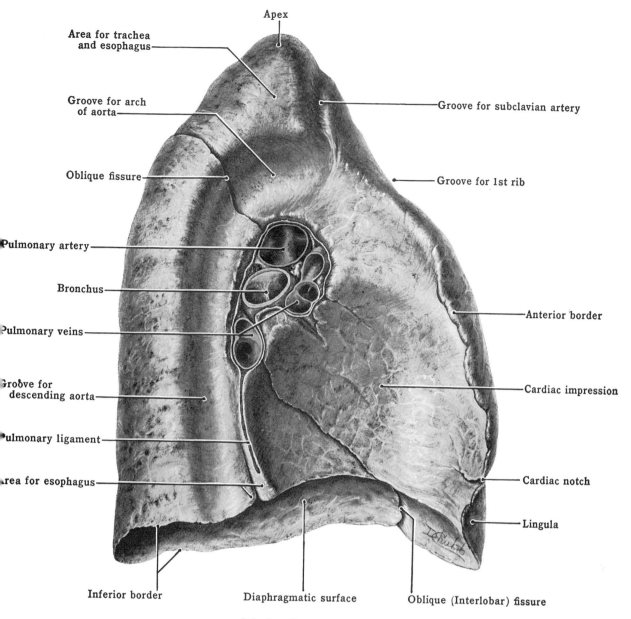

Apex

Area for trachea
and esophagus

Groove for subclavian artery

Groove for arch
of aorta

Oblique fissure

Groove for 1st rib

Pulmonary artery

Bronchus

Anterior border

Pulmonary veins

Groove for
descending aorta

Cardiac impression

Pulmonary ligament

Area for esophagus

Cardiac notch

Lingula

Inferior border

Diaphragmatic surface

Oblique (Interlobar) fissure

416   Mediastinal Surface of the Left Lung

Observe:

1. Near the centre, the root and the pulmonary ligament descending from it.
2. The site of contact with the esophagus, between the aorta and the lower end of the ligament.
3. The oblique (interlobar) fissure, cutting completely through the lung substance.
4. In both the right root and the left—the artery is above; the bronchus is behind; one vein is in front, and the other is below. In the right root, the bronchus (eparterial) to the upper lobe is the highest structure.

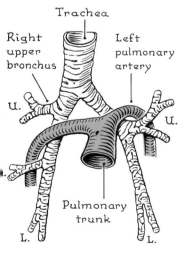

Trachea

Right
upper
bronchus

Left
pulmonary
artery

U.

U.

Pulmonary
trunk

L.

L.

416.1

Diagram. The gross difference between right and left roots is that: on the right, the upper and middle bronchi are spread apart by the artery, and on the left, pressed together.

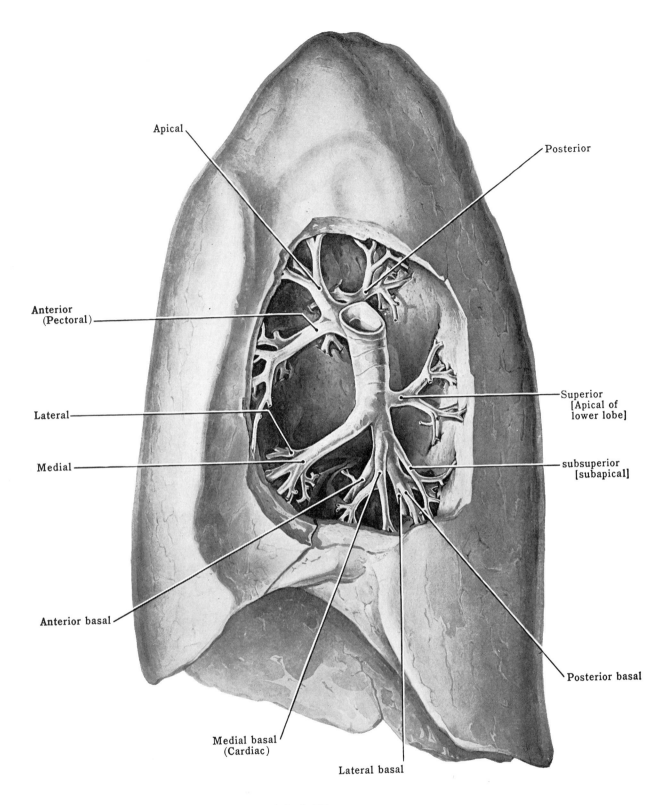

Apical

Posterior

Anterior
(Pectoral)

Superior
[Apical of
lower lobe]

Lateral

Medial

subsuperior
[subapical]

Anterior basal

Posterior basal

Medial basal
(Cardiac)

Lateral basal

417 Right Bronchial Tree

Fresh lungs were kept inflated with air under low pressure until thoroughly dry (about a week) and their natural form thereby assured. The tissues surrounding the bronchi were then moistened and cut away.

Terminology (after Jackson and Huber). There are usually 10 right and 8 left tertiary or segmental bronchi. They are approximately symmetrical in the two lungs. The reduced number in the left lung is accounted for by the fact that the left apical and posterior bronchi arise from a common stem, as do also the left anterior basal and medial basal.

18 Right Bronchi and Pulmonary Veins

The veins of fresh lungs were filled with blue latex and the bronchi kept inflated and treated as figure 417. (Dissected by Dr. C. W. Hill.)

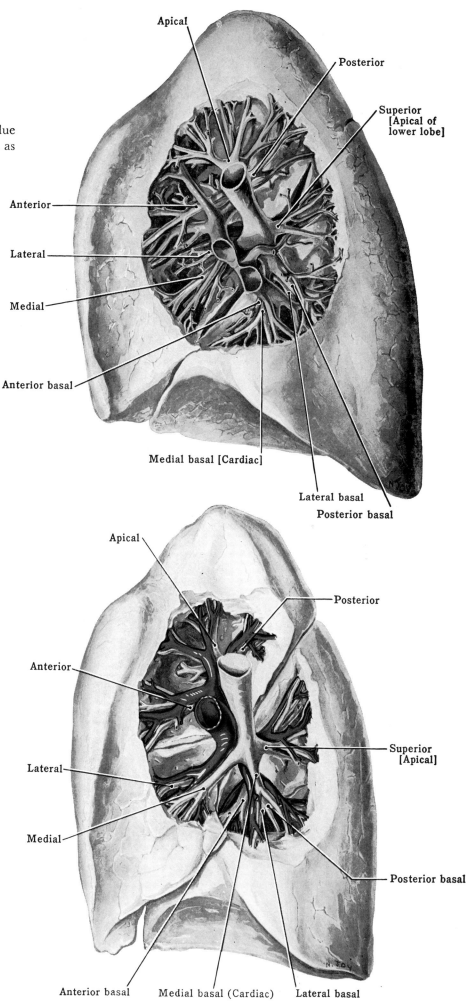

Apical

Posterior

Superior [Apical of lower lobe]

Anterior

Lateral

Medial

Anterior basal

Medial basal [Cardiac]

Lateral basal

Posterior basal

Apical

Posterior

Anterior

Superior [Apical]

Lateral

Medial

Posterior basal

9 Right Bronchi and Pulmonary Arteries

The arteries of fresh lungs were filled with latex and the bronchi kept inflated and treated as for figure 417.

Anterior basal

Medial basal (Cardiac)

Lateral basal

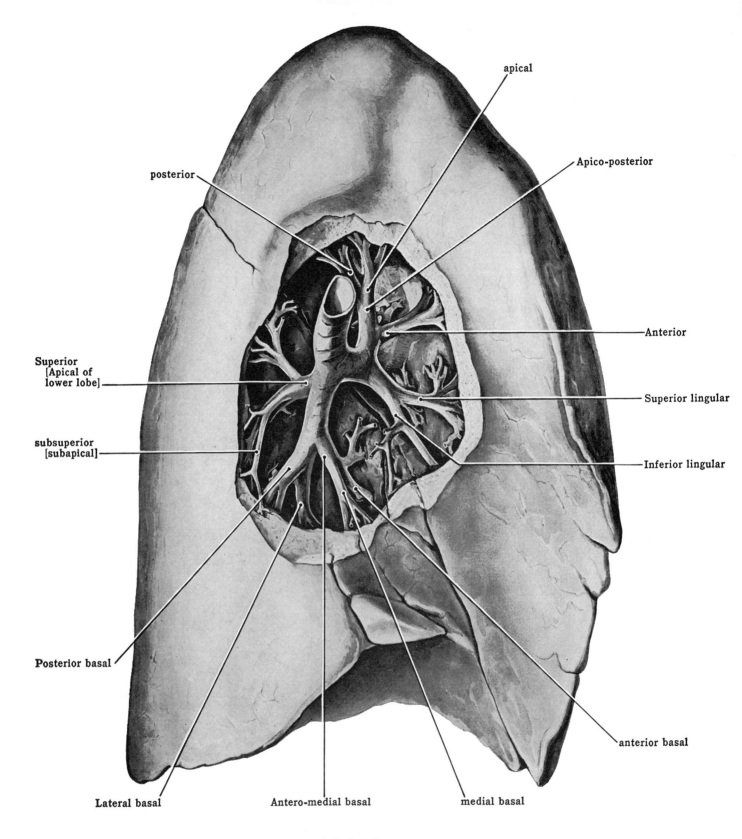

apical

Apico-posterior

posterior

Anterior

Superior
[Apical of
lower lobe]

Superior lingular

subsuperior
[subapical]

Inferior lingular

Posterior basal

anterior basal

Lateral basal   Antero-medial basal   medial basal

420 Left Bronchial Tree

Fresh lungs were kept inflated with air under low pressure until thoroughly dry (about a week) and their natural form thereby assured. The tissues surrounding the bronchi were then moistened and cut away.

Terminology (after Jackson and Huber). There are usually 10 right and 8 left tertiary or segmental bronchi. They are approximately symmetrical in the two lungs. The reduced number in the left lung is accounted for by the fact that the left apical and posterior bronchi arise from a common stem, as do also the left anterior basal and the medial basal.

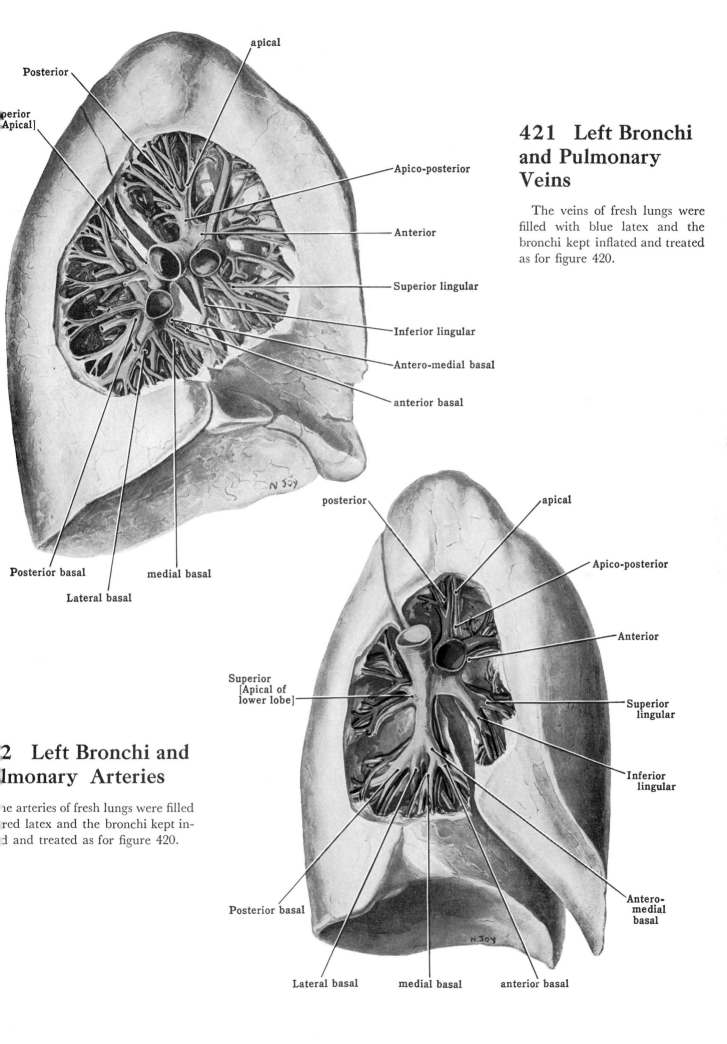

Posterior

uperior
[Apical]

apical

Apico-posterior

Anterior

Superior lingular

Inferior lingular

Antero-medial basal

anterior basal

421 Left Bronchi and Pulmonary Veins

The veins of fresh lungs were filled with blue latex and the bronchi kept inflated and treated as for figure 420.

Posterior basal

Lateral basal

medial basal

2 Left Bronchi and lmonary Arteries

he arteries of fresh lungs were filled
red latex and the bronchi kept in-
d and treated as for figure 420.

posterior

apical

Apico-posterior

Anterior

Superior
[Apical of
lower lobe]

Superior
lingular

Inferior
lingular

Antero-
medial
basal

Posterior basal

Lateral basal

medial basal

anterior basal

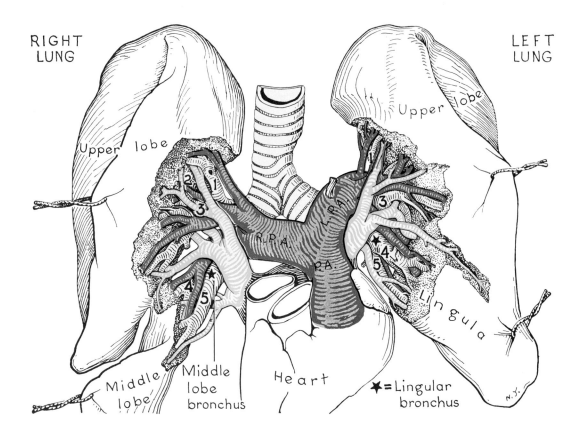

RIGHT
LUNG

LEFT
LUNG

Upper lobe

Upper lobe

2 1

3

3

R.P.A.

L.P.A.

P.A.

4

4

5

5

Lingula

Middle
lobe

Middle
lobe
bronchus

Heart

★ = Lingular
bronchus

423   Dissection of the Hili of the Lungs, from the front

(The bronchi and the pulmonary veins and arteries were injected.)

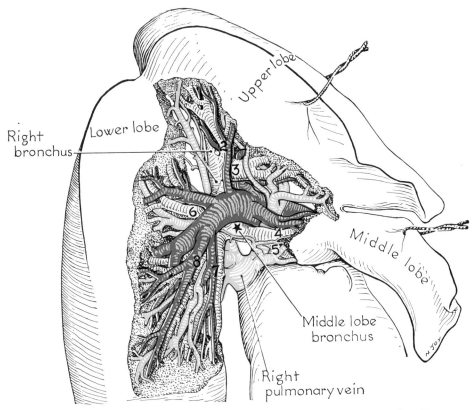

Upper lobe

Right
bronchus

Lower lobe

2

3

6

4

5

8 7

Middle lobe

Middle lobe
bronchus

Right
pulmonary vein

423.1   Dissection of the Hilus of the Right Lung, after opening the oblique fissure

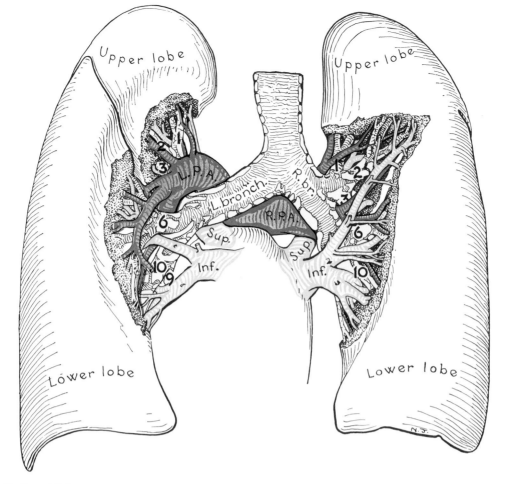

423.2   Dissection of the Hili of the Lungs, from behind

(The bronchi and the pulmonary veins and arteries were injected.)

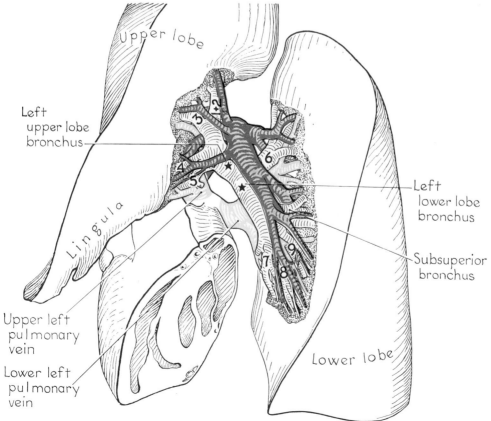

Left
upper lobe
bronchus

Lingula

Upper left
pulmonary
vein

Lower left
pulmonary
vein

Left
lower lobe
bronchus

Subsuperior
bronchus

423.3   Dissection of the Hilus of the Left Lung, after opening the oblique fissure

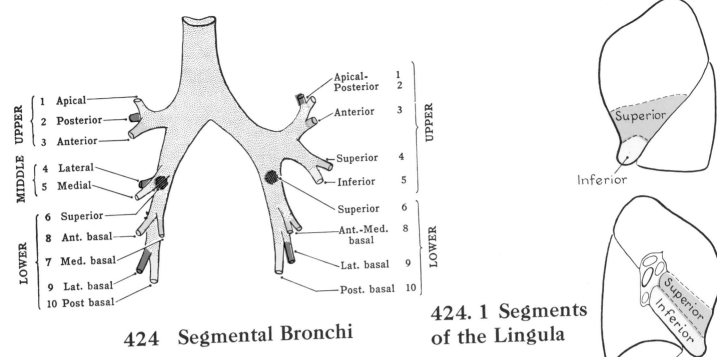

			Apical-Posterior	1 2	
MIDDLE / UPPER	1	Apical			
	2	Posterior	Anterior	3	UPPER
	3	Anterior			
	4	Lateral	Superior	4	
	5	Medial	Inferior	5	
LOWER	6	Superior	Superior	6	LOWER
	8	Ant. basal	Ant.-Med. basal	8	
	7	Med. basal	Lat. basal	9	
	9	Lat. basal	Post. basal	10	
	10	Post basal			

424   Segmental Bronchi

The 10 right and 8 left segmental bronchi. (After Jackson and Huber.) The numerals applied to these bronchi were suggested by the Thoracic Society.

424. 1 Segments of the Lingula

This is the usual pattern. Compare with figure 427. (After Jackson and Huber.)

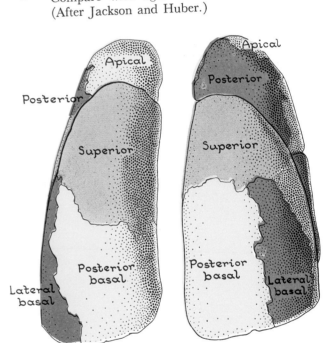

Right lung — ANTERIOR VIEW — Left lung

Left lung — POSTERIOR VIEW — Right lung

425   Broncho-pulmonary Segments

(All specimens were prepared by Dr. J. Callaghan, Dr. K. Nancekivell, C. E. Storton.)

The tertiary bronchi of fresh lungs were isolated within the hili of the lungs and injected with latex of various colours. Ten such bronchi may be recognized in each lung. Usually there are ten in the right lung, but in the left lung only eight, due to the fact that the left apical and posterior arise from a single stem, as do the left ante-

rior basal and medial basal. Each tertiary or segmental bronchus and the portion of lung it ventilates is called a broncho-pulmonary segment. Minor variations in the branching of the bronchi make for variations in the surface pattern.

For detailed information see "Segmental Anatomy of the Lungs" by E. A. Boyden.

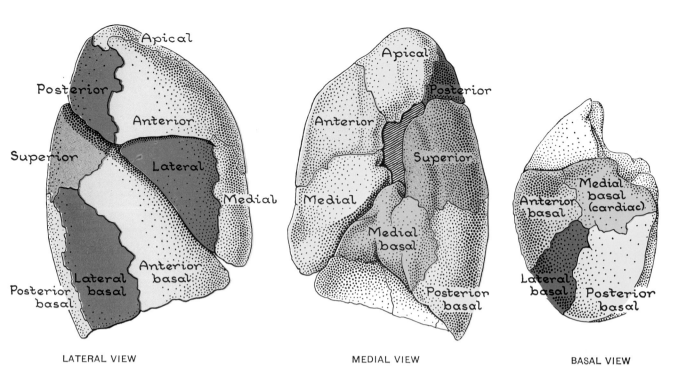

LATERAL VIEW   MEDIAL VIEW   BASAL VIEW

426   Right Broncho-pulmonary Segments

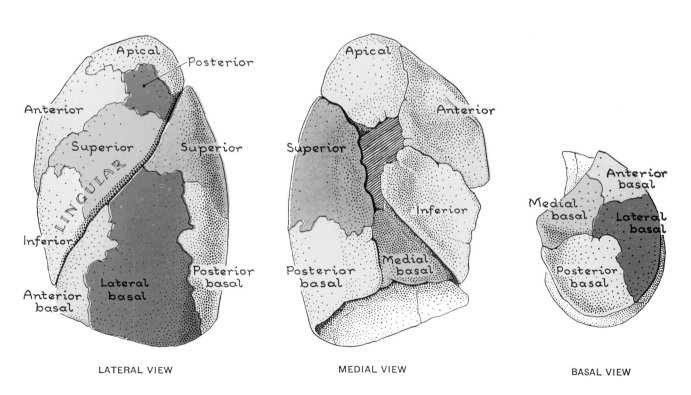

LATERAL VIEW   MEDIAL VIEW   BASAL VIEW

427   Left Broncho-pulmonary Segments

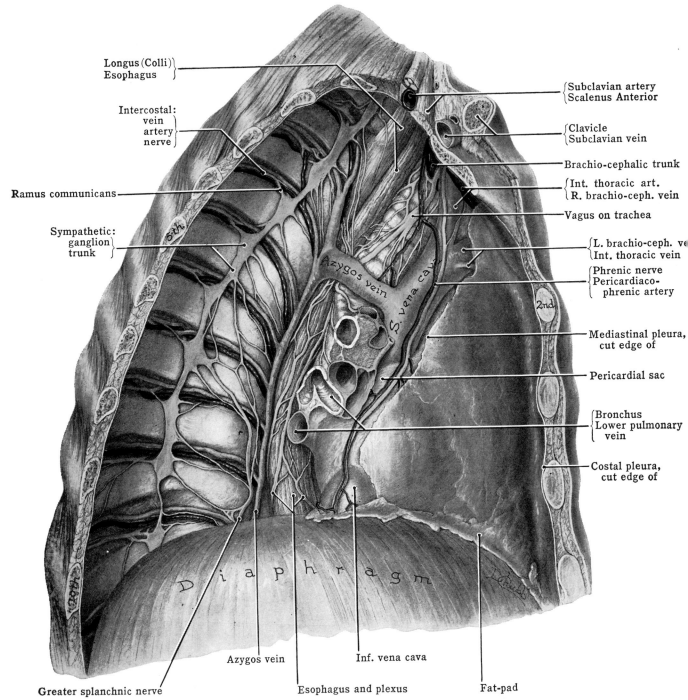

Longus (Colli)
Esophagus

Subclavian artery
Scalenus Anterior

Intercostal:
vein
artery
nerve

Clavicle
Subclavian vein

Brachio-cephalic trunk

Ramus communicans

Int. thoracic art.
R. brachio-ceph. vein

Vagus on trachea

Sympathetic:
ganglion
trunk

L. brachio-ceph. ve
Int. thoracic vein

Phrenic nerve
Pericardiaco-
phrenic artery

Mediastinal pleura,
cut edge of

Pericardial sac

Bronchus
Lower pulmonary
vein

Costal pleura,
cut edge of

Azygos vein

S. vena cava

2nd

5th

Diaphragm

Greater splanchnic nerve

Azygos vein

Inf. vena cava

Esophagus and plexus

Fat-pad

428 Right Side of the Mediastinum

(From a dissection by Major B. L. Guyatt.)

The costal and mediastinal pleura is largely removed and the underlying structures are thereby exposed.

428.1

Diagram. Great vessels of superior mediastinum, front view.

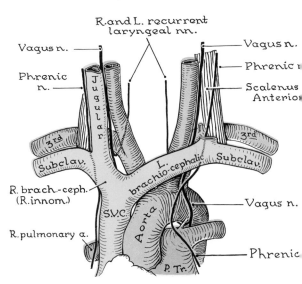

R. and L. recurrent
laryngeal nn.

Vagus n.

Vagus n.

Phrenic
n.

Phrenic n

Scalenus
Anterior

Jugular

3rd

3rd

Subclav.

L.
brachio-cephalic

Subclav.

R. brach.-ceph.
(R. innom.)

Vagus n.

S.V.C.

Aorta

R. pulmonary a.

Phrenic

P. Tr.

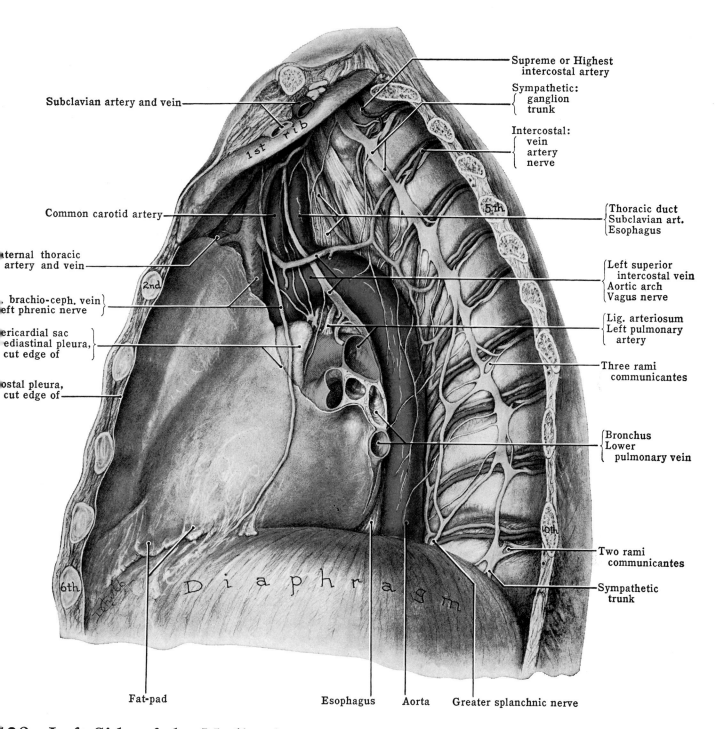

Subclavian artery and vein

Supreme or Highest intercostal artery

Sympathetic: { ganglion trunk

Common carotid artery

Intercostal: { vein artery nerve

1st rib

2nd

5th

{ Thoracic duct Subclavian art. Esophagus

ternal thoracic artery and vein

brachio-ceph. vein } eft phrenic nerve }

{ Left superior intercostal vein Aortic arch Vagus nerve

ericardial sac ediastinal pleura, cut edge of }

{ Lig. arteriosum Left pulmonary artery

ostal pleura, cut edge of

Three rami communicantes

{ Bronchus Lower pulmonary vein

6th

Two rami communicantes

10th

Sympathetic trunk

Diaphragm

Fat-pad   Esophagus   Aorta   Greater splanchnic nerve

429   Left Side of the Mediastinum

From a dissection by Major B. L. Guyatt.)

The costal and mediastinal pleura is largely removed and the nderlying structures are thereby exposed.

429.1

Diagram of an intercostal space. The artery arises nearer the median plane than where the vein ends, which is nearer than where the nerve enters.

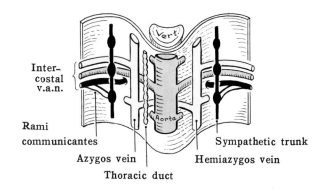

Inter-costal v.a.n.

Vert.

Aorta

Rami communicantes

Sympathetic trunk

Azygos vein

Hemiazygos vein

Thoracic duct

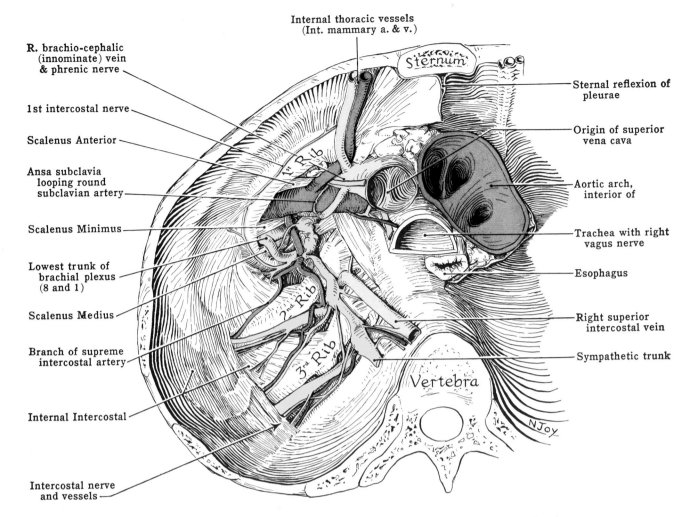

Internal thoracic vessels
(Int. mammary a. & v.)

R. brachio-cephalic
(innominate) vein
& phrenic nerve

1st intercostal nerve

Scalenus Anterior

Ansa subclavia
looping round
subclavian artery

Scalenus Minimus

Lowest trunk of
brachial plexus
(8 and 1)

Scalenus Medius

Branch of supreme
intercostal artery

Internal Intercostal

Intercostal nerve
and vessels

Sternum

Sternal reflexion of
pleurae

Origin of superior
vena cava

Aortic arch,
interior of

Trachea with right
vagus nerve

Esophagus

Right superior
intercostal vein

Sympathetic trunk

Vertebra

430 Cupola of right Pleura, from below

The cupola of the pleura (also called the cervical pleura, dome of the pleura, and apical pleura) is removed. It forms, so to speak, both the roof of the pleural cavity and the floor of the root of the neck—see figure 536.

Observe:

1. The first part of the subclavian artery, arching over the cupola and disappearing between Scalenus Anterior and Scalenus Minimus, which is an occasional muscle.
2. The internal thoracic artery and the supreme intercostal branch of the costo-cervical trunk.
3. Two nerves—the ansa subclavia from the sympathetic trunk and the recurrent laryngeal nerve from the vagus—looping round the subclavian artery.
4. The supreme intercostal artery crossing the neck of the 1st rib between the sympathetic trunk, which is on its medial side, and the ventral ramus of T. 1 to the brachial plexus, which is on its lateral side.

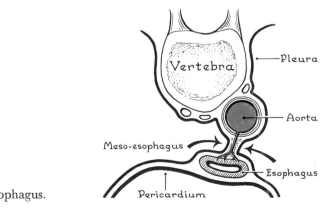

431.1

Diagram of meso-esophagus.

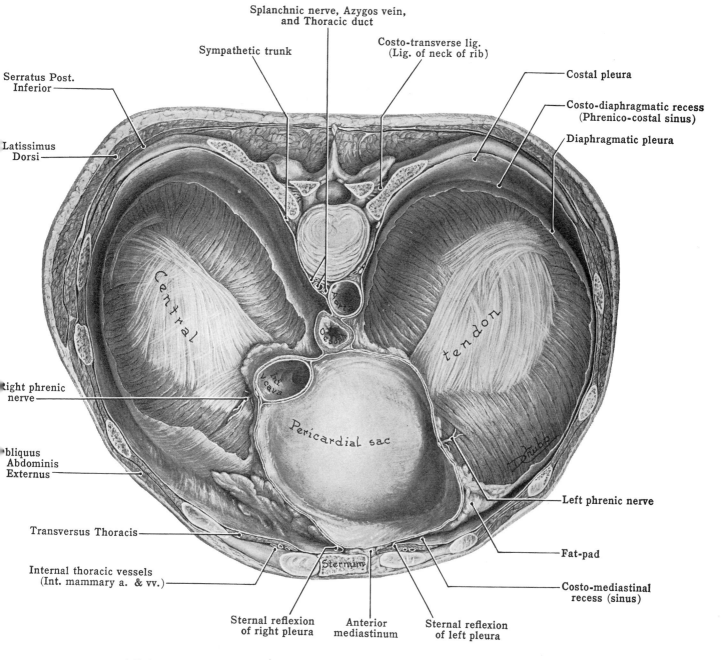

Labels on figure:

Splanchnic nerve, Azygos vein, and Thoracic duct

Sympathetic trunk

Costo-transverse lig. (Lig. of neck of rib)

Serratus Post. Inferior

Costal pleura

Costo-diaphragmatic recess (Phrenico-costal sinus)

Diaphragmatic pleura

Latissimus Dorsi

Central

tendon

Right phrenic nerve

Aorta

esoph.

Int. vcava

Pericardial sac

Obliquus Abdominis Externus

Left phrenic nerve

Transversus Thoracis

Fat-pad

Internal thoracic vessels (Int. mammary a. & vv.)

Sternum

Costo-mediastinal recess (sinus)

Sternal reflexion of right pleura

Anterior mediastinum

Sternal reflexion of left pleura

431 Diaphragm and the Pericardial Sac, from above

The diaphragmatic pleura is mostly removed.

Observe:

1. The pericardial sac, situated on the ventral half of the diaphragm; one third being to the right of the median plane and two thirds being to the left; the most caudal point being ventrally and to the left—like the apex of the heart.

2. The mouths of the large hepatic veins, opening into the inferior vena cava and directed upwards, towards the heart.

3. The sternal reflexion of the left pleural sac, failing to meet that of the right sac in the median plane, ventral to the pericardium.

4. The right and left pleural sacs almost meeting between esophagus and aorta to form a mesoesophagus.

5. The coston-diaphragmatic recess, deepest about the mid-lateral line (fig. 125).

6. The costal pleura, on reaching the vertebral column imperceptibly becoming the mediastinal pleura.

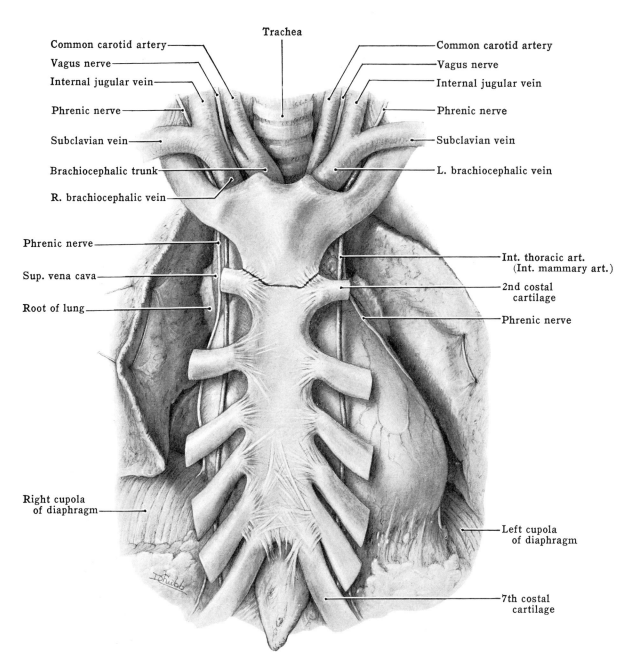

Trachea

Common carotid artery
Vagus nerve
Internal jugular vein
Phrenic nerve
Subclavian vein
Brachiocephalic trunk
R. brachiocephalic vein

Phrenic nerve
Sup. vena cava
Root of lung

Right cupola
of diaphragm

Common carotid artery
Vagus nerve
Internal jugular vein
Phrenic nerve
Subclavian vein
L. brachiocephalic vein

Int. thoracic art.
(Int. mammary art.)
2nd costal
cartilage
Phrenic nerve

Left cupola
of diaphragm

7th costal
cartilage

432 Pericardial Sac in Relation to the Sternum

Observe:

1. The internal thoracic arteries lying a finger's breadth from the borders of the sternum.

2. The pericardial sac, extending in the median plane from just above the level of the sterno-manubrial joint to the level of the xiphi-sternal junction; i.e., practically co-extensive with the body of the sternum, but one third lying to the right of the median plane and two thirds to the left.

3. The right and left phrenic nerves applied to the pericardial sac.

Note, the sterno-manubrial joint was divided preparatory to turning the body of the sternum downwards in order to permit of dissection.

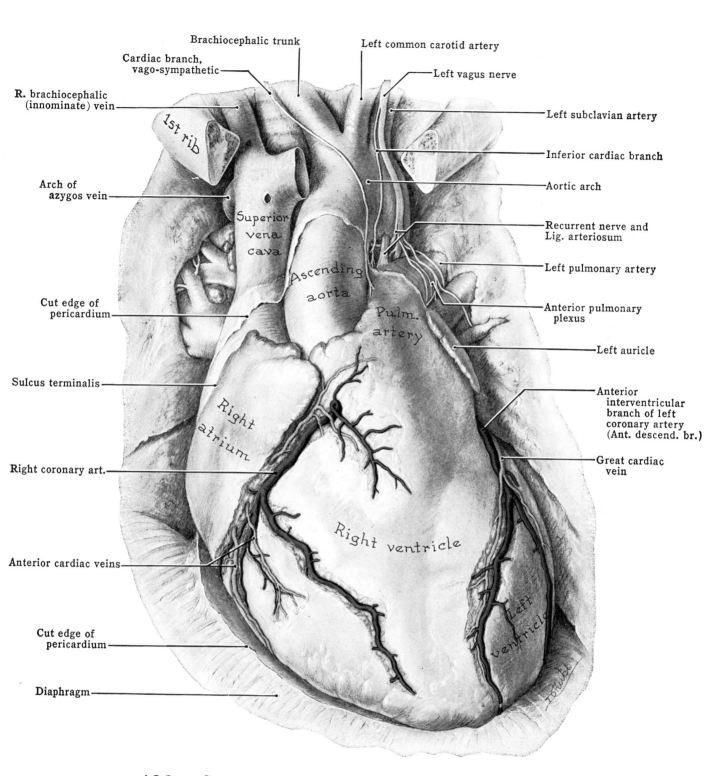

Brachiocephalic trunk

Cardiac branch,
vago-sympathetic

Left common carotid artery

Left vagus nerve

R. brachiocephalic
(innominate) vein

Left subclavian artery

1st rib

Inferior cardiac branch

Arch of
azygos vein

Aortic arch

Superior
vena
cava

Recurrent nerve and
Lig. arteriosum

Ascending
aorta

Left pulmonary artery

Pulm.
artery

Anterior pulmonary
plexus

Cut edge of
pericardium

Left auricle

Sulcus terminalis

Right
atrium

Anterior
interventricular
branch of left
coronary artery
(Ant. descend. br.)

Right coronary art.

Great cardiac
vein

Anterior cardiac veins

Right ventricle

Left
ventricle

Cut edge of
pericardium

Diaphragm

**433   Sternocostal Surface of the Heart and
Great Vessels, in situ**

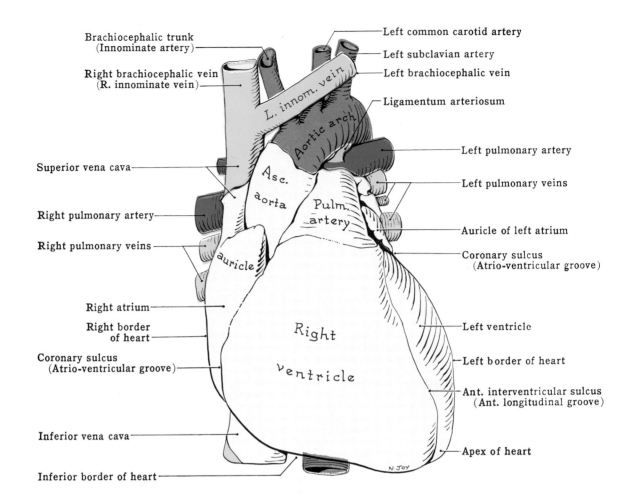

Brachiocephalic trunk
(Innominate artery)

Right brachiocephalic vein
(R. innominate vein)

Left common carotid artery

Left subclavian artery

Left brachiocephalic vein

Ligamentum arteriosum

Superior vena cava

Right pulmonary artery

Right pulmonary veins

Left pulmonary artery

Left pulmonary veins

Auricle of left atrium

Coronary sulcus
(Atrio-ventricular groove)

Right atrium

Right border
of heart

Coronary sulcus
(Atrio-ventricular groove)

Left ventricle

Left border of heart

Ant. interventricular sulcus
(Ant. longitudinal groove)

Inferior vena cava

Inferior border of heart

Apex of heart

L. innom. vein

Aortic arch

Asc. aorta

Pulm. artery

auricle

Right ventricle

N. JOY

434   Heart and Great Vessels, hardened in situ and removed en masse, sternocostal aspect

The pericardium is colored yellow.

Observe:

1. In shape and in size the heart resembles a closed right fist, the apex being the proximal interphalangeal joint of the index.

2. The right border, formed by the right atrium, slightly convex and almost in line with the superior and inferior caval veins. The inferior border (margo acutus), formed by the right ventricle and slightly by the left ventricle. The left border, formed by the left ventricle and very slightly by the left auricle.

3. The entire right auricle and much of the right atrium are visible from the front, but only a slight portion of the left auricle is visible. The auricles, like two closing claws, grasping the pulmonary artery and ascending aorta from behind.

4. The anterior interventricular sulcus, about a thumb's breadth from the left border.

5. The pulmonary trunk (artery), bifurcating below the aortic arch into the right and the left pulmonary artery.

6. The ligamentum arteriosum, continuing the direction of the pulmonary trunk (artery), and passing from the root of the left pulmonary artery to the aortic arch beyond the site of origin of the left subclavian artery.

7. The three branches of the aortic arch, crossed anteriorly by the left brachio-cephalic (innominate) vein.

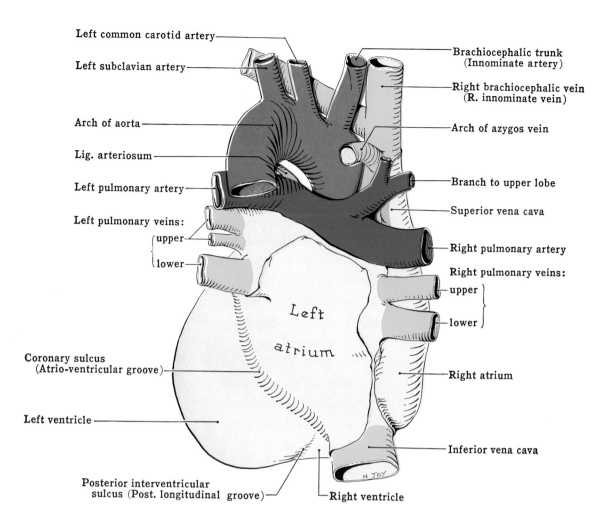

Left common carotid artery

Left subclavian artery

Arch of aorta

Lig. arteriosum

Left pulmonary artery

Left pulmonary veins:
  upper
  lower

Coronary sulcus
(Atrio-ventricular groove)

Left ventricle

Posterior interventricular
sulcus (Post. longitudinal groove)

Brachiocephalic trunk
(Innominate artery)

Right brachiocephalic vein
(R. innominate vein)

Arch of azygos vein

Branch to upper lobe

Superior vena cava

Right pulmonary artery

Right pulmonary veins:
  upper
  lower

Right atrium

Inferior vena cava

Right ventricle

Left atrium

N JOY

435 Heart and Great Vessels, hardened in situ and removed en masse, posterior aspect

Observe:

1. Visible from behind: most of the left atrium, much of the left ventricle, a little of the right atrium, and almost none of the right ventricle.

2. The right and left pulmonary veins, converging to open into the left atrium. The part of the atrium between them lies to the left of the line of the i. vena cava, occupies the median plane, and forms the anterior wall of the pericardial cul-de-sac called the oblique pericardial sinus, which admits two fingers (fig. 440).

   (Compare this with figures 177 and 136 of the caudate lobe of the liver, which likewise lies to the left of the line of the i. vena cava, occupies the median plane and forms the anterior wall of the peritoneal cul-de-sac called the upper recess of the omental bursa (lesser sac), which admits two fingers.)

3. The right and left pulmonary arteries, just above and parallel to the pulmonary veins and inclining from the left side downwards and to the right. Hence, the root of the right lung is lower than that of the left.

4. The aorta, arching over the left pulmonary vessels (and bronchus); the azygos vein arching over the right pulmonary vessels (and bronchus).

5. The aortic arch, arched in two planes: (a) upwards, (b) to the left. The convexity to the left is moulded on the esophagus and trachea.

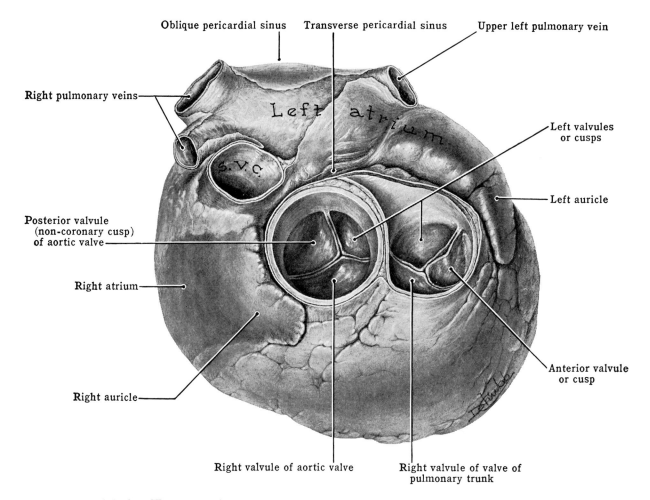

Oblique pericardial sinus   Transverse pericardial sinus   Upper left pulmonary vein

Right pulmonary veins

Left atrium

Left valvules or cusps

Left auricle

Posterior valvule (non-coronary cusp) of aortic valve

S.V.C.

Right atrium

Right auricle

Anterior valvule or cusp

Right valvule of aortic valve   Right valvule of valve of pulmonary trunk

436 Excised Heart, viewed from above

Observe:

1. The anterior position of the ventricles; the posterior position of the atria.
2. The ascending aorta and the pulmonary trunk, which conduct blood from the ventricles, accordingly placed anterior to the atria and to the s. vena cava and pulmonary veins, which conduct blood to the atria.
3. These two stems, enclosed within a common tube of serous pericardium; and partly embraced by the auricles of the atria.
4. The transverse pericardial sinus, curving behind the enclosed stems of the aorta and pulmonary trunk, and in front of the s. vena cava and upper limits of the atria.

Note: (a) The upper border of the atria is also the upper border of the heart.

(b) The names of the semilunar cusps or valvules of the aortic valve and valve of the pulmonary trunk have a developmental origin, as explained in figure 446.3.

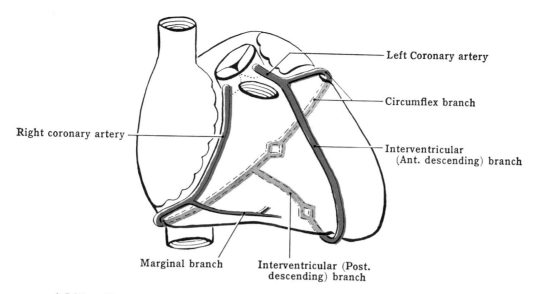

Left Coronary artery

Circumflex branch

Right coronary artery

Interventricular
(Ant. descending) branch

Marginal branch

Interventricular (Post.
descending) branch

437   Diagram of the Coronary (Cardiac) Arteries

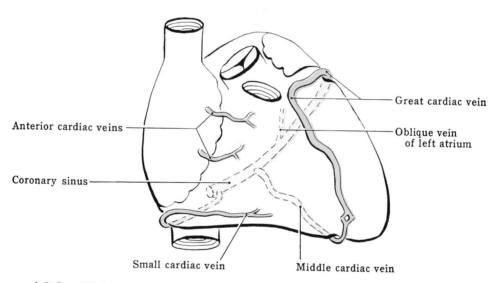

Anterior cardiac veins

Great cardiac vein

Oblique vein
of left atrium

Coronary sinus

Small cardiac vein

Middle cardiac vein

438   Diagram of the Cardiac Veins

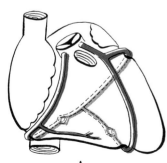

A.
Left coronary artery supplying
part of right coronary artery
territory.

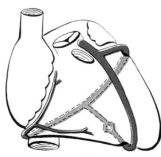

B.
A single coronary artery.

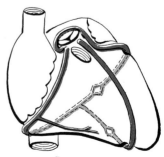

C.
Circumflex branch springing
from right aortic sinus.

439   Some Varieties of Coronary Arteries

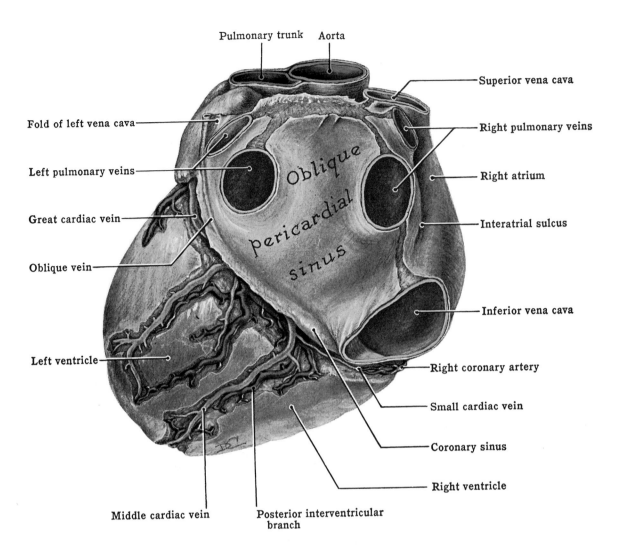

Pulmonary trunk   Aorta

Superior vena cava

Fold of left vena cava

Right pulmonary veins

Left pulmonary veins

Right atrium

Oblique pericardial sinus

Great cardiac vein

Interatrial sulcus

Oblique vein

Inferior vena cava

Left ventricle

Right coronary artery

Small cardiac vein

Coronary sinus

Right ventricle

Middle cardiac vein   Posterior interventricular branch

440 Heart, viewed from behind

This heart was excised from specimen 441, on the opposite page

Observe:

1. The entire base, or posterior surface, and part of the diaphragmatic surface are in view.
2. The slight appearance made by the right atrium.
3. The superior and the much larger inferior caval vein joining the upper and lower limits of the right atrium.
4. The left atrium, forming the greater part of the posterior surface.
5. The coronary arteries, here irregular in that the left one supplies the posterior interventricular branch.
6. Branches of the cardiac veins, when crossing branches of the coronary arteries, mostly do so superficially.
7. The fold of the left caval vein. For its significance consult figure 456.
8. The right pulmonary artery (removed) lay on the bare strip at the upper border of the atria, and intervened between the oblique sinus and the transverse sinus (not labelled).

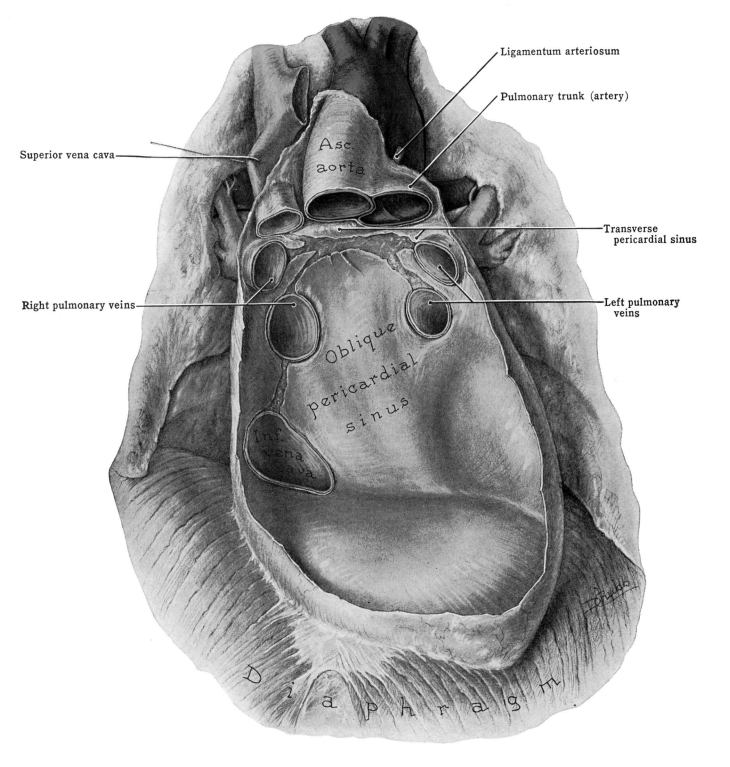

Ligamentum arteriosum

Pulmonary trunk (artery)

Superior vena cava

Asc. aorta

Transverse pericardial sinus

Right pulmonary veins

Oblique pericardial sinus

Left pulmonary veins

Inf. vena cava

Diaphragm

441 Interior of the Pericardial Sac, anterior view

Observe:

1. The 8 vessels severed on excising a heart—2 caval veins, 4 pulmonary veins, and 2 arteries.

2. The oblique sinus, circumscribed by 5 veins; open below and to the left; and rising to the level of the right pulmonary artery which separates it from the transverse sinus.

3. The peak of the pericardial sac, near the junction of the ascending aorta and the aortic arch.

4. The superior vena cava, partly inside and partly outside the pericardium, and the ligamentum arteriosum entirely outside.

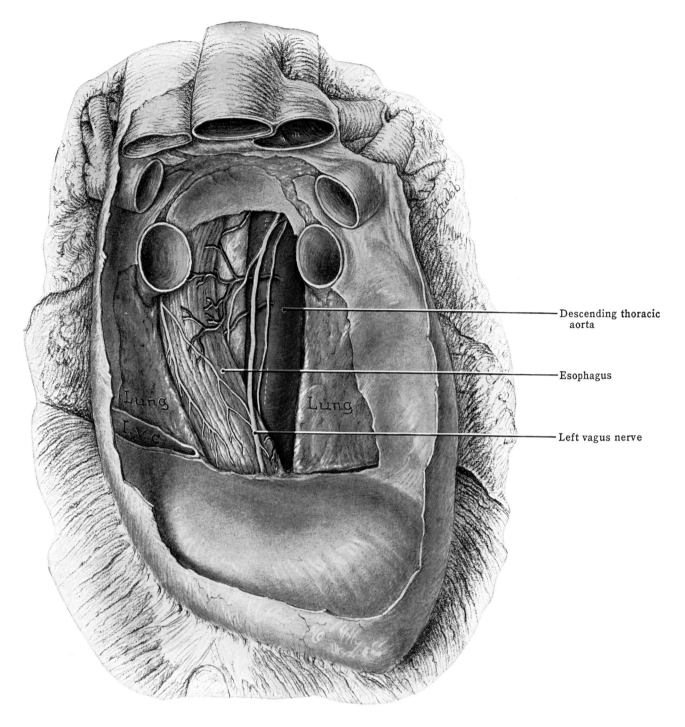

Descending **thoracic** aorta

Esophagus

Left vagus nerve

Lung

Lung

I.V.C

442 Posterior Relations of the Heart and Pericardium

The parietal pericardium (fibrous and serous layers) has been removed behind the oblique sinus and also on each side of it.

Observe:

1. The posterior relations are:—part of the right lung and the esophagus grooving it; part of the left lung and the aorta grooving it; and the vagus nerves forming a plexus on the esophagus.

2. The esophagus is here unduly deflected to the right. It usually lies in contact with the aorta.

(For abdominal relations of pericardium and heart, see fig. 125.)

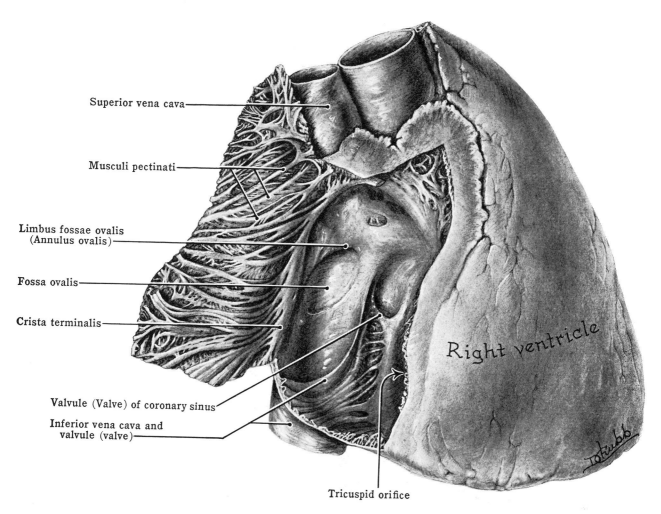

Superior vena cava

Musculi pectinati

Limbus fossae ovalis
(Annulus ovalis)

Fossa ovalis

Crista terminalis

Valvule (Valve) of coronary sinus

Inferior vena cava and
valvule (valve)

Right ventricle

Tricuspid orifice

443 Interior of the Right Atrium, antero-lateral view

Observe:

1. The smooth part of the atrial wall (primitive sinus venarum) and the rough part (primitive atrium).

2. Crista terminalis, the valvule of the i.v. cava, and the valvule of the coronary sinus, separating the smooth from the rough.

3. The 2 caval veins and the coronary sinus opening on to the smooth part.

4. That blunt forceps, passed upwards through the i.v. cava and in contact with its posterior wall, would catch on the limbus fossae ovalis; and, if the foramen ovale were patent (25 per cent), would pass through the interatrial septum into the left atrium.

5. The crista terminalis, descending from the front of the s. v. cava to the front of the i. v. cava; and the musculi pectinati, passing forwards from the crista like teeth from the back of a comb. The crista underlies the sulcus terminalis (fig. 433).

6. The right atrio-ventricular or tricuspid orifice, situated at the anterior aspect of the atrium.

7. The anterior cardiac veins (fig. 433) and the venae minimae (Thebesian veins) not visible, also open into the atrium.

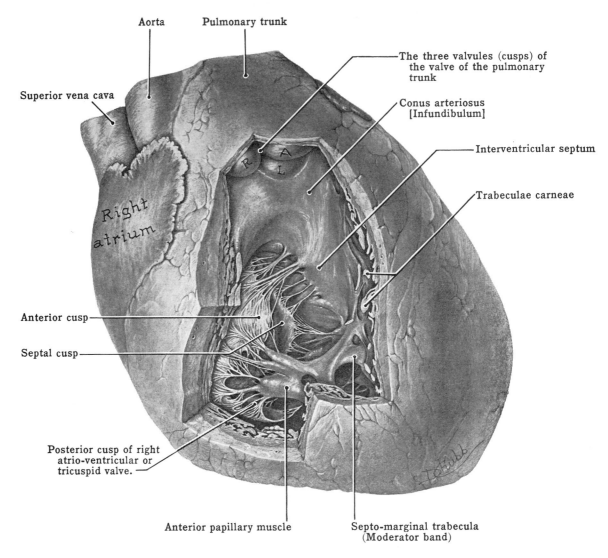

Aorta   Pulmonary trunk

The three valvules (cusps) of
the valve of the pulmonary
trunk

Superior vena cava

Conus arteriosus
[Infundibulum]

Interventricular septum

Right atrium

Trabeculae carneae

Anterior cusp

Septal cusp

Posterior cusp of right
atrio-ventricular or
tricuspid valve.

Anterior papillary muscle

Septo-marginal trabecula
(Moderator band)

444   Interior of the Right Ventricle

Observe:

1. The entrance to this chamber (right atrio-ventricular or tricuspid orifice), situated be
the exit (orifice of the pulmonary trunk) situated above.

2. The smooth funnel-shaped wall (conus arteriosus) below the pulmonary orifice; th
mainder of the ventricle, rough with fleshy trabeculae.

3. Three types of trabeculae—(a) mere ridges, (b) bridges, attached only at each end, ar
finger-like projections called papillary muscles. The anterior papillary muscle rising
the anterior wall; the posterior (not labelled) from the posterior wall; and a series of
septal papillae from the septal wall.

4. The septo-marginal trabecula, here very thick, extending from the septum to the b.
the anterior papillary muscle. It is a bridge.

5. The chordae tendineae (not labelled), passing from the tips of the papillary muscles
free margins and ventricular surfaces of the three cusps of the tricuspid valve.

6. Each papillary muscle controlling the adjacent sides of two cusps (fig. 446).

(*For names given to valvules or cusps of pulmonary trunk, see fig. 446.3.*)

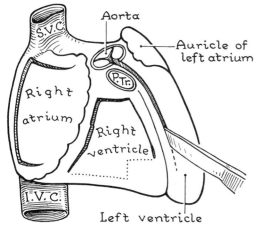

444.1

Suitable incisions for opening the chambers of the heart.
For guidance a finger, or a pencil, may be passed
through a caval or a pulmonary vein into an atrium
and onwards through an atrioventricular orifice into a
ventricle.

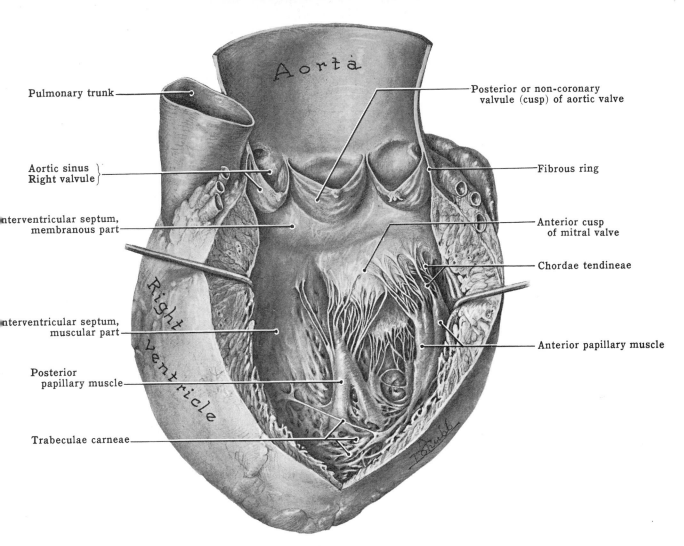

Pulmonary trunk

Aortic sinus ⎱
Right valvule ⎰

Interventricular septum,
membranous part

Interventricular septum,
muscular part

Posterior
papillary muscle

Trabeculae carneae

Aorta

Posterior or non-coronary
valvule (cusp) of aortic valve

Fibrous ring

Anterior cusp
of mitral valve

Chordae tendineae

Anterior papillary muscle

Right Ventricle

445 Interior of the Left Ventricle

Observe:

1. The conical shape of the left chamber.

2. The entrance (left atrio-ventricular, bicuspid, or mitral orifice), situated posteriorly. The exit (aortic orifice), situated superiorly.

3. The wall, thin and muscular near the apex; thick and muscular above; thin and fibrous (nonelastic) at the aortic orifice.

4. Trabeculae carneae, as in the right ventricle, forming ridges, bridges, and papillary muscles.

5. Two large papillary muscles—the anterior from the anterior wall and the posterior from the posterior wall—each controlling, via chordae tendineae, the adjacent halves of two cusps of the mitral valve.

6. The anterior cusp of the mitral valve intervening between the inlet (mitral orifice) and the outlet (aortic orifice).

Note the structure of the mitral and of the aortic valves (fig. 446).

445.1

Diagram of the impulse conducting system of the heart, after *J. W. A. Duckworth.*

The ventricles have been opened and the tricuspid valve has been removed.

Note the sinu-atrial node (S-A. node) at the upper end of the sulcus terminalis, and the atrio-ventricular node (A-V. node) in the lower part of the interatrial septum becoming the A-V. bundle which divides into a right and a left limb.

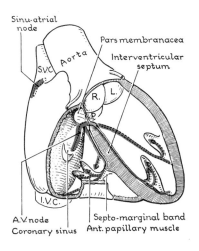

Sinu-atrial
node

Pars membranacea

Interventricular
septum

SVC

Aorta

R.   L.
B.

I.V.C.

A.V. node
Coronary sinus

Septo-marginal band
Ant. papillary muscle

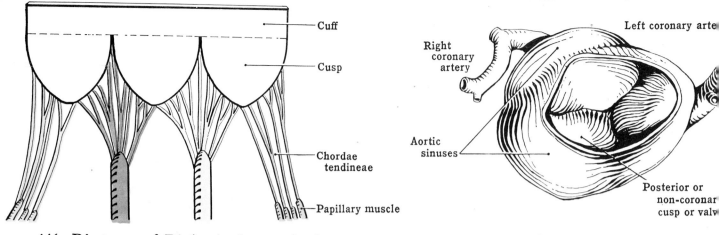

Cuff

Cusp

Chordae tendineae

Papillary muscle

446 Diagram of Right Atrioventricular Valve, spread out

Left coronary arte

Right coronary artery

Aortic sinuses

Posterior or non-coronar cusp or valv

446.1 Aortic Valve, closed ventricular aspect

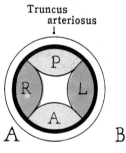
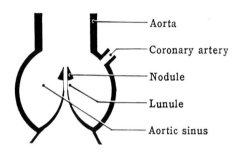

Aorta

Coronary artery

Nodule

Lunule

Aortic sinus

A. Closed, on longitudinal section.

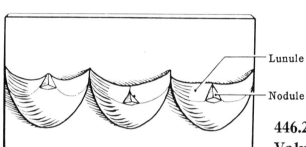
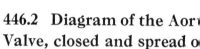

Lunule

Nodule

B. Spread out.

446.2 Diagram of the Aor Valve, closed and spread o

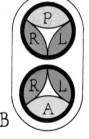

Truncus arteriosus

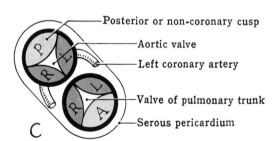

Posterior or non-coronary cusp

Aortic valve

Left coronary artery

Valve of pulmonary trunk

Serous pericardium

446.3 Names applied to the V vules, or cusps, of the Aortic Va and Valve of the Pulmonary Tru explained on a development ba

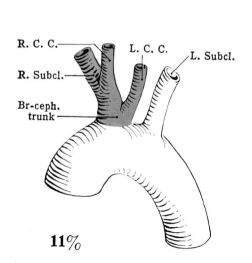

R. C. C.

R. Subcl.

Br-ceph. trunk

L. C. C.

L. Subcl.

11%

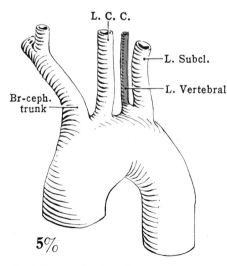

L. C. C.

Br-ceph. trunk

L. Subcl.

L. Vertebral

5%

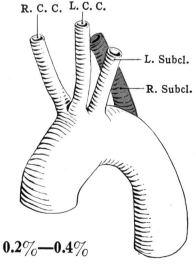

R. C. C. L. C. C.

L. Subcl.

R. Subcl.

0.2%—0.4%

446.4 Variations in the Origins of the Branches of the Aortic Arch

Approximate incidence: 11% of 1220 arches, 5% of 1000 arches, and 0.2% — 0.4% of 1500 arches. (Data on British and Japanese after Quain; Thomson; Adachi; and Loth.)

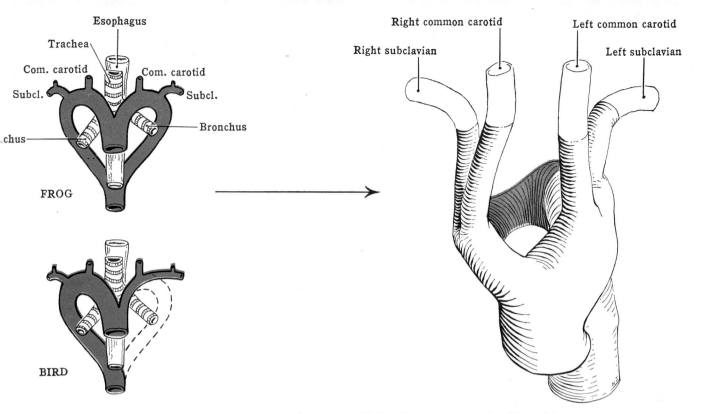

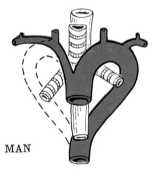

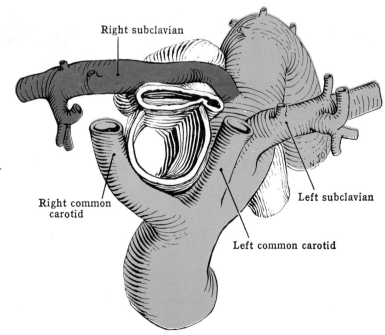

447.1   Specimen of a Double Aortic Arch, in an adult

Note: Both the right and the left aortic arch persist completely, as in the frog. The esophagus and trachea pass through the "aortic ring" so-formed. The condition is rare, and rarely do cases survive childhood.

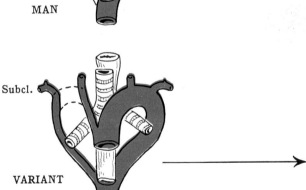

447   Scheme of Varieties of Aortic Arches

Note: The double aortic arch of the frog; the right aortic arch of the bird; the left aortic arch of the mammal, including man; and a variant.

447.2   Retro-esophageal Right Subclavian Artery

Note: The artery arises as the last branch of the aortic arch. It passes behind the esophagus and trachea. The right recurrent laryngeal nerve, having no vessel around which to recur, takes a direct course to the larynx, as in figure 532 drawn from the same subject. This condition was found in 14 or about 1% of 1,453 White, Negro, and Japanese cadavera (J. J. McDonald and Barry J. Anson).

VARIATIONS AND ANOMALIES

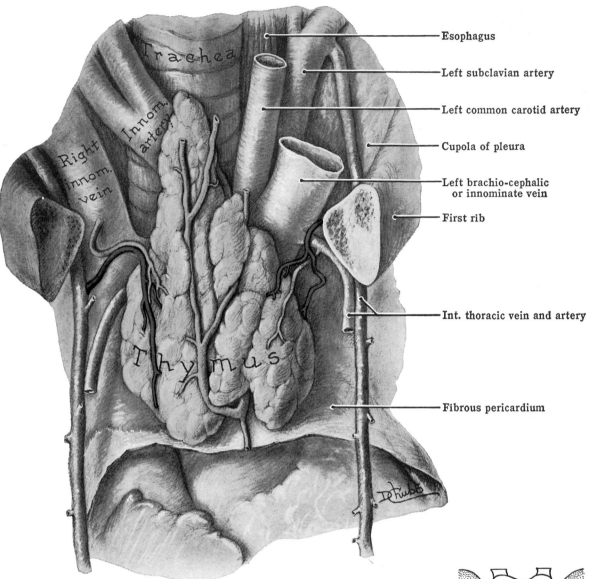

Esophagus

Left subclavian artery

Left common carotid artery

Cupola of pleura

Left brachio-cephalic
or innominate vein

First rib

Int. thoracic vein and artery

Fibrous pericardium

(labels within image: Trachea, Innom. artery, Right Innom. vein, Thymus)

448   Thymus: Superior Mediastinum—I

The sternum and ribs have been excised and the pleurae removed.

Observe:

1. The thymus lying in the superior mediastinum; overlapping the upper limit of the pericardial sac below; and extending into the neck, here farther than usual, above.

2. The longitudinal fissure that divides the thymus into two asymmetrical lobes, a larger right and a smaller left. These two developmentally separate parts are easily separated from each other by blunt dissection.

3. The blood supply—arteries from the internal thoracic arteries; veins to the brachio-cephalic and internal thoracic veins and communicating above with the inferior thyroid veins.

4. The posterior relations, shown in figure 449.

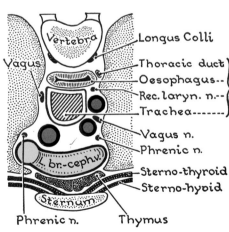

(labels within image: Vertebra, Longus Colli, Vagus, Thoracic duct, Oesophagus, Rec. laryn. n., Trachea, Vagus n., Phrenic n., L. br-cephv., Sterno-thyroid, Sterno-hyoid, Sternum, Phrenic n., Thymus)

448.1

Diagram of the superior mediastinum, cross-section, above the level of the aort arch.

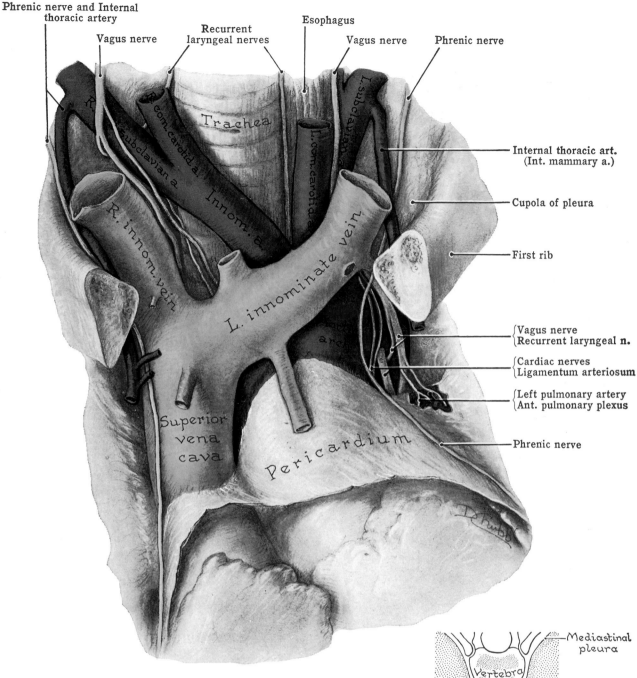

Phrenic nerve and Internal thoracic artery
Vagus nerve
Recurrent laryngeal nerves
Esophagus
Vagus nerve
Phrenic nerve

Trachea

R. subclavian a.
R. com. carotid a.
Innom. a.
L. com. carotid a.
L. subclavian a.

R. innom. vein

L. innominate vein

Internal thoracic art. (Int. mammary a.)

Cupola of pleura

First rib

Vagus nerve
Recurrent laryngeal n.

Cardiac nerves
Ligamentum arteriosum

Left pulmonary artery
Ant. pulmonary plexus

Superior vena cava

Pericardium

Phrenic nerve

49 Root of the Neck: Superior Mediastinum—II

This is figure 448 with the thymus removed.

Observe:

The great veins, anterior to the great arteries.

The backward direction of the aortic arch and the nerves crossing its left side.

The lig. arteriosum, outside the pericardial sac and having the left recurrent nerve on its left side and the vagal and sympathetic branches to the superficial cardiac plexus on its right.

The right vagus, crossing the right subclavian a. (4th right primitive aortic arch), there giving off its recurrent branch, and passing medially to reach the trachea and esophagus.

The left vagus, crossing the aortic arch (4th left primitive aortic arch), there giving off its recurrent branch, and passing medially to reach the esophagus (fig. 450).

The left phrenic nerve, crossing the path of the vagus, but ½″ anterior to it.

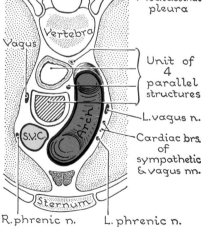

Mediastinal pleura

Vertebra

Vagus

Unit of 4 parallel structures

L. vagus n.

Cardiac brs. of sympathetic & vagus nn.

S.V.C.

Arch

Sternum

R. phrenic n.
L. phrenic n.

449.1

Diagram of the superior mediastinum, on cross-section, at the level of the aortic arch.

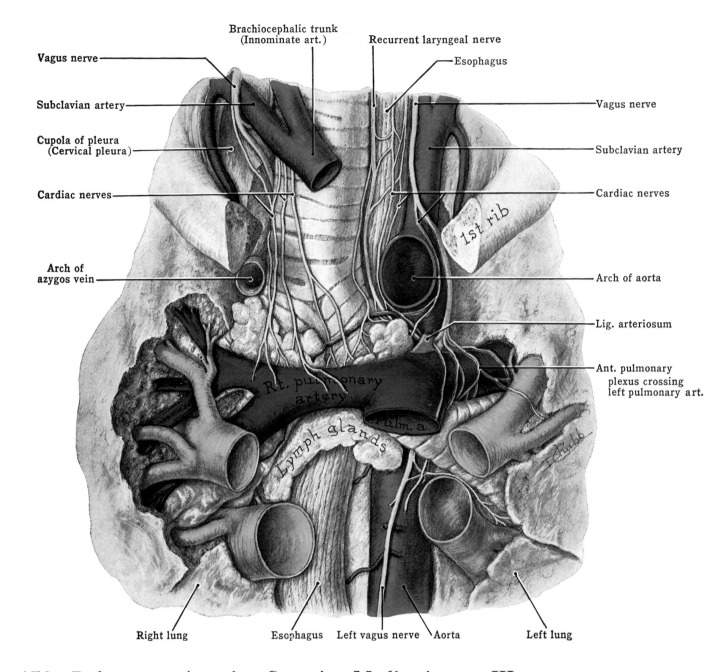

Vagus nerve

Brachiocephalic trunk
(Innominate art.)

Recurrent laryngeal nerve

Esophagus

Subclavian artery

Vagus nerve

Cupola of pleura
(Cervical pleura)

Subclavian artery

Cardiac nerves

Cardiac nerves

1st rib

Arch of
azygos vein

Arch of aorta

Lig. arteriosum

Rt. pulmonary artery

Lymph glands

L. pulm. a.

Ant. pulmonary
plexus crossing
left pulmonary art.

L. Schlabb

Right lung　　Esophagus　Left vagus nerve　Aorta　　Left lung

450　Pulmonary Arteries: Superior Mediastinum—III

Observe:

1. The pulmonary trunk, dividing into right and left pulmonary arteries, which run an oblique course (fig. 434). The right artery crossing below the bifurcation of the trachea and separated from the esophagus by lymph nodes (glands).
2. Cardiac branches of the vagus and sympathetic, streaming down the sides of the trachea and forming the cardiac plexuses.

450.1

Diagram. Relationships at bifurcation of trachea in 3 stages.

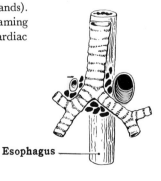

Esophagus

A. Lymph
nodes

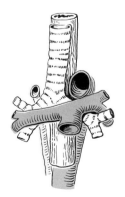

B. Pulmonary
arteries

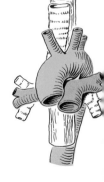

C. Asc. aorta an
arch

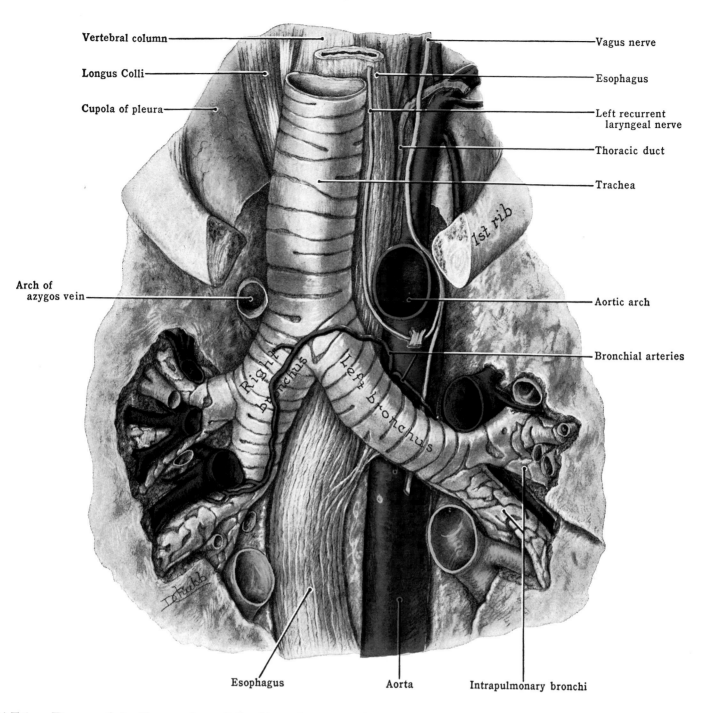

Vertebral column

Longus Colli

Cupola of pleura

Arch of
azygos vein

Vagus nerve

Esophagus

Left recurrent
laryngeal nerve

Thoracic duct

Trachea

1st rib

Aortic arch

Bronchial arteries

Right bronchus

Left bronchus

Esophagus   Aorta   Intrapulmonary bronchi

451   Bronchi: Superior Mediastinum—IV

Observe:

Four parallel structures—trachea, esophagus, left recurrent laryngeal nerve, and thoracic duct. The esophagus bulges to the left of the trachea; the recurrent nerve lies in the angle between the trachea and esophagus; and the duct is at the side of the esophagus.

The aortic arch runs backwards on the left of these 4 structures, and the arch of the azygos vein passing forwards on the right.

The trachea inclining to the right, hence the right bronchus is more vertical that the left, and its stem is shorter and wider, its first branch arising about 1″ from the bifurcation, whereas the first left branch arises about 2″ from the bifurcation.

The U-shaped rings of the trachea, commonly bifurcated; the ring at the bifurcation of the trachea being V-shaped; the intrapulmonary rings forming a mosaic around the bronchi.

The occasional broncho-esophageal muscle, attaching the esophagus to the left bronchus.

451.1

Scheme to explain asymmetrical courses of right and left recurrent laryngeal nerves. (III, IV and VI = embryonic aortic arches.)

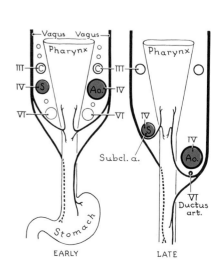

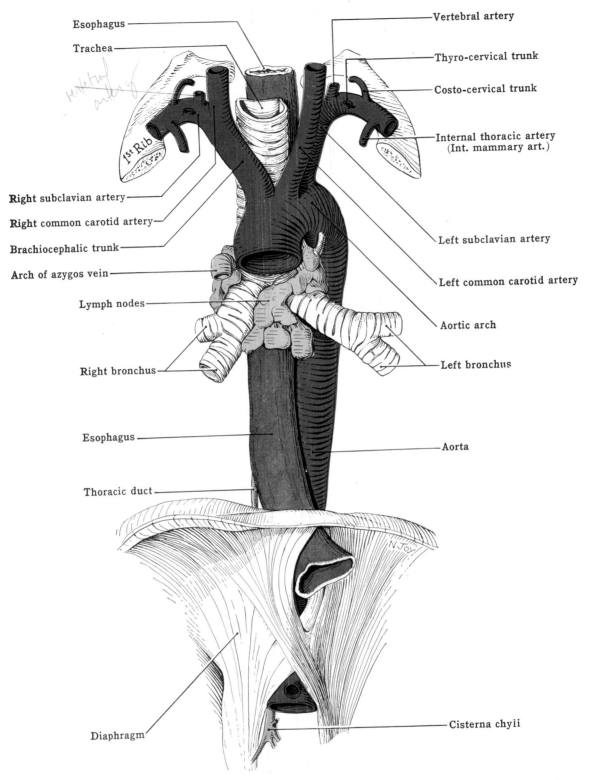

Esophagus

Trachea

Vertebral artery

Thyro-cervical trunk

Costo-cervical trunk

Internal thoracic artery
(Int. mammary art.)

1st Rib

Right subclavian artery

Right common carotid artery

Brachiocephalic trunk

Arch of azygos vein

Lymph nodes

Right bronchus

Left subclavian artery

Left common carotid artery

Aortic arch

Left bronchus

Esophagus

Aorta

Thoracic duct

N. Joy

Diaphragm

Cisterna chyli

452 Esophagus, Trachea and Aorta, thoracic parts, anterior view

Observe:

1. The arch of the aorta, arching backwards on the left side of the trachea and esophagus, and the arch of the azygos vein arching forwards on their right sides. Each arches above the root of a lung (figs. 415 and 416).

2. The posterior relation of the trachea is—esophagus.

3. The anterior relations of the thoracic part of the esophagus from above downwards are: trachea (throughout its entire length), left recurrent nerve; right and left bronchi, the inferior tracheobronchial lymph nodes (in front of which lies the right pulmonary artery, fig. 450), the pericardium (removed, in front of which lies the oblique pericardial sinus and the left atrium of the heart, figs. 441 & 442), and finally, the diaphragm.

4. Above the level of the aortic arch, the esophagus bulges to the left beyond the trachea.

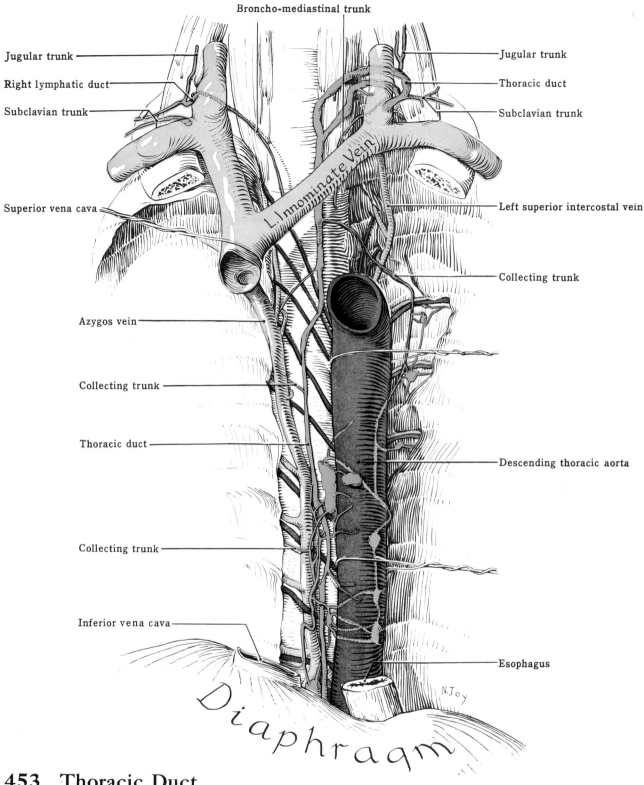

Jugular trunk

Right lymphatic duct

Subclavian trunk

Broncho-mediastinal trunk

Jugular trunk

Thoracic duct

Subclavian trunk

Superior vena cava

L. Innominate Vein

Left superior intercostal vein

Collecting trunk

Azygos vein

Collecting trunk

Thoracic duct

Descending thoracic aorta

Collecting trunk

Inferior vena cava

Esophagus

N. Joy

Diaphragm

453   Thoracic Duct

(A composite sketch made from photographs of two specimens dissected by Miss M. G. Gray.)

Observe

1. The thoracic duct (a) ascending on the vertebral column between the azygos vein and the descending aorta; and (b) at the junction of the posterior and superior mediastina, passing to the left and continuing its ascent to the neck where (c) it arches laterally to open near, or at, the angle of union of the internal jugular and subclavian veins.

2. The duct, here, as commonly, (a) plexiform in the posterior mediastinum and (b) splitting in the neck.

3. The duct receiving branches from the intercostal spaces of both sides via several collecting trunks and also branches from posterior mediastinal structures.

4. The duct finally receiving the jugular, subclavian, and broncho-mediastinal trunks.

5. The right lymph duct, very short and formed by the union of the right jugular, subclavian, and broncho-mediastinal trunks.

For origin of duct in cisterna chyli see figure 452; for termination of duct in the neck see figures 533 and 536.

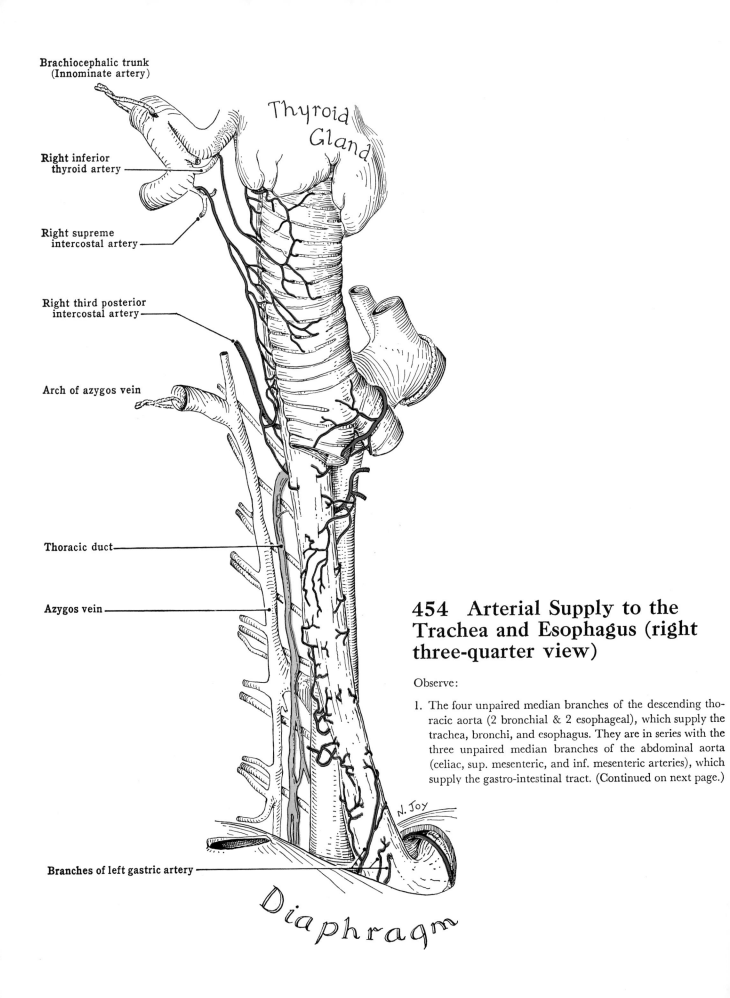

Brachiocephalic trunk
(Innominate artery)

Thyroid Gland

Right inferior
thyroid artery

Right supreme
intercostal artery

Right third posterior
intercostal artery

Arch of azygos vein

Thoracic duct

Azygos vein

N. Joy

Branches of left gastric artery

Diaphragm

454 Arterial Supply to the Trachea and Esophagus (right three-quarter view)

Observe:

1. The four unpaired median branches of the descending thoracic aorta (2 bronchial & 2 esophageal), which supply the trachea, bronchi, and esophagus. They are in series with the three unpaired median branches of the abdominal aorta (celiac, sup. mesenteric, and inf. mesenteric arteries), which supply the gastro-intestinal tract. (Continued on next page.)

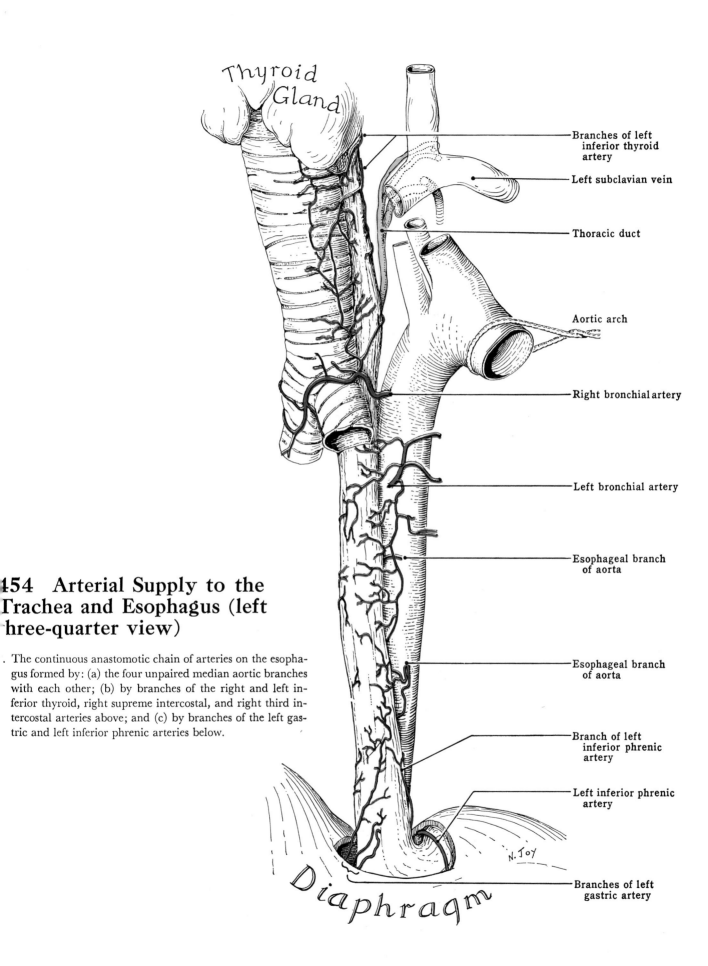

Thyroid Gland

Branches of left inferior thyroid artery

Left subclavian vein

Thoracic duct

Aortic arch

Right bronchial artery

Left bronchial artery

Esophageal branch of aorta

Esophageal branch of aorta

Branch of left inferior phrenic artery

Left inferior phrenic artery

Branches of left gastric artery

Diaphragm

N. Joy

454 Arterial Supply to the Trachea and Esophagus (left three-quarter view)

. The continuous anastomotic chain of arteries on the esophagus formed by: (a) the four unpaired median aortic branches with each other; (b) by branches of the right and left inferior thyroid, right supreme intercostal, and right third intercostal arteries above; and (c) by branches of the left gastric and left inferior phrenic arteries below.

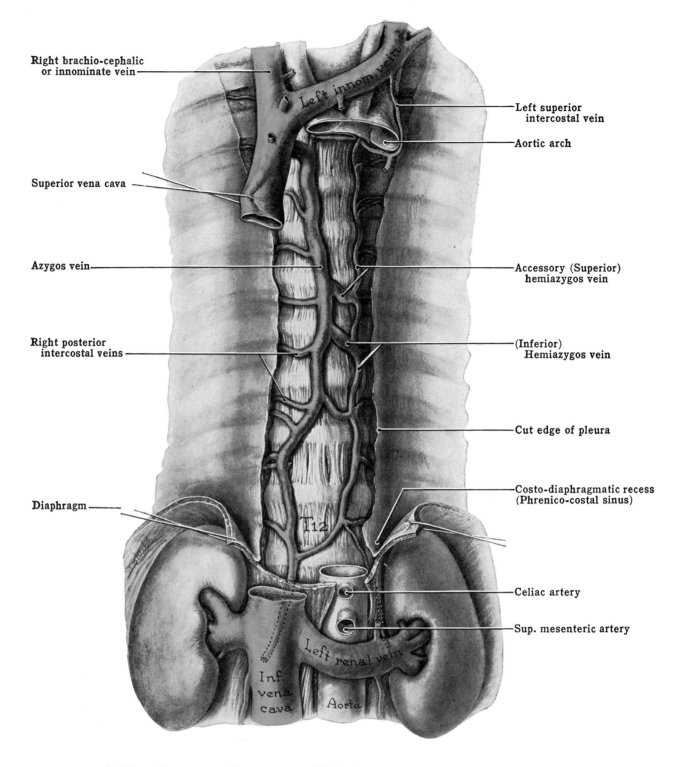

Right brachio-cephalic or innominate vein

Superior vena cava

Azygos vein

Right posterior intercostal veins

Diaphragm

Left innom. vein

Left superior intercostal vein

Aortic arch

Accessory (Superior) hemiazygos vein

(Inferior) Hemiazygos vein

Cut edge of pleura

Costo-diaphragmatic recess (Phrenico-costal sinus)

Celiac artery

Sup. mesenteric artery

T 12

Inf. vena cava

Left renal vein

Aorta

455   Azygos System of Veins

Observe:

1. The left renal vein ventral to the aorta; the left brachiocephalic (innominate) vein ventral to the three branches of the aortic arch. These two cross-channels conduct blood from the left side of the body to the right side—and so to the right atrium.

2. The paired and approximately symmetrical, right and left, longitudinal veins ventral to the vertebral column. The right, or azygos, vein communicating caudally with the i.v. cava; the left vein communicating with the left renal vein; and each receiving the respective right and left posterior intercostal veins. The right vein ending cranially in the s.v. cava; the left in the left brachio-cephalic, or innominate, vein.

3. The left vein being a chain of veins—hemiazygos, accessory hemiazygos, and left superior intercostal—which here are continuous, but commonly are discontinuous. It is united to the right, or azygos, vein by several (here 4) cross-connecting channels. (Sieb.)

56 Persisting Left superior Vena Cava

The vessel connecting the left brachiocephalic or innominate vein to the coronary sinus is the primitive left superior vena cava. It has 3 component segments: (1) an upper, the stem of the left superior intercostal vein; (2) a lower, the oblique vein of the left atrium; and (3) a middle, the vein uniting the intercostal vein to the oblique vein.

This channel to the right atrium functioned until the left superior vena cava established connection with the right by means of the left brachiocephalic vein, after which the blood was re-routed, and the middle segment disappeared, though it may persist as a vestigial thread within the fold of the left vena cava. (fig. 440).

(for persisting left inf. vena cava, see figs. 185 and 185.1.)

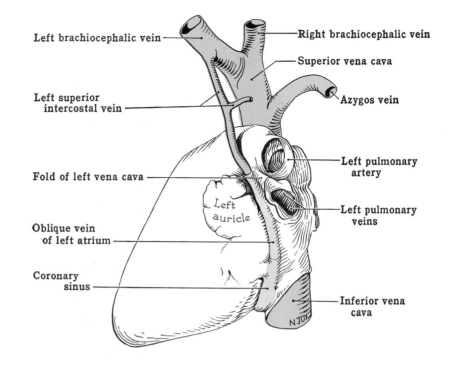

55.1

Diagram of the azygos system of veins.

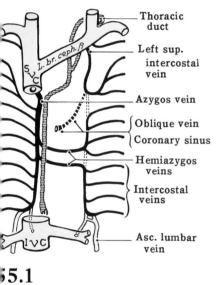

57 Lobe of the Azygos Vein

This lobe, said to be constant in the porpoise, really part of a bifid apex. It results during embryonic life when the apex of a developing right lung encounters the arch of the azygos vein and is cleft by it, a portion of the apex coming to lie on each side of the venous arch. The venous arch is suspended, so to speak, within a pleural mesentery.

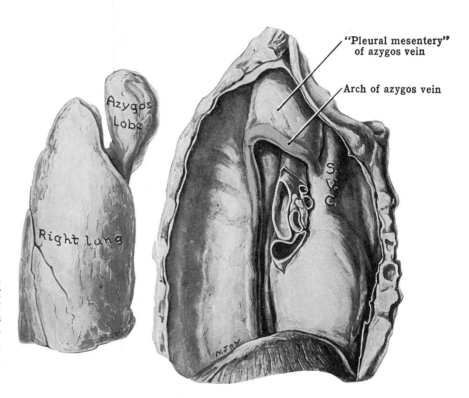

Variation and Anomaly

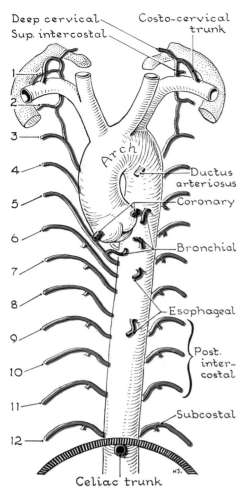

Deep cervical
Sup. intercostal
Costo-cervical trunk

1
2
3
4
5
6
7
8
9
10
11
12

Arch

Ductus arteriosus
Coronary
Bronchial
Esophageal
Post. inter- costal
Subcostal

Celiac trunk

457.1 Thoracic Aorta and its Branches

From the Ascending Aorta:
    Right coronary
    Left coronary
From the Arch of the Aorta:
    Brachiocephalic trunk
      Right subclavian
      Right common carotid
    Left common carotid
    Left subclavian
    (ductus arteriosus)
From the Descending Thoracic Aorta:
    Visceral branches:
      Esophageal
      Bronchial, left upper & lower
      Right bronchial
      Pericardial
      Mediastinal
    Parietal branches, paired:
      Posterior intercostal (Th. 3–11)
      Subcostal (Th. 12)
      Superior phrenic

Note:
The right bronchial artery arises from either the upper left bronchial or third right posterior inter-costal artery (here the fifth) or the aorta direct. The small arteries to pericardium, tissues in posterior mediastinum, and upper surface of diaphragm are not shown.

(*For abdominal aorta and its branches, see fig. 188.*)

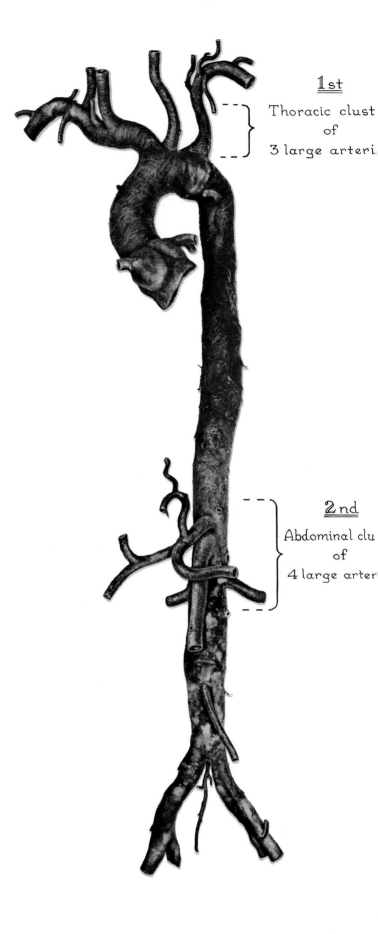

1st
Thoracic clust
of
3 large arteri

2nd
Abdominal clu
of
4 large arter

457.2 Aorta

The entire aorta, showing the 2 sites (aortic arch upper limit of abdominal aorta) where the large bran cluster.

The Head and Neck

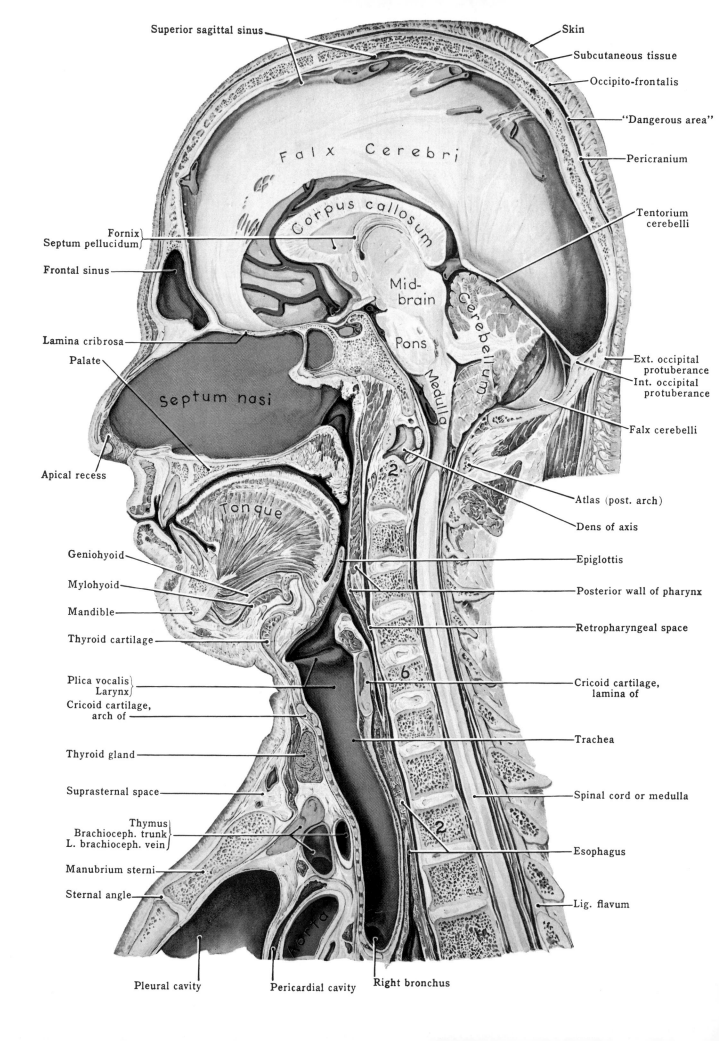

Superior sagittal sinus

Skin

Subcutaneous tissue

Occipito-frontalis

"Dangerous area"

Pericranium

Falx Cerebri

Corpus callosum

Tentorium cerebelli

Fornix
Septum pellucidum

Mid-brain

Cerebellum

Frontal sinus

Pons

Medulla

Lamina cribrosa

Ext. occipital protuberance
Int. occipital protuberance

Palate

Septum nasi

Falx cerebelli

Apical recess

2

Tongue

Atlas (post. arch)

Dens of axis

Geniohyoid

Epiglottis

Mylohyoid

Posterior wall of pharynx

Mandible

Retropharyngeal space

Thyroid cartilage

6

Cricoid cartilage, lamina of

Plica vocalis
Larynx

Cricoid cartilage, arch of

Thyroid gland

Trachea

Suprasternal space

Spinal cord or medulla

Thymus
Brachioceph. trunk
L. brachioceph. vein

2

Esophagus

Manubrium sterni

Sternal angle

Aorta

Lig. flavum

Pleural cavity

Pericardial cavity

Right bronchus

458 Head and Neck, on median section

Observe:

1. The 3 adherent layers of the scalp—skin, subcutaneous tissue, and occipito-frontalis muscle—separated from the pericranium by loose areolar tissue (the dangerous area) in which, following injury, blood or pus may collect.

2. The tentorium cerebelli suspended by the falx cerebri, sloping to the internal occipital protuberance, and forming a floor for the cerebrum (removed) and a roof for the cerebellum. The external occipital protuberance, nearly level with the internal protuberance, marking the line between scalp and thick bone above and nuchal muscles and thin bone below.

3. Behind the tip or apex of the nose, a shelf above which is the apical recess of the nasal cavity.

4. The nasal septum extending from the apical recess in front to the nasopharynx behind, where it ends in a free posterior border, and from the sieve-like lamina cribrosa (cribriform plate) above to the palate below.

5. The palate, the anterior $\frac{2}{3}$ of which contains bone and is known as the hard palate, and the posterior $\frac{1}{3}$ which contains gland and muscle and is called soft palate. The Levator Palati (in contraction, as it is during the act of swallowing) pulling the soft palate upward and backward (it retracts as well as elevates) thereby closing the oral pharynx (not labelled), which lies below the soft palate, from the nasopharynx which lies above. A small mass, the pharyngeal tonsil, projecting from the roof of the nasopharynx.

6. The Orbicularis Oris in the upper and lower lips, with free margins curved forward. The incisor teeth in modern man, not biting edge to edge but edge to lingual surface.

7. The Geniohyoid passing from the mental spine (genial tubercle) of the mandible to the hyoid bone (not labelled), and above it the Genioglossus (not labelled) radiating into the tongue. The anterior $\frac{2}{3}$ of the tongue forming part of the floor of the mouth; the posterior $\frac{1}{3}$ forming the anterior wall of the oral pharynx. Behind the tongue, the epiglottis.

8. The larynx, guarded in front by the thyroid cartilage and extending from the tip of the epiglottis above to the lower border of the cricoid cartilage below, where it becomes the trachea. A horizontal slit that runs posteriorly from the thyroid cartilage separating an upper or false cord from a lower or true vocal cord, the plica vocalis.

9. The 4″ to 4$\frac{1}{2}$″ long trachea, half in the neck and half in the thorax, bifurcating below into a right and a left bronchus, the mouth of the right bronchus being in view.

10. The cut ends of 19 tracheal rings (they may be counted) below the arch of the cricoid cartilage which always projects in front of the rings and is therefore palpable and readily identified. It is a valuable landmark. It is also a guide to the level of the 6th cervical vertebra which lies behind it. The isthmus of the thyroid gland crossing several tracheal rings, but leaving the upper one or two uncovered. The brachio-cephalic trunk (innominate artery), here as commonly, impressing the trachea.

11. The cricoid cartilage lying at the level of the body of the 6th cervical vertebra. At the lower border of this cartilage the larynx becoming the trachea and the pharynx becoming the esophagus. The diameter of the alimentary canal is here at its narrowest and least dilatable part. In the neck the esophagus projects to the left of the trachea, hence the right wall of the upper part of the esophagus is cut longitudinally and no lumen is seen.

12. The retropharyngeal space extending from the level of the atlas downward into the superior mediastinum.

13. The manubrium sterni is 2″ in length and is its own length of 2″ from the body of the 2nd thoracic vertebra.

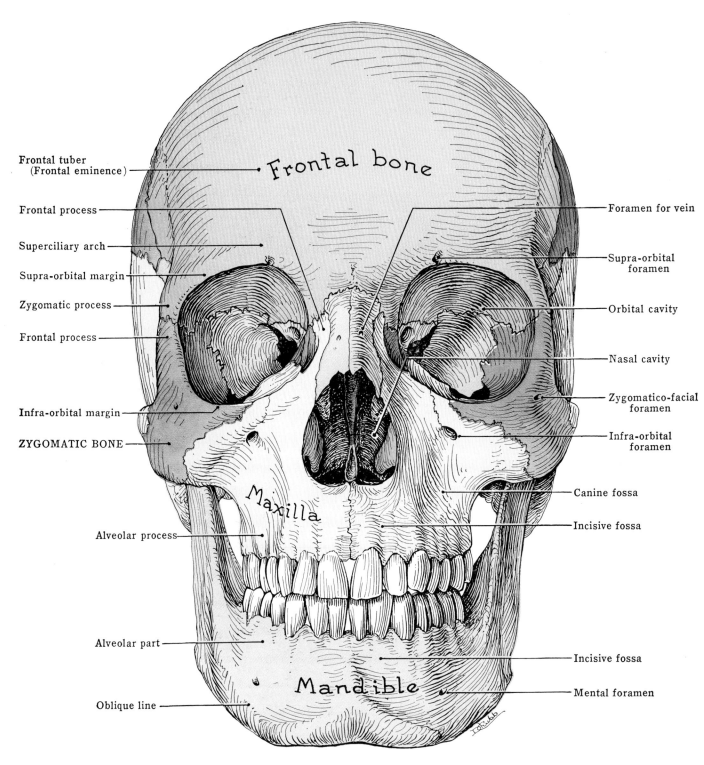

Frontal tuber
(Frontal eminence)

Frontal process

Superciliary arch

Supra-orbital margin

Zygomatic process

Frontal process

Infra-orbital margin

ZYGOMATIC BONE

Alveolar process

Alveolar part

Oblique line

Frontal bone

Foramen for vein

Supra-orbital
foramen

Orbital cavity

Nasal cavity

Zygomatico-facial
foramen

Infra-orbital
foramen

Canine fossa

Incisive fossa

Maxilla

Incisive fossa

Mandible

Mental foramen

459   Skull, front view (Norma Frontalis)

On the right side of the skull—surface features.

On the left side—foramina, fossae, and cavities.

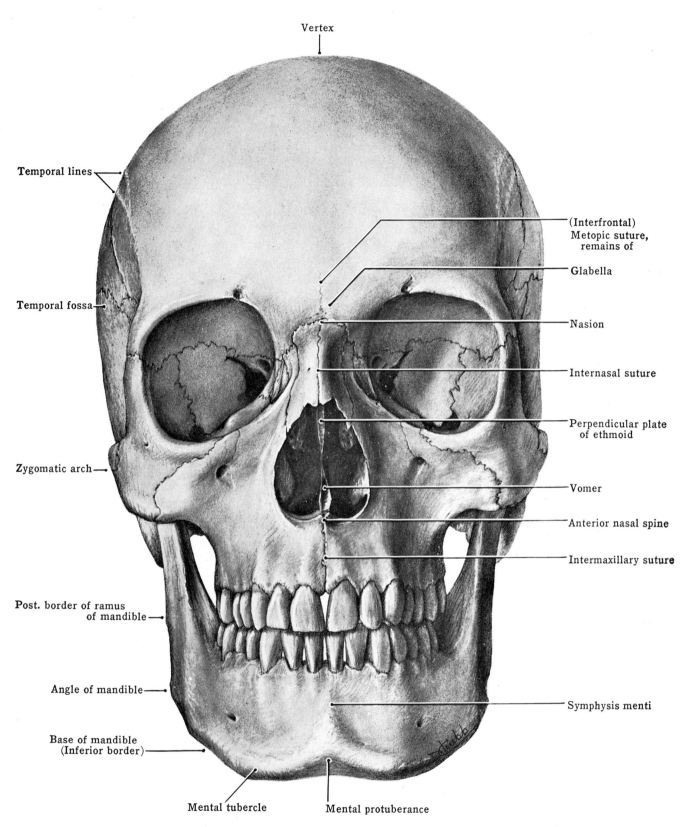

Vertex

Temporal lines

Temporal fossa

Zygomatic arch

Post. border of ramus of mandible

Angle of mandible

Base of mandible (Inferior border)

Mental tubercle

(Interfrontal) Metopic suture, remains of

Glabella

Nasion

Internasal suture

Perpendicular plate of ethmoid

Vomer

Anterior nasal spine

Intermaxillary suture

Symphysis menti

Mental protuberance

460 Skull, front view (Norma Frontalis)

On the right side of the skull—marginal or outline features.

On the left side—median line features.

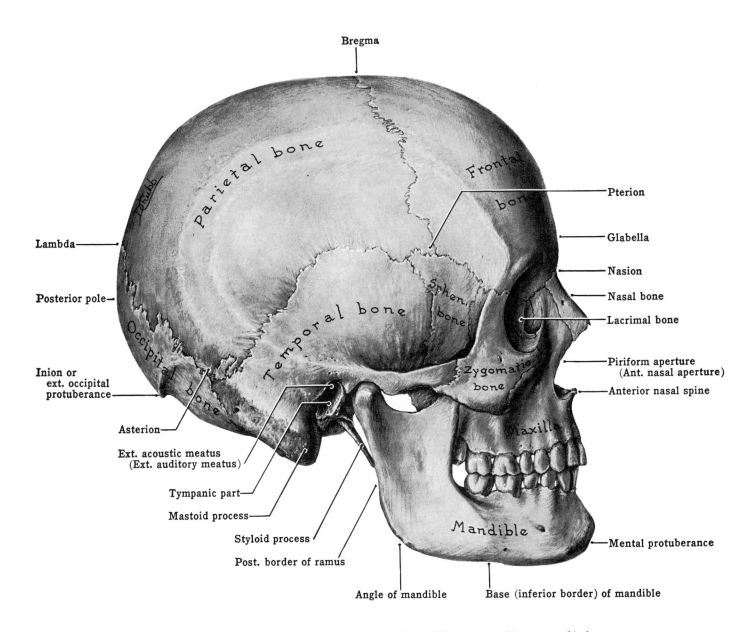

Bregma

Parietal bone

Frontal bone

Pterion

Glabella

Nasion

Nasal bone

Lacrimal bone

Sphen. bone

Temporal bone

Piriform aperture
(Ant. nasal aperture)

Zygomatic bone

Anterior nasal spine

Lambda

Posterior pole

Occipital bone

Maxilla

Inion or
ext. occipital
protuberance

Asterion

Mandible

Ext. acoustic meatus
(Ext. auditory meatus)

Tympanic part

Mental protuberance

Mastoid process

Styloid process

Post. border of ramus

Angle of mandible

Base (inferior border) of mandible

461 Skull, from the side (Norma Lateralis)

Names of bones, outline features, and anthropological points.

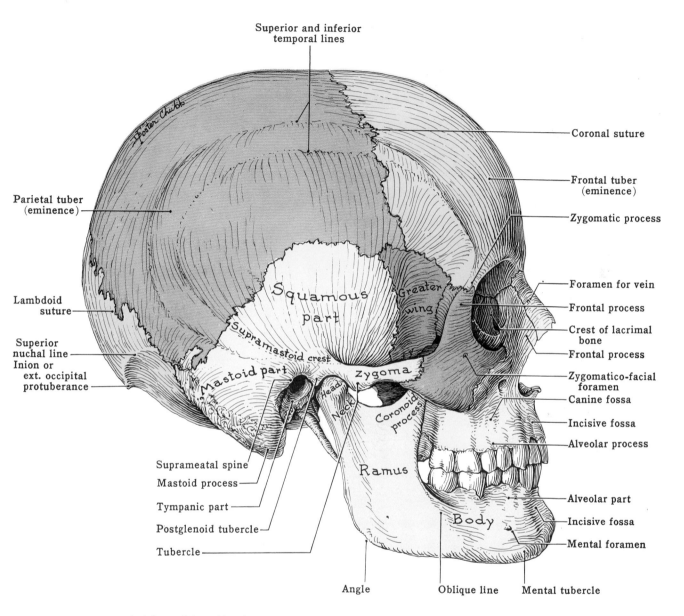

Superior and inferior
temporal lines

Coronal suture

Frontal tuber
(eminence)

Zygomatic process

Parietal tuber
(eminence)

Foramen for vein

Frontal process

Crest of lacrimal
bone

Frontal process

Lambdoid
suture

Squamous
part

Greater
wing

Supramastoid crest

Mastoid part

zygoma

Zygomatico-facial
foramen

Canine fossa

Incisive fossa

Alveolar process

Superior
nuchal line
Inion or
ext. occipital
protuberance

Head

Neck

Coronoid
process

Ramus

Body

Alveolar part

Incisive fossa

Mental foramen

Suprameatal spine

Mastoid process

Tympanic part

Postglenoid tubercle

Tubercle

Angle

Oblique line

Mental tubercle

462   Skull, from the side (Norma Lateralis)

Names of parts of bones and surface features.
(Zygoma is short for zygomatic process of the temporal bone.)

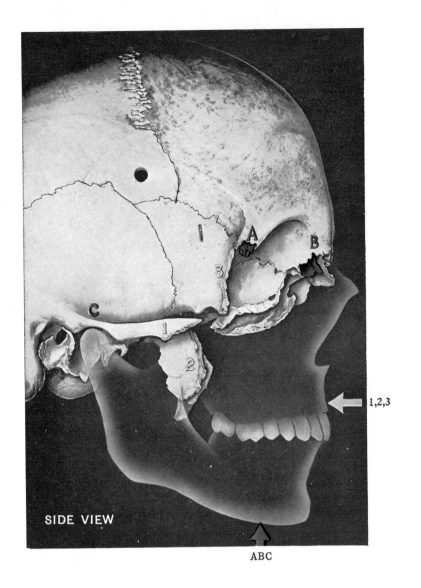

SIDE VIEW

1,2,3

ABC

463   The Buttresses of the Face

The mandible and the maxillae and the zygomatic bones are removed together with the smaller fragile bones of the face (nasal, lacrimal, inferior concha, vomer, and palatine).

Observe:

1. The three buttresses (yellow) on each side that prevent the bones of the face from being driven or displaced backward under the cranium are:
   (1) the zygomatic process of the temporal bone—horizontal,
   (2) the pterygoid process of the sphenoid bone—oblique,
   (3) the greater wing of the sphenoid bone—vertical.

2. The three buttresses (red) on each side that prevent the bones of the face from being driven or displaced upward are
   (A) the zygomatic process of the frontal bone,
   (B) the nasal part of the frontal bone
   (C) the roof of the mandibular fossa for what it is worth—thin and translucent and easily fractured (see fig. 619.2.)

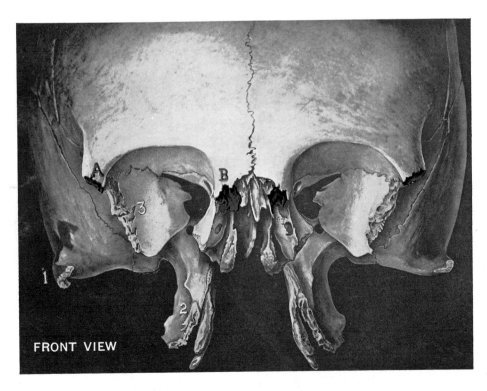

FRONT VIEW

64 Buttresses of ıe Nose

A. The margin of the Piriform erture, or Bony Anterior Nasal erture, is sharp and is formed the maxillae and the nasal nes.

B. On Removing the Nasal nes the areas on the frontal ocesses of the maxillae (yellow) d on the frontal bone (blue) t articulate with and buttress nasal bones are seen; so is the al septum (fig. 605).

B 1. Postero-superior view of Nasal Bones in Articulation h each other shows the median st which forms part of the al septum, the surfaces covered h mucous membrane (pink) l the grooves for the internal al nerves.

C. On Removing the Frontal ocesses of the Maxillae and ng the specimen, one sees:

The areas of the frontal bone yellow) against which the ontal processes of the maxil- e abut,

The areas of the labyrinths of e fragile ethmoid bone and e thin anterior borders of the crimal bones with which the axillae articulate (red), and so

The delicate and narrow lam- a cribrosa (cribriform plate) the ethmoid bone, which parates the roof of the nasal vities from the floor of the terior cranial fossa.

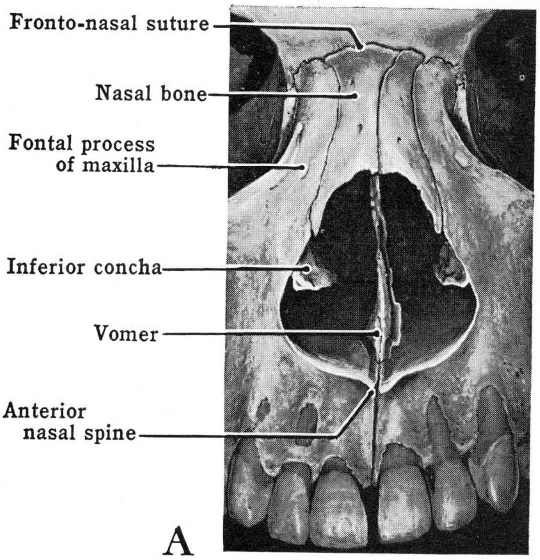

Fronto-nasal suture
Nasal bone
Fontal process of maxilla
Inferior concha
Vomer
Anterior nasal spine

A

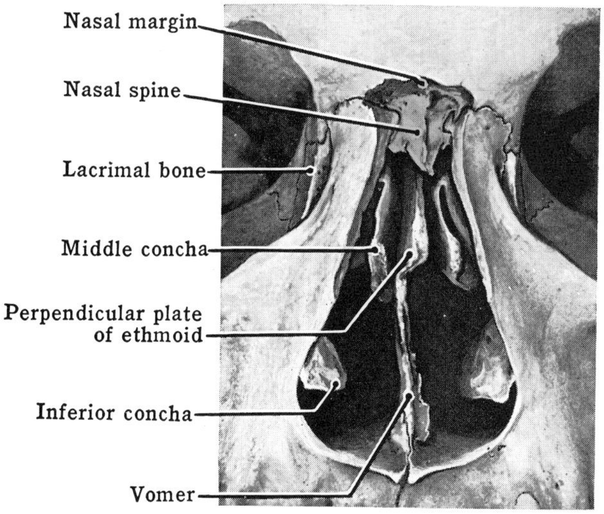

Nasal margin
Nasal spine
Lacrimal bone
Middle concha
Perpendicular plate of ethmoid
Inferior concha
Vomer

B

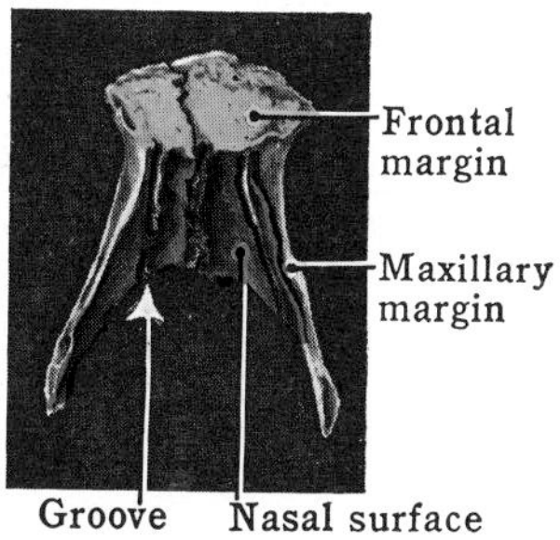

Frontal margin
Maxillary margin
Groove
Nasal surface

B 1

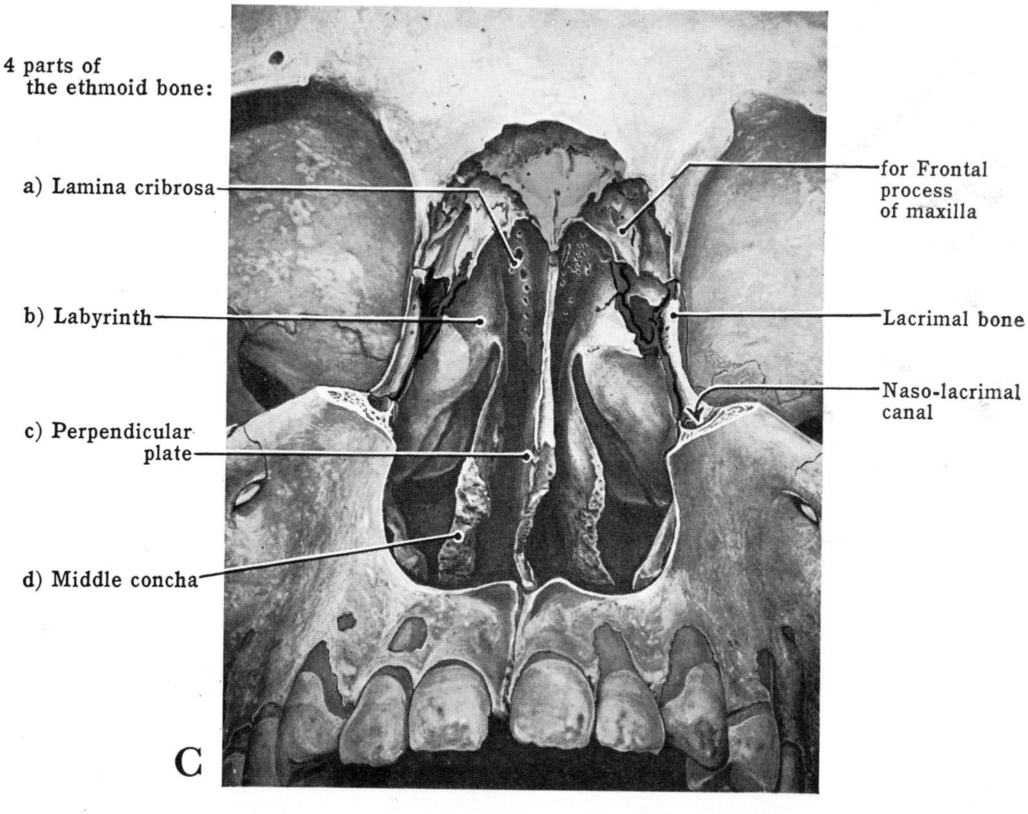

4 parts of the ethmoid bone:
a) Lamina cribrosa
b) Labyrinth
c) Perpendicular plate
d) Middle concha
for Frontal process of maxilla
Lacrimal bone
Naso-lacrimal canal

C

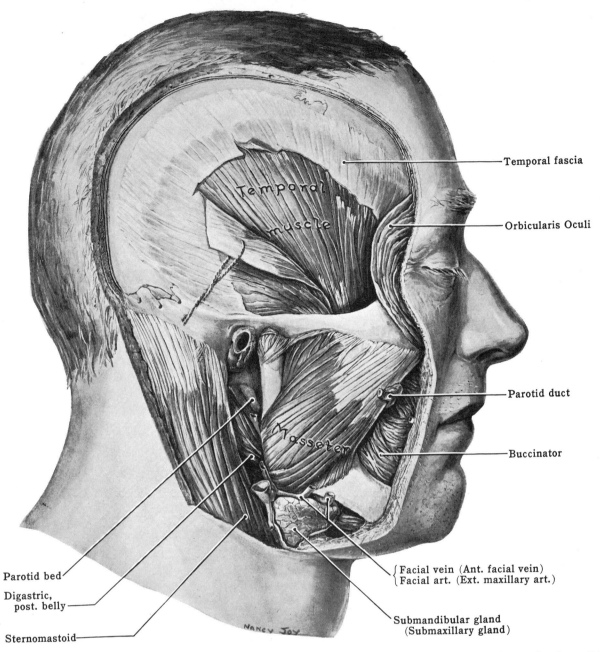

Temporal fascia

Orbicularis Oculi

Parotid duct

Buccinator

Facial vein (Ant. facial vein)
Facial art. (Ext. maxillary art.)

Submandibular gland
(Submaxillary gland)

Parotid bed

Digastric,
post. belly

Sternomastoid

465 Great Muscles on the Side of the Skull

Observe:

1. The temporal and masseteric muscles, both are supplied by the trigeminal nerve a
   both close the jaw. Temporalis, arising in part from the overlying fascia, c.f. Tibi
   Anterior (fig. 305).

2. Orbicularis Oculi and Buccinator, both are supplied by the facial nerve. One clo
   the eye; the other prevents food from collecting between cheeks and teeth.

3. Sternomastoid, which is the chief flexor of the head and neck, forming the poster
   boundary of the parotid region; and Digastric which limits this region below.

4. The submandibular gland, with the facial artery passing deep to it and the facial v
   passing superficial.

(For other facial muscles, figs. 466 and 470.)

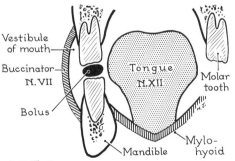

Vestibule
of mouth

Buccinator
N. VII

Bolus

Tongue
N. XII

Molar
tooth

Mandible

Mylo-
hyoid

465.1

Diagram: The Tongue and the
Buccinator retain food between the
molar teeth during the act of chewing.

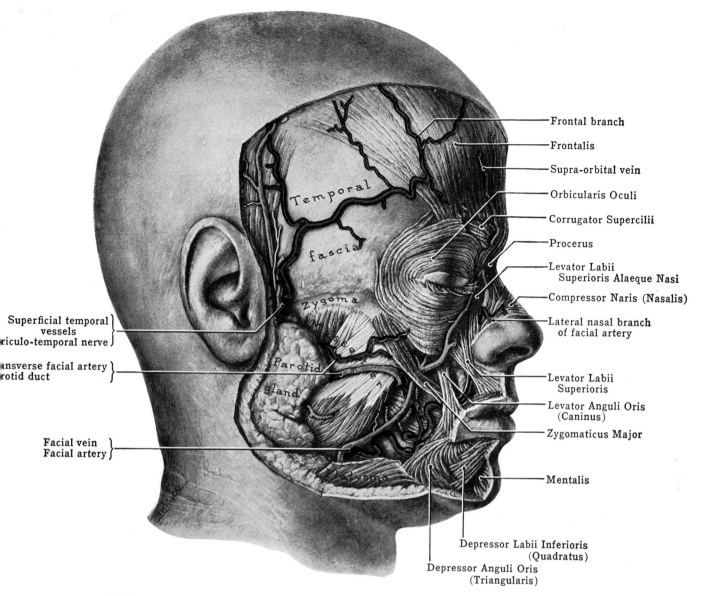

Labels on figure:
- Frontal branch
- Frontalis
- Supra-orbital vein
- Orbicularis Oculi
- Corrugator Supercilii
- Procerus
- Levator Labii Superioris Alaeque Nasi
- Compressor Naris (Nasalis)
- Lateral nasal branch of facial artery
- Levator Labii Superioris
- Levator Anguli Oris (Caninus)
- Zygomaticus Major
- Mentalis
- Depressor Labii Inferioris (Quadratus)
- Depressor Anguli Oris (Triangularis)
- Superficial temporal vessels
- riculo-temporal nerve
- ansverse facial artery
- rotid duct
- Facial vein
- Facial artery
- Temporal fascia
- Zygoma
- Parotid gland

466 Muscles of Expression; Arteries of Face, side view

Observe:

1. Around the eye—Orbicularis Oculi, Corrugator Supercilii, also Frontalis.

2. Around the nose—Compressor Naris, Procerus, and Levator Labii Superioris Alaeque Nasi.

3. Around the mouth—Orbicularis Oris (see fig. 470):
   In upper lip {Levator Labii Superioris Alaequae Nasi, Levator Labii Superioris, Zygomaticus Minor, Zygomaticus Major, Levator Anguli Oris.
   In cheek—Buccinator (fig. 559).
   In lower lip {Platysma (fig. 526), Risorius (not shown), Depressor Anguli Oris, and Depressor Labii Inferioris.
   In chin—Mentalis (fig. 470).

4. Around the Ear—Auriculares Anterior, Superior et Posterior (see fig. 467).
   All the above named muscles are supplied by the facial (VII) nerve.

5. The facial artery, usually sinuous but here tortuous, crossing the base of the mandible at the anterior border of Masseter, passing within half an inch of the angle of the mouth, and lying in front of the facial vein which takes a straight and more superficial course.

6. The transverse facial artery, crossing Masseter between the zygoma and the parotid duct.

Note: Assisting the facial and transverse facial arteries to supply the face are branches or twigs that accompany each branch of the trigeminal (V) nerve, shown in figure 470. Those accompanying V^1 are derived from the ophthalmic branch of the internal carotid artery; those accompanying V^2 and V^3, from the maxillary branch of the external carotid artery.

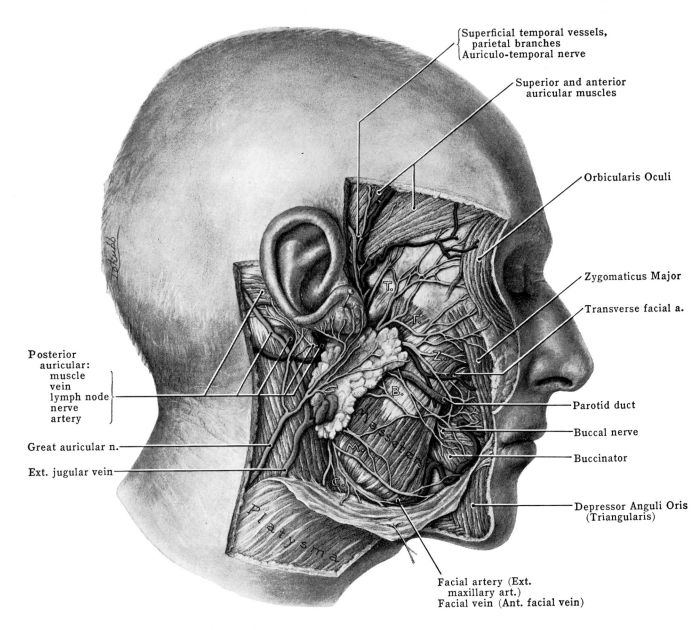

Superficial temporal vessels,
 parietal branches
Auriculo-temporal nerve

Superior and anterior
 auricular muscles

Orbicularis Oculi

Zygomaticus Major

Transverse facial a.

Posterior
auricular:
 muscle
 vein
 lymph node
 nerve
 artery

Great auricular n.—

Ext. jugular vein—

Parotid duct

Buccal nerve

Buccinator

Depressor Anguli Oris
 (Triangularis)

Facial artery (Ext.
 maxillary art.)
Facial vein (Ant. facial vein)

467 Face: Terminal Branches of the Facial Nerve, side view

General: Deep fascia is absent from the face, but present over Temporalis and Masseter.

The facial nerve supplies the muscles of expression and, though motor, is superficial. Masseter is a muscle of mastication and is supplied by the trigeminal nerve.

Observe:

1. The parotid gland, and the parotid duct crossing Masseter a finger's breadth below the zygomatic arch and turning medially to pierce Buccinator (fig. 574).

2. The branches of the facial nerve, radiating from under cover of the margin of the parotid gland like digits from an out-stretched hand, anastomosing with each other and with the branches of the trigeminal nerve, and entering the muscles on their deep surfaces except where the muscles are two layers thick, when the deeper layer is entered on its superficial surface, e.g., Buccinator, Levator Anguli Oris. The nerve is divided somewhat arbitrarily into T = temporal, Z = zygomatic, B = Buccal, M = Mandibular, and C = cervical branches.

3. The cervical branch, running less than a finger's breadth below the angle of the jaw and, after supplying branches to Platysma, crossing the base of the jaw at the anterior border of Masseter, crossing superficial to the facial vein and facial artery, anastomosing with the mandibular branch, and supplying the muscles of the lower lip and chin.

4. The buccal branch, which is motor to Buccinator, anastomosing with the buccal nerve (a branch of the trigeminal nerve) which is sensory.

5. The great auricular nerve (C. 2, 3), here lying ½" behind the external jugular vein, but commonly in contact with it (fig. 472), and dividing into facial, auricular, and mastoid branches.

6. The posterior auricular nerve (a branch of the facial nerve), which is motor to Auricularis Posterior and Occipitalis, joined by a twig from the great auricular nerve.

7. The retro-auricular (posterior auricular) and superficial parotid lymph nodes.

8. The auriculo-temporal nerve, ascending with the superficial temporal vessels. Their relationships vary (fig. 466); when the nerve is deep, a layer of fascia commonly separates it from the vessels.

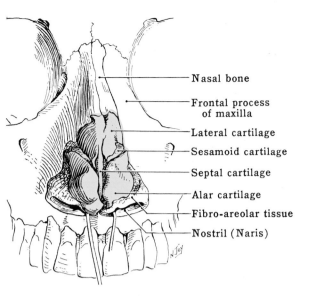

- Nasal bone
- Frontal process of maxilla
- Lateral cartilage
- Sesamoid cartilage
- Septal cartilage
- Alar cartilage
- Fibro-areolar tissue
- Nostril (Naris)

r cartilages pulled down in order to expose the moid cartilages.

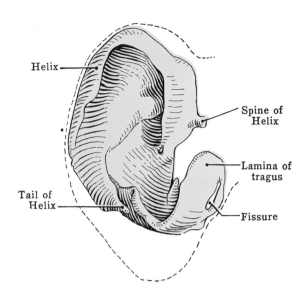

- Helix
- Spine of Helix
- Tail of Helix
- Lamina of tragus
- Fissure

Cartilage of Right Auricle.

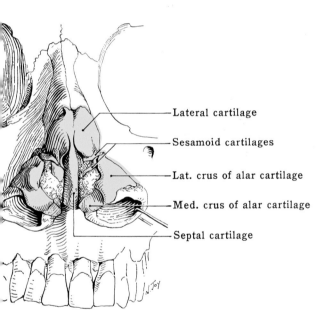

- Lateral cartilage
- Sesamoid cartilages
- Lat. crus of alar cartilage
- Med. crus of alar cartilage
- Septal cartilage

r cartilages separated by dissection and retracted to t and left.

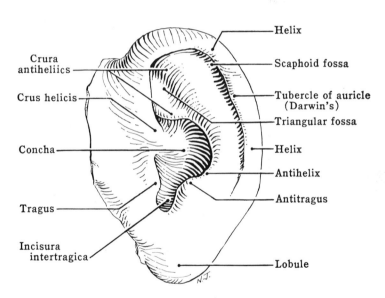

- Crura antiheliics
- Crus helicis
- Concha
- Tragus
- Incisura intertragica
- Helix
- Scaphoid fossa
- Tubercle of auricle (Darwin's)
- Triangular fossa
- Helix
- Antihelix
- Antitragus
- Lobule

Auricle of Opposite Side.

468 Cartilages of the Nose

Observe:

1. The lateral nasal cartilages, fixed by suture to the nasal bones and continuous with the septal cartilage.
2. The alar nasal cartilages, free, movable, and U-shaped.
3. The medial crus of the right and of the left U, when in apposition, forming part of the septum of the nose.
4. The lower part of the ala of the nose, formed of fibro-areolar tissue, cf. the lobule of the auricle.

Note: The nasal cartilages are hyaline cartilage; the cartilage of the auricle is elastic cartilage.

469 The Auricle

Note:

The cartilage of the auricle is yellow or elastic cartilage. It is continuous with the cartilage of the external acoustic meatus. It does not extend into the lobule, the basis of which is fibro-areolar tissue.

There being very little subcutaneous tissue on the lateral surface of the auricle, the skin adheres to the cartilage and follows its irregularities. On the cranial surface, there being fine muscles and more subcutaneous tissue, the skin is movable.

The foramen at the root of the crus of the cartilage of the helix transmits an artery (fig. 551); the fissure in the cartilage of the external meatus is an unchondrified area, closed with fibrous tissue (fig. 577). (For arteries & nerves, see fig. 551.)

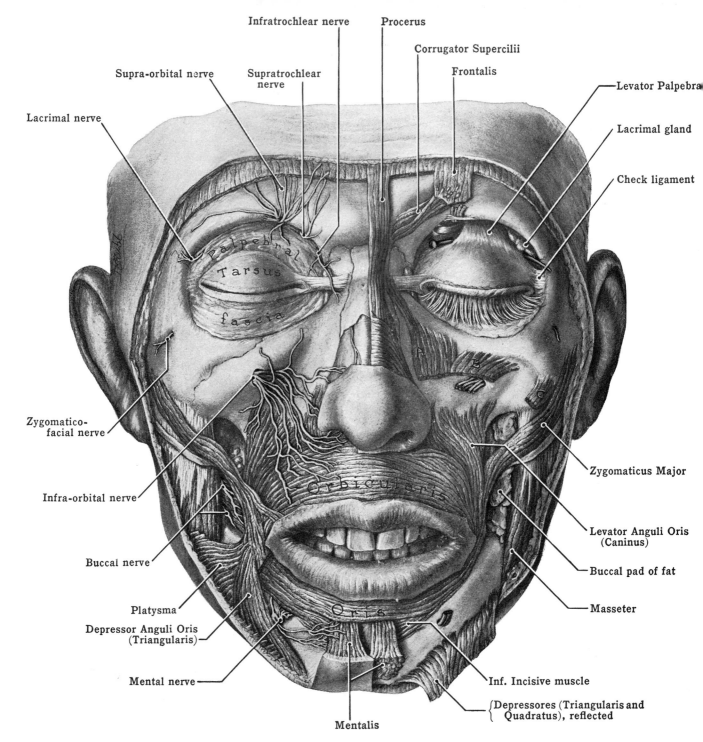

Infratrochlear nerve

Procerus

Corrugator Supercilii

Frontalis

Supra-orbital nerve

Supratrochlear nerve

Lacrimal nerve

Levator Palpebra

Lacrimal gland

Check ligament

Palpebral

Tarsus

fascia

Zygomatico-facial nerve

Zygomaticus Major

Infra-orbital nerve

Orbicularis

Levator Anguli Oris (Caninus)

Buccal nerve

Buccal pad of fat

Platysma

Masseter

Depressor Anguli Oris (Triangularis)

Oris

Inf. Incisive muscle

Mental nerve

Depressores (Triangularis and Quadratus), reflected

Mentalis

470 Cutaneous Branches of Trigeminal Nerve; Muscles; Eyelid

Observe:

1. The 5 cutaneous branches of the ophthalmic nerve (V¹). Of these, the external nasal branch is shown but not labelled; and a sixth set of branches, for the supply of the cornea, is not shown, viz., the ciliary branches of the naso-ciliary nerve (fig. 520).

2. The 3 cutaneous branches of the maxillary nerve (V²):—(a) The infra-orbital branch, appearing through the infra-orbital foramen, 1 cm. below the orbital margin, between Levator Labii Superioris and Levator Anguli Oris; its branches radiating to the lower eyelid, dorsum of the nose, the vestibule of nose and upper lip. (b) The zygomatico-facial; and (c) the zygomatico-temporal (fig. 551).

3. The 3 cutaneous branches of the mandibular nerve (V³):— (a) The mental branch, appearing through the mental foramen, deep to Depressor Anguli Oris, and spreading out in the lower lip and chin. (b) The buccal branch, appearing at the anterior border of Masseter, below the level of the parotid duct, applied to Buccinator, and piercing it to supply the mucous membrane of the cheek; and (c) the auriculo-temporal branch (fig. 466).

4. A = Levator Labii Superioris Alaeque Nasi; B = Levator Labii Superioris B = Levator Labii Superioris; C = Zygomaticus Minor.

5. The buccal pad of fat, filling the space between Buccinator medially and the ramus of the jaw and Masseter laterally.

Continued on page facing

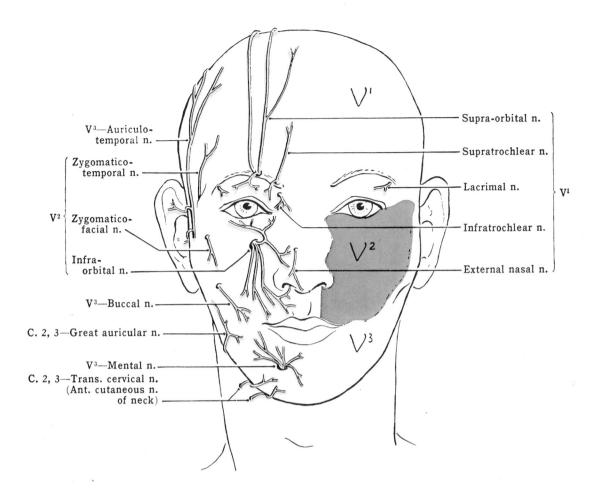

V³—Auriculo-
temporal n.

Zygomatico-
temporal n.

V² Zygomatico-
facial n.

Infra-
orbital n.

V³—Buccal n.

C. 2, 3—Great auricular n.

V³—Mental n.
C. 2, 3—Trans. cervical n.
(Ant. cutaneous n.
of neck)

Supra-orbital n.

Supratrochlear n.

Lacrimal n.

Infratrochlear n.

External nasal n.

V^1

V^1

V^2

V^3

470.1   Diagram of Sensory Nerves of Face, front view

The 3 divisions of the trigeminal nerve (N.V.) correspond in their distribution, nearly but not absolutely, to the 3 embryological regions of the face. Thus, the ophthalmic nerve (V^1) supplies the fronto-nasal process; the maxillary nerve (V^2), the maxillary process (colored pink); and the mandibular nerve (V^3), the mandibular process. And, they supply the whole thickness of the processes—from skin to mucous surface—indeed, to the median plane (i.e., falx cerebri, nasal septum, & septum of tongue).

Cutaneous branches (supra-orbital and auriculo-temporal) have spread backwards in the scalp beyond a line that joins the auricles across the vertex, and there they meet the greater and lesser occipital nerves (fig. 500). The great auricular nerve has spread into the parotid region. The buccal nerve supplies the skin and mucous membrane of the cheek, reaching to the angle of the mouth.

470   Cutaneous Branches of the Trigeminal Nerve: Dissection of the Eyelid

Continued from page facing

6. Levator Anguli Oris, continuous medially with the nasal muscles (Depressor Alae Nasi and Depressor Septi Nasi—not in view).

7. The orbital septum (palpebral fascia), attached to the orbital margin and, medially, passing behind the lacrimal sac to the crest of the lacrimal bone (post. lacrimal crest).

8. The medial palpebral ligament, crossing in front of the lacrimal sac, and attaching the elliptical upper and the rod-like lower tarsus to the frontal process of the maxilla.

9. The fan-shaped aponeurosis of Levator Palpebrae Superioris, attached to the front of the superior tarsus. Its medial edge, which is attached behind the lacrimal sac, and its lateral edge, which is attached to a tubercle within the orbital margin, are said to check the over-action of Levator Palpebrae.

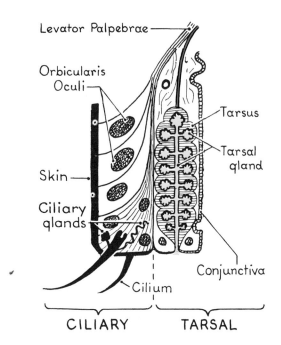

Levator Palpebrae

Orbicularis
Oculi

Skin

Ciliary
glands

Cilium

Tarsus

Tarsal
gland

Conjunctiva

CILIARY — TARSAL

471 Diagram of the Superior Palpebra or Eyelid, on sagittal section

(*After Whitnall.*)

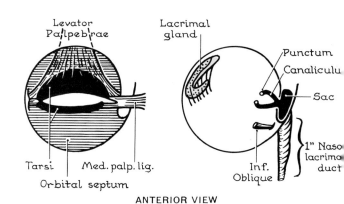

Levator
Palpebrae

Lacrimal
gland

Punctum

Caniculu

Sac

Tarsi   Med. palp. lig.

Orbital septum

Inf.
Oblique

1" Naso
lacrima
duct

ANTERIOR VIEW

Zygomatic bone   Pars lacrimalis

EYE
BALL

Tarsus
&
Palpebral liqs.

Tear sac

HORIZONTAL SECTION

471.1 Diagram of the Lacrimal Apparatus

Note:

lacrimal gland and its ductules; conjunctival sac; lacrimal puncta, canaliculi and sac, and nasolacrimal duct. Also Pars lacrimalis of the Orbicularis Oculi. (*After Whitnall.*)

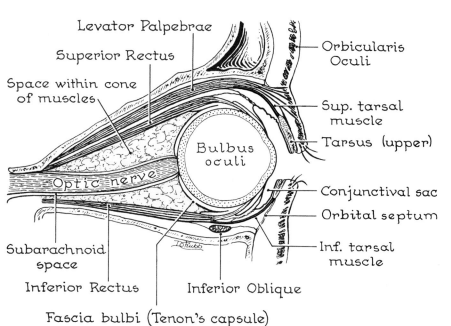

Levator Palpebrae

Superior Rectus

Space within cone
of muscles

Optic nerve

Bulbus
oculi

Orbicularis
Oculi

Sup. tarsal
muscle

Tarsus (upper)

Conjunctival sac

Orbital septum

Inf. tarsal
muscle

Subarachnoid
space

Inferior Rectus   Inferior Oblique

Fascia bulbi (Tenon's capsule)

471.2 Diagram of th Orbital Contents, on sagittal section

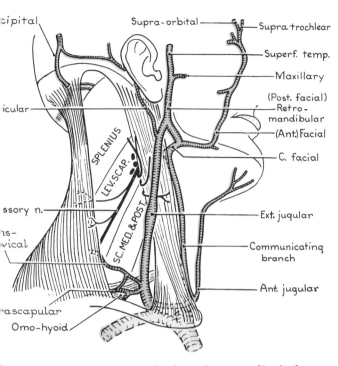

1.3 Diagram of the Superficial Veins of the Head and Neck

Labels on figure 1.3: cipital, Supra-orbital, Supra-trochlear, Superf. temp., Maxillary, (Post. facial) Retro-mandibular, (Ant.) Facial, C. facial, icular, Ext. jugular, ssory n., Communicating branch, ns-vical, Ant. jugular, rascapular, Omo-hyoid, SPLENIUS, LEV. SCAP., SC. MED. & POST.

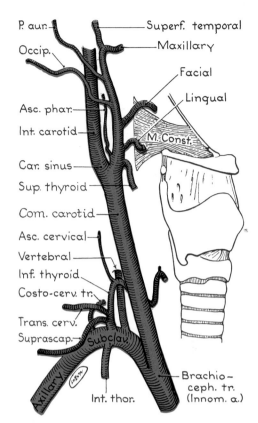

471.4 Diagram of the Subclavian and Carotid Arteries and their Branches

Labels on figure 471.4: P. aur., Occip., Superf. temporal, Maxillary, Facial, Lingual, Asc. phar., Int. carotid, M. Const., Car. sinus, Sup. thyroid, Com. carotid, Asc. cervical, Vertebral, Inf. thyroid, Costo-cerv. tr., Trans. cerv., Suprascap., Subclav., Axillary, Int. thor., Brachio-ceph. tr. (Innom. a.)

1.5 Branches of the Third Part the Subclavian Artery

lmost as a rule some branch springs from the 3rd part of
artery, or else from its short 2nd part, and passes laterally
ough the brachial plexus, usually behind nerve segments
6 or 5, 6 & 7 (figs. 531, 536 both sides, & 537).

is:

a) "The dorsal scapular art." (art. to Rhomboids, or de-
ding branch of trans. cervical art.) so behaves in about
% of cases;

b) the transverse cervical art. in about 20% of cases, when
hay be said to spring from the dorsal scapular art. rather
n vice versa; and

c) the suprascapular art. in about 10% of cases. (For details,
D. F. Hulke; and D. MacIntosh and G. G. Smith.)

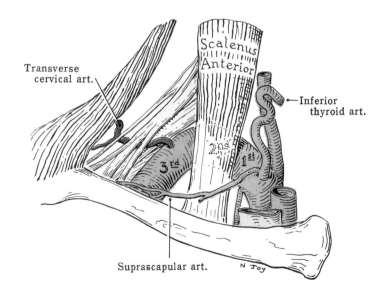

Labels on figure: Transverse cervical art., Scalenus Anterior, Inferior thyroid art., 1st, 2nd, 3rd, Suprascapular art., N JOY

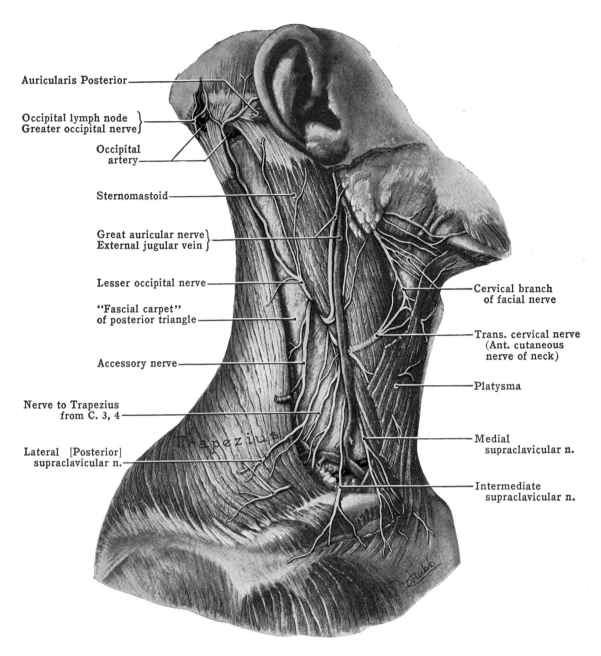

Auricularis Posterior

Occipital lymph node
Greater occipital nerve

Occipital
artery

Sternomastoid

Great auricular nerve
External jugular vein

Lesser occipital nerve

"Fascial carpet"
of posterior triangle

Accessory nerve

Nerve to Trapezius
from C. 3, 4

Lateral [Posterior]
supraclavicular n.

Trapezius

Cervical branch
of facial nerve

Trans. cervical nerve
(Ant. cutaneous
nerve of neck)

Platysma

Medial
supraclavicular n.

Intermediate
supraclavicular n.

472 Posterior Triangle of the Neck: Superficial Structures—I

Observe:

1. The 3 sides of the triangle—Trapezius, Sternomastoid, middle third of the clavicle—the apex being where the aponeuroses of the two muscles blend a little below the superior nuchal line.

2. Platysma (partly cut away), covering the lower part of the triangle. (For entire Platysma, fig. 526.)

3. The external jugular vein, descending vertically from behind the angle of the jaw, across Sternomastoid to its posterior border where, an inch above the clavicle, it pierces the investing deep fascia.

4. The "fascial carpet" that covers the muscular floor.

5. The accessory nerve—the only motor nerve superficial to the "fascial carpet"—descending within the deep fascia, and disappearing 2 fingers' breadth or more above the clavicle.

6. The cutaneous nerves (C. 2, 3, 4), radiating from the posterior border of Sternomastoid, below the accessory nerve.

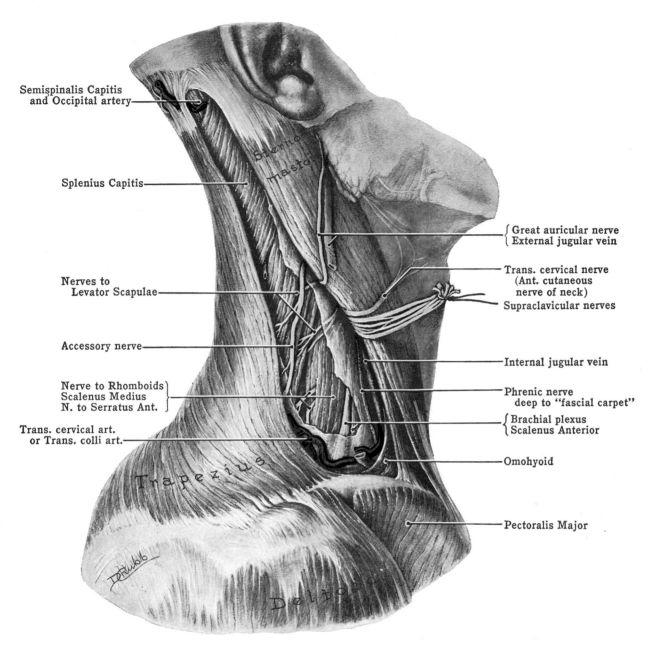

Semispinalis Capitis and Occipital artery

Splenius Capitis

Nerves to Levator Scapulae

Accessory nerve

Nerve to Rhomboids
Scalenus Medius
N. to Serratus Ant.

Trans. cervical art. or Trans. colli art.

Sterno Mastoid

Trapezius

Deltoid

Great auricular nerve
External jugular vein

Trans. cervical nerve (Ant. cutaneous nerve of neck)
Supraclavicular nerves

Internal jugular vein

Phrenic nerve deep to "fascial carpet"

Brachial plexus
Scalenus Anterior

Omohyoid

Pectoralis Major

473 Posterior Triangle of the Neck: Motor Nerves deep to Fascial Carpet—II

Observe:

1. The muscles forming the floor of the upper part of the triangle (Semispinalis Capitis, Splenius, Levator Scapulae); those forming the lower part are shown in figure 475.

2. The accessory nerve (i.e., nerve to Sternomastoid and Trapezius), (fig. 661) lying along Levator Scapulae but separated by the "fascial carpet".

3. Three motor nerves to upper limb muscles, lying (a) in the plane between the facial carpet and the muscular floor, and (b) between the accessory nerve above and the brachial plexus below. They are:—nerves to Levator Scapulae (C. 3, 4), to Rhomboids (C. 5), and to Serratus Anterior (C. 5, 6—the branch from C. 7 lies protected behind the plexus, fig. 23).

4. Two structures of surgical importance, situated just beyond the geometrical confines of the triangle: (a) a fourth motor nerve, viz the phrenic nerve to the Diaphragm (C. 3, 4, 5), placed between carpet and floor; (b) the internal jugular vein, superficial to the carpet.

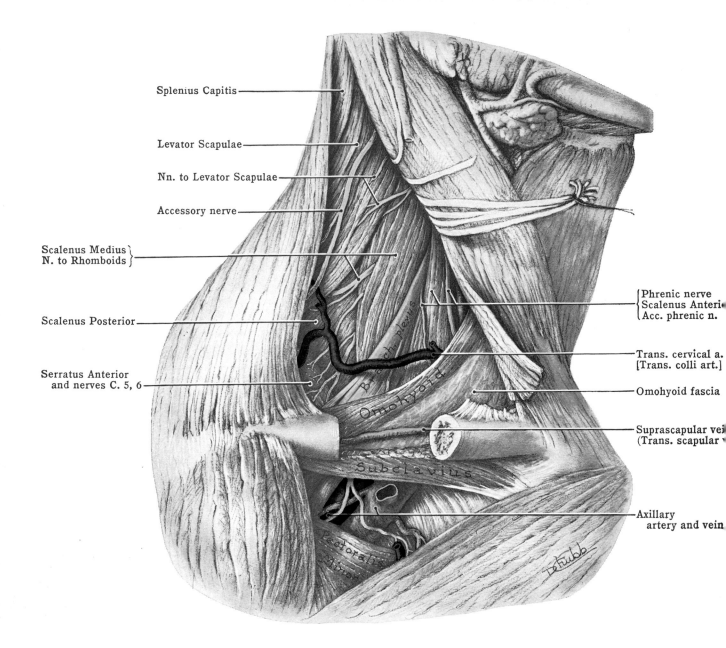

Splenius Capitis

Levator Scapulae

Nn. to Levator Scapulae

Accessory nerve

Scalenus Medius
N. to Rhomboids

Scalenus Posterior

Serratus Anterior
and nerves C. 5, 6

Phrenic nerve
Scalenus Anteri‹
Acc. phrenic n.

Trans. cervical a.
[Trans. colli art.]

Omohyoid fascia

Suprascapular vei‹
(Trans. scapular ‹

Axillary
artery and vein

Brachial plexus

Omohyoid

Subclavius

Pectoralis Minor

474 Posterior Triangle of the Neck: Omohyoid and its Fascia—III

The clavicular head of Pectoralis Major and part of the clavicle have been excised.

Observe:

1. The posterior belly of Omohyoid, held down by a sheet of "Omo-hyoid" fascia to the fascia ensheathing Subclavius; and the resulting pocket between this fascia posteriorly and the investing deep fascia and Sternomastoid anteriorly (fig. 542).
2. The brachial plexus, appearing between Scalenus Anterior and Scalenus Medius and here, as commonly, giving off an accessory phrenic nerve (see next figure) from C. 5.
3. The posterior border of Scalenus Anterior, nearly parallel to the posterior border of Sterno-mastoid, and slightly behind it; hence one is a guide to the other.

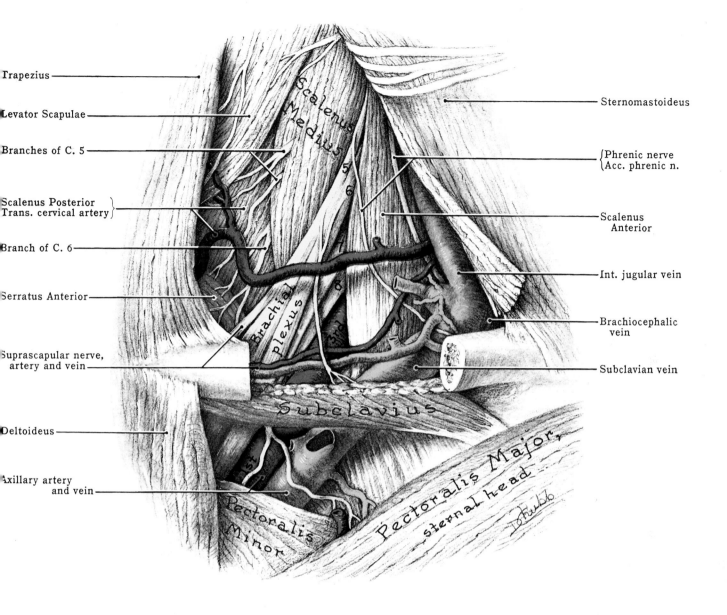

Trapezius

Levator Scapulae

Branches of C. 5

Scalenus Posterior
Trans. cervical artery

Branch of C. 6

Serratus Anterior

Suprascapular nerve,
artery and vein

Deltoideus

Axillary artery
and vein

Scalenus Medius

5

6

Brachial plexus

3rd part of

Subclavius

1st

Pectoralis Minor

Pectoralis Major, sternal head

Sternomastoideus

{Phrenic nerve
{Acc. phrenic n.

Scalenus Anterior

Int. jugular vein

Brachiocephalic vein

Subclavian vein

475 Posterior Triangle of the Neck: Brachial Plexus and Subclavian Vessels—IV

The 3rd part of the subclavian artery and the 1st part of the axillary artery are labelled.

Observe:

1. The muscles forming the floor of the lower part of the triangle (Scaleni Posterior, Medius et Anterior and Serratus Anterior).

2. The brachial plexus and subclavian artery, appearing between Scalenus Medius and Scalenus Anterior; the lowest root of the plexus (T. 1), concealed by the 3rd part of the artery.

3. The suprascapular nerve, found by following the lateral border of the plexus caudally.

4. The subclavian vein, hardly rising above the level of the clavicle, and separated from the 2nd part of the subclavian artery by Scalenus Anterior.

5. Subclavius, unimportant as a muscle, but valuable as a buffer between a fractured clavicle and the subclavian vessels.

Note how, by voluntarily forcing the upper limb backwards and downwards, the clavicle and Subclavius compress the subclavian vessels against the first rib and so arrest the pulse.

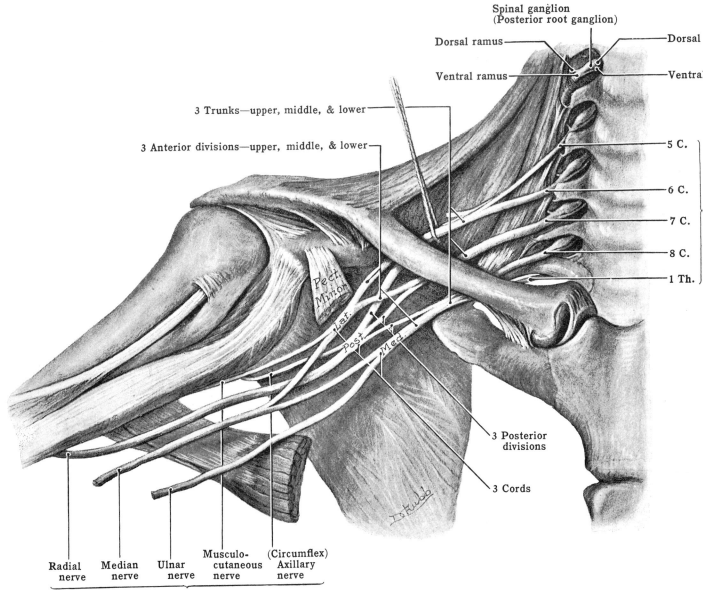

Spinal ganglion
(Posterior root ganglion)

Dorsal ramus —

Ventral ramus —

— Dorsal

— Ventral

3 Trunks—upper, middle, & lower —

3 Anterior divisions—upper, middle, & lower —

— 5 C.

— 6 C.

— 7 C.

— 8 C.

— 1 Th.

Pect.
Minor

Lat.

Post.

Med.

3 Posterior
divisions

3 Cords

Radial
nerve

Median
nerve

Ulnar
nerve

Musculo-
cutaneous
nerve

(Circumflex)
Axillary
nerve

5 Terminal Branches

476 Brachial Plexus

Observe:

1. A dorsal (sensory) root of a spinal nerve larger than a ventral (motor) root.

2. The 2 roots uniting beyond the ganglion to form a very short mixed spinal nerve.

3. The mixed nerve at once dividing into a small dorsal ramus and a large ventral ramus.

4. The 5 ventral rami forming the brachial plexus (of these the middle ramus, C.7, is the largest, and C.5 and Th.I the smallest).

5. The 5 rami uniting to form the 3 trunks of the plexus.

6. Each trunk dividing into 2 divisions, an anterior and a posterior.

7. From the divisions 3 cords resulting.

8. The 3 cords lying behind Pectoralis Minor.

9. The posterior cord and the radial nerve derived from segments C. 5, 6, 7 and 8, and slightly from Th.I.

10. The median nerve derived from segments C. 6, 7, 8 and Th.I, and slightly from C. 5.

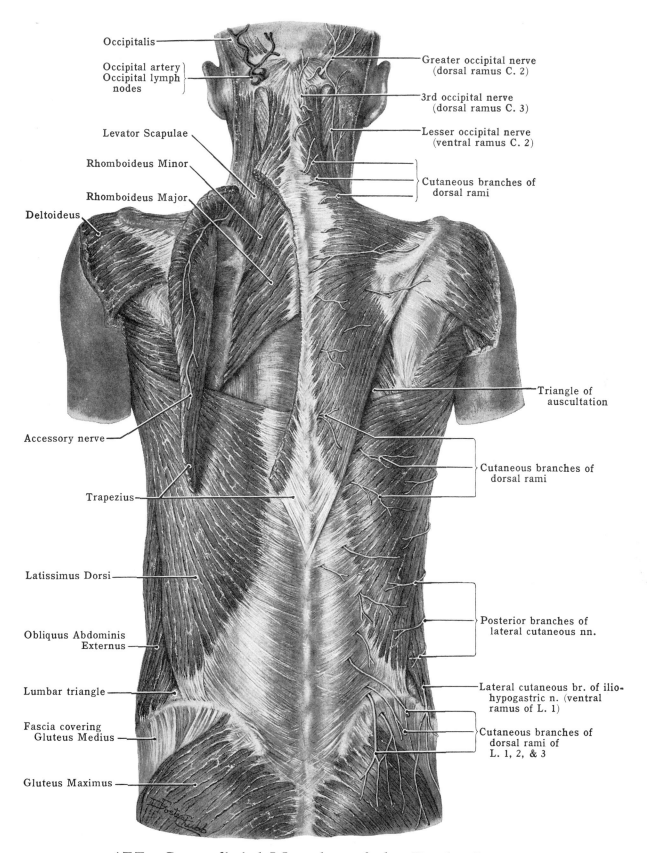

Occipitalis

Occipital artery
Occipital lymph
nodes

Levator Scapulae

Rhomboideus Minor

Rhomboideus Major

Deltoideus

Accessory nerve

Trapezius

Latissimus Dorsi

Obliquus Abdominis
Externus

Lumbar triangle

Fascia covering
Gluteus Medius

Gluteus Maximus

Greater occipital nerve
(dorsal ramus C. 2)

3rd occipital nerve
(dorsal ramus C. 3)

Lesser occipital nerve
(ventral ramus C. 2)

Cutaneous branches of
dorsal rami

Triangle of
auscultation

Cutaneous branches of
dorsal rami

Posterior branches of
lateral cutaneous nn.

Lateral cutaneous br. of ilio-
hypogastric n. (ventral
ramus of L. 1)

Cutaneous branches of
dorsal rami of
L. 1, 2, & 3

477 Superficial Muscles of the Back—I

On the left side, Trapezius is reflected.

Note: 1st layer—Trapezius and Latissimus Dorsi.
2nd layer—Levator Scapulae and Rhomboidei Minor et Major.

These muscles help to attach the upper limb to the trunk.

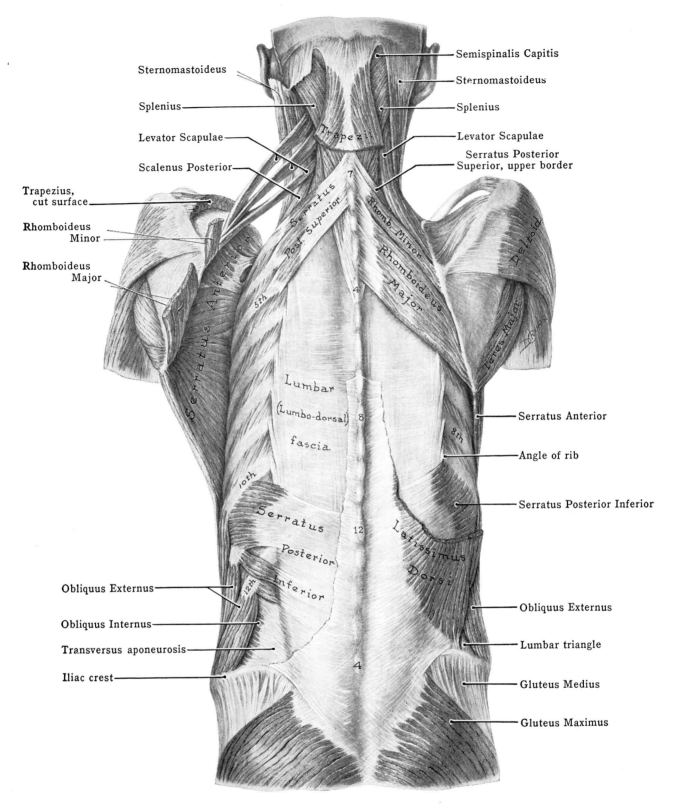

Sternomastoideus

Splenius

Levator Scapulae

Scalenus Posterior

Trapezius, cut surface

Rhomboideus Minor

Rhomboideus Major

Obliquus Externus

Obliquus Internus

Transversus aponeurosis

Iliac crest

Semispinalis Capitis

Sternomastoideus

Splenius

Levator Scapulae

Serratus Posterior Superior, upper border

Serratus Anterior

Angle of rib

Serratus Posterior Inferior

Obliquus Externus

Lumbar triangle

Gluteus Medius

Gluteus Maximus

Trapezii

Serratus Post. Superior

Rhomb. Minor

Rhomboideus Major

Serratus Anterior

Deltoid

Teres Major

Lumbar (Lumbo-dorsal) fascia

Serratus Posterior Inferior

Latissimus Dorsi

5th

7

4

8

8th

10th

12

12th

4

478 Intermediate Muscles of the Back—II

Trapezius and Latissimus Dorsi are largely cut away on both sides.

Observe:

1. On the right side—Levator Scapulae and Rhomboidei, in situ. Serratus Superior, rising above Rhomboideus Minor. It is apt to be divided when Rhomboidei are severed.

2. On the left side—Rhomboidei, severed and allowing the vertebral border of the scapula to part from the thoracic wall. The 3 (usually 4) digitations of Levator Scapulae.

3. Serrati Posteriores Superior et Inferior—the 3rd or intermediate layer of muscles—bridging the deep muscles, passing from spines to ribs, and sloping in opposite directions. These are muscles of inspiration.

4. The thoraco-lumbar (lumbo-dorsal) fascia, extending laterally to the angles of the ribs, becoming thin superiorly, passing deep to Serratus Superior, and reinforced inferiorly by Latissimus Dorsi and Serratus Inferior.

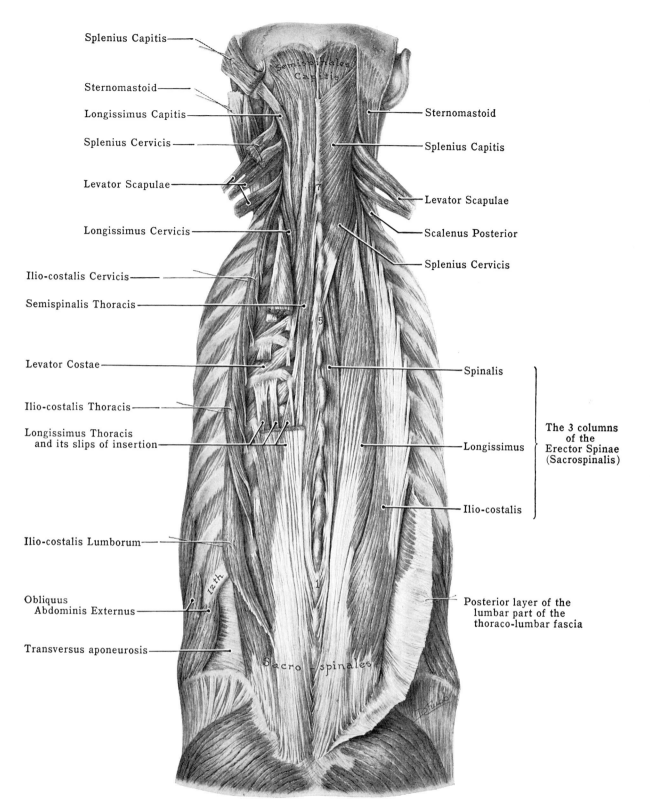

Splenius Capitis

Sternomastoid

Longissimus Capitis

Splenius Cervicis

Levator Scapulae

Longissimus Cervicis

Ilio-costalis Cervicis

Semispinalis Thoracis

Levator Costae

Ilio-costalis Thoracis

Longissimus Thoracis
and its slips of insertion

Ilio-costalis Lumborum

Obliquus
Abdominis Externus

Transversus aponeurosis

Semispinales
Capitis

Sternomastoid

Splenius Capitis

Levator Scapulae

Scalenus Posterior

Splenius Cervicis

Spinalis

Longissimus

Ilio-costalis

The 3 columns
of the
Erector Spinae
(Sacrospinalis)

Posterior layer of the
lumbar part of the
thoraco-lumbar fascia

Sacro-spinales

479 Deep Muscles of the Back—III

Observe:

1. Splenius Capitis et Cervicis—the 4th layer of muscles—in situ on the right side; reflected on the left side and attached (Splenius Capitis) to the mastoid process deep to Sternomastoid and (Splenius Cervicis) to 1st, 2nd (and 3rd) transverse processes deep to Levator Scapulae.

2. Erector Spinae—the 5th layer of muscles—in situ on the right side, lying between the spines medially and the angles of the ribs laterally, and splitting into 3 columns—lateral, middle, and medial. On the left side, the lateral column is everted, a section is taken from the middle column, the medial column is in situ. Only the middle or Longissimus column extends to the skull, and is there inserted into the mastoid process deep to Splenius Capitis.

3. Semispinalis (thoracis, cervicis et capitis) in situ and belonging to the 6th, or transverso-spinalis, group of muscles.

4. For suboccipital muscles see figs. 490 & 491.

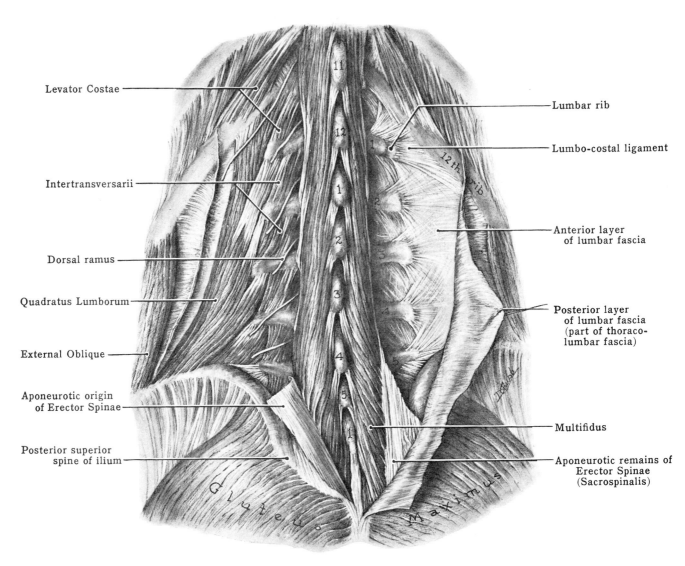

Levator Costae

Intertransversarii

Dorsal ramus

Quadratus Lumborum

External Oblique

Aponeurotic origin
of Erector Spinae

Posterior superior
spine of ilium

Lumbar rib

Lumbo-costal ligament

Anterior layer
of lumbar fascia

Posterior layer
of lumbar fascia
(part of thoraco-
lumbar fascia)

Multifidus

Aponeurotic remains of
Erector Spinae
(Sacrospinalis)

480 Multifidus: Quadratus Lumborum:
Lumbar Fascia—IV

Semispinalis, Multifidus, and Rotatores constitute the transverso-spinalis group
deep muscles. In general, their bundles pass obliquely upwards and medially, fro
transverse processes to spines, in successively deeper layers.

The bundles of Semispinalis span about 5 interspaces, those of Multifidus about
and those of Rotatores, 1 or 2.

(a) Semispinalis extends from the lower thoracic region to the skull (figs. 47
490).

(b) Multifidus extends from the sacrum to the spine of the axis (fig. 493).

(c) Rotatores are well developed only in the thoracic region (fig. 411).

Observe:

1. Multifidus in the lumbo-sacral region, arising from the aponeurosis of Erector Spinae, fro
   dorsum sacri (not seen), and from mammillary processes (fig. 371), and inserted into spino
   processes several segments higher up.

2. On the right side, after removal of Erector Spinae—the anterior layer of lumbar fasc
   [thoraco-lumbar] attached in fan-shaped manner to the tips of transverse processes. Als
   a short lumbar rib.

3. On the left side, after removal of the anterior layer of lumbar fascia—the lateral border
   Quadratus Lumborum to be oblique, and the medial border to be in continuity wi
   Intertransversarii.

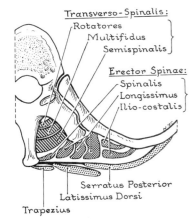

Transverso-Spinalis:
Rotatores
Multifidus
Semispinalis
Erector Spinae:
Spinalis
Longissimus
Ilio-costalis

Serratus Posterior
Latissimus Dorsi
Trapezius

480.1

Diagram of the muscles of back,
thoracic region, on cross section, to
show Erector Spinae (in 3 columns)
and Transverso-spinalis (in 3 layers).

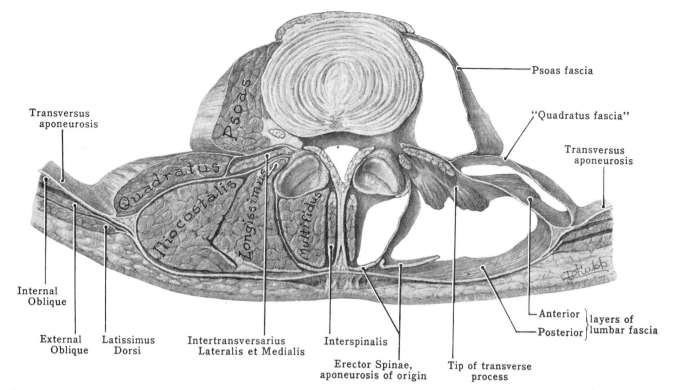

Transversus aponeurosis

Internal Oblique

External Oblique

Latissimus Dorsi

Intertransversarius Lateralis et Medialis

Interspinalis

Erector Spinae, aponeurosis of origin

Tip of transverse process

Anterior } layers of
Posterior } lumbar fascia

Transversus aponeurosis

"Quadratus fascia"

Psoas fascia

481 Muscles of the Back, on cross section—V

On the left side, the muscles are seen within their sheaths or compartments. On the right side, the empty sheaths are seen.

Observe:

1. The posterior aponeurosis of Transversus Abdominis, splitting into two strong sheets—the anterior and the posterior layer of the lumbar fascia (being part of the thoracolumbar fascia) which enclose the deep muscles of the back.

2. The posterior layer, reinforced by Latissimus Dorsi and at a higher level (fig. 478) by Serratus Posterior Inferior.

3. The weak areolar layer covering Quadratus Lumborum and that covering Psoas.

4. Ends of Intertransversarius, Longissimus, and Quadratus Lumborum, attached to a transverse process.

482 Spinal Cord within Its Membranes, from behind

Observe:

1. The denticulate lig., running like a band along each side of the spinal cord and, by means of strong tooth-like processes, anchoring the cord to the dura between successive nerve roots. (For highest tooth, fig. 564.)

2. The ventral nerve roots, lying in front of the denticulate lig. and the dorsal nerve roots lying behind it.

3. The ventral and the dorsal root of each nerve, leaving the dura by a separate opening. The lowest right dorsal root in this specimen leaves by three openings.

4. The fila of the various dorsal roots, having a linear attachment to the cord.

5. One filum of the lowest left dorsal root, deserting its own root and joining the root above.

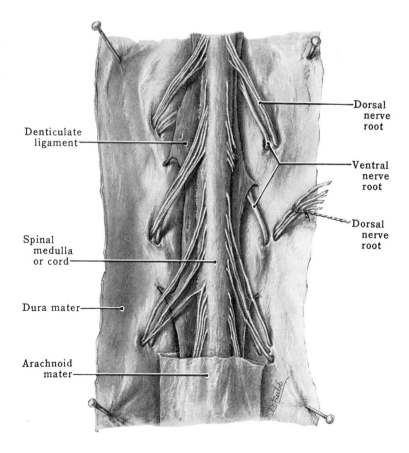

Denticulate ligament

Spinal medulla or cord

Dura mater

Arachnoid mater

Dorsal nerve root

Ventral nerve root

Dorsal nerve root

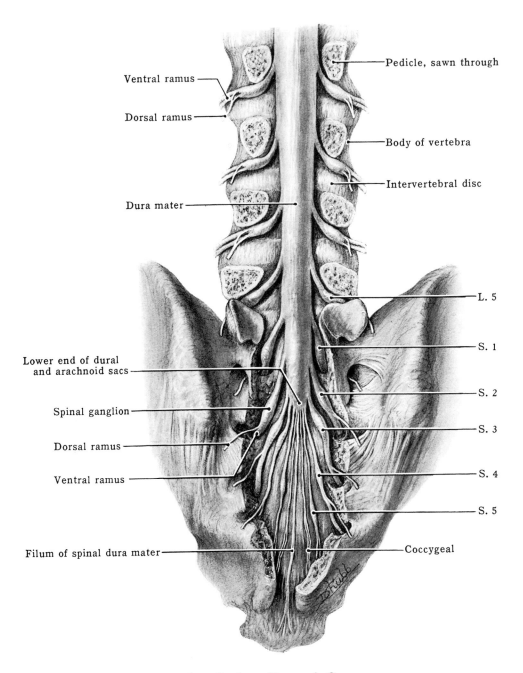

Ventral ramus

Dorsal ramus

Dura mater

Lower end of dural
and arachnoid sacs

Spinal ganglion

Dorsal ramus

Ventral ramus

Filum of spinal dura mater

Pedicle, sawn through

Body of vertebra

Intervertebral disc

L. 5

S. 1

S. 2

S. 3

S. 4

S. 5

Coccygeal

483 Lower End of the Dural Sac, from behind—I

The posterior parts of the lumbar and sacral vertebrae are sawn and nibbled away

Observe:

1. The lower limit of the dural (and the contained arachnoid) sac, at the level of the posterior superior iliac spine (= body of 2nd sacral vertebra), and the continuation of the dura as the filum of spinal dura mater.
2. The lumbar spinal ganglia in the intervertebral foramina; the sacral spinal ganglia, somewhat asymmetrical, within the sacral canal.
3. The dorsal nerve rami, smaller than ventral rami, and having both efferent and afferent components.
4. The superior articular processes of the sacrum, asymmetrical.

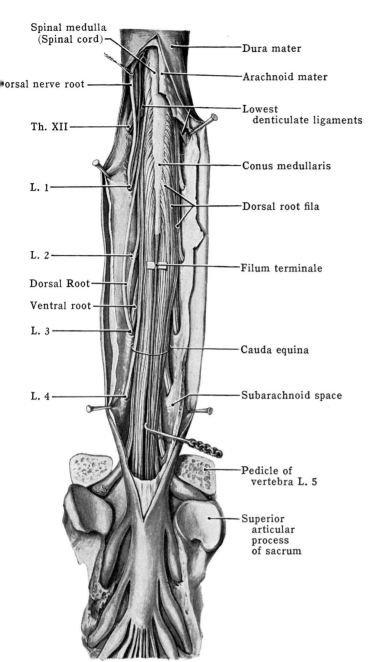

Spinal medulla (Spinal cord)

Dorsal nerve root

Th. XII

L. 1

L. 2

Dorsal Root

Ventral root

L. 3

L. 4

Dura mater

Arachnoid mater

Lowest denticulate ligaments

Conus medullaris

Dorsal root fila

Filum terminale

Cauda equina

Subarachnoid space

Pedicle of vertebra L. 5

Superior articular process of sacrum

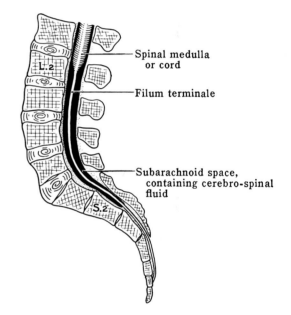

Spinal medulla or cord

Filum terminale

Subarachnoid space, containing cerebro-spinal fluid

484.1

Diagram of the Spinal Cord or Medulla, in situ

Note:

1. The spinal cord ends at the level of the disc between the 1st and 2nd lumbar vertebrae.

2. The subarachnoid space ends at the level of the disc between the 1st and 2nd sacral vertebrae—but it may be lower (figs. 203 & 236).

3. Variations: 95% of 801 cords ended within the limits of the bodies of vertebrae L.1 and L.2; whereas 3% ended behind the lower half of vertebra T.12, and 2% behind vertebra L.3. (Observations and collected data after Reimann, A. F. and Anson, B. J.; also Jit, I. and Charnalia, V. M.).

**84   Lower Ends of the Dural
nd Arachnoid Sacs, opened,
om behind—II**

serve:

The lowest tooth or dens of the denticulate ligament, variable in level and asymmetrical (MacDonald, I. B. et al.).

A radicular branch of a spinal vein accompanying the dorsal root of nerve L. 1.

There are only four or five radicular veins and arteries on each side of the cord to accompany the 31 pairs of spinal nerves. (Suh, T. H. and Alexander, L.)

The conus medullaris, or conical lower end of the spinal medulla, continued as a glistening thread, the filum terminale, which descends with the dorsal and ventral nerve roots. These constitute the cauda equina.

The hook retracting the elongated nerve roots, which surround a tubular space.

The subarachnoid space enclosed by arachnoid mater; the subdural space, which is the potential space between the dural and arachnoid maters.

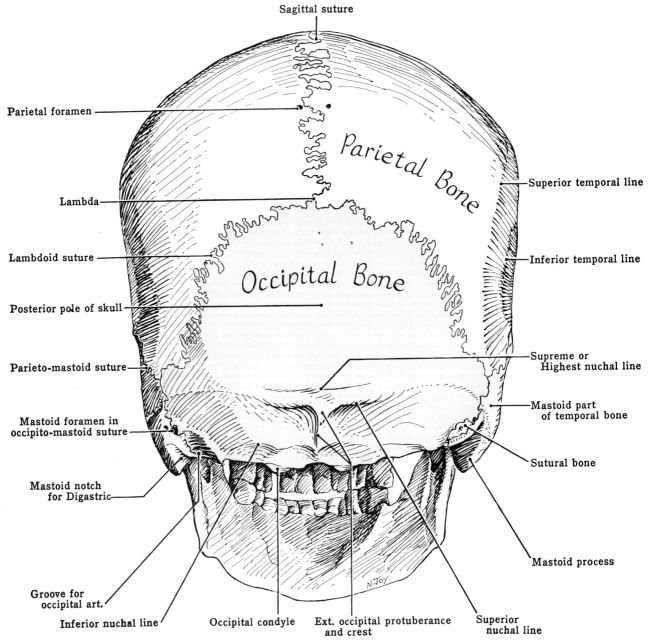

Sagittal suture

Parietal foramen

Parietal Bone

Superior temporal line

Lambda

Inferior temporal line

Lambdoid suture

Occipital Bone

Posterior pole of skull

Supreme or
Highest nuchal line

Parieto-mastoid suture

Mastoid part
of temporal bone

Mastoid foramen in
occipito-mastoid suture

Sutural bone

Mastoid notch
for Digastric

Mastoid process

Groove for
occipital art.

Inferior nuchal line

Occipital condyle

Ext. occipital protuberance
and crest

Superior
nuchal line

485 Skull from behind—Norma Occipitalis

The outline is horseshoe-shaped from the tip of one mastoid process, over the vertex to the tip of the other.
1. At the base of the skull, the outline is nearly straight (slightly convex) from one mastoid process to the other, except where the occipital condyles project downwards. On each side, it crosses two grooves (for the origin of the posterior belly of Digastric laterally, and for the occipital artery medially). Between the condyles is the foramen magnum.
2. The surface is convex. Near the centre is the lambda. From it a triradiate suture runs: the sagittal (interparietal) upwards in the median plane, and the lambdoid (parieto-occipital) infero-laterally to the blunt postero-inferior angles of the parietal bones where it bifurcates.
3. On each side are three inconstant foramina for emissary veins and meningeal arteries:—parietal and mastoid foramina, and condylar canal (fig. 569).
    Midway between lambda and foramen magnum is the ext. occipital protuberance or (inion.) From it the superior nuchal line curves laterally and crosses the lateral aspect

of the mastoid, dividing it into a smooth upper an rough lower part.
    The surface below the superior nuchal line is nuchal area for the muscles of the neck or nucha.

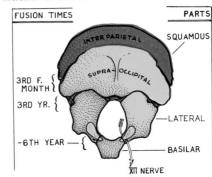

485.1 Occipital Bone at Birth

At birth the bone is in 4 parts. Blue areas develop cartilage; the red area develops in membrane. T squama has a double origin.

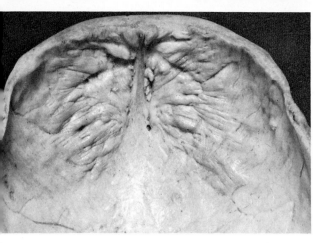

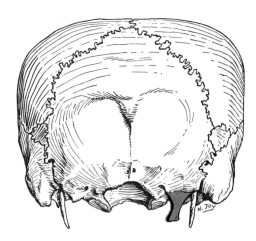

486 Hyperostosis Frontalis Interna

This symmetrical bony overgrowth of transverse ridges and furrows has been found, in institutions and the dissecting room, to occur in less than 0.5% of men and 6.0% of women, over middle age.

(*See Hawkins & Martin.*)

487 Paramastoid Process

Rarely, a process descends from the jugular process of the occipital bone towards, or to, the transverse process of the atlas.

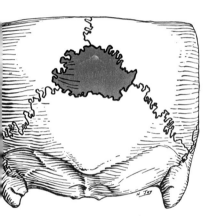

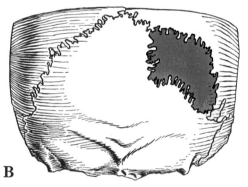

488 Interparietal Bone (Os Incae)

Occasionally, the several centres of ossification of the interparietal part of the occipital bone fail (A and B) in part or (C) in whole to coalesce with the supra-occipital part (fig. 486). The result is an independent interparietal bone.

Sutural bones (yellow) are commonly present, as in this specimen and in figure 487, notably at the inferior angles of the parietal bone.

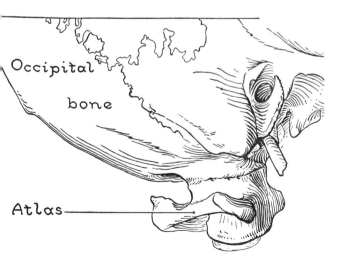

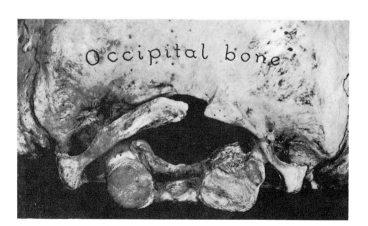

489   Two Varieties of Occipitalization of Atlas

VARIATIONS and ANOMALIES

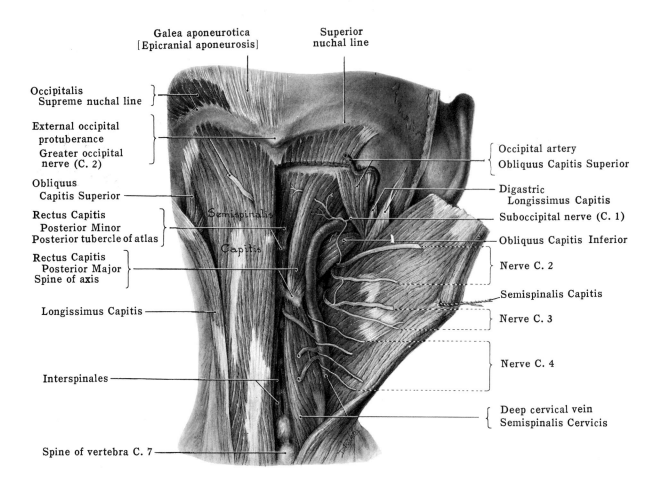

Galea aponeurotica
[Epicranial aponeurosis]

Superior
nuchal line

Occipitalis
Supreme nuchal line

External occipital
protuberance
Greater occipital
nerve (C. 2)

Obliquus
Capitis Superior

Rectus Capitis
Posterior Minor
Posterior tubercle of atlas

Rectus Capitis
Posterior Major
Spine of axis

Longissimus Capitis

Interspinales

Spine of vertebra C. 7

Semispinalis

Capitis

Occipital artery
Obliquus Capitis Superior

Digastric
Longissimus Capitis

Suboccipital nerve (C. 1)

Obliquus Capitis Inferior

Nerve C. 2

Semispinalis Capitis

Nerve C. 3

Nerve C. 4

Deep cervical vein
Semispinalis Cervicis

490 Suboccipital Region—I

Trapezius, Sternomastoid, and Splenius are removed.
   Observe:

1. Semispinalis Capitis, the great extensor of the head and neck, forming the posterior wall of the suboccipital region, pierced by the greater occipital nerve (C. 2, post. ramus), and having free medial and lateral borders at this high level. The right Semispinalis is divided and turned laterally.

2. The greater occipital nerve, when followed caudally, leading to the lower border of Obliquus Capitis Inferior around which it turns and to which it is the guide.

3. This border of Obliquus Inferior, followed medially, leading to spine of axis, and, followed laterally, to transverse process of atlas.

4. Five muscles (all paired) attached to spine of axis:— Obliquus Capitis Inferior, Rectus Capitis Posterior Major, Semispinalis Cervicis which largely conceals Multifidus, and Interspinalis.

5. Occipital veins emerging through suboccipital triangle to join the deep cervical vein and, with it, the suboccipital nerve (C. 1, post. ramus).

6. The suboccipital triangle, bounded by 3 muscles: Obliquus Inferior, Obliquus Superior, and Rectus Major.

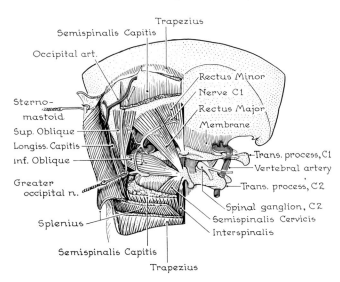

Trapezius

Semispinalis Capitis

Occipital art.

Sterno-
mastoid

Sup. Oblique

Longiss. Capitis

Inf. Oblique

Greater
occipital n.

Splenius

Semispinalis Capitis

Trapezius

Rectus Minor
Nerve C1
Rectus Major
Membrane

Trans. process, C1
Vertebral artery
Trans. process, C2
Spinal ganglion, C2
Semispinalis Cervicis
Interspinalis

490.1 Diagram of the Suboccipital Region

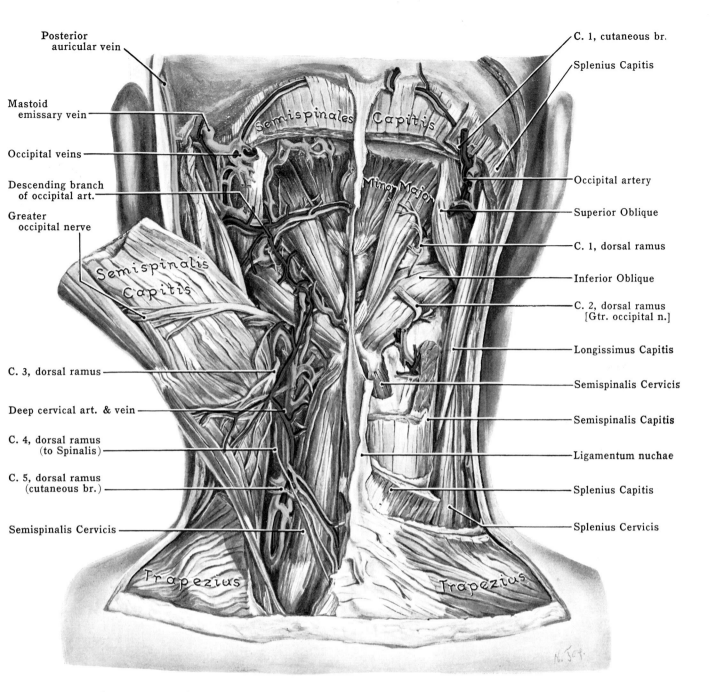

Posterior auricular vein

Mastoid emissary vein

Occipital veins

Descending branch of occipital art.

Greater occipital nerve

Semispinalis Capitis

C. 3, dorsal ramus

Deep cervical art. & vein

C. 4, dorsal ramus (to Spinalis)

C. 5, dorsal ramus (cutaneous br.)

Semispinalis Cervicis

Semispinales Capitis

Minor Major

Trapezius

C. 1, cutaneous br.

Splenius Capitis

Occipital artery

Superior Oblique

C. 1, dorsal ramus

Inferior Oblique

C. 2, dorsal ramus [Gtr. occipital n.]

Longissimus Capitis

Semispinalis Cervicis

Semispinalis Capitis

Ligamentum nuchae

Splenius Capitis

Splenius Cervicis

Trapezius

491   Suboccipital Region—II

Observe:

1. The ligamentum nuchae, which represents the cervical part of the supraspinous ligament, as a median, thin, fibrous partition attached to the spines of the cervical vertebrae and the external occipital crest. Its posterior border gives origin to Trapezius and extends upward to the inion or external occipital protuberance.

2. Rectus Capitis Posterior Minor (paired), the only muscle attached to the posterior tubercle of the atlas, which accordingly is upturned. (The atlas has no spine.)

3. The suboccipital nerve (C. 1, post. ramus) supplying the 3 muscles bounding the suboccipital triangle, also Rectus

Capitis Minor, and communicating with the greater occipital nerve.

4. The 1st cervical nerve, here delivering a cutaneous branch —which is unusual.

5. The descending branch of the occipital artery anastomosing with the deep cervical artery (a branch of the subclavian).

6. The posterior vertebral venous plexus. This plexus is largely imbedded in fascia, is usually empty and therefore inconspicuous, and hence is removed unnoticed with the fascia unless specially injected, as here, or engorged with blood.

7. Longissimus Capitis being the only section of Erector Spinae to reach the skull.

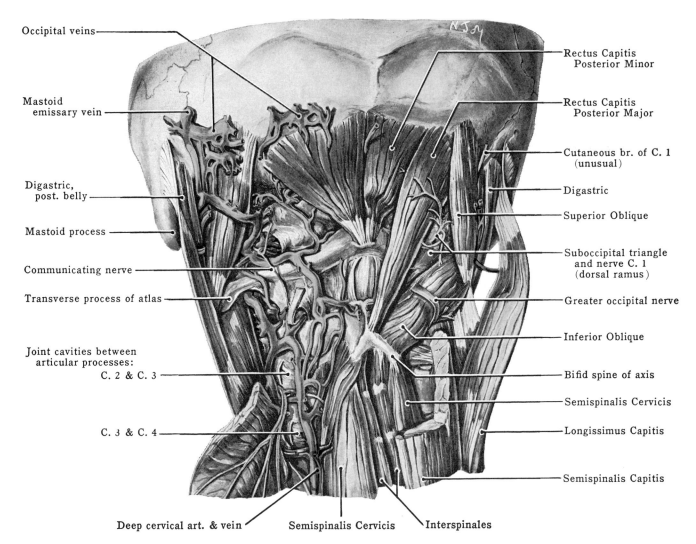

Occipital veins

Mastoid emissary vein

Digastric, post. belly

Mastoid process

Communicating nerve

Transverse process of atlas

Joint cavities between articular processes:
C. 2 & C. 3

C. 3 & C. 4

Deep cervical art. & vein   Semispinalis Cervicis   Interspinales

Rectus Capitis Posterior Minor

Rectus Capitis Posterior Major

Cutaneous br. of C. 1 (unusual)

Digastric

Superior Oblique

Suboccipital triangle and nerve C. 1 (dorsal ramus)

Greater occipital nerve

Inferior Oblique

Bifid spine of axis

Semispinalis Cervicis

Longissimus Capitis

Semispinalis Capitis

492 Suboccipital Region—III

On the left side, Rectus Capitis Posterior Major and Obliquus Capitis Inferior are removed.

Observe:

1. Rectus Capitis Posterior Major ascending from the spine of the axis to the occipital bone. Obliquus Capitis Superior ascending from the tip of the transverse process of the atlas to the occipital bone. Obliquus Capitis Inferior passing from spine of axis to tip of transverse process of atlas.

2. The foregoing 3 muscles, (viz. Inf. Oblique, Rectus Major, and Sup. Oblique), forming the sides of the suboccipital triangle, which lies within the suboccipital region, whose lower limit is the axis.

3. Rectus Capitis Posterior Minor arising from the posterior tubercle of the atlas and therefore lying on a deeper plane than the Posterior Major, which arises from a spine.

4. The posterior arch of the atlas forming the floor of the suboccipital triangle. The posterior atlanto-occipital membrane (not labelled) passing from that arch to the margin of the foramen magnum above, and the posterior atlanto-axial membrane passing to the lamina of the axis below. The vertebral artery lying on the arch; the suboccipital nerve (i.e., dorsal ramus of C. 1) appearing between arch and artery and supplying the two straight muscles (minor and major) and the two oblique muscles (superior and inferior).

5. The gaps in these membranes through which pass nerve C. 1, the vertebral artery, the veins accompanying this artery, and nerve C. 2.

6. A branch connecting the dorsal rami of nerves C. 1 and C. 2 behind the posterior arch of the atlas.

In figure 561 the ventral rami of these nerves are seen in communication.

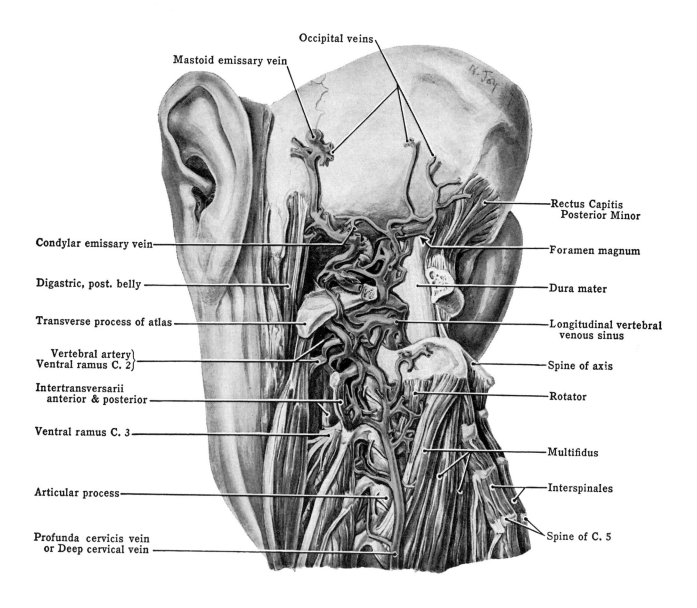

Occipital veins

Mastoid emissary vein

Condylar emissary vein

Digastric, post. belly

Transverse process of atlas

Vertebral artery
Ventral ramus C. 2

Intertransversarii
anterior & posterior

Ventral ramus C. 3

Articular process

Profunda cervicis vein
or Deep cervical vein

Rectus Capitis
Posterior Minor

Foramen magnum

Dura mater

Longitudinal vertebral
venous sinus

Spine of axis

Rotator

Multifidus

Interspinales

Spine of C. 5

493 Suboccipital Region—IV

(Postero-lateral view.)

The posterior arch of the atlas is removed and also the atlanto-occipital and atlanto-axial membranes.

Observe:

1. The vertebral venous system of veins and its numerous intercommunications·and connections, e.g., through the foramen magnum and the mastoid foramen and condylar canal with the intracranial venous sinuses; between the laminae and through the intervertebral foramina with the longitudinal vertebral venous sinuses (figs. 390 and 494); communicating with the veins of the scalp above, with the veins around the vertebral artery and, via the deep cervical vein, with brachio-cephalic vein below.

2. The Interspinales and the Multifidi extending up to, but not above, the spine of the axis.

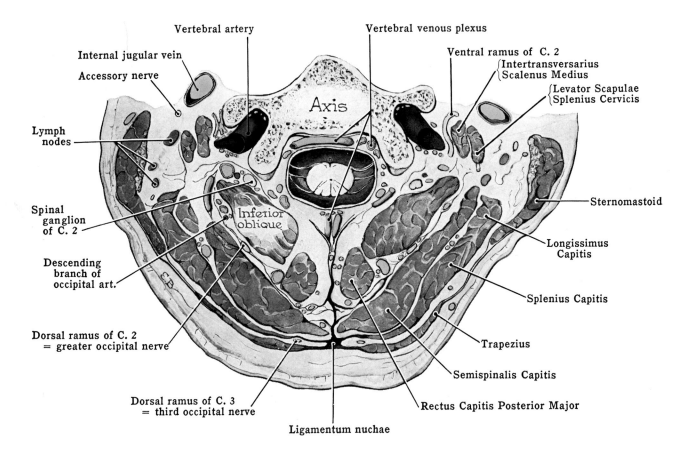

Vertebral artery

Internal jugular vein

Accessory nerve

Vertebral venous plexus

Ventral ramus of C. 2
{ Intertransversarius
{ Scalenus Medius
{ Levator Scapulae
{ Splenius Cervicis

Axis

Lymph nodes

Spinal ganglion of C. 2

Inferior oblique

Sternomastoid

Descending branch of occipital art.

Longissimus Capitis

Splenius Capitis

Dorsal ramus of C. 2 = greater occipital nerve

Trapezius

Semispinalis Capitis

Dorsal ramus of C. 3 = third occipital nerve

Rectus Capitis Posterior Major

Ligamentum nuchae

494 Cross Section of the Nuchal Region, at the level of the axis

Level—The section, clearly, passes above the level of the spine and laminae of the axis, for Obliquus Inferior and Rectus Capitis Major are present, whereas Semispinalis Cervicis and Multifidus are not. Clearly, also, it passes below the posterior arch of the atlas, for Obliquus Superior and Rectus Capitis Minor do not appear.

Observe:

1. Trapezius, Splenius, and Semispinalis Capitis forming a covering or roof for the suboccipital region.
2. The two muscles that ascend from the spine of the axis divided, viz., Inferior Oblique and Rectus Capitis Posterior Major.
3. Many anastomosing veins: (a) those around the vertebral artery unite, before leaving the 6th cervical transverse foramen to form the vertebral vein (fig. 567); (b) the vertebral venous plexus, which followed cranially communicates through the foramen magnum with the basilar and occipital venous sinuses.
4. The ventral ramus of C. 2 passing forwards lateral to the vertebral artery; and the dorsal ramus ascending behind Inferior Oblique.
5. The spinal cord having plenty of room at this high level.

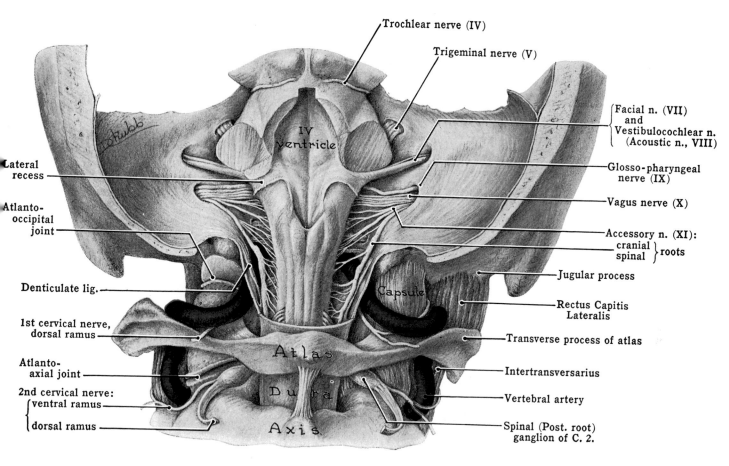

Trochlear nerve (IV)

Trigeminal nerve (V)

Facial n. (VII) and Vestibulocochlear n. (Acoustic n., VIII)

Glosso-pharyngeal nerve (IX)

Vagus nerve (X)

Accessory n. (XI): cranial } roots spinal }

Jugular process

Rectus Capitis Lateralis

Transverse process of atlas

Intertransversarius

Vertebral artery

Spinal (Post. root) ganglion of C. 2.

Lateral recess

Atlanto-occipital joint

Denticulate lig.

1st cervical nerve, dorsal ramus

Atlanto-axial joint

2nd cervical nerve: { ventral ramus { dorsal ramus

IV ventricle

Capsule

Atlas

Dura

Axis

495 Cranial Nerves, exposed from behind

The cerebellum is removed.

Observe:

1. The trochlear (IV) nerves, arising from the dorsal aspect of midbrain just below the inferior colliculi; the trigeminal (V) nerves, ascending to enter the mouths of the trigeminal caves (Meckel's caves); the facial (VII) and vestibulo-cochlear (VIII) nerves ascending to enter the internal acoustic meatuses; the glossopharyngeal (IX) nerves, piercing the dura mater separately and passing with the vagus (X) and accessory (XI) nerves through the jugular foramina; the fila of the accessory nerves of opposite sides, leaving the medulla and spinal cord asymmetrically; and the gnarled appearance of the spinal roots.

2. The abducent (VI) nerves are not in view; the hypoglossal (XII) nerves are seen vaguely in front of the spinal roots of nerves XI and just above the vertebral arteries.

3. The transverse process of the atlas, joined to the jugular process (i.e., transverse process) of the occipital bone by Rectus Capitis Lateralis, which morphologically is an Intertransverse muscle.

4. The vertebral arteries, raised from their beds on the posterior arch of the atlas.

5. The 1st cervical or suboccipital nerve, here having no sensory component. Its dorsal ramus or suboccipital nerve) passing between the vertebral artery and the posterior arch of the atlas. Its ventral ramus (not labelled), curving around the atlanto-occipital joint.

6. The 2nd cervical nerve (largely sensory), having a large spinal ganglion, a large dorsal ramus (or greater occipital nerve), and a smaller ventral ramus. The fila of its dorsal root are seen just above the cut edge of the dura and behind the spinal root of nerve XI.

(For front view, fig. 506.)

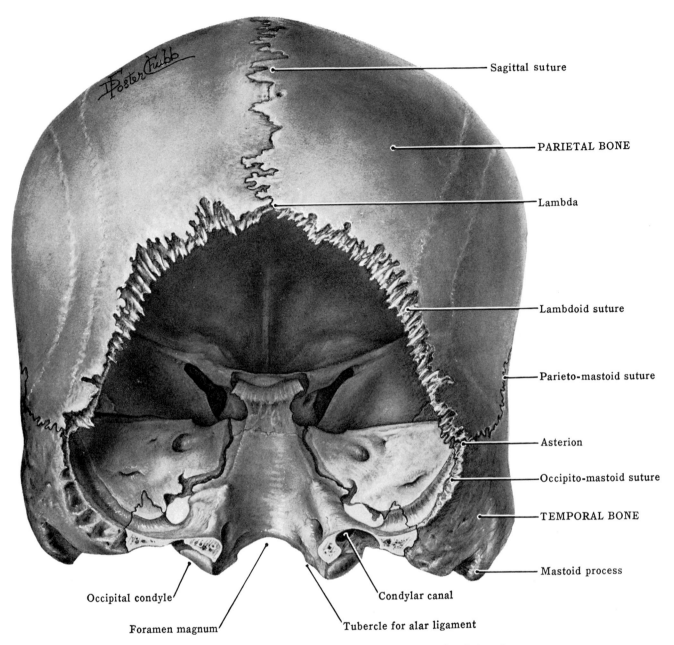

Sagittal suture

PARIETAL BONE

Lambda

Lambdoid suture

Parieto-mastoid suture

Asterion

Occipito-mastoid suture

TEMPORAL BONE

Mastoid process

Occipital condyle

Foramen magnum

Condylar canal

Tubercle for alar ligament

496 Posterior Cranial Fossa, from behind

The squamous part of the occipital bone was removed, after the right and left lateral parts had been sawn through. (Figure 497 is a key to this figure.)

Note:

1. The *Dorsum Cellae* is the squarish plate of bone rising from the body of the sphenoid. At its superior angles are the posterior clinoid processes.

2. The *Clivus* is the sloping surface between the dorsum sellae and the foramen magnum. It is formed by the basilar part of the occipital bone (basi-occipital) with some assistance from the body of the sphenoid, as figure 511 makes clear.

3. The *Sulci*, or grooves, for the sigmoid sinus and the inferior petrosal sinus both lead downwards to the jugular foramen.

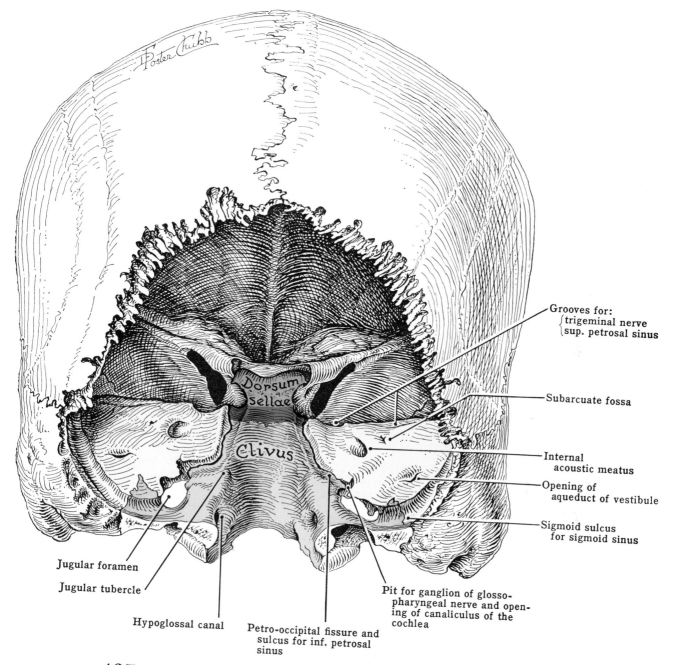

Grooves for:
{trigeminal nerve
{sup. petrosal sinus

Subarcuate fossa

Internal
acoustic meatus

Opening of
aqueduct of vestibule

Sigmoid sulcus
for sigmoid sinus

Pit for ganglion of glossopharyngeal nerve and opening of canaliculus of the
cochlea

Jugular foramen

Jugular tubercle

Hypoglossal canal

Petro-occipital fissure and
sulcus for inf. petrosal
sinus

Dorsum sellae

Clivus

497 Posterior Cranial Fossa, from behind

Note: (1) That at birth the subarcuate fossa was large and extended laterally, under the arc of the anterior semicircular canal (see fig. 645.1).

2. That the aqueduct of the vestibule opened under the arc of the posterior semicircular canal. This aqueduct transmits the endolymphatic duct (see figs. 644 and 650).

3. That the perilymphatic duct (within the canaliculus of the cochlea, figs. 633 & 644) opens at the bottom of the pyramidal pit for the glossopharyngeal ganglion. This capillary aqueduct is said to allow the perilymph of the internal ear to mix with the cerebrospinal fluid in the posterior cranial fossa; but there is evidence that it ends as a closed sac. (*Wharton Young.*)

(*For posterior cranial fossa from above, see figs. 508 & 512.*)

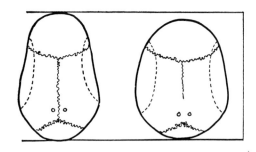

DOLICHOCEPHALIC SKULL.   BRACHYCEPHALIC SKULL.

498   Skulls, viewed from above

When the maximum width of a skull is less than 75% of the maximum length, the skull is called dolichocephalic or long headed; when more than 80%, it is brachycephalic or broad headed; and when between 75% and 80%, it is mesaticephalic.

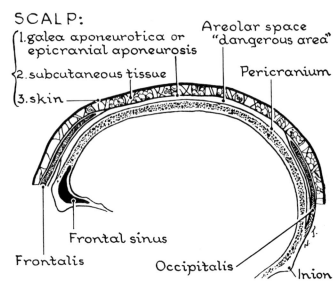

SCALP:
1. galea aponeurotica or epicranial aponeurosis
2. subcutaneous tissue
3. skin
Areolar space "dangerous area"
Pericranium
Frontal sinus
Frontalis
Occipitalis
Inion

498.1   Diagram of skull cap and its coverings, on paramedian section, to show the 3 layers of the scalp and the subaponeurotic, areolar space. (Also fig. 458.)

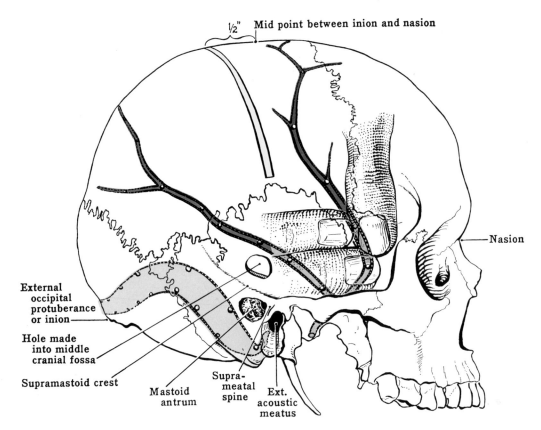

½"   Mid point between inion and nasion

Nasion

External occipital protuberance or inion
Hole made into middle cranial fossa
Supramastoid crest
Mastoid antrum
Supra-meatal spine
Ext. acoustic meatus

499   Surface Anatomy of the Cranium

The artery and the venous sinus were related to the outside of the skull by drilling holes along the grooves on the inside.

Note: The pterion, two fingers' breadth above the zygomatic arch and a thumb's breadth behind the frontal process of the zygomatic bone. The ant. branch of the middle meningeal a. crosses the pterion; the post. branch curves backwards less than a finger's breadth above the zygomatic arch and supramastoid crest; the stem of the artery traverses the foramen spinosum medial to the head of the mandible (fig. 508).

The lesser wing of the sphenoid extends almost to the pterion (fig. 508); hence, the pterion marks also the stem of the lateral cerebral fissure, the ant. perforated substance, etc. (fig. 506).

The central sulcus (yellow) has its upper end where indicated: its lower end lies 2″ above the external acoustic meatus.

The supramastoid crest approximately at the level of the floor of the middle cranial fossa; hence, a hole drilled below the crest and behind the suprameatal spine enters the mastoid antrum; whereas one drilled above the crest enters the middle cranial fossa.

The transverse and sigmoid sinuses (blue) curve from the inion, across the asterion, to a point less than ¾″ behind the ext. meatus, and thence forwards and downwards to a point in front of the mastoid process and below the ext. meatus where (on the post. transverse line, fig. 571.2) it becomes the jugular vein.

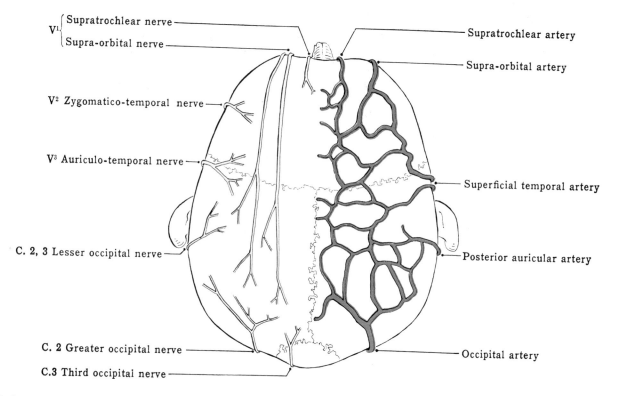

500 Diagram of the Arteries and Nerves of the Scalp

Observe:

1. The arteries, anastomosing freely. The supra-orbital and supratrochlear are derived from the internal carotid artery via the ophthalmic artery; the three others are branches of the external carotid artery.

2. The nerves, appearing in sequence:—V^1, V^2, V^3, ventral rami of C. 2 & 3 and dorsal rami of C.2 & 3 (C. 1 has no cutaneous branch.)

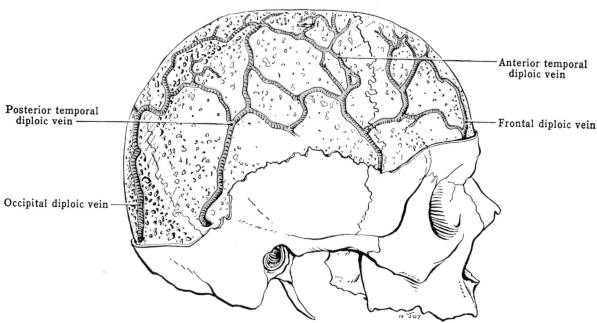

501 Diploic Veins

The outer table of the skull has been filed away and the channels for the diploic veins thereby opened.

Note:

Of the four (paired) diploic veins, the frontal opens into the supra-orbital vein at the supra-orbital notch; the anterior temporal opens into the spheno-parietal sinus; the posterior temporal and the occipital both open into the transverse sinus—but they may open into surface veins.

There are no accompanying diploic arteries; the meningeal and pericranial arteries provide the arterial blood.

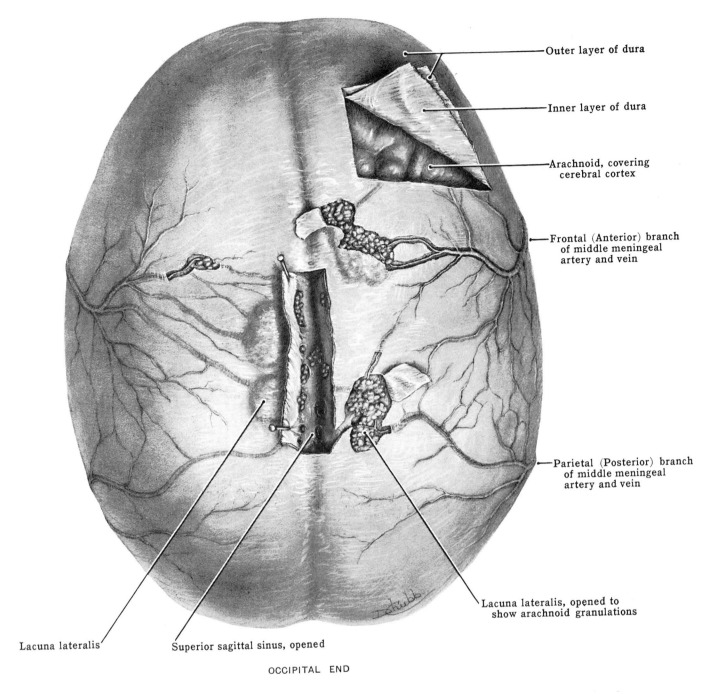

Outer layer of dura

Inner layer of dura

Arachnoid, covering cerebral cortex

Frontal (Anterior) branch of middle meningeal artery and vein

Parietal (Posterior) branch of middle meningeal artery and vein

Lacuna lateralis, opened to show arachnoid granulations

Lacuna lateralis

Superior sagittal sinus, opened

502 External Surface of the Dura Mater: Arachnoid Granulations

The skull cap is removed. In the median plane, the thick roof of the superior sagittal dural sinus is partly pinned aside and, laterally, the thin roofs of two lacunae laterales are reflected.

At the right front, an angular flap of both layers of dura is turned forwards; the subdural space is thereby opened; and the convolutions of the cerebral cortex are visible through the cobweb-like arachnoid mater.

Observe:

1. The frontal and parietal branches of the middle meningeal artery, arborising and anastomosing within the external or periosteal layer of the dura.

2. Each artery lying in a venous channel (middle meningeal veins) which enlarges above into a lake, lacuna lateralis.

3. Cauliflower-like masses, arachnoid granulations, dangling in the lakes, cf. chorionic villi of the placenta.

4. A channel or channels, draining the lake into the superior sagittal sinus which is triangular on cross section and has many discrete granulations protruding into it.

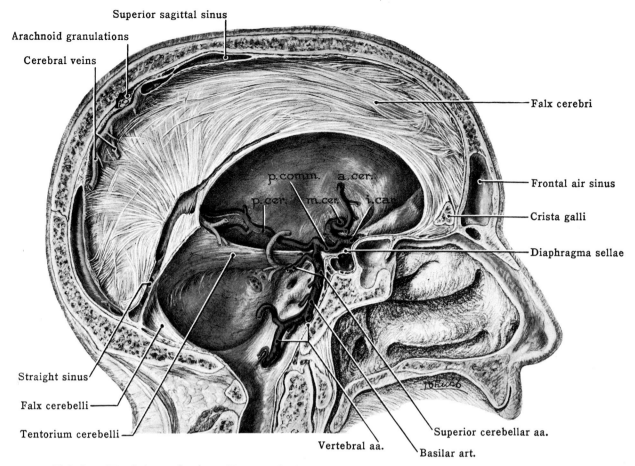

Superior sagittal sinus
Arachnoid granulations
Cerebral veins

Falx cerebri

p.comm. a.cer.
p.cer. m.cer. i.car.

Frontal air sinus
Crista galli
Diaphragma sellae

Straight sinus
Falx cerebelli
Tentorium cerebelli

Vertebral aa.
Basilar art.
Superior cerebellar aa.

503 Folds of the Dura Mater

Observe:

1. The 4 reduplications of the inner layer of the dura mater, namely:—2 sickle shaped folds, (a) falx cerebri and (b) falx cerebelli, which lie vertically in the median plane; and the 2 roof-like folds, (c) tentorium cerebelli and (d) diaphragma sellae, which lie horizontally.
   The tentorium is perforated by the mid brain; the diaphragma, by the stalk of the hypophysis cerebri.
2. The 2 paired arteries that supply the brain—internal carotid and vertebral.

4 Diagram of (Venous) Sinuses of Dura Mater

erve:

) The superior sagittal sinus at the upper or onvex border of the falx cerebri; (b) the ferior sagittal sinus in the concave or free rder; (c) the great cerebral vein joining the f. sagittal sinus to form (d) the straight sinus hich runs obliquely in the junction between lx cerebri and tentorium; (e) the occipital nus in the attached border of the falx cerebelli. he sup. sagittal sinus usually becomes—right ansverse sinus—right sigmoid sinus—right t. jugular vein; the straight sinus behaves milarly on left side. (Variations, see Brown- g.)

ne cavernous sinus communicating with the ins of the face via the ophthalmic veins and e pterygoid plexus, and emptying via the o petrosal sinuses (fig. 643).

e basilar sinus connecting the inf. petrosal uses of opposite sides and, like the occipital us, communicating below with the vertebral exus (fig. 493).

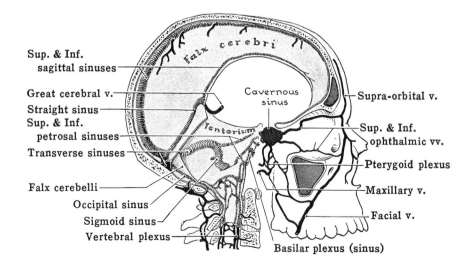

Sup. & Inf. sagittal sinuses
Great cerebral v.
Straight sinus
Sup. & Inf. petrosal sinuses
Transverse sinuses
Falx cerebelli
Occipital sinus
Sigmoid sinus
Vertebral plexus
Falx cerebri
Cavernous sinus
Tentorium
Supra-orbital v.
Sup. & Inf. ophthalmic vv.
Pterygoid plexus
Maxillary v.
Facial v.
Basilar plexus (sinus)

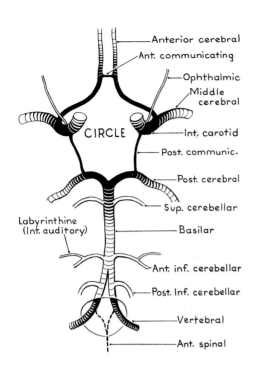

Anterior cerebral
Ant. communicating
Ophthalmic
Middle cerebral
CIRCLE
Int. carotid
Post. communic.
Post. cerebral
Sup. cerebellar
Labyrinthine (Int. auditory)
Basilar
Ant. inf. cerebellar
Post. Inf. cerebellar
Vertebral
Ant. spinal

505 Key to figure 505.1

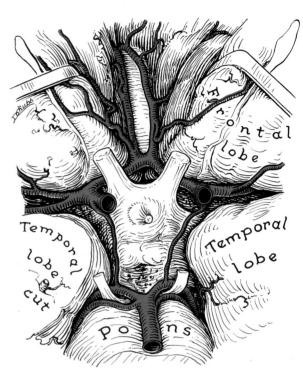

Frontal lobe
Temporal lobe cut
Temporal lobe
Pons

505.1 Cerebral Arterial Circle (of Willis)

Two arteries (paired) enter the skull to supply the brain:
Internal carotid at foramen lacerum (fig. 514) and
vertebral at foramen magnum (fig. 495).

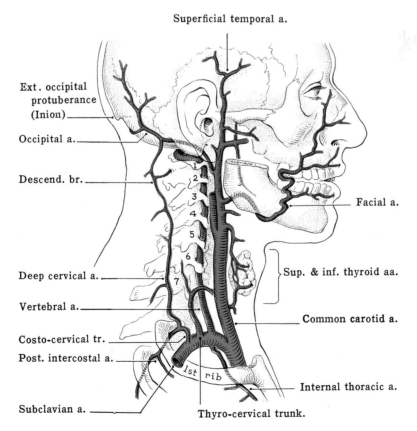

Superficial temporal a.

Ext. occipital protuberance (Inion)

Occipital a.

Descend. br.

Deep cervical a.

Vertebral a.

Costo-cervical tr.

Post. intercostal a.

Subclavian a.

Facial a.

Sup. & inf. thyroid aa.

Common carotid a.

Internal thoracic a.

Thyro-cervical trunk.

1st rib

505.2 Diagram. The four chief Arterial Connections (paired) between the Aortic Arch and the Head.

(Based on Jones and Shepard. Manual of Surgical Anatomy, Saunders, and arteries in this Atlas.)

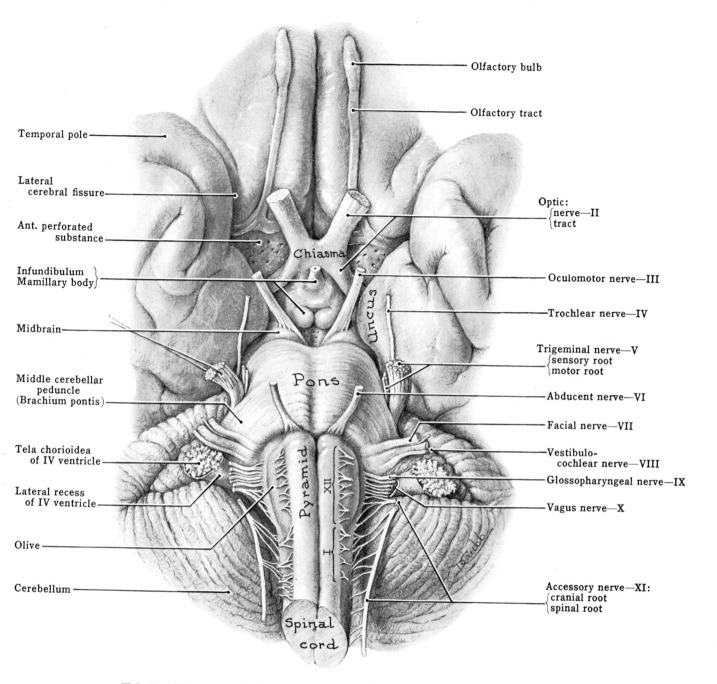

Olfactory bulb

Olfactory tract

Temporal pole

Lateral
cerebral fissure

Ant. perforated
substance

Infundibulum
Mamillary body

Midbrain

Middle cerebellar
peduncle
(Brachium pontis)

Tela chorioidea
of IV ventricle

Lateral recess
of IV ventricle

Olive

Cerebellum

Chiasma

Uncus

Pons

Pyramid

XII

I

Spinal
cord

Optic:
nerve—II
tract

Oculomotor nerve—III

Trochlear nerve—IV

Trigeminal nerve—V
sensory root
motor root

Abducent nerve—VI

Facial nerve—VII

Vestibulo-
cochlear nerve—VIII

Glossopharyngeal nerve—IX

Vagus nerve—X

Accessory nerve—XI:
cranial root
spinal root

506 Base of the Brain: The Superfical Origins of the Cranial Nerves

Note:

1. The olfactory bulb, in which the olfactory (1) nerves (not shown) end.
2. The superficial origin of the trochlear (IV) nerve is shown in figure 495.
3. The slender nervus intermedius, or so-called sensory root of the facial nerve (seen, but not labelled) between the facial (VII) and vestibulo-cochlear (acoustic, VIII) nerves.
4. The fila of the hypoglossal (XII) nerve, arising between the pyramid and the olive, and in line with the ventral root of the 1st cervical nerve.

(For dorsal view, fig. 495.)

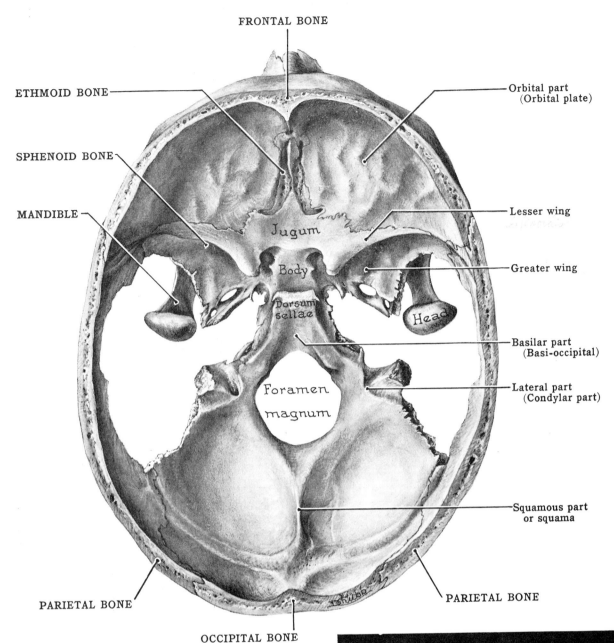

FRONTAL BONE

ETHMOID BONE

SPHENOID BONE

MANDIBLE

Orbital part
(Orbital plate)

Lesser wing

Greater wing

Jugum

Body

Dorsum
sellae

Head

Basilar part
(Basi-occipital)

Lateral part
(Condylar part)

Foramen
magnum

Squamous part
or squama

PARIETAL BONE

PARIETAL BONE

OCCIPITAL BONE

507 Interior of the Base of the Skull

The temporal bones are removed, but the heads of the mandible remain in situ.

Observe:

1. The head of the mandible, lying lateral to the spine of the sphenoid, at which there is a perforation, the foramen spinosum, for the transmission of the middle meningeal vessels.
2. The long axes of the right and left heads, when produced medially, meet near the anterior border of the foramen magnum.
3. The 3 bones contributing to the anterior cranial fossa.
4. The 4 parts of the occipital bone—basilar, right and left lateral, and squamous.

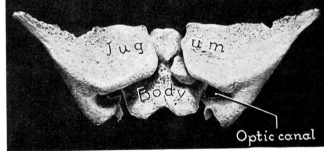

Jug um

Body

Optic canal

507.1 Lesser Wings of Sphenoid, before birth, posterior view

Note:

1. These wings, like sliding doors, close above the body of the sphenoid to form the jugum or yoke.
2. The posterior edge of the jugum becomes the anterior edge of the chiasmatic sulcus, which leads to the optic canals.
3. The left canal is not yet pinched off from the superior orbital fissure, but the right is.

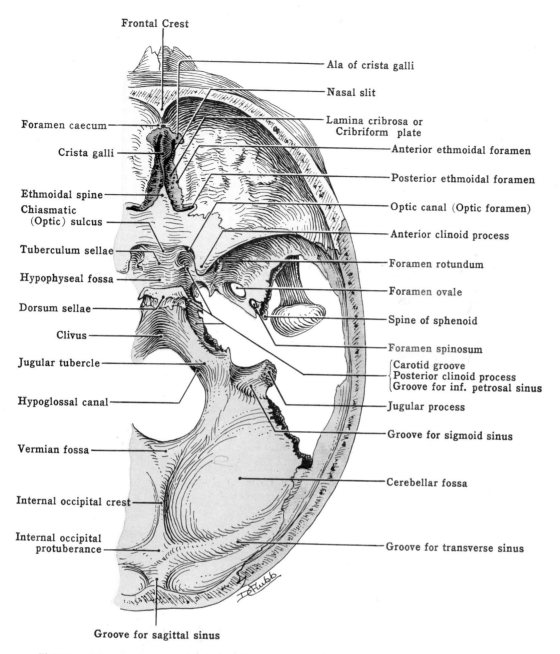

Frontal Crest

Ala of crista galli

Nasal slit

Lamina cribrosa or
Cribriform plate

Foramen caecum

Anterior ethmoidal foramen

Crista galli

Posterior ethmoidal foramen

Optic canal (Optic foramen)

Ethmoidal spine

Anterior clinoid process

Chiasmatic
(Optic) sulcus

Tuberculum sellae

Foramen rotundum

Hypophyseal fossa

Foramen ovale

Dorsum sellae

Spine of sphenoid

Clivus

Foramen spinosum

Jugular tubercle

Carotid groove
Posterior clinoid process
Groove for inf. petrosal sinus

Hypoglossal canal

Jugular process

Groove for sigmoid sinus

Vermian fossa

Internal occipital crest

Cerebellar fossa

Internal occipital
protuberance

Groove for transverse sinus

Groove for sagittal sinus

508   Interior of the Base of the Skull

(Key to facing figure, 507.)

Features in the median plane:

of the anterior cranial fossa—frontal crest and crista galli (for attachment of falx cerebri) with foramen caecum in between, and jugum whose free posterior edge limits this fossa posteriorly.

of the middle cranial fossa—chiasmatic sulcus (leading from one optic canal to the other, but not lodging the chiasma, see fig. 521), tuberculum sellae, hypophyseal fossa, and dorsum sellae which limits this fossa posteriorly.

of the posterior cranial fossa—dorsum sellae, clivus, foramen magnum, vermian fossa (below vermis of cerebellum), internal occipital crest (for falx cerebelli), and internal occipital protuberance from which the sulci for the transverse sinuses curve laterally, limiting this fossa postero-superiorly.

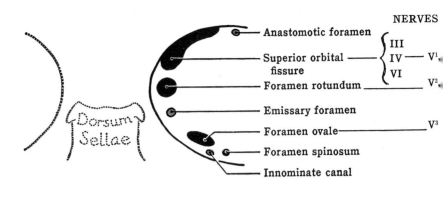

Anastomotic foramen

Superior orbital fissure — { III, IV — V¹, VI }

Foramen rotundum — V²

Emissary foramen

Foramen ovale — V³

Foramen spinosum

Innominate canal

509 Crescent of Foramina in the Middle Cranial Fossa

Note: Seven paired foramina, of which 4 (black) are constant and 3 (red) are inconstant, open from the sphenoid bone into the middle cranial fossa. Because of the crescentic design made by these foramina, it is simple to relate one foramen to another.

Anastomotic foramen transmits a branch from middle meningeal art. to lacrimal art. (fig. 524). *Emissary foramen* transmits a vein from cavernous sinus to pterygoid plexus. *Innominate canal*, in lieu of foramen ovale, transmits lesser petrosal nerve to otic ganglion.

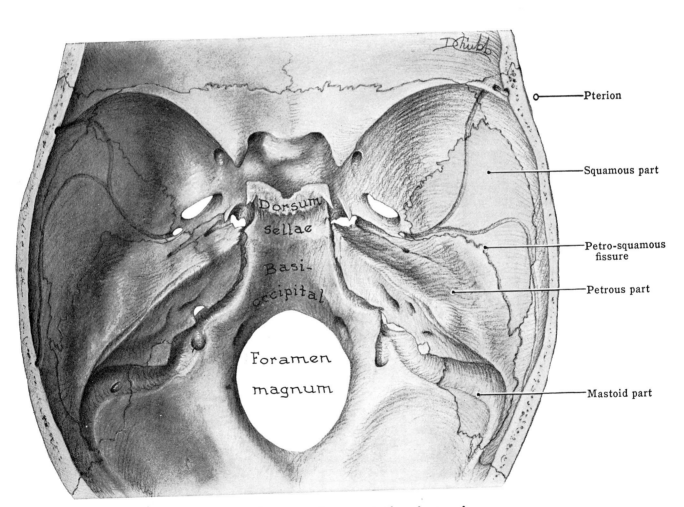

Pterion

Squamous part

Petro-squamous fissure

Petrous part

Mastoid part

510 Temporal Bone, in its setting, at the interior of the base of the skull

(*Figures 509 and 512 are keys to figure 510.*)

1 Spheno-occipital ynchondrosis (Basilar Suture), paramedian section, aged out ten years

This synchondrosis is usually obliterated (becomes a synostosis) the 17th or 18th year, and always by the 21st year (McKern & wart).

Note the right sphenoidal sinus, like an inflated rubber balloon, ading the cancellous bone.

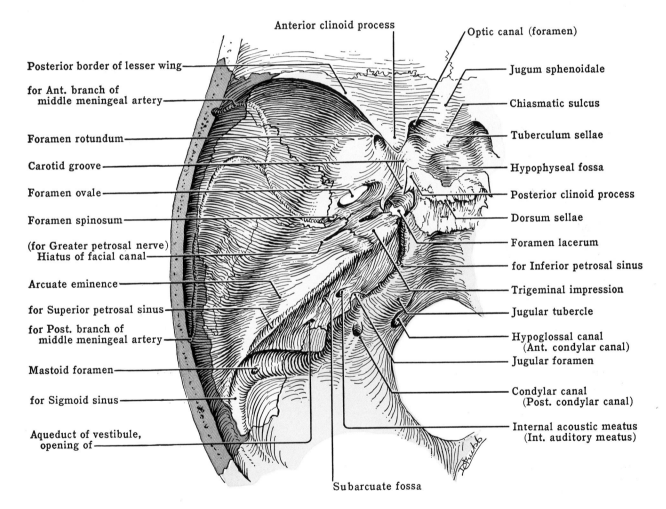

512 **Middle and Posterior Cranial Fossae, from above**

Note:

1. Three features—tuberculum sellae, hypophyseal fossa, and dorsum sellae—constitute the sella turcica or Turkish saddle.

2. Of the two, paired clinoid processes (for the attachment of the tentorium, fig. 514) the anterior, on the lesser wing of the sphenoid, is conical; the posterior, on the angle of the dorsum sellae, is beak-like.

3. The foramen lacerum is situated between the hypophyseal fossa and the apex of the petrous bone. There the carotid canal discharges the internal carotid art. into the upper half of the foramen lacerum.

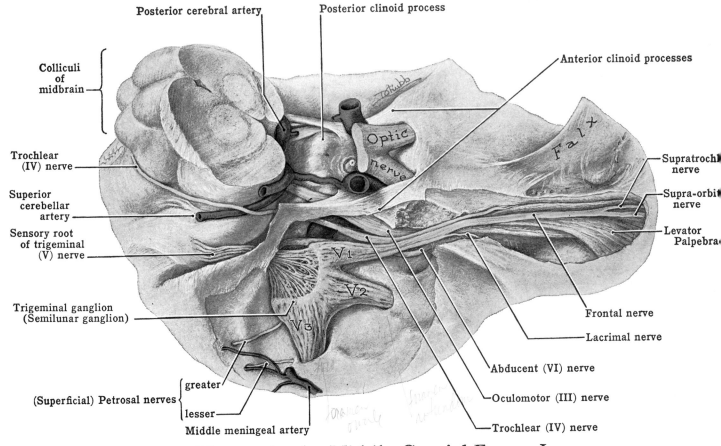

Colliculi of midbrain

Posterior cerebral artery

Posterior clinoid process

Anterior clinoid processes

Trochlear (IV) nerve

Superior cerebellar artery

Sensory root of trigeminal (V) nerve

Optic nerve

Falx

Supratrochlear nerve

Supra-orbital nerve

Levator Palpebra

V_1

V_2

V_3

Trigeminal ganglion (Semilunar ganglion)

(Superficial) Petrosal nerves { greater / lesser }

Middle meningeal artery

Frontal nerve

Lacrimal nerve

Abducent (VI) nerve

Oculomotor (III) nerve

Trochlear (IV) nerve

513   Nerves in the Middle Cranial Fossa—I

The tentorium cerebelli is cut away to reveal the courses of the trochlear and trigeminal nerves in the posterior cranial fossa, i.e., below the tentorium. The dura is largely removed from the middle fossa; the roof of the orbit is partly removed.

Observe:

1. The trigeminal (semilunar) ganglion and its 3 divisions.
2. The mandibular nerve (V^3), dropping down through the foramen ovale (into the infratemporal fossa).
3. The maxillary nerve (V^2), passing forwards through the foramen rotundum (into the pterygo-palatine fossa).
4. The ophthalmic nerve (V^1), ascending slightly, closely applied to the trochlear (IV) nerve, and dividing into frontal and lacrimal branches. These 3 (trochlear, frontal, lacrimal) nerves, running forwards through the superior orbital fissure and applied to the roof of the orbital cavity (removed).

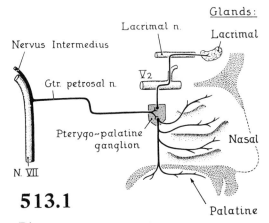

Glands:

Lacrimal n.

Lacrimal

Nervus Intermedius

Gtr. petrosal n.

V_2

Pterygo-palatine ganglion

Nasal

N. VII

Palatine

513.1

Diagram

The Greater Petrosal Nerve brings secreto-motor fibers to the pterygopalatine ganglion for relay and distribution, via branches of the maxillary nerve, to glands (lacrimal, nasal, and palatine) in maxillary territory (figs. 470.1, pink, and 560.2).

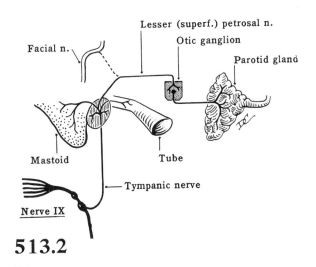

Lesser (superf.) petrosal n.

Facial n.

Otic ganglion

Parotid gland

Mastoid

Tube

Tympanic nerve

Nerve IX

513.2

Diagram:

1. The Lesser Petrosal Nerve brings secreto-motor fibers to the otic ganglion for relay and distribution to the parotid gland.

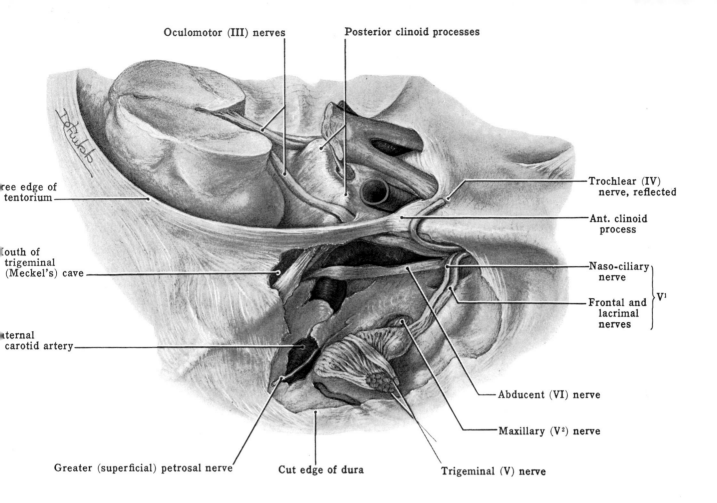

Oculomotor (III) nerves

Posterior clinoid processes

[ree] edge of tentorium

Trochlear (IV) nerve, reflected

Ant. clinoid process

[M]outh of trigeminal (Meckel's) cave

Naso-ciliary nerve

Frontal and lacrimal nerves } V¹

[In]ternal carotid artery

Abducent (VI) nerve

Maxillary (V²) nerve

Greater (superficial) petrosal nerve

Cut edge of dura

Trigeminal (V) nerve

514   Nerves in the Middle Cranial Fossa—II

The trigeminal nerve is divided, withdrawn from the mouth of the trigeminal cave, and turned forwards. The trochlear nerve also is turned forwards.

Observe:

1. The bed of the trigeminal ganglion partly formed by the greater petrosal nerve and the internal carotid artery, dura intervening.

2. The motor root of nerve V (the nerve to the muscles of mastication), crossing the ganglion diagonally, from medial to lateral side, to join V³.

3. V¹, giving off the naso-ciliary nerve, and crowding with nerves III, IV, and VI through the superior orbital fissure.

4. The anterior clinoid process, "pulled backwards" by the free edge of the tentorium between the optic nerve and internal carotid artery medially, and the oculo-motor nerve below.

5. The abducent (VI) nerve, making a right-angled turn at the apex of the petrous bone and then, as it runs horizontally forwards, hugging the internal carotid artery which flattens it.

6. The sinuous course of the internal carotid artery.

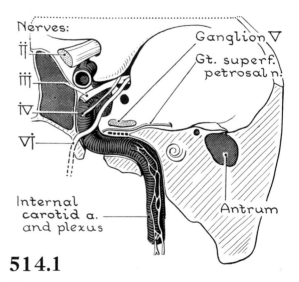

Nerves:
II
III
IV
VI

Ganglion V
Gt. superf. petrosal n.

Internal carotid a. and plexus

Antrum

514.1

Diagram:
1. The Internal Carotid Artery takes an (inverted) L-shape course from the under surface of the petrous bone to its apex. There, at upper end of foramen lacerum, it enters the cranial cavity and takes an S-shape course. Note its contacts.

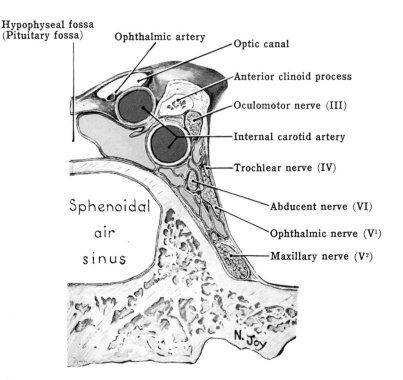

Hypophyseal fossa (Pituitary fossa)
Ophthalmic artery
Optic canal
Anterior clinoid process
Oculomotor nerve (III)
Internal carotid artery
Trochlear nerve (IV)
Abducent nerve (VI)
Ophthalmic nerve (V¹)
Maxillary nerve (V²)
Sphenoidal air sinus
N. Joy

515 Cavernous Sinus, on coronal section

Observe:

1. This venous sinus, situated at the side of the sp_
noidal air sinus and of the hypophyseal fossa.
2. The internal carotid artery, surrounded by the _
ternal carotid plexus (not drawn), and the ab__
cent nerve (fig. 643), passing through the sinus.
3. The internal carotid artery, having made an acu_
bend, is cut twice. This artery and the oculomot_
nerve grooving the anterior clinoid process.

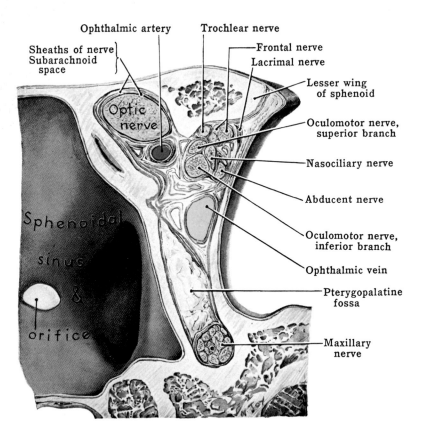

Ophthalmic artery
Trochlear nerve
Sheaths of nerve
Subarachnoid space
Frontal nerve
Lacrimal nerve
Lesser wing of sphenoid
Optic nerve
Oculomotor nerve, superior branch
Nasociliary nerve
Abducent nerve
Oculomotor nerve, inferior branch
Ophthalmic vein
Sphenoidal sinus & orifice
Pterygopalatine fossa
Maxillary nerve

516 Nerves and Vessels at the Apex of the Orbital Cavity on coronal section

Observe:

1. The optic nerve within its pial, arachnoid, a_
dural sheaths and the subarachnoid space. The op_
thalmic artery emerging from the optic canal.
2. Other nerves crowded together, tightly pack_
passing through the medial end of the superior orbi_
fissure. They are: the upper and the lower branch_
the oculomotor nerve (III), the trochlear nerve (IV
the frontal, lacrimal and naso-ciliary branches of t_
ophthalmic nerve (V¹); and the abducent nerve (V_
3. The ophthalmic vein, about to open into the ca_
ernous sinus, in turn to be drained by the super_
and inferior petrosal sinuses (fig. 643).

*(For posterior half of orbital cavity on coronal section,
see figures 591 & 592.)*

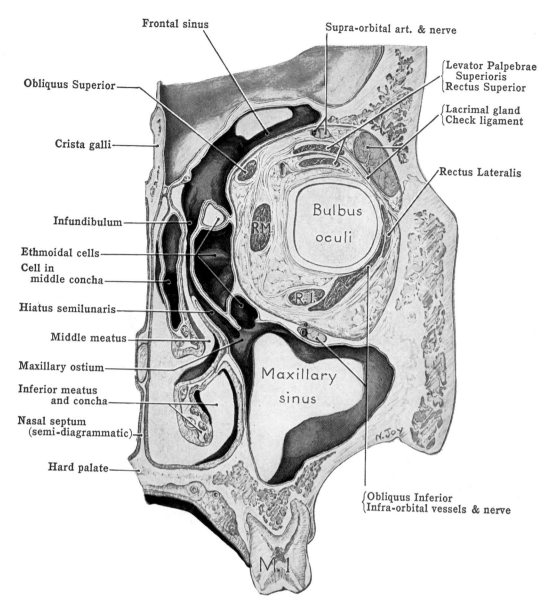

Frontal sinus

Supra-orbital art. & nerve

Obliquus Superior

Levator Palpebrae
Superioris
Rectus Superior

Crista galli

Lacrimal gland
Check ligament

Rectus Lateralis

Bulbus

oculi

R M.

Infundibulum

Ethmoidal cells

R. I.

Cell in
middle concha

Hiatus semilunaris

Middle meatus

Maxillary ostium

Inferior meatus
and concha

Maxillary

sinus

N. JOY

Nasal septum
(semi-diagrammatic)

Hard palate

Obliquus Inferior
Infra-orbital vessels & nerve

M. I.

517 Right Side of the Head, on coronal section, viewed from behind

Observe:

1. The bulbus oculi (eyeball) within the somewhat circular orbital cavity. The stout, thick lateral bony wall; the thin, papery roof, medial wall, and floor surrounded with air sinuses—frontal, ethmoidal, and maxillary.

2. The 4 Recti Oculi and 2 Obliqui Oculi arranged around the bulb, Obliquus Inferior inserted by tendon. Levator Palpebrae Superioris above Rectus Superior, and the check ligament passing from it.

3. The lacrimal gland lying between the check ligament and the frontal bone.

4. The 4 Recti and the fascia uniting them forming a circle around the bulb—it is a section of the cone of muscles.

5. The nasal septum (semidiagrammatic). The middle concha, here, containing an air cell. The entrance to the frontal sinus through the infundibulum, which is at the lowest point of the sinus.

6. The entrance to the maxillary sinus through the hiatus semilunaris, which is at the level of the roof of the sinus. The lowest point of the sinus, here as commonly, below the level of the floor of the nasal cavity. The nasal wall of the sinus is very thin in the inferior meatus, well above the floor of the nose.

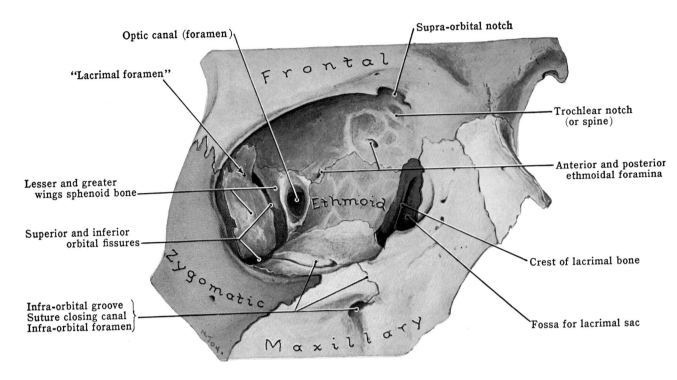

Optic canal (foramen)

"Lacrimal foramen"

Supra-orbital notch

Frontal

Trochlear notch
(or spine)

Anterior and posterior
ethmoidal foramina

Lesser and greater
wings sphenoid bone

Ethmoid

Superior and inferior
orbital fissures

Crest of lacrimal bone

Zygomatic

Infra-orbital groove
Suture closing canal
Infra-orbital foramen

Maxillary

Fossa for lacrimal sac

518 Orbital Cavity

Observe:

1. The quadrangular orbital margin, at the base of the cavity, to which the frontal, maxillary, and zygomatic bones contribute.

2. The spiral form of the medial part of this margin. It is spiral since the supra-orbital margin leads to the crest of the lacrimal bone (post. lacrimal crest); whereas the infra-orbital margin is continuous with the crest on the frontal process of the maxilla (ant. lacrimal crest).

3. The fossa for the lacrimal sac, between these two crests.

4. The optic canal, situated at the apex of the pear-shaped orbital cavity, and placed between the body of the sphenoid and the two roots of the lesser wing. A straight probe must pass along the lateral wall of the cavity, if it is to traverse the canal.

5. The superior wall or roof, formed by the orbital plate of the frontal bone.

6. The inferior wall or floor, formed by the orbital plate of the maxilla and slightly by the zygomatic bone, and crossed by the infra-orbital groove, the anterior end of which is converted into the infra-orbital canal which ends at the infra-orbital foramen.

7. The stout lateral wall, formed by the frontal process of the zygomatic bone and by the greater wing of the sphenoid. The superior and inferior orbital fissures, together forming a V-shaped fissure which limits the greater wing of the sphenoid.

8. The fragile medial wall, formed by the papery lacrimal bone and the papery orbital plate (lamina papyracea) of the ethmoid bone. The anterior and posterior ethmoidal foramina, which developed in the suture between the frontal and ethmoidal bones, but are now, in this specimen, enveloped by the frontal bone.

9. The "lacrimal foramen", just beyond the supero-lateral end of the superior orbital fissure, for the anastomosis between the middle meningeal and lacrimal arteries. The zygomatic foramen on the orbital surface of the zygomatic bone is not in view.

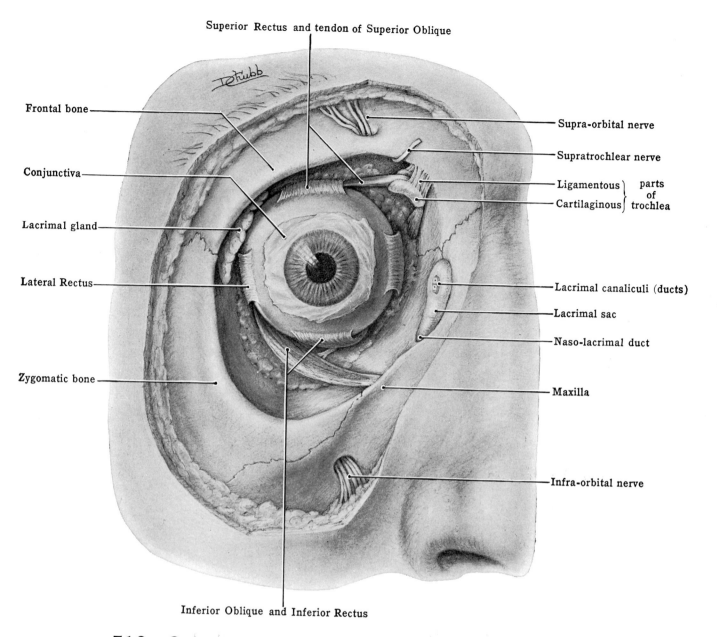

Superior Rectus and tendon of Superior Oblique

Frontal bone

Conjunctiva

Lacrimal gland

Lateral Rectus

Zygomatic bone

Supra-orbital nerve

Supratrochlear nerve

Ligamentous ⎫ parts
Cartilaginous ⎭ of trochlea

Lacrimal canaliculi (ducts)

Lacrimal sac

Naso-lacrimal duct

Maxilla

Infra-orbital nerve

Inferior Oblique and Inferior Rectus

519 Orbital Cavity, dissected from the front

The eyelids, orbital septum, Levator Palpebrae Superioris, and some fat are removed.

Observe:

1. The ocular conjunctiva, loose and wrinkled over the sclera, but adherent to the cornea.
2. The aponeurotic insertions of the four Recti, inserted 6 to 8 mm. behind the sclero-corneal junction.
3. The superior and inferior oblique muscles, crossing below the corresponding superior and inferior straight muscles.
4. The tendon of Obliquus Superior, playing in a cartilaginous pulley or trochlea, which is fixed by ligamentous fibres just behind the supero-medial angle of the orbital margin.
5. The nerve to Obliquus Inferior entering its posterior border.
6. The lacrimal gland, placed between the bony orbital wall laterally and the eyeball and Rectus Lateralis medially.
7. The lacrimal sac, receiving the superior and inferior lacrimal canaliculi (ducts) and becoming the naso-lacrimal duct which traverses the (bony) naso-lacrimal canal to open into the nose (fig. 610).

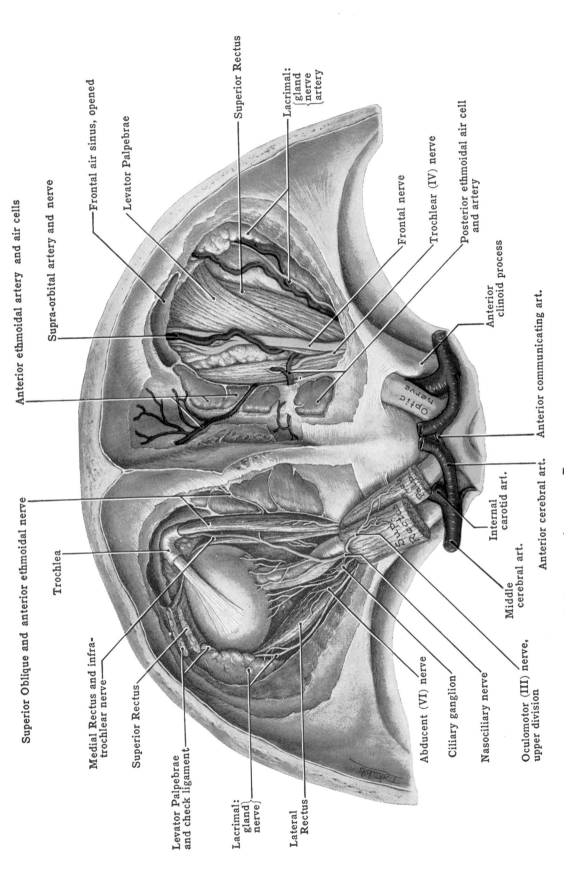

Anterior ethmoidal artery and air cells

Supra-orbital artery and nerve

Frontal air sinus, opened

Levator Palpebrae

Superior Rectus

Lacrimal: { gland { nerve { artery

Frontal nerve

Trochlear (IV) nerve

Posterior ethmoidal air cell and artery

Anterior clinoid process

Anterior communicating art.

Optic nerve

Internal carotid art.

Middle cerebral art.

Anterior cerebral art.

Oculomotor (III) nerve, upper division

Nasociliary nerve

Ciliary ganglion

Abducent (VI) nerve

Lateral Rectus

Lacrimal: { gland { nerve

Levator Palpebrae and check ligament

Superior Rectus

Medial Rectus and infra-trochlear nerve

Trochlea

Superior Oblique and anterior ethmoidal nerve

520 Orbital Cavity, dissected from above—I

On the right side—The orbital plate of the frontal bone is removed.
On the left side—Levator Palpebrae and Rectus Superior are reflected.

Observe, on the right side:

1. Levator Palpebrae Superioris, overlying Rectus Superior.
2. The 3 nerves applied to the roof of the orbital cavity—trochlear, frontal, lacrimal.
3. Four of the branches of the ophthalmic artery.

Observe, on the left side:

4. The superior division nerve III, supplying Rectus Superior and Levator Palpebrae.
5. The entire course of Obliquus Superior, and the trochlear (IV) nerve supplying it.
6. Rectus Lateralis and the abducent (VI) nerve supplying it.
7. Rectus Medialis and a branch of the oculomotor (III) nerve supplying it.
8. The lacrimal nerve, running above Rectus Lateralis to the lacrimal gland.
9. The ciliary ganglion, placed between Rectus Lateralis and the optic nerve and giving off many short ciliary nerves. The nasociliary nerve, giving off of 2 long ciliary nerves

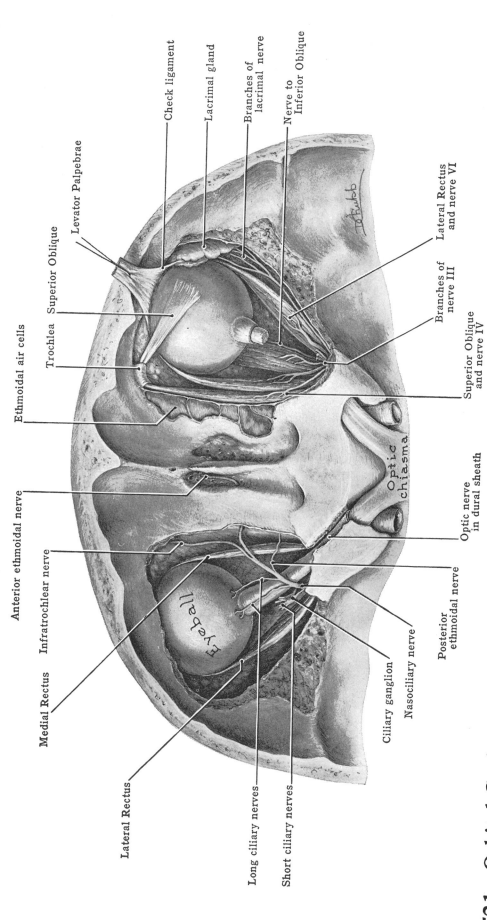

Ethmoidal air cells

Trochlea Superior Oblique

Levator Palpebrae

Check ligament

Lacrimal gland

Branches of lacrimal nerve

Nerve to Inferior Oblique

Lateral Rectus and nerve VI

Branches of nerve III

Superior Oblique and nerve IV

Optic chiasma

Optic nerve in dural sheath

Posterior ethmoidal nerve

Nasociliary nerve

Ciliary ganglion

Short ciliary nerves

Long ciliary nerves

Lateral Rectus

Medial Rectus

Infratrochlear nerve

Anterior ethmoidal nerve

Eyeball

521 Orbital Cavity, dissected from above—II

Observe, on the right side:

1. The nerves to the six ocular muscles—4 Recti and 2 Obliqui—the trochlear to Obliquus Superior, the abducent to Rectus Lateralis, and the oculomotor to the remaining four and also to Levator Palpebrae Superioris.

2. The four Recti (Superior, Medialis, Inferior, Lateralis), supplied on their ocular surfaces; the two Obliqui (Superior, Inferior) near their borders. Rectus Superior and Obliquus Inferior are not in view.

Observe, on the left side:

3. The eyeball, occupying the anterior half of the 2″ long orbital cavity.

4. The ciliary ganglion, faintly brownish in colour, lying far back between Rectus Lateralis and the sheath of the optic nerve, receiving a twig (sensory and sympathetic) from the nasociliary nerve and a twig (motor to Sphincter Pupillae and Ciliary muscle) from the nerve to Obliquus Inferior, and giving off short ciliary nerves (cut short).

5. The nasociliary nerve, sending a twig to the ciliary ganglion, crossing the optic nerve, giving off two long ciliary nerves (sensory to the eyeball and cornea), and the posterior ethmoidal nerve (to the sphenoidal sinus and posterior ethmoidal cells), and dividing into the anterior ethmoidal and infratrochlear nerves.

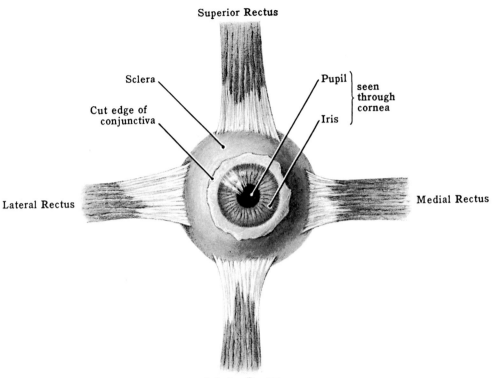

522 Eyeball and Insertions of the Four Recti Oculi, front view

The 4 Recti are spread out to show the insertions of their aponeuroses into the anterior half of the bulb or eyeball, 6 to 8 mm. behind the sclero-corneal junction.

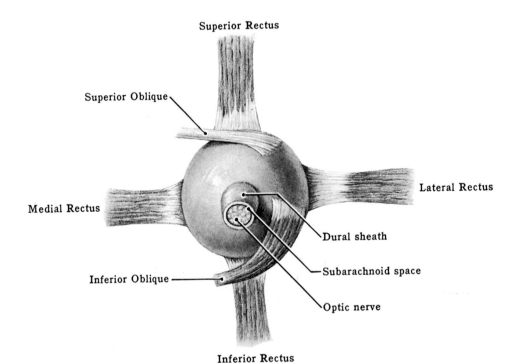

522.1 Eyeball and Insertions of the Two Obliqui Oculi, posterior view

The 2 Obliques are inserted by aponeuroses into the postero-lateral quadrant of the eyeball.

When in situ, Inferior Rectus passes above Inferior Oblique, as in figure 519.

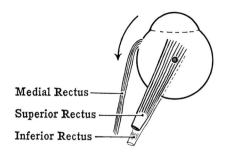

Medial Rectus

Superior Rectus

Inferior Rectus

Inferior Oblique

Superior Oblique

Lateral Rectus

ADDUCTORS **VERTICAL AXIS** ABDUCTORS

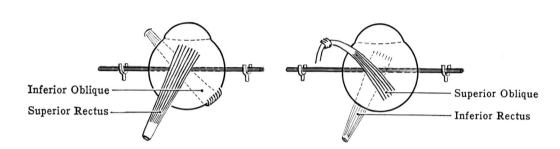

Inferior Oblique

Superior Rectus

Superior Oblique

Inferior Rectus

ELEVATORS **HORIZONTAL AXIS** DEPRESSORS

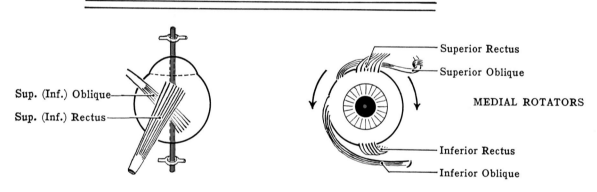

Sup. (Inf.) Oblique

Sup. (Inf.) Rectus

Superior Rectus

Superior Oblique

MEDIAL ROTATORS

Inferior Rectus

Inferior Oblique

MED. (LAT.) ROTATORS LATERAL ROTATORS

SAGITTAL AXIS

523 Actions of the Six Ocular Muscles

In each instance it is the right eyeball that is represented

Note: Of the 6 ocular muscles, the Medial Rectus and the Lateral Rectus move the eyeball on one axis only; each of the four other muscles moves it on all three axes.

Rectus Superior   elevates,   adducts,   and rotates medially.
Rectus Inferior   depresses,   adducts,   and rotates laterally.
Obliquus Superior depresses,   abducts,   and rotates medially.
Obliquus Inferior elevates,   abducts,   and rotates laterally.

The 2 Obliqui also protract (protrude) the eyeball, whereas the 4 Recti retract it.

Clinical tests: It is true that Superior Rectus turns the eye up and, along with Inferior Rectus, assists Medial Rectus to turn the eye in. Clinical evidence, however, proves that the greatest upward action of Superior Rectus is when the eye is turned out—it is then working directly over the centre of rotation. Therefore, the test for the efficiency of Superior Rectus is to look up and out; whereas for Inferior Rectus it is to look down and out.

Similarly, the greatest upward action of Inferior Oblique is when the eye is turned up and in; whereas the greatest downwards action of Superior Oblique is when the eye is turned down and in. Hence, the test for the efficiency of these two muscles is to look in these directions.

523.1 Diagram of the Eyeball, on horizontal section

The Eyeball or Bulbus Oculi has 3 coats.
1. External or fibrous coat:
   sclera and *cornea.*
2. Middle or vascular coat:
   choroid, ciliary body, and *iris.*
3. Internal or retinal coat:
   (a) *outer layer* of pigmented cells,
   (b) *inner layer* of cells which are optic (visual) behind the ora serrata; thin and mostly pigmented in front of it. These extend to the pupillary margin

The 4 Refractive Media are: (1) Cornea; and behind it (2) Aqueous Humor, which fills two chambers or cameras—an anterior in front of the iris and a posterior behind the iris; (3) Lens; and (4) Vitreous Body, a jellylike substance within a capsule, the vitreous (hyaloid) membrane, and occupying the vitreous chamber.

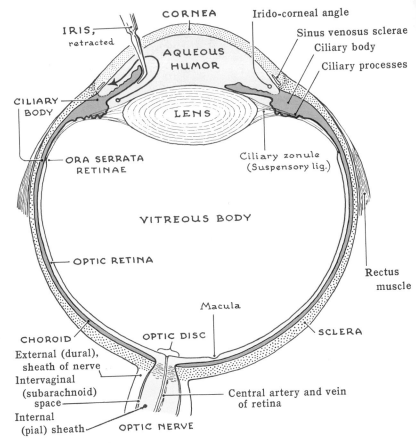

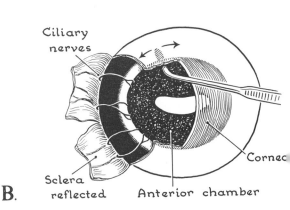

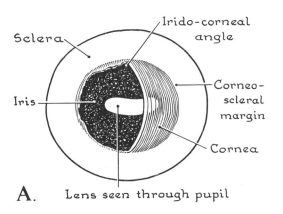

A.

B.

523.2 Eyeball of an Ox

Its anterior half is dissected from the front in 3 stages (A, B, and C) and viewed from behind (D).

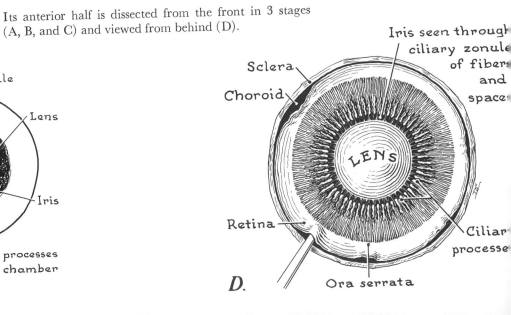

C.

D.

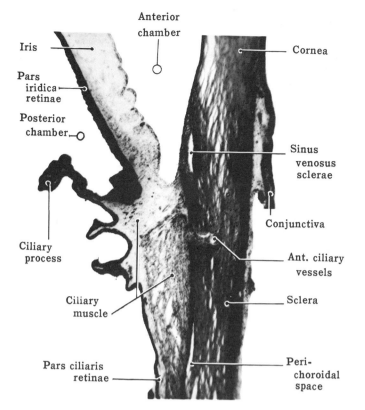

Iris

Pars iridica retinae

Posterior chamber

Ciliary process

Ciliary muscle

Pars ciliaris retinae

Anterior chamber

Cornea

Sinus venosus sclerae

Conjunctiva

Ant. ciliary vessels

Sclera

Peri-choroidal space

523.3   Irido-corneal Region, on microscope section

(Courtesy of Dr. Sylvia Bensley.)

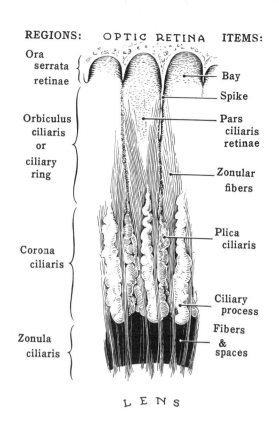

REGIONS: OPTIC RETINA   ITEMS:

Ora serrata retinae

Orbiculus ciliaris or ciliary ring

Corona ciliaris

Zonula ciliaris

Bay

Spike

Pars ciliaris retinae

Zonular fibers

Plica ciliaris

Ciliary process

Fibers & spaces

LENS

523.4   Ciliary and Zonular Regions, viewed from behind, a composite of two illustrations

(Courtesy of Dr. Clement McCulloch.)

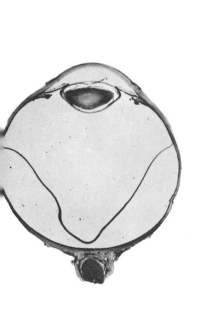

523.5

Section through eyeball in which retina is partially detached. Note varying thicknesses of structures.

(Courtesy of Dr. Sylvia Bensley.)

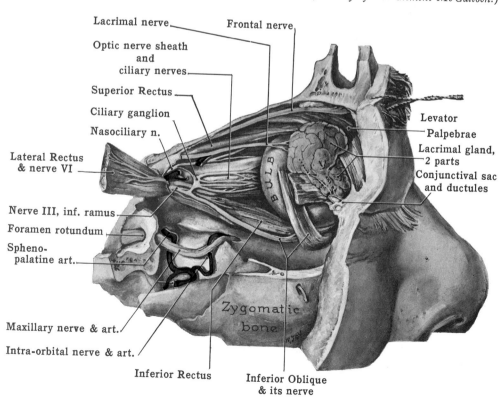

Lacrimal nerve

Frontal nerve

Optic nerve sheath and ciliary nerves

Superior Rectus

Ciliary ganglion

Nasociliary n.

Lateral Rectus & nerve VI

Nerve III, inf. ramus

Foramen rotundum

Spheno-palatine art.

Maxillary nerve & art.

Intra-orbital nerve & art.

Inferior Rectus

Inferior Oblique & its nerve

Levator Palpebrae

Lacrimal gland, 2 parts

Conjunctival sac and ductules

BULB

Zygomatic bone

523.6   Ciliary Ganglion: Dissection of Orbit from lateral approach

(Courtesy of K. O. McCuaig.)

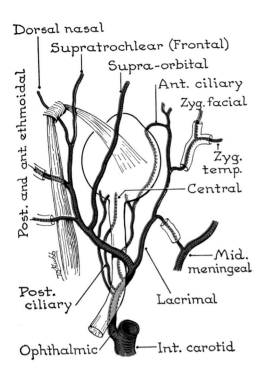

Dorsal nasal

Supratrochlear (Frontal)

Supra-orbital

Ant. ciliary

Zyg. facial

Post. and ant. ethmoidal

Zyg. temp.

Central

Mid. meningeal

Post. ciliary

Lacrimal

Ophthalmic

Int. carotid

524 Diagram of the Ophthalmic Artery

Note:

1. This branch of the internal carotid artery enters the orbit via the optic canal within the dural sheath of the optic nerve shown in figure 516. It supplies the contents of the orbit.
2. Of its branches: the central a. to the retina is an end artery. Of the 8 or so posterior ciliary arteries, 6 supply the choroid which in turn nourishes the outer non-vascular layer of the retina; whereas 2 long posterior ciliary arteries, one on each side of the eyeball, run between sclera and choroid to anastomose with anterior ciliary arteries, which are derived from muscular branches.
3. Six branches pass beyond the orbit (a) supratrochlear a. and (b) supraorbital a. to the forehead, (c) dorsal nasal a. to the face, (d) lacrimal a. to the eyelid and, via its zygomatic branches, to the cheek and the temporal region, and (e and f) anterior and posterior ethmoidal aa. to the nasal cavity. These 6 arteries which extend beyond the orbit anastomose freely with branches of the external carotid artery.
4. The lacrimal artery commonly anastomoses with the middle meningeal artery, via the foramen lacrimale (fig. 509), and may be derived from it.

(For ophthalmic veins, see fig. 504.)

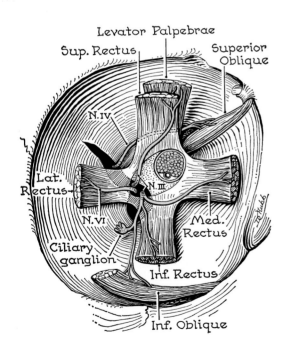

Levator Palpebrae

Sup. Rectus

Superior Oblique

N. IV

Lat. Rectus

N. III

N. VI

Med. Rectus

Ciliary ganglion

Inf. Rectus

Inf. Oblique

525 Diagram of the Motor Nerves of the Orbit

Observe:

1. The optic nerve within its pial, arachnoid, and dural sheaths.
2. The 4 Recti arising from a fibrous cuff, called the anulus tendineus, that encircles:—the dural sheath of the optic nerve, nerve VI (abducent n.), and the upper and lower divisions of nerve III (oculomotor n.). The naso-ciliary nerve (not shown) also passes through this cuff, but nerve IV (trochlear n.) clings to the bony roof of the cavity.
3. Nerves IV and VI supplying one muscle each, and nerve III supplying the remaining five orbital muscles—2 via its upper division; 3 via its lower division and, via the ciliary ganglion, it supplies parasympathetic fibres to the ciliary muscle and sphincter iridis.

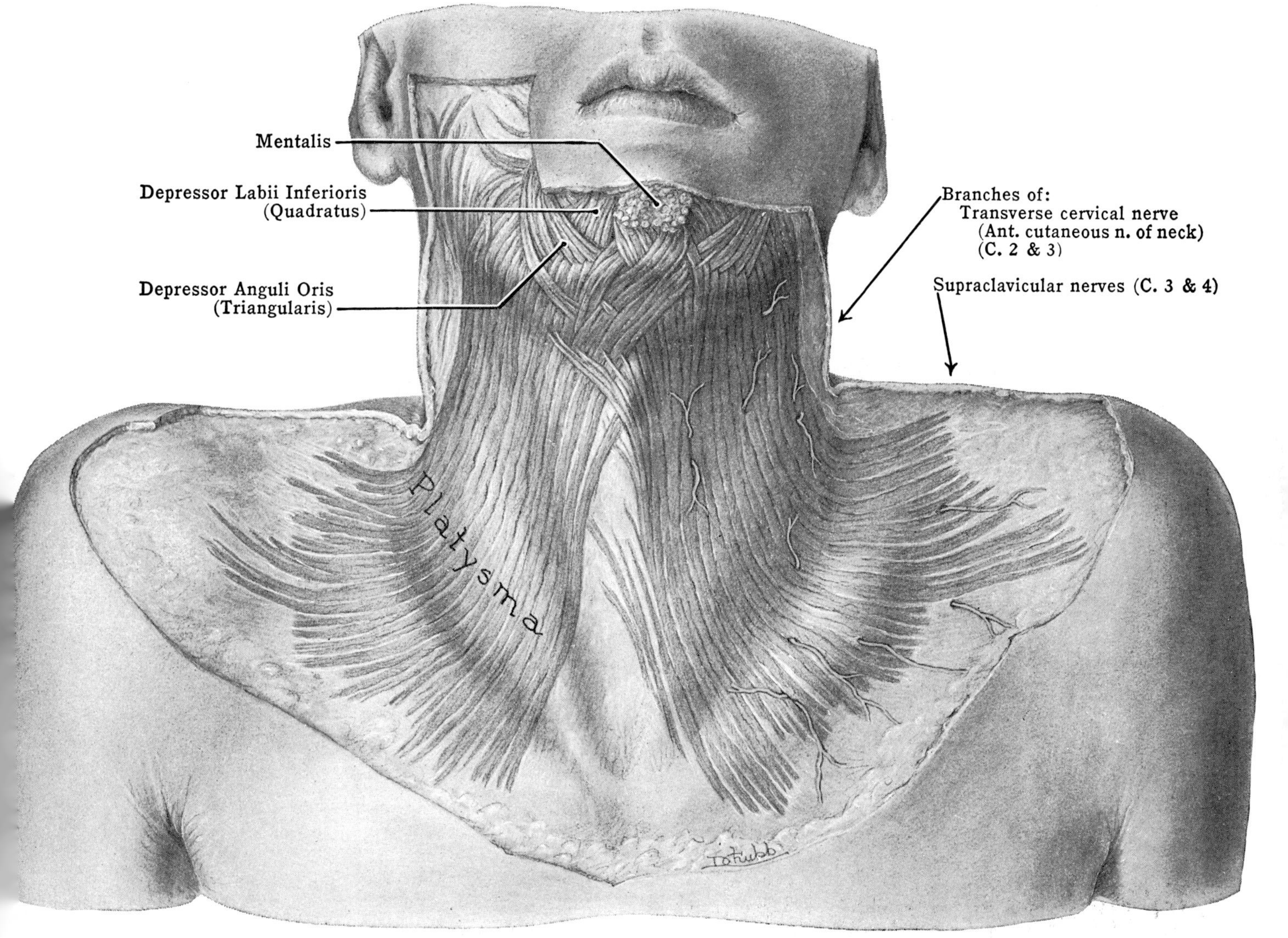

Mentalis

Depressor Labii Inferioris
(Quadratus)

Depressor Anguli Oris
(Triangularis)

Branches of:
Transverse cervical nerve
(Ant. cutaneous n. of neck)
(C. 2 & 3)

Supraclavicular nerves (C. 3 & 4)

Platysma

526   Platysma, front view

Observe:

1. The platysma, spreading subcutaneously like a sheet, pierced by cutaneous nerves, crossing the whole length of the lower border of the mandible above, crossing the whole length of the clavicle below, and extending downwards to the level of the 1st or 2nd rib and to (or towards) the acromion.

2. The anterior borders of the two Platysmas, decussating behind the chin (in the submental region) and, below that, free and diverging, and so leaving the median part of the neck uncovered.

3. Its posterior border, free, covering the antero-inferior part of the posterior triangle, and continuing upwards across the lower border of the jaw to the angle of the mouth.

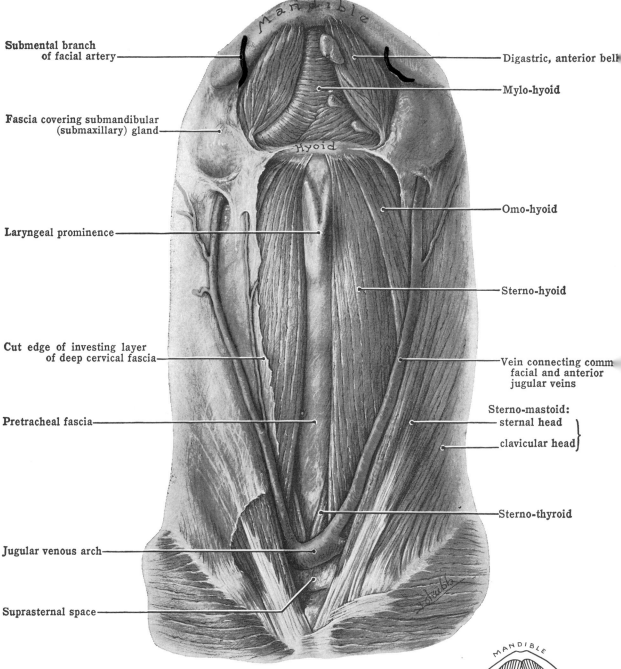

Submental branch
of facial artery

Digastric, anterior bell[y]

Mylo-hyoid

Fascia covering submandibular
(submaxillary) gland

Omo-hyoid

Laryngeal prominence

Sterno-hyoid

Cut edge of investing layer
of deep cervical fascia

Vein connecting comm[on]
facial and anterior
jugular veins

Sterno-mastoid:
sternal head

clavicular head

Pretracheal fascia

Sterno-thyroid

Jugular venous arch

Suprasternal space

527 Median Part of the Front of the Neck—I

Observe:

1. This region, extending from the mandible above to the sternum below; and divided by the hyoid bone into a suprahyoid and an infrahyoid part.

2. The suprahyoid part or submental triangle, having the Digastrics (anterior bellies) for its sides, the hyoid bone for its base, the Mylohyoid for its floor, and some submental lymph nodes for contents. Actually, the submental triangle is part of the floor of the mouth. (Fig. 595).

3. The infrahyoid part, shaped like an elongated diamond, and bounded on each side by Sterno-hyoid above and Sterno-thyroid below.

4. The suprasternal (fascial) space, containing a cross-connecting vein called the jugular venous arch. In this specimen the anterior jugular veins were absent, as such, in the median part of the neck, but were present above the clavicles.

5. The connecting vein along the anterior border of Sternomastoid.

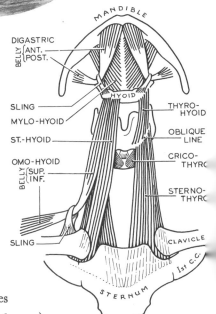

DIGASTRIC
BELLY { ANT.
POST.

SLING

MYLO-HYOID

ST.-HYOID

OMO-HYOID
BELLY { SUP.
INF.

SLING

MANDIBLE

HYOID

THYRO-
HYOID

OBLIQUE
LINE

CRICO-
THYRO[ID]

STERNO-
THYRO[ID]

CLAVICLE

1st C.C.

STERNUM

527.1 Diagram of the Infrahyoid Muscles

(Strap muscles or depressors of hyoid bone and larynx).

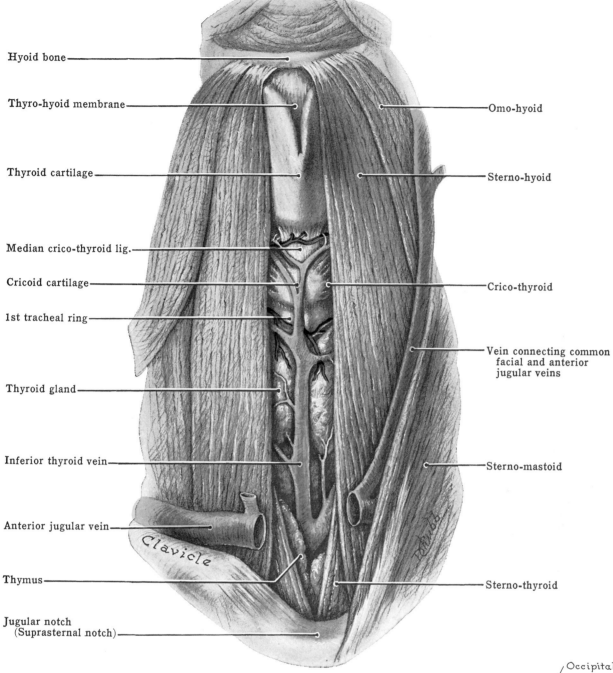

Hyoid bone

Thyro-hyoid membrane

Thyroid cartilage

Median crico-thyroid lig.

Cricoid cartilage

1st tracheal ring

Thyroid gland

Inferior thyroid vein

Anterior jugular vein

Clavicle

Thymus

Jugular notch
(Suprasternal notch)

Omo-hyoid

Sterno-hyoid

Crico-thyroid

Vein connecting common
facial and anterior
jugular veins

Sterno-mastoid

Sterno-thyroid

528　Median Part of the Front of the Neck: Depressors of the Larynx—II

Observe:

1. The structures in the median plane, labelled on the left side of the picture; also the un-labelled anastomoses between the crico-thyroid arteries, between the superior thyroid arteries, and between the anterior jugular veins (excised). Also, the thymus (enlarged) projecting upwards from the thorax. On looking behind it, you might see, peeping above the jugular notch, the left brachiocephalic (innominate) vein and the trunk. (Figs. 449 & 529).

2. The two superficial Depressors of the larynx or "strap muscles"—Omo-hyoid (superior belly) and Sterno-hyoid.

528.1　Diagram of the Ansa Cervicalis

(The upper branch of this nerve to Sterno-hyoid is not usually present.)

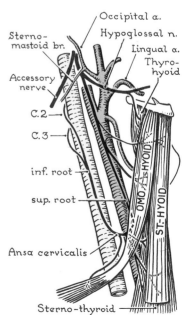

Occipital a.

Sterno-mastoid br.

Hypoglossal n.

Lingual a.

Thyro-hyoid

Accessory nerve

C.2

C.3

inf. root

sup. root

Ansa cervicalis

OMO-HYOID

ST-HYOID

Sterno-thyroid

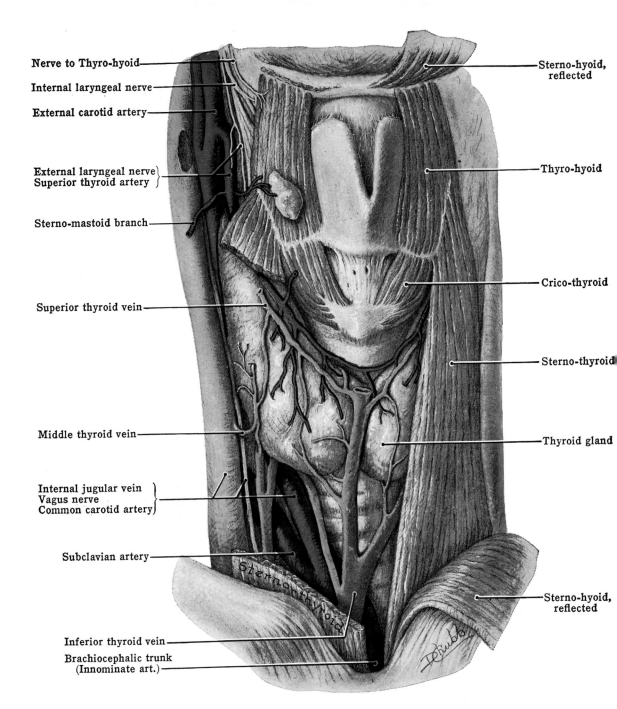

Nerve to Thyro-hyoid

Internal laryngeal nerve

External carotid artery

External laryngeal nerve }
Superior thyroid artery

Sterno-mastoid branch

Superior thyroid vein

Middle thyroid vein

Internal jugular vein }
Vagus nerve
Common carotid artery

Subclavian artery

Inferior thyroid vein

Brachiocephalic trunk
(Innominate art.)

Sterno-hyoid,
reflected

Thyro-hyoid

Crico-thyroid

Sterno-thyroid

Thyroid gland

Sterno-hyoid,
reflected

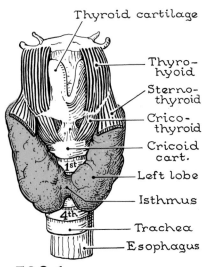

Thyroid cartilage

Thyro-hyoid

Sterno-thyroid

Crico-thyroid

Cricoid cart.

Left lobe

Isthmus

Trachea

Esophagus

529.1

Diagram. Thyroid Gland, in situ

529 Front of the Neck: Depressors of the Larynx: Thyroid Gland—III

On left side the two superficial Depressors (Sternohyoid and Omo-hyoid) are reflected and the two deep Depressors (Sterno-thyroid and Thyro-hyoid) are thereby uncovered. On right side, Sterno-thyroid is largely excised.

Observe:

1. The two lobes of the thyroid gland, united across the median plane by an isthmus.
2. The surface network of veins on the gland, drained by the superior, middle, and inferior thyroid veins.
3. The right lobe of the gland, overlying the common carotid artery.
4. The upper pole of the right lobe, pushing the superior thyroid artery into the angle between the attachments of Sterno-thyroid and Inferior Constrictor to the thyroid cartilage, and therefore, against the external laryngeal nerve (see also figs. 530 and 534).
5. An accessory thyroid gland, or detached lobule, occasionally present.

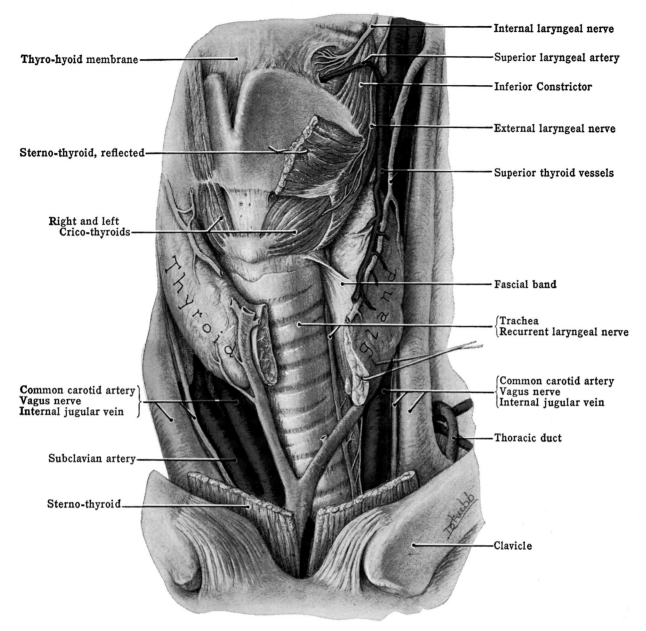

Thyro-hyoid membrane

Sterno-thyroid, reflected

Right and left
Crico-thyroids

Common carotid artery
Vagus nerve
Internal jugular vein

Subclavian artery

Sterno-thyroid

Internal laryngeal nerve

Superior laryngeal artery

Inferior Constrictor

External laryngeal nerve

Superior thyroid vessels

Fascial band

Trachea
Recurrent laryngeal nerve

Common carotid artery
Vagus nerve
Internal jugular vein

Thoracic duct

Clavicle

530   Front of the Neck: Thyroid Gland—IV

The isthmus of the thyroid gland is divided; and the left lobe is retracted.

Observe:

1. The retaining fascial band, attaching the capsule of the
thyroid gland to the crico-tracheal ligament and cricoid
cartilage.

2. The left recurrent laryngeal nerve, on the side of the
trachea, just in front of the angle between the trachea and
esophagus, and behind the retaining band.

3. The internal laryngeal nerve, running along the upper

border of Inferior Constrictor, and piercing the thyro-
hyoid membrane as several branches.

4. The external laryngeal nerve, applied to Inferior Constrictor, running along the anterior border of the superior
thyroid artery, passing deep to the insertion of Sterno-
thyroid, and giving twigs to Inferior Constrictor and
piercing it before ending in Crico-thyroid.

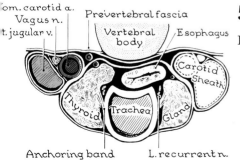

om. carotid a.
Vagus n.
t. jugular v.
Prevertebral fascia
Vertebral body
Esophagus
Carotid Sheath
Thyroid
Trachea
Gland
Anchoring band
L. recurrent n.

530.1

Diagram. Relations of Thyroid Gland,

530.2

Diagram to explain how Crico-thyroids,
acting on the crico-thyroid joints,
render taut the vocal cords.

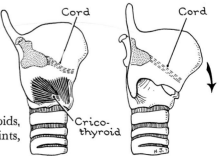

Cord

Cord

Crico-thyroid

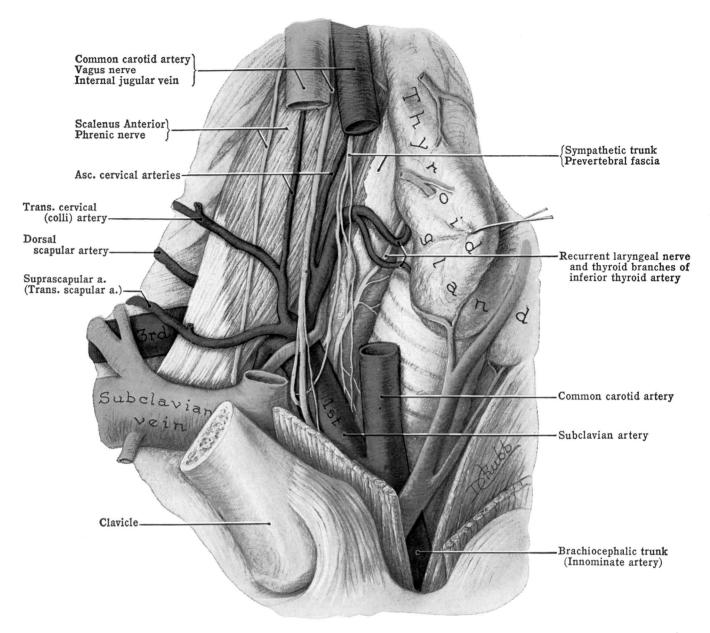

Common carotid artery
Vagus nerve
Internal jugular vein

Scalenus Anterior
Phrenic nerve

Asc. cervical arteries

Trans. cervical (colli) artery

Dorsal scapular artery

Suprascapular a. (Trans. scapular a.)

3rd

Subclavian vein

1st

Clavicle

Thyroid gland

Sympathetic trunk
Prevertebral fascia

Recurrent laryngeal nerve and thyroid branches of inferior thyroid artery

Common carotid artery

Subclavian artery

Brachiocephalic trunk (Innominate artery)

531 Root of the Neck, right side

The clavicle is removed; sections are taken from the common cartoid art. and int. jugular vein; the right lobe of the thyroid gland is retracted.

Observe:

1. The brachiocephalic trunk dividing behind the sterno-clavicular joint into the right common carotid and right subclavian arteries.

2. Scalenus Anterior, dividing the subclavian artery into three parts—1st, 2nd, and 3rd—and separating the 2nd part from the subclavian vein. This vein, lying antero-inferior to the artery, and joining the internal jugular vein at the medial border of Scalenus Anterior to form the brachiocephalic vein.

3. Running vertically on the obliquely placed Scalenus Anterior: (a) the common carotid artery, internal jugular vein, and vagus nerve (inside the carotid sheath); (b) the sympathetic trunk behind the common carotid artery (outside the sheath); (c) the ascending cervical artery (here represented by two vessels); and (d) most lateral of all, the phrenic nerve which is clamped down by two arteries and, therefore cannot be mistaken for the vagus nerve.

4. The vagus, crossing the 1st part of the subclavian artery, and giving off an (inferior) cardiac branch and the recurrent laryngeal nerve. The latter (a) recurring below the artery, (b) crossing behind the common carotid artery on its way to the side of the trachea, and (c) giving twigs to the trachea and esophagus, and receiving twigs from the sympathetic.

5. The sympathetic trunk, throwing a fine loop, the ansa sub-clavia, around the 1st part of the artery. The middle cervical ganglion is not labelled.

6. The thyro-cervical trunk (not labelled), dividing into the inferior thyroid artery which takes an S-shaped course, and the transverse cervical and suprascapular arteries which cross Scalenus Anterior.

7. The deep or dorsal scapular branch of the trans. cervical artery, here and commonly, springing from the 2nd or 3rd part of the subclavian artery. The vertebral vein (not labelled) crossing the 1st part of the artery.

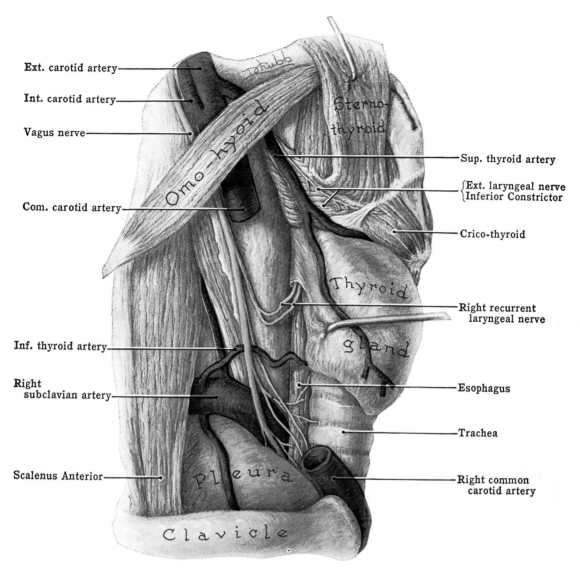

Ext. carotid artery

Int. carotid artery

Vagus nerve

Com. carotid artery

Inf. thyroid artery

Right subclavian artery

Scalenus Anterior

Sup. thyroid artery

Ext. laryngeal nerve
Inferior Constrictor

Crico-thyroid

Right recurrent laryngeal nerve

Esophagus

Trachea

Right common carotid artery

532 Anomalous Right Recurrent Laryngeal Nerve

From the same subject as figure 447.2

Occasionally the right subclavian artery springs directly from the aortic arch, as its fourth branch, and passes behind the trachea and esophagus. For embryological reasons, shown in figure 447, the right recurrent nerve, having then no artery around which to recur, takes an almost direct course to the larynx. As would be expected, many of its esophageal and tracheal branches then spring directly from the parent vagus nerve.

Note: The inferior thyroid artery here springs directly from the subclavian artery. The vertebral and internal thoracic arteries are not labelled.

ANOMALY

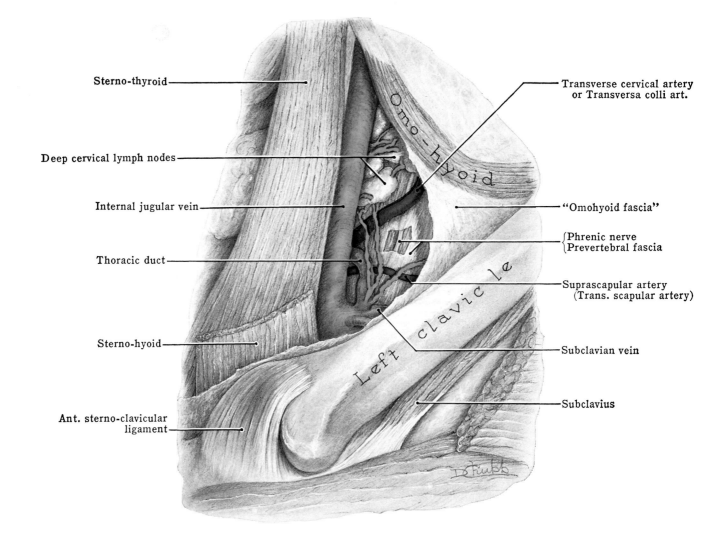

Sterno-thyroid

Deep cervical lymph nodes

Internal jugular vein

Thoracic duct

Sterno-hyoid

Ant. sterno-clavicular ligament

Omo-hyoid

Left clavicle

Transverse cervical artery or Transversa colli art.

"Omohyoid fascia"

{ Phrenic nerve
{ Prevertebral fascia

Suprascapular artery (Trans. scapular artery)

Subclavian vein

Subclavius

533 Termination of the Thoracic Duct

Sternomastoid and the enveloping fascia of the neck are removed. The deeper layer of fascia, "the Omohyoid fascia", is partly snipped away.

Observe:

1. "The Omohyoid fascia", continuous in front of Sternohyoid and across the suprasternal space with the fascia of the opposite side.

2. The thoracic duct, receiving a tributary from the nodes of the neck (jugular trunk), another from the nodes of upper limb (subclavian trunk), and ending in the angle between the internal jugular and subclavian veins. (For thoracic course, figs. 453 and 429).

3. The phrenic nerve, descending in naked contact with Scalenus Anterior, i.e., deep to Scalenus Anterior fascia, which is a lateral prolongation of the prevertebral fascia, and clamped down by the 2 arteries labelled.

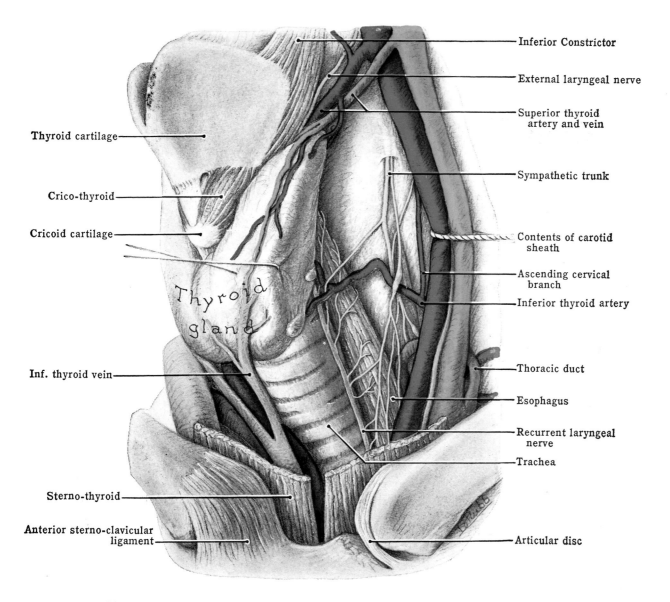

Thyroid cartilage

Crico-thyroid

Cricoid cartilage

Thyroid gland

Inf. thyroid vein

Sterno-thyroid

Anterior sterno-clavicular ligament

Inferior Constrictor

External laryngeal nerve

Superior thyroid artery and vein

Sympathetic trunk

Contents of carotid sheath

Ascending cervical branch

Inferior thyroid artery

Thoracic duct

Esophagus

Recurrent laryngeal nerve

Trachea

Articular disc

534 Root of the Neck, left side

(Esophagus, Trachea, Left Recurrent Laryngeal Nerve, Thoracic Duct.)

Observe:

1. The three structures contained in the carotid sheath (internal jugular vein, common carotid artery, and vagus nerve), retracted.

2. The esophagus, bulging to the left of the trachea. It does not bulge to the right.

3. The left recurrent nerve, ascending on the side of the trachea just in front of the angle between the trachea and esophagus, giving twigs to the esophagus and trachea (not in view), and receiving twigs from the sympathetic.

4. The thoracic duct, passing from the side of the esophagus to its termination (figs. 533 & 453) and, in so doing, arching immediately behind the 3 structures contained in the carotid sheath.

5. The middle cervical (sympathetic) ganglion, here in 2 parts: one in front of the inferior thyroid artery; the other, just above the thoracic duct, is called the vertebral ganglion.

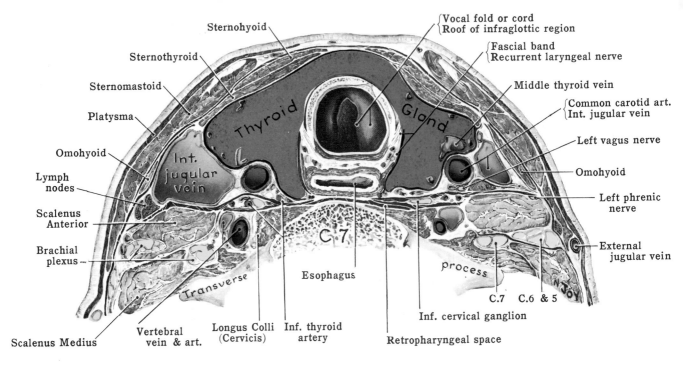

Cross section of Neck labels:
Sternohyoid — Vocal fold or cord / Roof of infraglottic region — Fascial band / Recurrent laryngeal nerve — Middle thyroid vein — Common carotid art. / Int. jugular vein — Left vagus nerve — Omohyoid — Left phrenic nerve — External jugular vein — Inf. cervical ganglion — C.7 — C.6 & 5 — Retropharyngeal space — Inf. thyroid artery — Esophagus — Longus Colli (Cervicis) — Vertebral vein & art. — Transverse — Scalenus Medius — Brachial plexus — Scalenus Anterior — Lymph nodes — Omohyoid — Platysma — Sternomastoid — Sternothyroid — Int. jugular vein — Thyroid Gland — process

535 Cross section of Neck, at the level of the Thyroid Gland, from below

Observe:

1. The thyroid gland, within its sheath, asymmetrically enlarged and overflowing the carotid sheath and its contents (common carotid artery, internal jugular vein and vagus nerve) on one side and thrusting it laterally on the other.

2. The internal jugular veins, of unequal size, as sometimes happens; and usually unequal vertebral arteries.

3. The retropharyngeal space of loose areolar tissue, extending far laterally behind the carotid sheath. The approach to the space is from the posterior border to Sternomastoid.

4. Scalenus Anterior deep to the posterior border to Sternomastoid.

5. The vertebral artery and vein near the apex of the "Triangle of the Vertebral Artery" (fig. 536A) between Longus Colli and Scalenus Anterior.

6. The brachial plexus passing infero-laterally between Scalenus Anterior and Scalenus Medius (see fig. 475).

7. The inferior thyroid artery (divided twice) and the middle cervical ganglion on a plane between the carotid sheath and the vertebral artery.

8. The fascial band that retains the thyroid gland and, behind it, the recurrent laryngeal nerve and the inferior laryngeal artery (see fig. 530).

9. The vocal folds and the conus elasticus (crico-vocal membranes), covered with mucous membrane and having the same shape as the tentorium cerebelli (fig. 572), hence, air expelled forcibly from the lungs would blow the vocal folds apart.

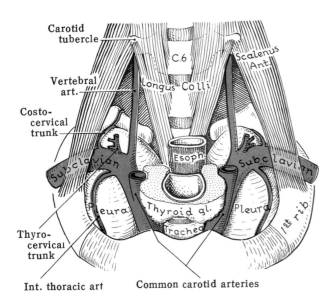

536A Triangle of the Vertebral Artery

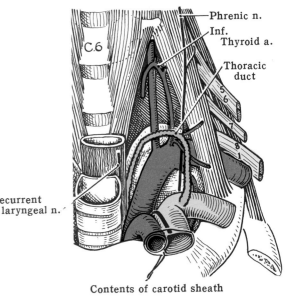

536B Course of the Thoracic Duct in Neck

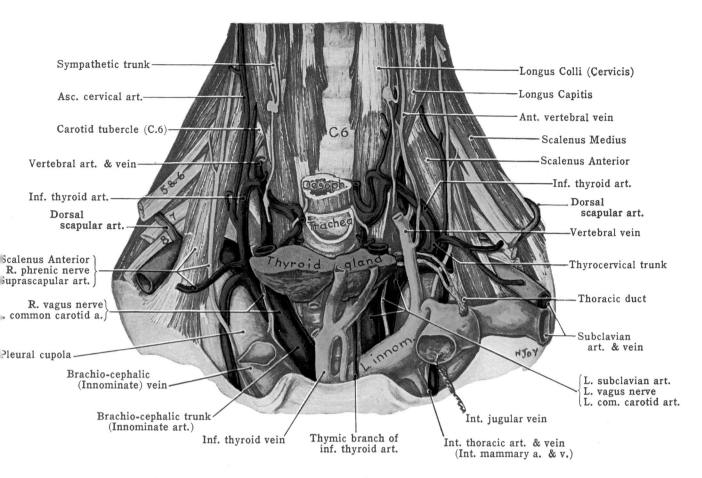

Sympathetic trunk
Asc. cervical art.
Carotid tubercle (C.6)
Vertebral art. & vein
Inf. thyroid art.
Dorsal scapular art.
Scalenus Anterior }
R. phrenic nerve }
Suprascapular art. }
R. vagus nerve }
common carotid a. }
Pleural cupola
Brachio-cephalic (Innominate) vein
Brachio-cephalic trunk (Innominate art.)
Inf. thyroid vein
Thymic branch of inf. thyroid art.
Int. jugular vein
Int. thoracic art. & vein (Int. mammary a. & v.)

Longus Colli (Cervicis)
Longus Capitis
Ant. vertebral vein
Scalenus Medius
Scalenus Anterior
Inf. thyroid art.
Dorsal scapular art.
Vertebral vein
Thyrocervical trunk
Thoracic duct
Subclavian art. & vein
{ L. subclavian art.
{ L. vagus nerve
{ L. com. carotid art.

C.6 — Oesoph. — Trachea — Thyroid gland — L. innom.

536 Root of the Neck, viewed obliquely from above

Observe:

1. *Laterally:* The pleural cupola, rising 1½ inches above the sternal end of the 1st rib. The subclavian artery, which arches over the pleura, divided into 3 unequal parts by Scalenus Anterior. The 3rd part of the artery and the brachial plexus appearing between Scalenus Anterior and Scalenus Medius, the lowest trunk of the plexus (C.8 & T.1) being behind the artery.

2. The phrenic nerve, descending almost vertically and crossing the obliquely running Scalenus Anterior to which it is clamped by the suprascapular artery and, on leaving Scalenus Anterior, lying on the pleura and crossing the internal thoracic artery before meeting the right brachio-cephalic vein.

3. *In the Median Plane:* The esophagus applied to the vertebral column, the trachea applied to the esophagus, the thyroid gland applied to the trachea and overlapping the common carotid arteries. The inferior thyroid veins descending to the left brachio-cephalic (innominate) vein, and an occasional branch of the inferior thyroid artery descending to the thymus).

4. *Lateral to these Median Structures:* "The Triangle of the Vertebral Artery" (see above, A & B) bounded laterally by Scalenus Anterior, and medially by Longus Colli. The apex where these 2 muscles meet at the carotid tubercle (ant. tubercle of trans. process of C.6); the base being the lst part

of the subclavian artery. The vertebral artery, which ascends from base to apex, dividing the triangle into 2 nearly equal parts.

Anterior to the triangle, the carotid sheath and its 3 contents (artery, vein and nerve). On the left side, between sheath and vertebral artery, and therefore below the level of the carotid tubercle, 2 vessels arching in opposite directions—the inferior thyroid artery and the thoracic duct. The artery of both sides arching medially, and on the left side the duct arching laterally. The artery reaching the thyroid gland as 2 branches, an upper and a lower. The recurrent laryngeal nerve bears a varying relationship to these 2 terminal arteries (being either anterior to, or posterior to, or between, them), here, between them.

The duct pulled down by the reflected internal jugular vein in which it ends. The arching duct lying immediately behind the carotid sheath and its 3 contents and sometimes, as here, a 4th structure, namely, the vertebral vein.

5. The right and left vagus nerves descending on the lateral side of the corresponding common carotid artery; the right vagus being conducted to the subclavian artery which it crosses, giving off its recurrent nerve (not labelled) as it does so; the left vagus being conducted to the aortic arch (not in view) where it behaves similarly. The vagus nerves, free, and not clamped down as are the phrenic nerves.

Scalenus Anterior intervening between the subclavian artery and vein.

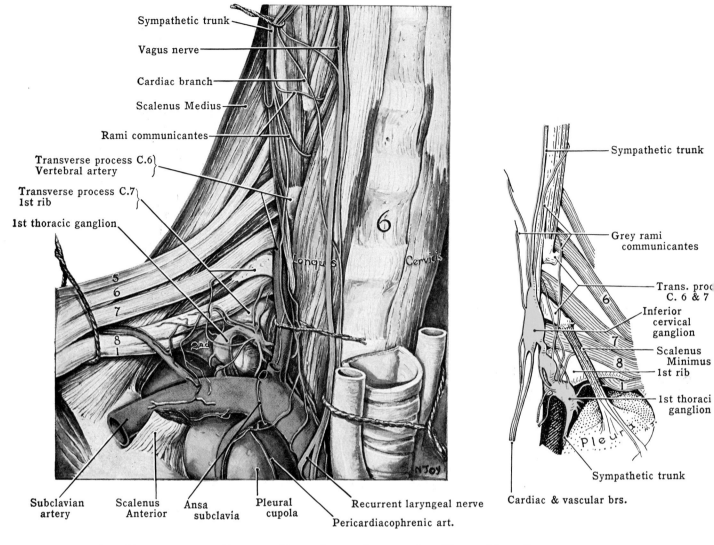

Sympathetic trunk

Vagus nerve

Cardiac branch

Scalenus Medius

Rami communicantes

Transverse process C.6
Vertebral artery

Transverse process C.7
1st rib

1st thoracic ganglion

Sympathetic trunk

Grey rami
communicantes

Trans. proc
C. 6 & 7

Inferior
cervical
ganglion

Scalenus
Minimus

1st rib

1st thoracic
ganglion

Sympathetic trunk

Subclavian
artery

Scalenus
Anterior

Ansa
subclavia

Pleural
cupola

Recurrent laryngeal nerve

Pericardiacophrenic art.

Cardiac & vascular brs.

537 Stellate Ganglion [Cervico-thoracic Ganglion]

The pleura has been depressed and the vertebral artery retracted. (Dissection by G. F. Lewis.)

Observe:

1. The lowest trunk of the brachial plexus (C. 8 & T. 1) raised from the groove it occupies on the 1st rib behind the sub-clavian artery; the dorsal scapular artery (not labelled) here arising from the 3rd part of the artery and passing through the plexus (fig. 471). (fig. 471.5).

2. The sympathetic trunk (retracted laterally) sending a communicating branch to the vagus, and gray rami communicantes (postganglionic fibres) to the roots of the cervical nerves, and cardiac branches.

3. The vertebral artery, retracted medially in order to uncover the stellate ganglion (i.e., the combined inferior cervical and 1st thoracic ganglia) which rests behind it on the 1st and 2nd ribs.

4. Fine branches passing from the ganglion to nerves C. 7, 8,

and T. 1, and to adjacent arteries.

5. The vertebral ganglion, quite small, just below the thread that retracts the vertebral artery. From this ganglion the sympathetic trunk passing behind the vertebral artery to join the stellate ganglion, but before so doing sending a slender branch around the subclavian artery as the ansa subclavia.

6. On the left side a pen and ink tracing of a photograph of a dissection of the left side of the same specimen, revealing a very different pattern. Thus, the inferior cervical ganglion occupies its more usual position between the transverse process of C. 7 and the 1st rib, ganglion T. 1 being on and below the 1st rib. Scalenus Minimus (Scalenus Pleuralis) here present (also in fig. 567).

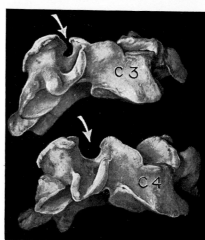

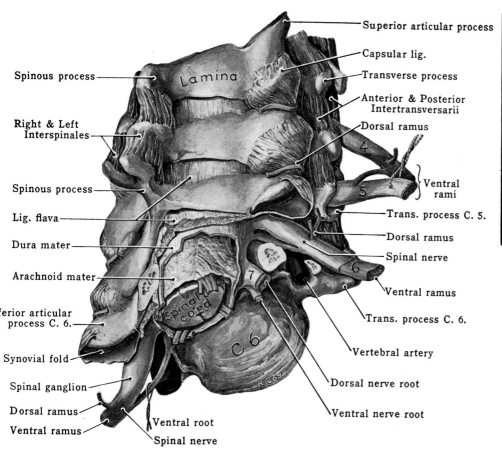

Superior articular process

Capsular lig.

Transverse process

Anterior & Posterior Intertransversarii

Dorsal ramus

Spinous process

Lamina

Right & Left Interspinales

Ventral rami

Spinous process

Trans. process C. 5.

Lig. flava

Dorsal ramus

Dura mater

Spinal nerve

Arachnoid mater

Ventral ramus

...ferior articular process C. 6.

Trans. process C. 6.

Synovial fold

Vertebral artery

Spinal ganglion

Dorsal nerve root

Dorsal ramus

Ventral nerve root

Ventral ramus

Ventral root

Spinal nerve

38   A Cervical Nerve, in situ

...serve:

Two paired Interspinales uniting the bifid ends of 3 spinous processes.
Capsular ligaments uniting articular processes.

Anterior and Posterior Intertransversarii uniting anterior and posterior tubercles of transverse processes.

The ligamentum flavum attached to the upper border of one lamina and to the ventral surface of the lamina next above, and extending transversely from one articular capsule to the other.

Dura mater applied to ligamentum flavum; arachnoid mater applied to dura and separated from pia mater, which clothes the medulla or cord, by cerebrospinal fluid, which has escaped.

The fila of the dorsal nerve roots (7th & 8th) leaving the spinal medulla in single file. One filum of C. 8 joining C. 7.

Dura (and arachnoid) carried distally as a covering for the roots, nerve, and rami and gradually fading away.

A dorsal nerve root (here 6th and 7th) larger than a ventral root; its swelling, the spinal ganglion. The 2 roots, each in a separate dural sheath, uniting beyond the ganglion to form a spinal nerve. The nerve, about 1 cm. long, dividing into a small dorsal and a large ventral ramus.

The roots and the nerve crossing behind the vertebral artery. The dorsal ramus of the spinal nerve curving dorsally, applied to the root of a superior articular process, and passing medial to a Posterior Intertransverse muscle. The ventral ramus resting on the transverse process, which is grooved to support it, and emerging between an anterior and a posterior intertransverse muscle. C. 5 raised from its grooved bed.

Inset: On vertebra C. 3, in contrast with C. 4, bony overgrowths at intervertebral foramen (on sup. articular process and body) may constrict the roots of the nerve. This condition is not uncommon in the cervical vertebrae of dissecting-room subjects.

Synovial folds projecting between articular surfaces, as they do elsewhere.

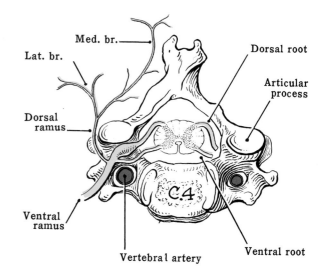

Med. br.

Lat. br.

Dorsal root

Articular process

Dorsal ramus

Ventral ramus

Vertebral artery

Ventral root

538.1

Semidiagram of the spinal, or central, end of a Segmental Nerve, after removal of the meninges, showing relationship to vertebral artery.

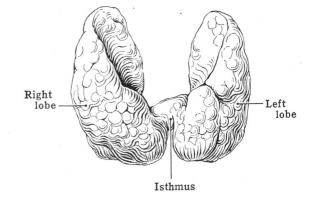

Right lobe — Left lobe

Isthmus

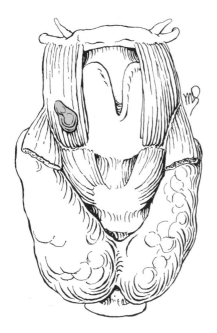

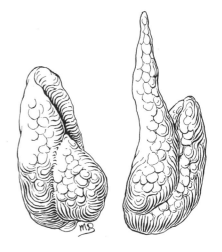

B **An Accessory Thyroid Gland** may occur between the levels of the suprahyoid region and the aortic arch. (See fig. 529.)

C **Pyramidal Lobe. Absence of Isthmus.** About 50% of glands have a pyramidal lobe which extends from near the isthmus to, or towards, the hyoid bone. The isthmus is occasionally absent, the gland being then in two parts.

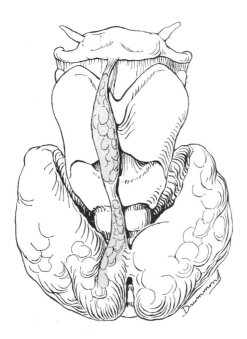

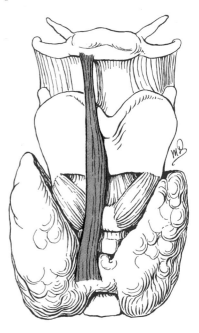

D **Accessory Thyroid Tissue** may occur along the course of the thyroglossal duct.

E **Levator Glandulae Thyroideae** sometimes present, is an errant slip of infrahyoid musculature.

539 Thyroid Gland

VARIATIONS AND ANOMALIES

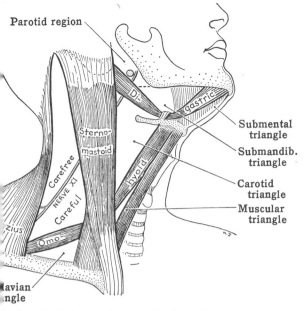

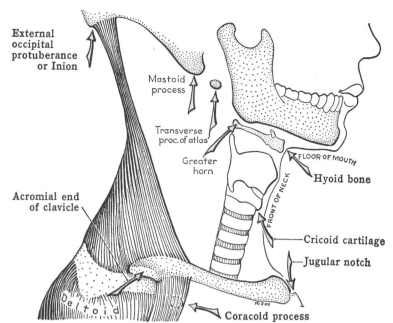

40 Triangles of the Neck

te:

The obliquely set Sternomastoid divides the side of the neck o an anterior and a posterior triangle.

The anterior triangle is bounded by Sternomastoid, the dian line of the neck, and the lower border of the mandible. is subdivided into 3 smaller triangles—submandibular, otid, and muscular. The posterior belly of Digastric (and lohyoid) separates the carotid triangle from the submandib- r triangle; the superior belly of Omohyoid separates the otid triangle from the muscular triangle. The region be- en the anterior bellies of the Digastrics and the body of hyoid bone is the (unpaired) submental triangle.

The posterior triangle is bounded by Trapezius, Sterno- stoid, and the middle third of the clavicle (figs. 472–475). is divisible into a subclavian (supraclavicular) and an oc- ital triangle by the inferior belly of Omohyoid, but of much ater significance is the fact that it is divided by the accessory ve (nerve XI) into nearly equal upper and lower parts. Of se, the upper contains little of importance, but the lower tains numerous structures of great importance. Hence, ve the nerve your dissection may be carefree, whereas ow it you must proceed very carefully.

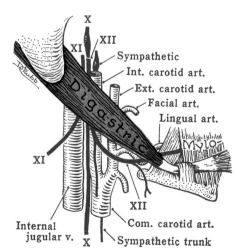

540.1 Bony Landmarks of the Neck

Note:

The inion and the mastoid process (and the superior nuchal line uniting them) are created by the downward pull of Trape- zius and Sternomastoid.

The transverse process of the atlas, being the most prominent of the cervical transverse processes, is felt with the finger-tip on pressing upwards between the angle of the jaw and the mastoid process.

The body of the hyoid bone lies at the angle between the floor of the mouth and the front of the neck.

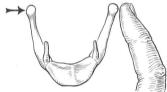

The greater horn of one side of the hyoid bone is palpable only when the greater horn of the opposite side is steadied.

The arch of the cricoid cartilage projects beyond the rings of the trachea (figs. 622, 623), and is thereby readily identified in life, on running the finger-tip upwards. It is the guide to the level of C.6, where so many things happen.

The jugular (suprasternal) notch is visible and palpable be- tween the medial ends of the clavicles.

The lateral end of the clavicle, being thicker than the acro- mium, is palpable on pressing medially, above the acromion.

The coracoid process, located 1″ below the clavicle, under the edge of the Deltoid, is palpable on pressing laterally with the finger in the deltopectoral triangle.

Note:

1. Except for:—(a) cervical brs. of the facial nerve, (b) facial brs. of the great auricular nerve, and (c) the ext. jugular vein and its connections (figs. 467 & 471.3), all vessels and nerves crossing this belly cross deep to it pathetic trunk (fig. 551).
2. This belly runs from mastoid process to hyoid bone, and crosses deep to the angle of the jaw.

.2

ram of the posterior belly of Digastric to demon- : its superficial and key position.

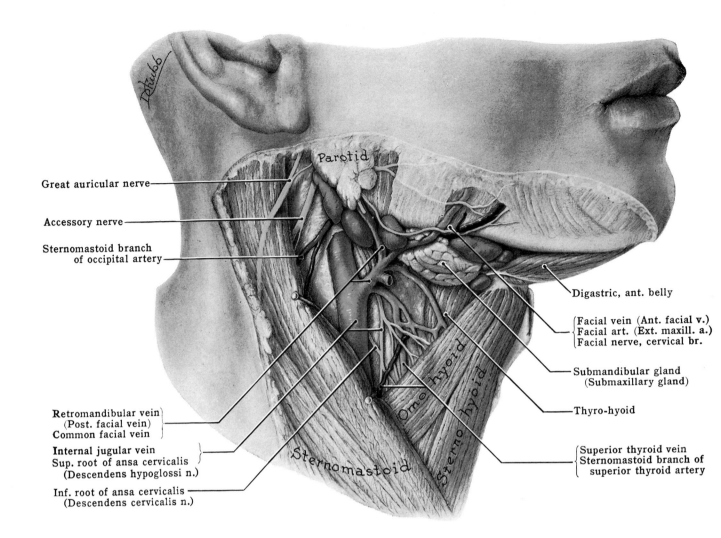

Great auricular nerve

Accessory nerve

Sternomastoid branch
of occipital artery

Parotid

Digastric, ant. belly

Facial vein (Ant. facial v.)
Facial art. (Ext. maxill. a.)
Facial nerve, cervical br.

Submandibular gland
(Submaxillary gland)

Thyro-hyoid

Retromandibular vein
(Post. facial vein)
Common facial vein

Internal jugular vein
Sup. root of ansa cervicalis
(Descendens hypoglossi n.)

Inf. root of ansa cervicalis
(Descendens cervicalis n.)

Superior thyroid vein
Sternomastoid branch of
superior thyroid artery

541 Anterior Triangle of the Neck, superficial dissection—I

Observe:

1. The accessory nerve entering the deep surface of Sternomastoid between $1\frac{1}{2}$ and $2\frac{1}{2}$ inches below the tip of the mastoid process, and joined along its lower border by the sternomastoid branch of the occipital artery.

2. The internal jugular vein joined in front by several veins, notably, common facial vein, about the level of the hyoid bone.

3. Branches of the ansa cervicalis (ansa hypoglossi) passing deep to Omohyoid.

4. The sternomastoid branch of the superior thyroid artery descending near the upper border of Omohyoid.

5. The submandibular gland and lymph nodes filling—and indeed overflowing—the submandibular triangle (digastric triangle). The retromandibular and facial veins running superficial to the gland.

Continued from page facing

border of Omohyoid; (b) the nerve to Thyrohyoid crossing the greater horn of the hyoid bone to enter the superficial surface of this muscle.

7. The internal and external laryngeal nerves appearing deep to the external carotid artery; the former following the upper border of Inferior Constrictor and piercing the thyrohyoid membrane; the latter applied to Inferior Constrictor and lying close to the superior thyroid artery and giving it twigs.

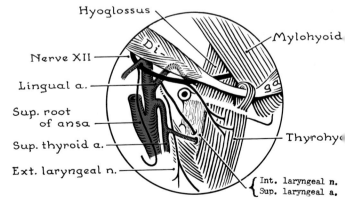

Hyoglossus

Mylohyoid

Nerve XII

Lingual a.

Sup. root
of ansa

Sup. thyroid a.

Ext. laryngeal n.

Thyrohyo[

Int. laryngeal n.
Sup. laryngeal a.

541.1

Diagram:

1. The tip of the greater horn is the reference point for ma[
structures—muscles, nerves, and arteries.

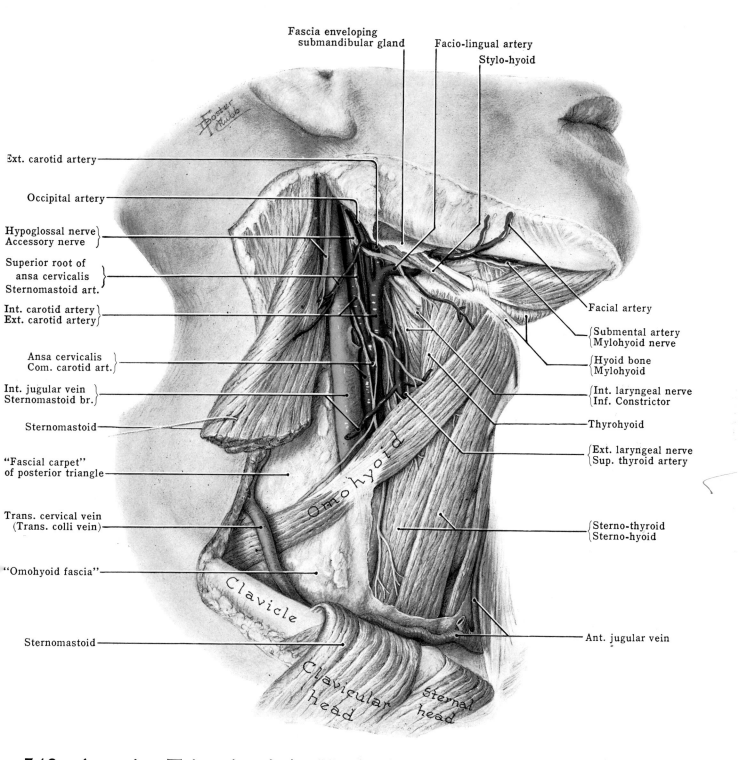

Fascia enveloping
submandibular gland

Facio-lingual artery
Stylo-hyoid

Ext. carotid artery

Occipital artery

Hypoglossal nerve }
Accessory nerve }

Superior root of
ansa cervicalis }
Sternomastoid art.

Int. carotid artery }
Ext. carotid artery }

Ansa cervicalis }
Com. carotid art. }

Int. jugular vein }
Sternomastoid br. }

Sternomastoid

"Fascial carpet"
of posterior triangle

Trans. cervical vein
(Trans. colli vein)

"Omohyoid fascia"

Sternomastoid

Facial artery

{ Submental artery
{ Mylohyoid nerve

{ Hyoid bone
{ Mylohyoid

{ Int. laryngeal nerve
{ Inf. Constrictor

Thyrohyoid

{ Ext. laryngeal nerve
{ Sup. thyroid artery

{ Sterno-thyroid
{ Sterno-hyoid

Ant. jugular vein

Omohyoid

Clavicle

Clavicular head

Sternal head

542 Anterior Triangle of the Neck, deeper dissection—II

Observe:

1. The intermediate tendon of Digastric held down to the hyoid bone by a fascial sling; the intermediate tendon of Omohyoid similarly held down to the clavicle.

2. The remains of the fascial sheath of the submandibular gland which posteriorly, as the stylo-mandibular ligament, separates this gland from the parotid gland.

3. The facial and lingual arteries, here arising by a common stem, passing deep to Stylohyoid and Digastric to enter the submandibular triangle The facial artery here giving off its submental branch, which accompanies the mylohyoid nerve.

4. Thyrohyoid and Inferior Constrictor forming the floor (more

literally, the medial wall) of the carotid triangle.

5. The hypoglossal nerve curving into the carotid triangle and curving out again; passing deep to Digastric twice; crossing the internal and external carotid arteries and giving off two branches from its convex side.

6. Of these branches, note (a) the superior root of the ansa cervicalis arising from the hypoglossal nerve where the sternomastoid artery arises from the occipital artery, descending superficial to the internal and common carotid arteries outside their fascial sheath, and joining the inferior root of ansa cervicalis (C.2 and 3) which appears on the medial side of the internal jugular vein (commonly on the lateral side) to form the ansa cervicalis near the upper

Continued on page opposite

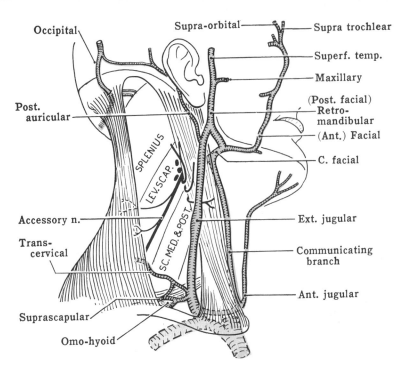

543   Diagram of the Superficial Veins of the Neck

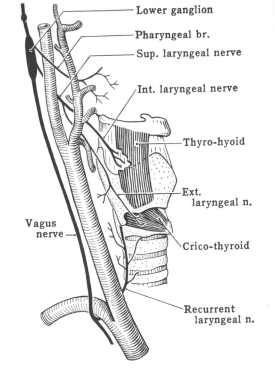

543.1   Diagram of the Laryngeal Branches of Right Vagus Nerve

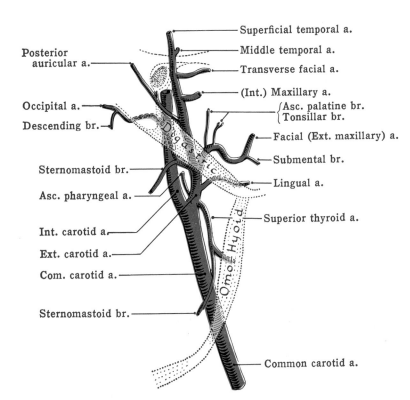

543.2   Diagram of the Carotid Arteries and their Branches in the Neck

Note: The common carotid divides into 2 terminal branches, the internal and the external, and neither the common carotid nor the internal carotid gives off collateral branches in the neck.

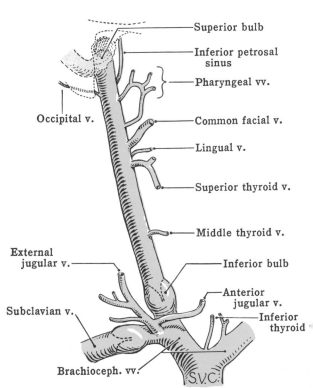

543.3   Diagram of the Internal Jugular Vein and its Tributaries

Note the dilatation or bulb at each end of the internal jugular vein. The superior jugular bulb is separated from the floor of the middle ear by a delicate bony plate. The inferior jugular bulb, like the corresponding bulb at the end of the subclavian vein, contains a bicuspid valve which permits the flow of blood towards the heart. There are no valves in the brachio-cephalic veins or in the superior vena cava.

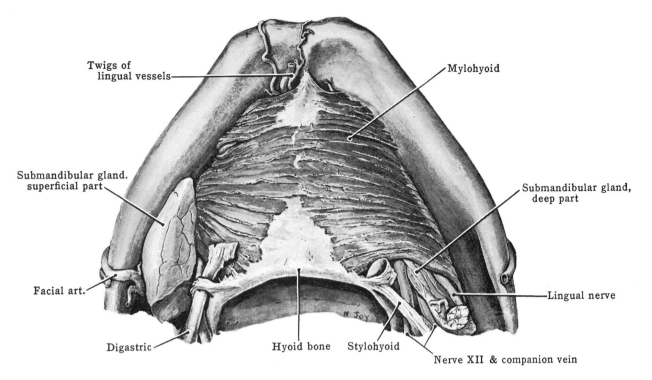

Twigs of
lingual vessels

Mylohyoid

Submandibular gland,
superficial part

Submandibular gland,
deep part

Facial art.

Lingual nerve

Digastric

Hyoid bone Stylohyoid

Nerve XII & companion vein

544 Floor of the Mouth, from below—Mylohyoids 1

(The anterior bellies of the Digastrics are removed, fig. 527.)

Observe:

1. The right and left Mylohyoids, which together form the "oral diaphragm", arising from the mylohyoid line of the jaw (fig. 553.1), and inserted into an indefinite median raphe and into the hyoid bone (fig. 596).

2. The submandibular gland turning round the posterior border of Mylohyoid.

3. The hypoglossal nerve and its companion vein passing deep to the same posterior border; and high up the lingual nerve applied to the jaw.

5   Floor of the Mouth,
·m below—Geniohyoids II

· left Mylohyoid and part of the right are
·cted.)

·rve:

·he Geniohyoid, triangular, in contact
·ith its fellow, and extending from the
·ental spine of the jaw to the front of the
·ody of the hyoid bone.

·he structures seen in figure 544 followed
·orwards: companion vein (distended),
·ypoglossal nerve, deep part of gland, and
·ngual nerve (appearing at anterior
·order of Medial Pterygoid).

·he areolar covered sublingual gland, and
·ateral to it the mucous membrane of the
·outh with twigs of the sublingual artery.

·For mouth from medial side and from
·bove, see figs. 597, 598, & 599.)

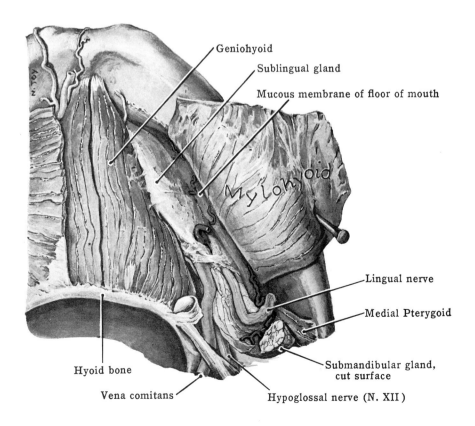

Geniohyoid

Sublingual gland

Mucous membrane of floor of mouth

Mylohyoid

Lingual nerve

Medial Pterygoid

Submandibular gland,
cut surface

Hyoid bone

Vena comitans

Hypoglossal nerve (N. XII)

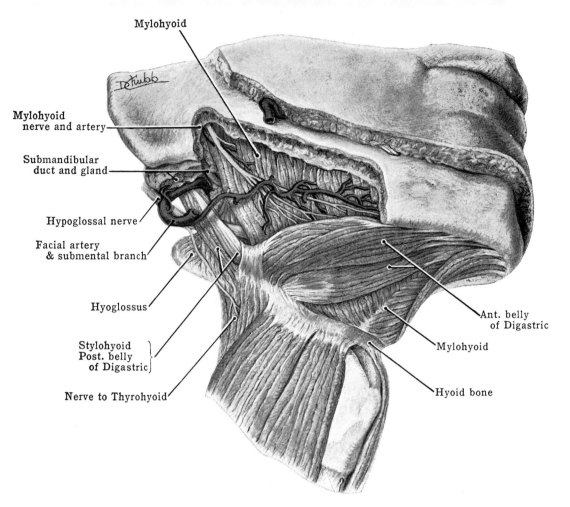

Mylohyoid

Mylohyoid
nerve and artery

Submandibular
duct and gland

Hypoglossal nerve

Facial artery
& submental branch

Hyoglossus

Stylohyoid
Post. belly
of Digastric

Nerve to Thyrohyoid

Ant. belly
of Digastric

Mylohyoid

Hyoid bone

546   Suprahyoid Region—I

Medial wall of submandibular (digastric) triangle

Observe:

1. Stylohyoid and the posterior belly of Digastric forming the posterior side of the triangle; the facial artery arching over these. The anterior belly of the Digastric forming the anterior side. Here this belly has an extra origin from the hyoid bone.

2. Mylohyoid forming the medial wall of the triangle and having a free, thick posterior border.

3. The mylohyoid nerve, which supplies Mylohyoid and anterior belly of Digastric, accompanied by the mylohyoid branch of the inferior alveolar artery posteriorly and by the submental branch of the facial artery anteriorly.

4. The hypoglossal nerve, the submandibular gland, and the submandibular duct passing forwards deep to the posterior border of Mylohyoid.

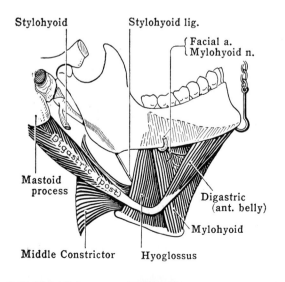

Stylohyoid

Stylohyoid lig.

Facial a.
Mylohyoid n.

Mastoid
process

Digastric (post.)

Middle Constrictor

Digastric
(ant. belly)

Mylohyoid

Hyoglossus

546.1

Diagram of 4 layers of suprahyoid muscles:—Digastric, Mylohyoid, Hyoglossus, and Middle Constrictor.

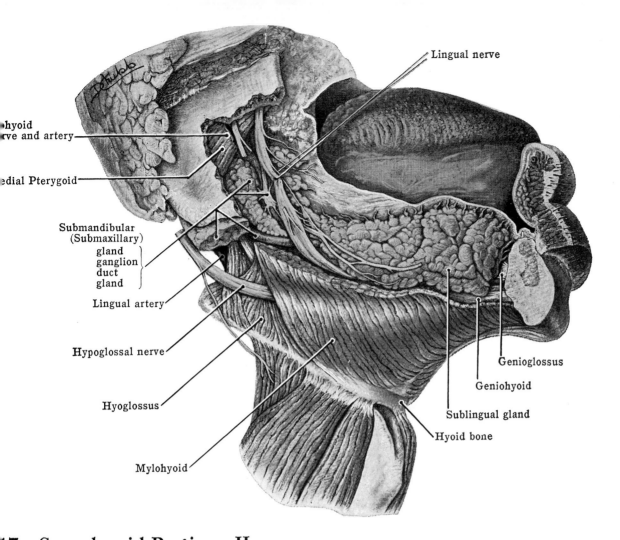

Lingual nerve

hyoid
rve and artery

edial Pterygoid

Submandibular
(Submaxillary)
gland
ganglion
duct
gland

Lingual artery

Hypoglossal nerve

Hyoglossus

Mylohyoid

Genioglossus

Geniohyoid

Sublingual gland

Hyoid bone

47 Suprahyoid Region—II

vary glands, on lateral view.

erve:

he cut surface of Mylohyoid becoming progressively thinner as traced for-
ards.

he sublingual salivary gland, almond-shaped, almost touching its fellow of
ie opposite side behind the symphysis menti and in contact with the deep part
f the submandibular gland posteriorly. (For medial view, fig. 597.)

he dozen or more fine ducts passing from the upper border of the sublingual
land to open on the plica sublingualis.

everal individual or detached lobules of the sublingual gland, each having a
ne duct, behind the main mass of the gland, and labial glands in the lip
unlabelled).

he mylohyoid nerve and artery (cut short) and the lingual nerve clamped
etween Medial Pterygoid and the ramus of the jaw.

he lingual nerve lying between the sublingual gland and the deep or oral
art of the submandibular gland; the submandibular ganglion suspended from
his nerve, and various sensory and secretory fibres leaving it.

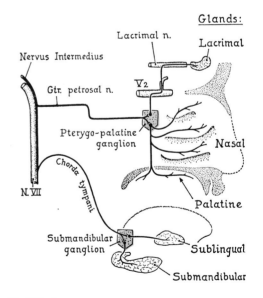

Glands:

Lacrimal n.

Lacrimal

Nervus Intermedius

Gtr. petrosal n.

V_2

Pterygo-palatine
ganglion

Nasal

Chorda
tympani

N. VII

Palatine

Submandibular
ganglion

Sublingual

Submandibular

547.1

Diagram: Nerve VII, via the greater petrosal
nerve brings secretomotor fibers to pterygo-
palatine ganglion and via chorda tympani to
submandibular ganglion; one to be relayed
and distributed to glands above the oral
cavity, the other to glands below it. (See
fig. 513.1.)

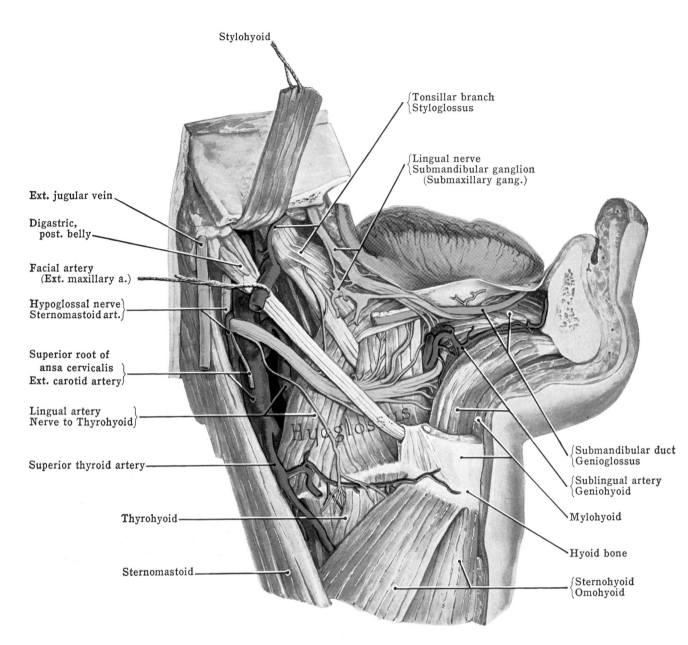

Stylohyoid

Tonsillar branch
Styloglossus

Lingual nerve
Submandibular ganglion
(Submaxillary gang.)

Ext. jugular vein

Digastric,
post. belly

Facial artery
(Ext. maxillary a.)

Hypoglossal nerve
Sternomastoid art.

Superior root of
ansa cervicalis
Ext. carotid artery

Lingual artery
Nerve to Thyrohyoid

Superior thyroid artery

Thyrohyoid

Sternomastoid

Hyoglossus

Submandibular duct
Genioglossus

Sublingual artery
Geniohyoid

Mylohyoid

Hyoid bone

Sternohyoid
Omohyoid

548 Suprahyoid Region—III

Relationships of Hyoglossus and of side of tongue.

Observe:

1. Stylohyoid pulled up. Posterior belly of Digastric left in situ, as a landmark.

2. Hyoglossus ascending from the greater horn and body of the hyoid bone to the side of the tongue; Styloglossus, postero-superiorly, crossed by the tonsillar branch of the facial artery and interdigitating with bundles of Hyoglossus; and Genioglossus, anteriorly, fanning out into the tongue.

3. The hypoglossal nerve, crossed twice by Digastric, crossing twice the lingual artery, and supplying all the muscles of the tongue, both extrinsic and intrinsic, Palatoglossus excepted. The branches of the hypoglossal nerve before the 2nd crossing of Digastric, leaving its lower border; hence, the wise dissector works along the upper border.

4. The submandibular duct running forwards, across Hyoglossus and Genioglossus, to its orifice.

5. The lingual nerve in contact with the jaw posteriorly, making a partial spiral around the submandibular duct, and ending in the tongue. The submandibular ganglion suspended from the nerve, and twigs leaving the nerve to supply mucous membrane.

6. The 1st part of the lingual artery behind Hyoglossus, and the 3rd part in front.

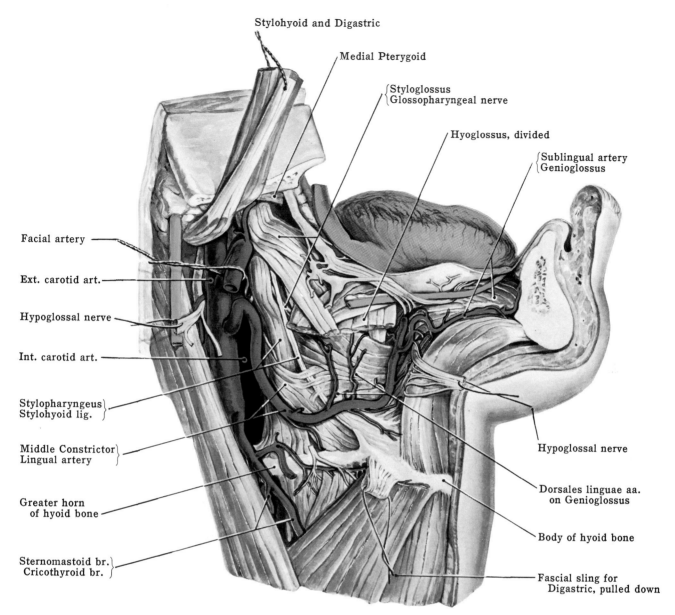

Stylohyoid and Digastric

Medial Pterygoid

Styloglossus
Glossopharyngeal nerve

Hyoglossus, divided

Sublingual artery
Genioglossus

Facial artery

Ext. carotid art.

Hypoglossal nerve

Int. carotid art.

Stylopharyngeus
Stylohyoid lig.

Middle Constrictor
Lingual artery

Greater horn
of hyoid bone

Sternomastoid br.
Cricothyroid br.

Hypoglossal nerve

Dorsales linguae aa.
on Genioglossus

Body of hyoid bone

Fascial sling for
Digastric, pulled down

549   Suprahyoid Region—IV

The lingual artery displayed

Stylohyoid and posterior belly of Digastric are pulled up; the hypoglossal nerve is divided and thrown backwards and forwards; and Hyoglossus is mostly removed, and the 2nd part of the lingual artery is thereby uncovered.

Observe:

1. The 1st part of the lingual artery, as in figure 548.

2. The 2nd part, deep to Hyoglossus, parallel to greater horn of hyoid bone, and lying on Middle Constrictor, stylohyoid ligament, and Genioglossus.

3. The 3rd part, ascending at the anterior border of Hyoglossus, which partly overlaps it, and turning into the tongue as the profunda linguae artery (see fig. 592).

4. The branches of the lingual artery:—(a) muscular, (b) dorsales linguae from the 2nd part which reach the tonsil bed, and (c) the sublingual artery which supplies the sublingual gland and the front of the floor of the mouth.

5. Stylopharyngeus, appearing deep to Styloglossus and disappearing deep to Middle Constrictor.

6. The glossopharyngeal nerve, not making the usual spiral descent lateral to Stylopharyngeus as in figure 574 but descending medial to it.

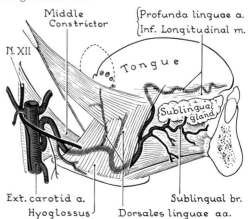

Middle Constrictor

Profunda linguae a.
Inf. Longitudinal m.

N. XII

Tongue

Sublingual Gland

Ext. carotid a.
Hyoglossus

Dorsales linguae aa.

Sublingual br.

549.1 Diagram of the Lingual Artery and its named branches

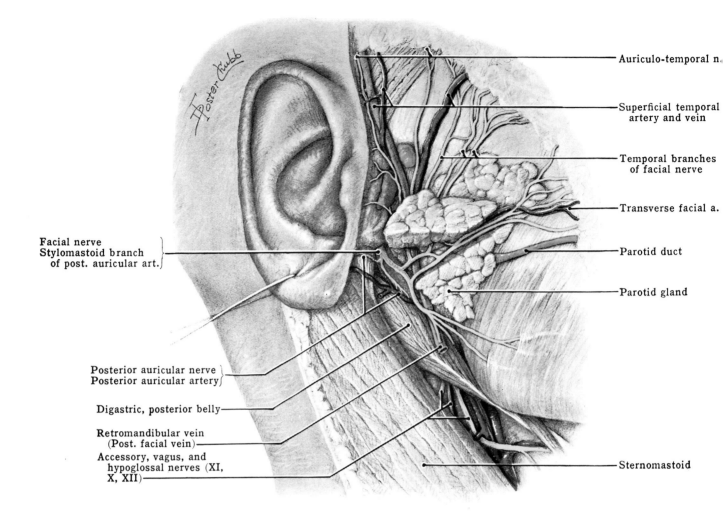

Auriculo-temporal n.

Superficial temporal artery and vein

Temporal branches of facial nerve

Transverse facial a.

Parotid duct

Parotid gland

Sternomastoid

Facial nerve
Stylomastoid branch
of post. auricular art.

Posterior auricular nerve
Posterior auricular artery

Digastric, posterior belly

Retromandibular vein
(Post. facial vein)

Accessory, vagus, and
hypoglossal nerves (XI,
X, XII)

550 Parotid Region—II

(Stage **I** is represented in figure 467.) The parotid gland is partly cut away.

Observe:

1. The stem of the facial nerve descending from the stylomastoid foramen for $\frac{1}{4}''$ to $\frac{1}{2}''$ before curving forwards to penetrate the deeper part of the parotid gland.

2. The nerve to the posterior belly of Digastric arising from the stem of the facial nerve.

3. The posterior auricular artery giving off a branch, the stylomastoid art., which accompanies the facial nerve through the stylomastoid foramen into the facial canal.

4. The relatively superficial position of the great landmark in the upper part of the neck, namely:—posterior belly of Digastric (fig. 540.2). Only three structures cross superficial to it: (a) the cervical branch of the facial nerve, (b) branches of the retromandibular vein, and (c) branches of the great auricular nerve shown in figure 467. All other crossing structures cross deep to it.

5. Preauricular lymph nodes.

6. Auricular and temporal branches of the auriculo-temporal nerve.

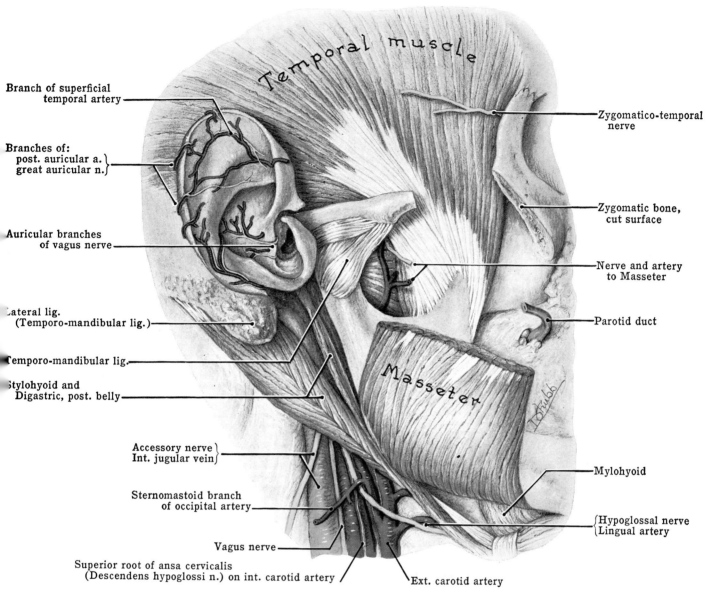

Branch of superficial
temporal artery

Temporal muscle

Zygomatico-temporal
nerve

Branches of:
post. auricular a.
great auricular n.

Zygomatic bone,
cut surface

Auricular branches
of vagus nerve

Nerve and artery
to Masseter

Lateral lig.
(Temporo-mandibular lig.)

Parotid duct

Temporo-mandibular lig.

Masseter

Stylohyoid and
Digastric, post. belly

Accessory nerve
Int. jugular vein

Mylohyoid

Sternomastoid branch
of occipital artery

Hypoglossal nerve
Lingual artery

Vagus nerve

Superior root of ansa cervicalis
(Descendens hypoglossi n.) on int. carotid artery

Ext. carotid artery

551 Parotid Bed: The Temporal Muscle:
Auricular Vessels and Nerves—III

Observe:

1. The mastoid process, rough where Sternomastoid (and also Splenius Capitis and Longissimus Capitis) has been removed from it.

2. The posterior belly of Digastric, arising deep to the mastoid process and passing deep to the angle of the jaw.

3. The vessels and nerves passing deep to Digastric—notably: the internal jugular vein, internal carotid artery, external carotid artery and its lingual, facial, and occipital branches, and the last three cranial nerves.

4. The Temporal muscle, inserted into the beak-shaped coronoid process.

5. The nerve and artery to Masseter, crossing the mandibular notch behind the Temporal muscle—the nerve appearing from above Lateral Pterygoid and the artery from below it.

6. Vessels and nerves of the auricle, mostly turning round the free borders of the cartilage, but some piercing the cartilage.

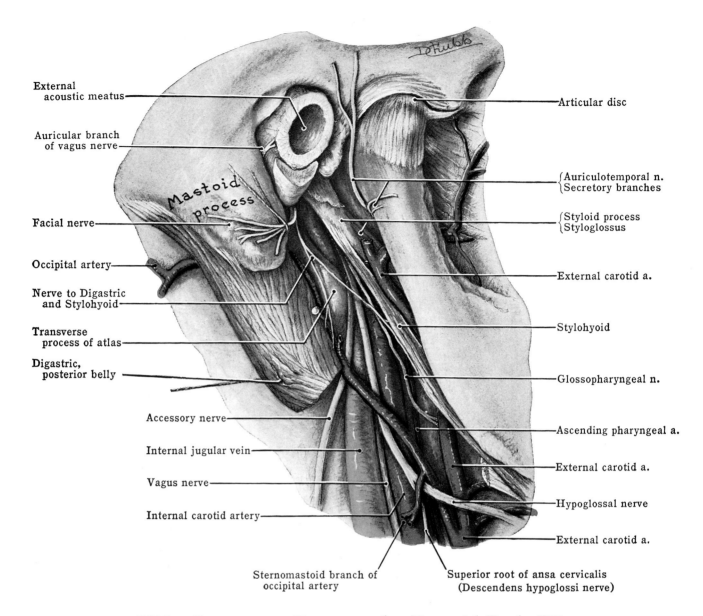

External acoustic meatus

Auricular branch of vagus nerve

Facial nerve

Occipital artery

Nerve to Digastric and Stylohyoid

Transverse process of atlas

Digastric, posterior belly

Accessory nerve

Internal jugular vein

Vagus nerve

Internal carotid artery

Mastoid process

Articular disc

Auriculotemporal n.
Secretory branches

Styloid process
Styloglossus

External carotid a.

Stylohyoid

Glossopharyngeal n.

Ascending pharyngeal a.

External carotid a.

Hypoglossal nerve

External carotid a.

Sternomastoid branch of occipital artery

Superior root of ansa cervicalis (Descendens hypoglossi nerve)

552   Structures Deep to the Parotid Bed—IV

The facial nerve, the posterior belly of Digastric and the nerve to this belly are retracted, whereas the external carotid artery, Stylohyoid and the nerve to Stylohyoid remain in situ.

Observe:

1. The tip of the transverse process of the atlas, about midway between the tip of the mastoid process and the angle of the jaw.

2. The internal jugular vein, the internal carotid artery, and the last four cranial nerves crossing in front of the transverse process and deep to the styloid process.

3. The strange impression made on the internal jugular vein by the transverse process.

4. The internal and external carotids separated from each other by the styloid process.

5. The last four cranial nerves (XII concealing X) starting to diverge from each other as they cross the transverse process.

6. The two nerves that pass forwards to the tongue (a) IX or glossopharyngeal being above the level of the angle of the jaw and passing between the two carotid arteries, and (b) XII or hypoglossal being below the angle of the jaw and passing superficial to both carotids, and indeed, to all the arteries it meets, except the occipital artery and its sternomastoid branch.

7. The thickness of the skin lining the cartilage of the meatus, and the stems of the two nerves— auricular branch of the vagus and auriculo-temporal—that supply the meatus and the outer surface of the tympanic membrane.

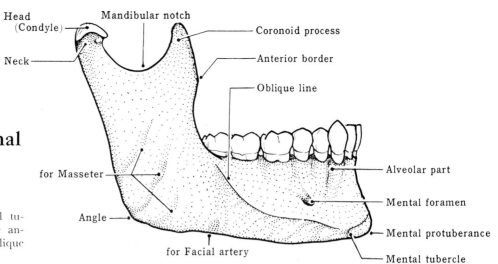

553 Mandible, external surface

Observe:

The coronoid process and the mental tubercle imperfectly connected by (a) the anterior border of the ramus, and (b) the oblique line that crosses the body diagonally.

Labels (external surface):
Head (Condyle) — Mandibular notch — Coronoid process — Neck — Anterior border — Oblique line — for Masseter — Alveolar part — Mental foramen — Angle — Mental protuberance — for Facial artery — Mental tubercle

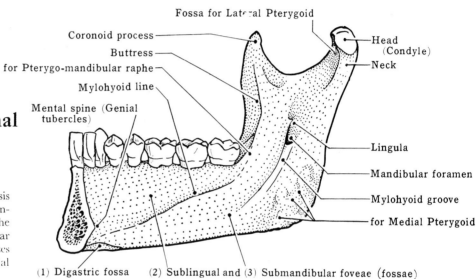

553.1 Mandible, internal surface

Observe:

The coronoid process and the symphysis menti (median plane of jaw) imperfectly connected by (a) the strengthening buttress, (b) the line of attachment of the pterygo-mandibular raphe, and (c) the mylohyoid line which crosses the body diagonally to end between the mental spine and the digastric fossa.

Labels (internal surface):
Fossa for Lateral Pterygoid — Coronoid process — Buttress — for Pterygo-mandibular raphe — Mylohyoid line — Mental spine (Genial tubercles) — Head (Condyle) — Neck — Lingula — Mandibular foramen — Mylohyoid groove — for Medial Pterygoid — (1) Digastric fossa — (2) Sublingual and (3) Submandibular foveae (fossae)

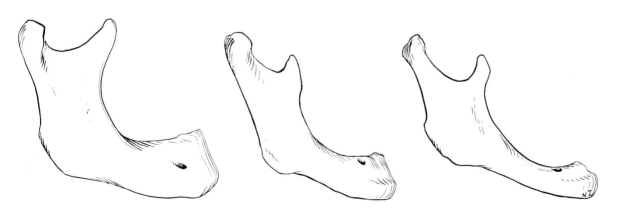

553.2 Mental Foramen, in edentulous jaws

Observe:

The position of the mental foramen in edentulous jaws varying with the extent of the absorption of the alveolus.

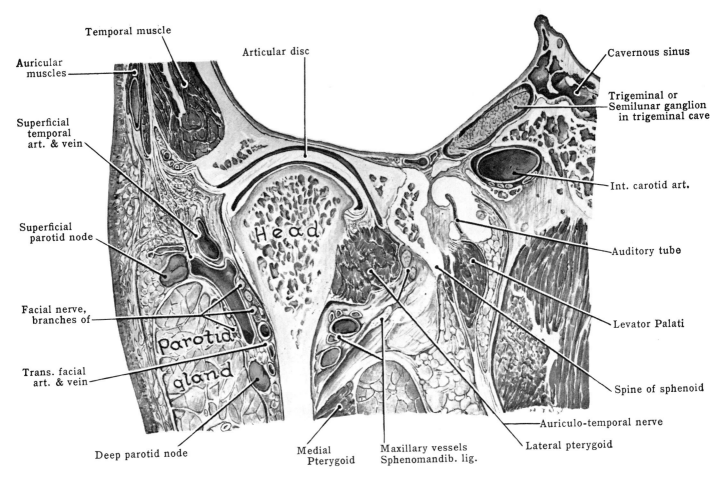

Temporal muscle

Auricular muscles

Superficial temporal art. & vein

Superficial parotid node

Facial nerve, branches of

Trans. facial art. & vein

Deep parotid node

Articular disc

Head

Parotid gland

Medial Pterygoid

Maxillary vessels
Sphenomandib. lig.

Cavernous sinus

Trigeminal or Semilunar ganglion in trigeminal cave

Int. carotid art.

Auditory tube

Levator Palati

Spine of sphenoid

Auriculo-temporal nerve

Lateral pterygoid

554 Temporo-mandibular Joint, on coronal section

Observe:

1. The articular disc attached to the neck of the jaw medially and laterally, partly in conjunction with the Lateral Pterygoid.
2. The roof of the mandibular fossa, which separates head and disc from the middle cranial fossa, to be thin centrally (fig. 619.2) but thick elsewhere, cf., the acetabulum.
3. The spine of the sphenoid (figs. 569 & 571.1) at the medial end of the fossa, and the two roots of the auriculo-temporal nerve crossing lateral to it (fig. 560).
4. The auditory tube with closed slit-like lumen, and the Levator Palati lying below it.
5. The trigeminal ganglion in its trigeminal cave, the mouth of which opens below the tentorium (fig. 565); and separated from the int. carotid artery by membrane (bone being deficient) and, therefore, subjected to the pulsations of that artery (figs. 513 & 514).
6. The maxillary vessels crossing the neck of the jaw on its medial side.
7. Superficial and deep parotid lymph nodes.
8. The "aponeurotic" tendon of Temporalis, buried in the muscle for it receives fleshy fibres from the temporal fossa on one side and from the temporal fascia on the other (figs. 465 & 591).

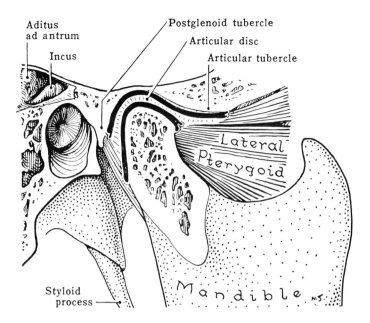

Aditus ad antrum
Incus
Postglenoid tubercle
Articular disc
Articular tubercle
Lateral Pterygoid
Styloid process
Mandible

555   Temporo-mandibular Joint, on sagittal section

Note the articular disc dividing the articular cavity into an upper and a lower compartment, and the Lateral Pterygoid inserted in part into the disc.

(For orientation of head of jaw, see figure 507; for articular part of mandibular fossa and articular tubercle, see figures 558 & 619.2; for lateral, or temporo-mandibular, lig., see figure 551.)

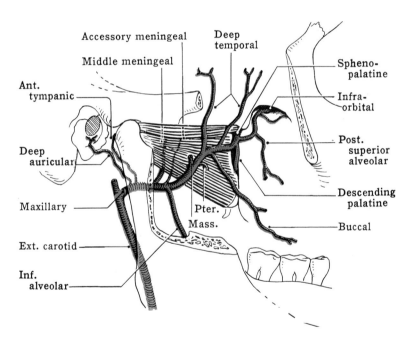

Accessory meningeal
Middle meningeal
Deep temporal
Ant. tympanic
Spheno-palatine
Infra-orbital
Deep auricular
Post. superior alveolar
Maxillary
Pter.
Mass.
Descending palatine
Ext. carotid
Buccal
Inf. alveolar

556   Diagram of the Maxillary Artery

Observe:

1. This, the larger of the two terminal branches of the ext carotid art., arising at neck of jaw and divided into three parts by Lateral Pterygoid.
2. The branches of the first pass through foramina or canals: (a) deep auricular a. to ext. acoustic meatus, (b) anterior tympanic a. to tympanum (c, d) middle and accessory meningeal aa. to cranial cavity, and (e) inf. alveolar a. to jaw and teeth.
3. The branches of the second part supply muscles—by masseteric, deep temporal, pterygoid and buccal branches.

4. The branches of the third part arise just before and within the pterygo-palatine fossa: (a) post superior alveolar a., (b) infra-orbital a., (c) descending palatine a., (d) art of pterygoid canal, (e) pharyngeal a., and (f) sphenopalatine a. These, accompanied by branches of the maxillary nerve, pass through bony canals or foramina. The descending palatine a. divides into a greater and 2 or 3 lesser palatine aa. (fig. 583). The sphenopalatine a. ends as the post. lateral nasal and post. nasal septal aa. (fig. 607) (Also figs. 559–560.3.)

(For variations, see Pearson, Mackenzie and Goodman.)

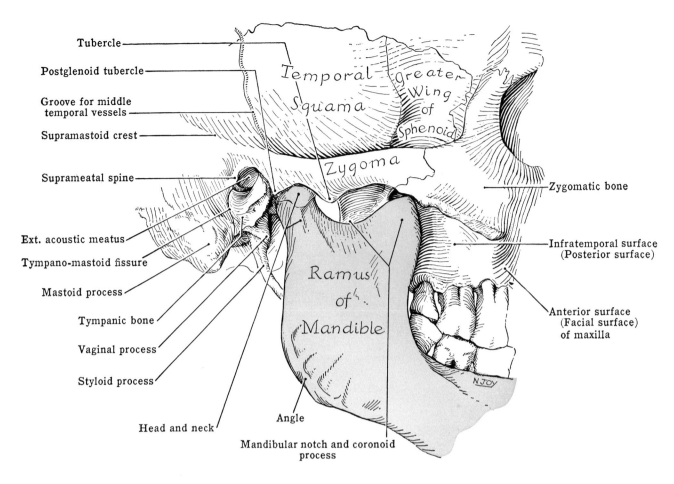

Tubercle
Postglenoid tubercle
Groove for middle temporal vessels
Supramastoid crest
Suprameatal spine
Ext. acoustic meatus
Tympano-mastoid fissure
Mastoid process
Tympanic bone
Vaginal process
Styloid process
Head and neck
Angle
Mandibular notch and coronoid process

Temporal Squama

Greater Wing of Sphenoid

Zygoma

Zygomatic bone

Ramus of Mandible

Infratemporal surface (Posterior surface)

Anterior surface (Facial surface) of maxilla

N JOY

557 Lateral Wall of the Infratemporal Fossa—I

That wall is the ramus of the mandible.

Note:

1. The zygoma [zygomatic process of the squamous part of the temporal bone] plus the zygomatic bone constitute the zygomatic arch. This arch is continued as a buttress downwards and forwards to the first or second molar tooth. The buttress forms the anterior limit of the infratemporal fossa and separates it from the facial aspect of the skull.
2. The zygoma lies at the boundary line between the temporal fossa above and the infratemporal fossa below.
3. Below the tubercle of the zygoma and in front of the neck of the jaw there is a clear passage across the base of the skull through which a pencil can be passed—see figure 571.
4. When in occlusion a tooth bites on two other teeth.

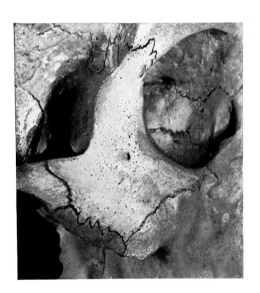

557.1 Bipartite Zygomatic Bone (Os Japonicum)

Rarely the zygomatic bone is divided either horizontally or vertically into two parts. In this instance the condition was bilateral and the subject an (Asiatic) Indian. (Courtesy of Dr. J. E. Anderson.)

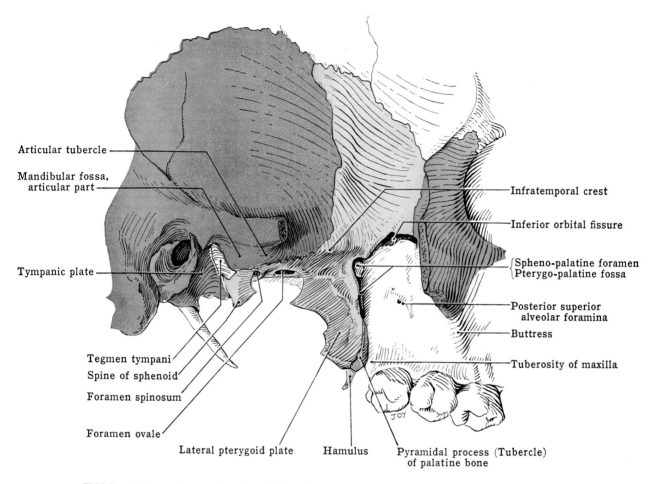

Articular tubercle

Mandibular fossa,
articular part

Tympanic plate

Tegmen tympani
Spine of sphenoid

Foramen spinosum

Foramen ovale

Lateral pterygoid plate   Hamulus

Infratemporal crest

Inferior orbital fissure

Spheno-palatine foramen
Pterygo-palatine fossa

Posterior superior
alveolar foramina

Buttress

Tuberosity of maxilla

Pyramidal process (Tubercle)
of palatine bone

558 Roof and the Medial and Anterior Walls of the Infratemporal Fossa, infero-lateral view—II

The jaw is removed and the zygomatic arch is cut away.

Note:

1. The medial wall of the fossa is formed by the lateral pterygoid plate.

2. The posterior free border of this plate, when followed upwards, leads to the foramen ovale in the roof of the fossa. Behind the foramen ovale, at the root of the spine of the sphenoid, is the foramen spinosum (Figs. 508 & 569). The roof is separated from the temporal fossa by the infratemporal crest.

3. Below, the anterior border of the lateral plate is separated from the maxilla by the pyramidal process of the palatine bone which is insinuated as a buffer between the two (figs. 569 & 570). Above, the border is free and forms the posterior limit of the pterygo-maxillary fissure, which is the entrance to the pterygo-palatine fossa on the medial wall of which can be seen the sphenopalatine foramen which leads to the nasal cavity.

4. The rounded anterior wall of the fossa is the infratemporal surface of the maxilla, which is of egg-shell thickness, is limited above by the inferior orbital fissure, and is pierced by two (or more) posterior superior alveolar (dental) foramina for the vessels and nerves of the same name.

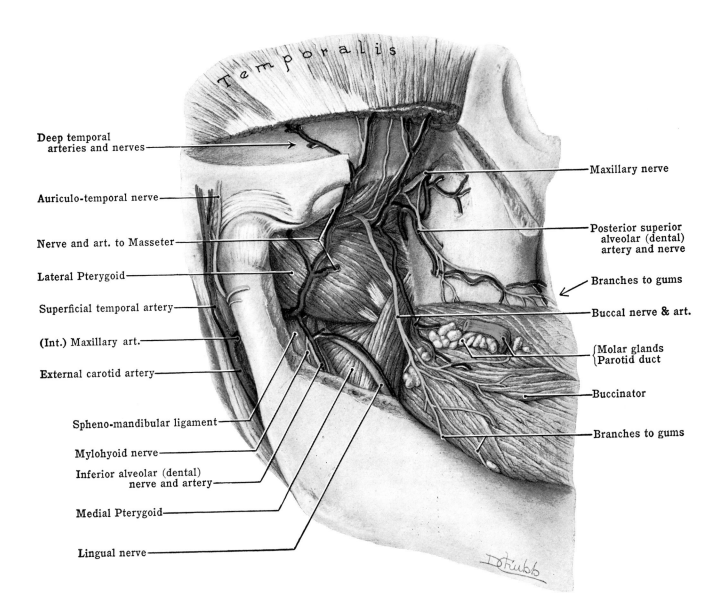

Deep temporal arteries and nerves

Auriculo-temporal nerve

Nerve and art. to Masseter

Lateral Pterygoid

Superficial temporal artery

(Int.) Maxillary art.

External carotid artery

Spheno-mandibular ligament

Mylohyoid nerve

Inferior alveolar (dental) nerve and artery

Medial Pterygoid

Lingual nerve

Temporalis

Maxillary nerve

Posterior superior alveolar (dental) artery and nerve

Branches to gums

Buccal nerve & art.

{Molar glands
{Parotid duct

Buccinator

Branches to gums

559   Infratemporal Region, superficial dissection—III

Observe:

1. Lateral Pterygoid, triangular in shape, arising from the medial wall and roof of the infratemporal fossa (fig. 558), the two heads being at a right angle to each other, and inserted into the articular disc of the temporo-mandibular joint and into the front of the neck of the jaw.

2. Below this, Medial Pterygoid is seen; in front of Medial Pterygoid, Buccinator is seen.

3. Appearing:—(a) between Lateral Pterygoid and the roof—nerves to Masseter and Temporalis; (b) between the heads of Lateral Pterygoid—buccal nerve and maxillary artery (the nerve here pierces Lateral Pterygoid); and (c) between Lateral and Medial Pterygoids—inferior alveolar and lingual nerves.

4. The maxillary nerve (V²) becoming the infra-orbital nerve and passing through the inferior orbital fissure, after giving off the posterior superior alveolar nerve which sends two (or more) branches into the foramina of the same name.

5. The maxillary artery, which is the larger of the two end branches of the external carotid, running forwards deep to the neck of the jaw, disappearing deep to Lateral Pterygoid, and reappearing between its two heads before plunging into the pterygo-palatine fossa. It is seen sending branches to accompany each nerve mentioned above.

6. Buccinator, pierced by:—(a) parotid duct, (b) ducts of the molar glands, and (c) branches (sensory) of the buccal nerve.

7. At the upper and lower borders of Buccinator, branches of the posterior superior alveolar and buccal nerves sending branches to the upper and lower gums respectively.

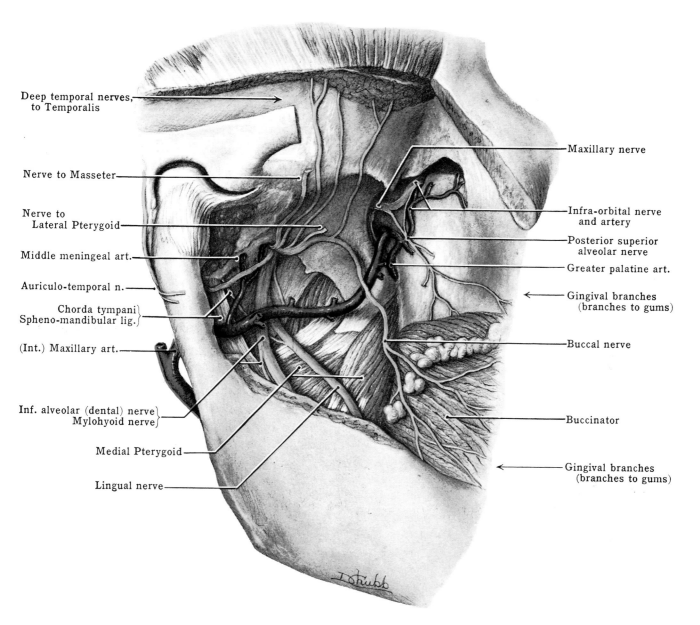

Deep temporal nerves, to Temporalis

Nerve to Masseter

Nerve to Lateral Pterygoid

Middle meningeal art.

Auriculo-temporal n.

Chorda tympani
Spheno-mandibular lig.

(Int.) Maxillary art.

Inf. alveolar (dental) nerve
Mylohyoid nerve

Medial Pterygoid

Lingual nerve

Maxillary nerve

Infra-orbital nerve and artery

Posterior superior alveolar nerve

Greater palatine art.

Gingival branches (branches to gums)

Buccal nerve

Buccinator

Gingival branches (branches to gums)

560   Infratemporal Region, deeper dissection—IV

Lateral Pterygoid is removed and so are most branches of the artery.

Observe:

1. Medial Pterygoid arising from the medial surface of the lateral pterygoid plate and having a small superficial head which arises from the pyramidal process of the palatine bone (fig. 558).

2. The spheno-mandibular ligament, which, as a fascial band, descends from near the spine of the sphenoid to the lingula of the mandible (fig. 553).

3. The maxillary artery and the auriculo-temporal nerve passing between the ligament and the neck of the jaw.

4. The mandibular nerve (V³) entering the infratemporal fossa through the roof, via the foramen ovale which also transmits the accessory meningeal artery (not labelled).

5. The middle meningeal artery and vein passing through the roof via the foramen spinosum.

6. The inferior alveolar and lingual nerves descending on Medial Pterygoid. The former giving off the mylohyoid nerve (to Mylohyoid and anterior belly of Digastric); the latter receiving the chorda tympani (which carries secretory fibres and fibres of taste).

7. The nerves to 4 muscles of mastication:—Masseter, Temporal, and Lateral Pterygoid, which are labelled, and the nerve to Medial Pterygoid which is not labelled. Note the buccal branch of the mandibular nerve is sensory; it is the buccal branch of the facial nerve that supplies Buccinator.

8. The maxillary nerve (V²) becoming the infra-orbital nerve which enters the infra-orbital groove at the inferior orbital fissure.

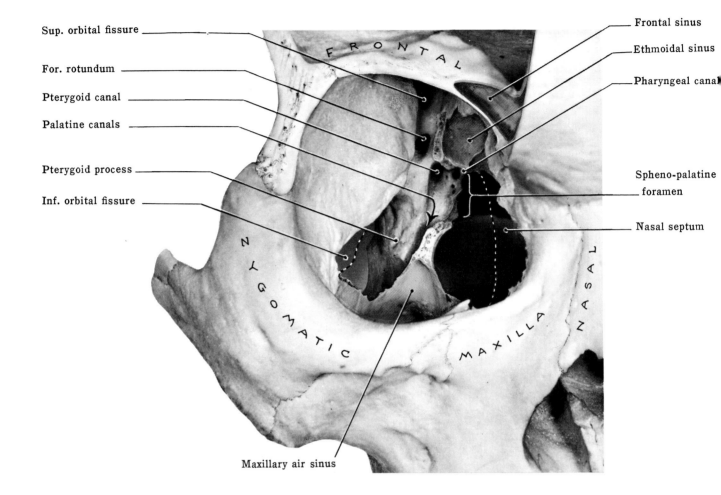

Sup. orbital fissure

For. rotundum

Pterygoid canal

Palatine canals

Pterygoid process

Inf. orbital fissure

Frontal sinus

Ethmoidal sinus

Pharyngeal canal

Spheno-palatine foramen

Nasal septum

Maxillary air sinus

560.1 Photograph of Pterygopalatine Fossa, front view

Exposed through floor of orbit and maxillary sinus.

For front view, see also figure 619.1. For lateral view (from infratemporal fossa); see figure 558. For medial view (from nasal cavity), see figure 608.1 where the spheno-palatine foramen, which is flush with the under surface sphenoidal sinus, is divided by attachment of middle concha into an upper part for the posterior nasal septal artery and a lower part for the posterior lateral nasal artery, and accompanying nerves.

50.2 Maxillary Nerve (Nerve V²)

This afferent nerve supplies territory extending from skin laterally (fig. 470.1, pink area) to nasal septum medially (see coronal section of head, fig. 591), the lateral and medial branches of the nerve being separated by the maxillary sinus. (For lateral branches, see fig. 5; medial branches, fig. 606.)

The greater petrosal nerve, via nerve of pterygoid canal, brings parasympathetic fibers to the (spheno-) pterygopalatine ganglion, there to be relayed and distributed, with branches of nerve V², as secreto-motor fibers (see fig. 513.1).

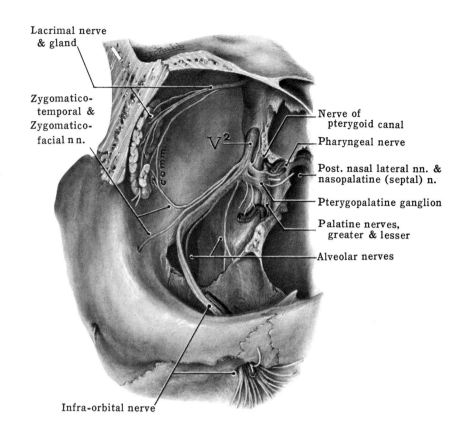

Lacrimal nerve & gland

Zygomatico-temporal & Zygomatico-facial n n.

Nerve of pterygoid canal

Pharyngeal nerve

Post. nasal lateral nn. & nasopalatine (septal) n.

Pterygopalatine ganglion

Palatine nerves, greater & lesser

Alveolar nerves

Infra-orbital nerve

50.3 Maxillary Artery, Third part

To serve:

The stem of this artery, arising at the neck of the jaw, is divided into 3 parts by Lateral Pterygoid (fig. 556).

The branches of 1st part pass through either foramina or canals.

The branches of 2nd part supply muscles of mastication (fig. 556).

The branches of 3rd part arise just before and within the pterygopalatine fossa:—(a) infra-orbital, (b) posterior superior alveolar, (c) descending palatine, (d) artery of pterygoid canal, (e) pharyngeal, and (f) spheno-palatine arteries. The descending palatine artery divides into the greater and lesser palatine arteries (fig. 583). The spheno-palatine artery divides into the posterior nasal septal and posterior lateral nasal arteries (fig. 607).

The 3rd part of the artery, often very tortuous, lies ventral to the maxillary nerve and its branches.

For variations, see Pearson, MacKenzie, and Goodman. In this particular specimen, the artery of pterygoid canal and the pharyngeal artery make unusually long ascents on the pterygoid process.

(Pharyngeal canal = palato-vaginal canal.)

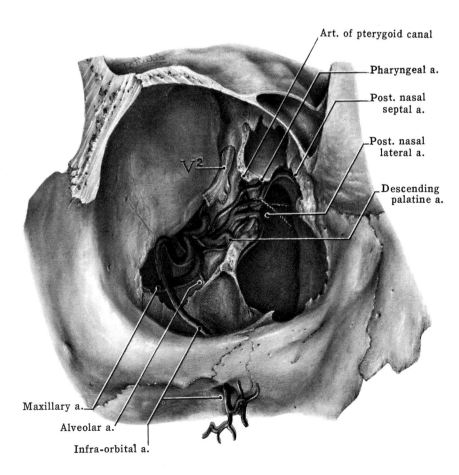

Art. of pterygoid canal

Pharyngeal a.

Post. nasal septal a.

Post. nasal lateral a.

Descending palatine a.

Maxillary a.

Alveolar a.

Infra-orbital a.

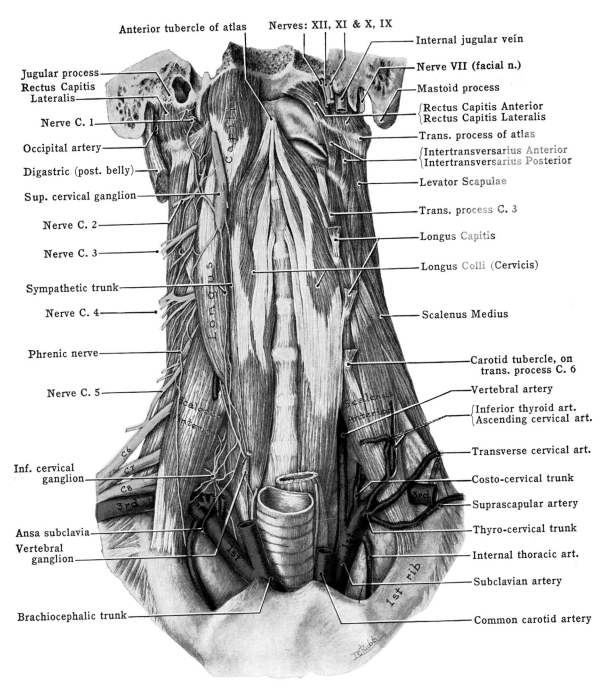

Anterior tubercle of atlas

Nerves: XII, XI & X, IX

Jugular process
Rectus Capitis Lateralis

Nerve C. 1

Occipital artery

Digastric (post. belly)

Sup. cervical ganglion

Nerve C. 2

Nerve C. 3

Sympathetic trunk

Nerve C. 4

Phrenic nerve

Nerve C. 5

Inf. cervical ganglion

Ansa subclavia
Vertebral ganglion

Brachiocephalic trunk

Internal jugular vein

Nerve VII (facial n.)

Mastoid process

Rectus Capitis Anterior
Rectus Capitis Lateralis

Trans. process of atlas

Intertransversarius Anterior
Intertransversarius Posterior

Levator Scapulae

Trans. process C. 3

Longus Capitis

Longus Colli (Cervicis)

Scalenus Medius

Carotid tubercle, on trans. process C. 6

Vertebral artery

Inferior thyroid art.
Ascending cervical art.

Transverse cervical art.

Costo-cervical trunk

Suprascapular artery

Thyro-cervical trunk

Internal thoracic art.

Subclavian artery

Common carotid artery

561 Prevertebral Region: Root of the Neck

On the right side, Longus Capitis is removed.

Observe:

1. The prevertebral and deep lateral muscles of the neck. Of these muscles, 3—Scalenus Anterior, Longus Capitis, and Longus Colli—are attached to the anterior tubercles of the transverse processes of vertebrae C. 3, 4, 5 and 6; hence, the prominence of these tubercles, as seen in figures 367 & 368.

2. The transverse process of the atlas joined to the transverse process of the axis by Intertransverse muscles; and joined similarly to the "transverse process" of the occipital bone (i.e., jugular process) by Rectus Capitis Lateralis which morphologically is an Intertransverse muscle. Note: the internal jugular vein crossing these structures.

3. The cervical plexus arising from ventral rami, C. 1, 2, 3 and 4; and the brachial plexus from C. 5, 6, 7, 8 and T. 1.

4. The sympathetic trunk and ganglia and its gray rami communicantes.

5. The subclavian artery and its branches.

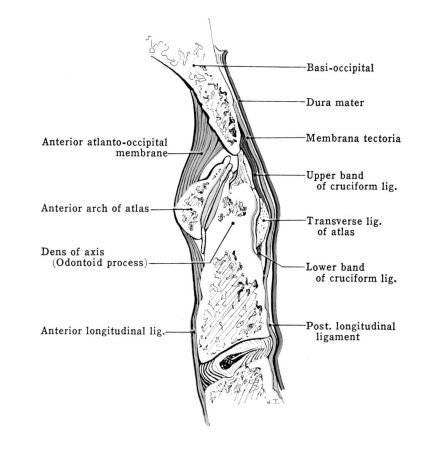

Basi-occipital

Dura mater

Membrana tectoria

Upper band
of cruciform lig.

Transverse lig.
of atlas

Lower band
of cruciform lig.

Post. longitudinal
ligament

Anterior atlanto-occipital
membrane

Anterior arch of atlas

Dens of axis
(Odontoid process)

Anterior longitudinal lig.

62   Ligaments of the atlanto-axial and atlanto-occipital Joints, in median section

Observe:

The layers of tissue encountered in the median plane. From behind forwards they are: (a) dura mater, (b) posterior longitudinal lig., continued upwards as the membrana tectoria, stretching from axis to occipital bone, (c) transverse ligament of the atlas and the upper and lower longitudinal bands, which, like the membrana, stretch from axis to occipital bone and (d) the lig. apicis dentis (not labelled), which is a vestigial filament stretching from the apex of the dens to the occipital bone.

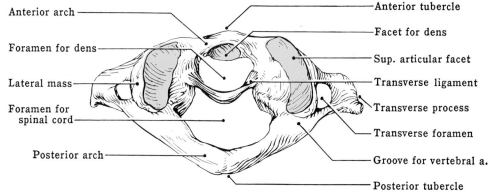

Anterior arch

Foramen for dens

Lateral mass

Foramen for
spinal cord

Posterior arch

Anterior tubercle

Facet for dens

Sup. articular facet

Transverse ligament

Transverse process

Transverse foramen

Groove for vertebral a.

Posterior tubercle

63   Atlas and its Transverse Ligament and the Axis, from above

Observe:

The large vertebral foramen of the atlas which is divided into two foramina by the transverse ligament of the atlas. In the larger, posterior foramen the spinal cord lies loosely. In the smaller, anterior foramen the dens of the axis fits tightly. It articulates in front with the anterior arch of the atlas and behind with the transverse ligament which, like the annular ligament of the radius, forms an arc of a circle.

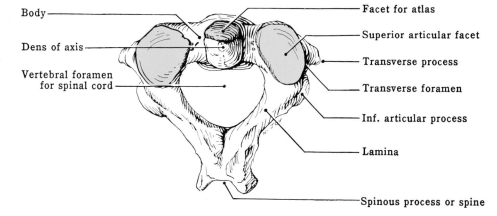

Body

Dens of axis

Vertebral foramen
for spinal cord

Facet for atlas

Superior articular facet

Transverse process

Transverse foramen

Inf. articular process

Lamina

Spinous process or spine

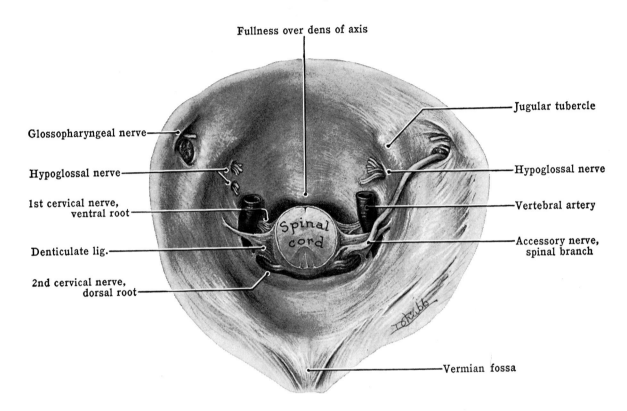

Fullness over dens of axis

Glossopharyngeal nerve

Hypoglossal nerve

1st cervical nerve, ventral root

Denticulate lig.

2nd cervical nerve, dorsal root

Spinal cord

Jugular tubercle

Hypoglossal nerve

Vertebral artery

Accessory nerve, spinal branch

Vermian fossa

564 Structures seen through the Foramen Magnum, from above

Observe:

1. In front, the fullness over the transverse ligament of the atlas (fig. 563), which curves tightly behind the dens of the axis.

2. Passing through the foramen magnum within the meninges:—(a) the spinal cord or medulla, (b) the vertebral arteries, (c) the spinal roots of the accessory nerves (XI), and (d) the highest tooth of the ligamentum denticulatum of each side. (For lower teeth, figs. 482 & 484.)

3. The hypoglossal nerves (XII) leaving the dura mater through two openings which are close together on the right side and separated on the left side.

4. In this specimen the first cervical nerve has no posterior (sensory) root.

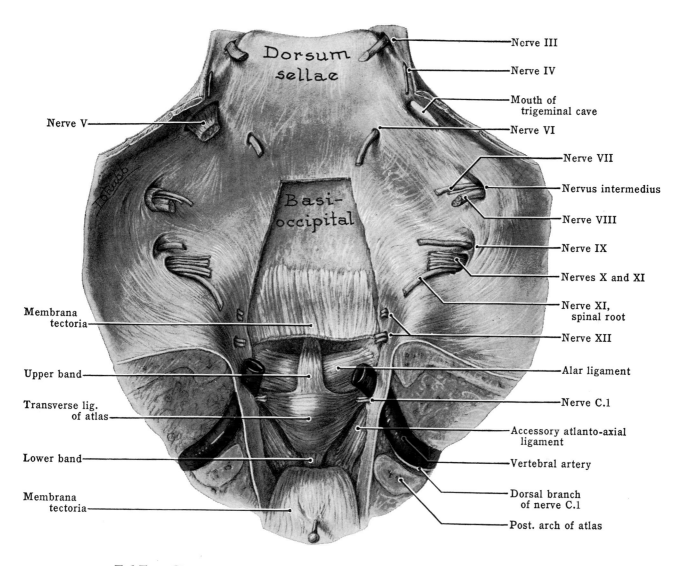

Dorsum sellae

Basi-occipital

Nerve V

Nerve III

Nerve IV

Mouth of trigeminal cave

Nerve VI

Nerve VII

Nervus intermedius

Nerve VIII

Nerve IX

Nerves X and XI

Nerve XI, spinal root

Nerve XII

Alar ligament

Nerve C.1

Accessory atlanto-axial ligament

Vertebral artery

Dorsal branch of nerve C.1

Post. arch of atlas

Membrana tectoria

Upper band

Transverse lig. of atlas

Lower band

Membrana tectoria

565 Cranio-vertebral Joints, dorsal view

Ligaments of atlanto-axial and atlanto-occipital joints.

Observe:

1. The bow-shaped transverse ligament of the atlas, which, by the addition of an upper and a lower longitudinal band, becomes a cruciform ligament.

2. The alar or check ligaments passing from the sides of the apex of the dens postero-laterally, above the transverse ligament, to the medial sides of the occipital condyles.

3. The sites where the last ten pairs of cranial nerves and the first pair of cervical nerves pass through the dura, noting:—(a) that they are in numerical sequence, cranio-caudally, and (b) that nerves III, IV and VI, which supply the muscles of the eye, and XII, which supplies the muscles of the tongue, are nearly in vertical line with each other and with the ventral or motor root of C. 1.

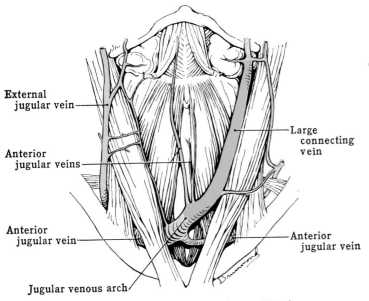

External jugular vein

Anterior jugular veins

Anterior jugular vein

Jugular venous arch

Large connecting vein

Anterior jugular vein

566　Large Connecting Vein

A small vein that lies along the anterior border of Sternomastoid and connects the common facial vein to the anterior jugular vein may attain great size. It may, indeed, be greater than even the internal jugular vein and it is at times mistaken for it.

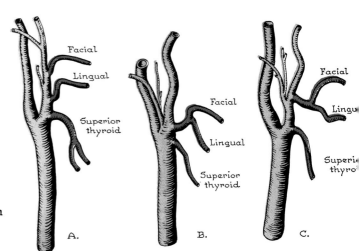

Facial

Lingual

Superior thyroid

Facial

Superior thyroid

Lingual

Superior thyroid

Facial

Lingual

Superior thyroid

A.　B.　C.

566.1　Variations in the Origin of the Lingual Artery

A. The superior thyroid, lingual, and facial arteries arose separately in 80% of 211 specimens.　B, C. In 20% the lingual and facial arteries arose from a common stem, either high or low. In one instance the superior thyroid and lingual arteries arose from a common stem. (*G. F. Lewis.*)

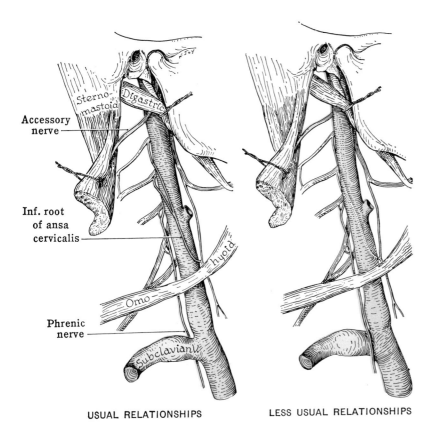

Accessory nerve

Inf. root of ansa cervicalis

Phrenic nerve

Sterno-mastoid　Digastric

Omo　hyoid

Subclavian V.

USUAL RELATIONSHIPS　　LESS USUAL RELATIONSHIPS

566.2　Variable Relationships of the Accessory, Ansa Cervicalis, and Phrenic Nerves to the Great Veins

The accessory nerve crossed anterior to the internal jugular vein in 70% of 188 instances, and posterior to it in 30%. (J. C. B. G.)

The inferior root of the ansa cervicalis, while on its way to join the superior root, passed round the medial side of the internal jugular vein in 43% of 118 instances, and round the lateral side in 57%. (D. L. MacIntosh and G. G. Smith.)

The phrenic nerve (C.3, 4, and 5) passes behind the site of union of the subclavian, internal, jugular, and brachiocephalic veins, but occasionally the branch from C.5, or less commonly the entire phrenic nerve, passes anterior to the subclavian vein.

VARIATIONS AND ANOMALIES

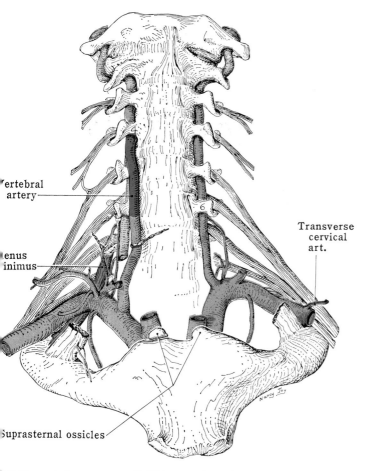

vertebral
artery

enus
inimus

Transverse
cervical
art.

Suprasternal ossicles

567 Abnormal Vertebral Artery: Suprasternal Ossicles: Scalenus Minimus

The Vertebral Artery, in 6.4% of 1,000 half heads (Japanese), enters not the foramen of the 6th cervical transverse process but another—the 5th in 4.5%, the 7th in 1.2%, and the 4th as here in 0.7% (Adachi).

Suprasternal Ossicles, which range in size between that of a small shot and an average female lunate bone, were found either paired or singly, and either separate from the manubrium or fused to it, in 6.8% of 544 white adult sterna examined by X-rays. (W. Montague Cobb.)

Scalenus Minimus, passing between subclavian artery and brachial plexus, is commonly present. (Also fig. 537.)

Aberrant Transverse Cervical Artery, see figure 471.5.

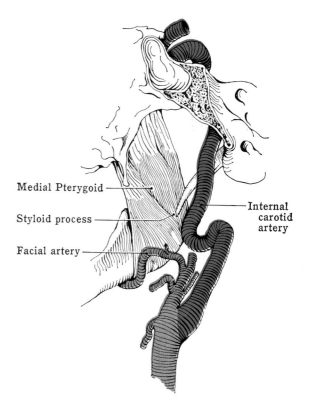

Medial Pterygoid

Styloid process

Facial artery

Internal
carotid
artery

567.1 Tortuous Internal Carotid Artery

This artery is always tortuous inside the skull. It may be tortuous outside also and come to lie close behind the tonsil.

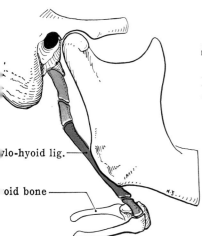

ylo-hyoid lig.

oid bone

568 Ossified Stylohyoid Ligament

here unites the styloid process (in 2 pieces) to the lesser horn. Thus, a chain of 4 bones with 4 joints attaches the body and greater horn of the hyoid to the skull.

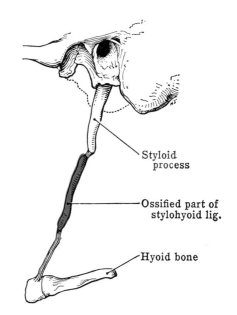

Styloid
process

Ossified part of
stylohyoid lig.

Hyoid bone

568.1 Partial Ossification of Stylohyoid Ligament, left side

VARIATIONS AND ANOMALIES

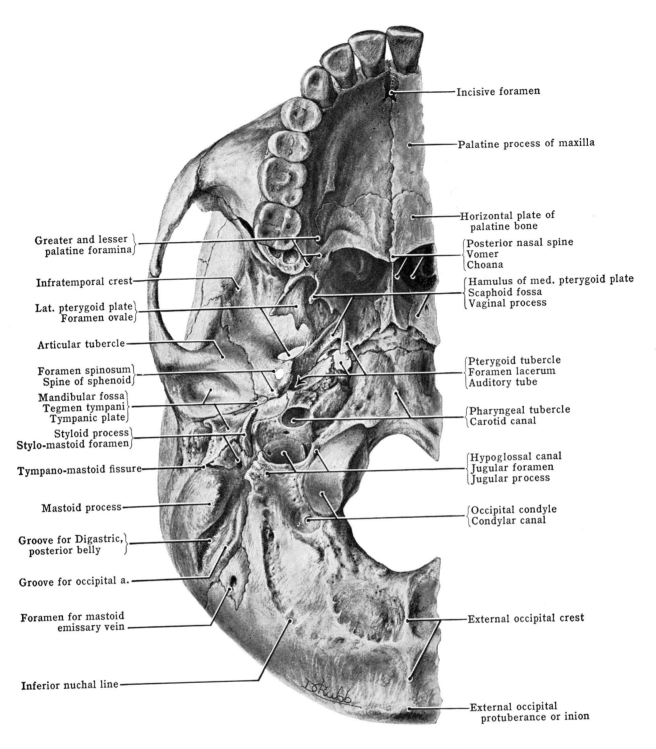

Incisive foramen

Palatine process of maxilla

Horizontal plate of palatine bone

Posterior nasal spine
Vomer
Choana

Hamulus of med. pterygoid plate
Scaphoid fossa
Vaginal process

Greater and lesser palatine foramina

Infratemporal crest

Lat. pterygoid plate
Foramen ovale

Articular tubercle

Pterygoid tubercle
Foramen lacerum
Auditory tube

Foramen spinosum
Spine of sphenoid

Mandibular fossa
Tegmen tympani
Tympanic plate

Pharyngeal tubercle
Carotid canal

Styloid process
Stylo-mastoid foramen

Hypoglossal canal
Jugular foramen
Jugular process

Tympano-mastoid fissure

Mastoid process

Occipital condyle
Condylar canal

Groove for Digastric, posterior belly

Groove for occipital a.

Foramen for mastoid emissary vein

External occipital crest

Inferior nuchal line

External occipital protuberance or inion

569   Exterior of the Base of the Skull

Note:

(1) The unlabelled foramen between the carotid canal and the jugular foramen which transmits the tympanic branch of the glosso-pharyngeal nerve (figs. 659 and 640.1).

(2) The unlabelled foramen on the lateral wall of the jugular foramen which transmits the auricular branch of the vague nerve, shown in figure 552. The auricular branch enters this foramen, crosses the stylomastoid foramen, and leaves through the tympano-mastoid fissure.

(3) The foramen for the mastoid emissary vein, in this specimen, lies in a sutural bone.

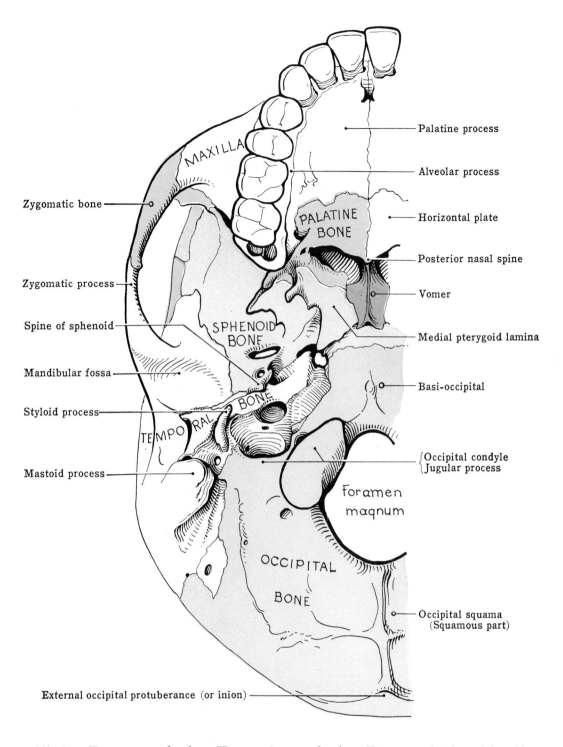

Palatine process

Alveolar process

Horizontal plate

Posterior nasal spine

Vomer

Medial pterygoid lamina

Basi-occipital

Occipital condyle
Jugular process

Foramen magnum

Occipital squama
(Squamous part)

Zygomatic bone

Zygomatic process

Spine of sphenoid

Mandibular fossa

Styloid process

Mastoid process

External occipital protuberance (or inion)

MAXILLA

PALATINE BONE

SPHENOID BONE

TEMPORAL BONE

OCCIPITAL BONE

570   Bones of the Exterior of the Base of the Skull

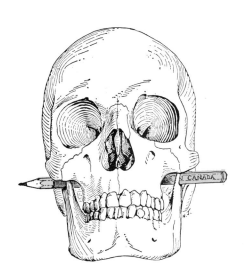

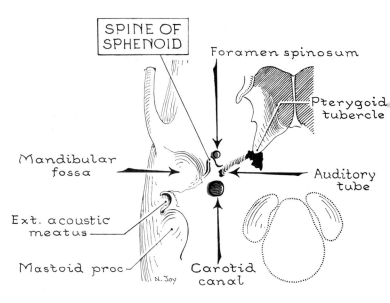

571   A Pencil Passed Across the Base of the Skull

(Anterior transverse line.)
Note:
There being nothing to stop it, a pencil can be passed through both mandibular notches and across the base of the skull; i.e., the pencil lies behind the pterygoid plates and occupies the anterior transverse line (see fig. 571.2, below).

571.1   Spine of the Sphenoid

Note: A blow delivered to the side of the jaw does not drive the jaw under the cranium, because the head of the jaw would require to descend the steep medial wall of the mandibular fossa and the spine of the sphenoid in which that wall ends. Like a sentinel, the spine "keeps guard over" 4 strategic points: (1) anteriorly, the foramen spinosum for the middle meningeal art.; (2) posteriorly, the entrance to the carotid canal; (3) medially, the entrance to the bony auditory tube; and (4) laterally, the mandibular fossa which lodges the head of the mandible, which therefore is the surface landmark to the spine.

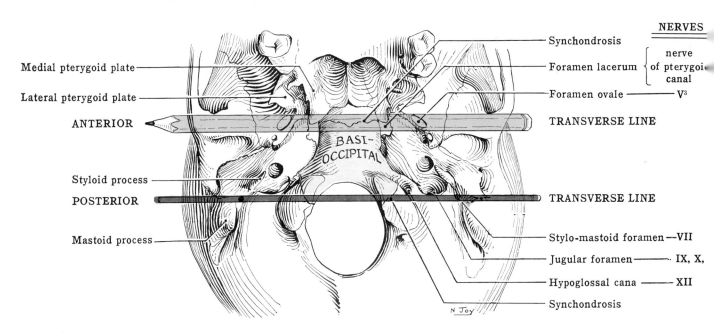

571.2   Anterior and Posterior Transverse Lines at the Base of the Skull

Note: (1) The foramen ovale at the root of the lateral pterygoid plate; the foramen lacerum at the root of the medial pterygoid plate; and the synchondrosis between the basi-occipital and the body of the sphenoid.
(2) The posterior transverse line stretches across the base of the skull between the mastoid and the styloid processes of the two sides. The features it crosses are labelled.
(3) It is to the nerves issuing from the foramina crossed by the transverse lines that the lines owe their importance.

THE 3 KEYS TO EXTERIOR OF BASE OF SKULL

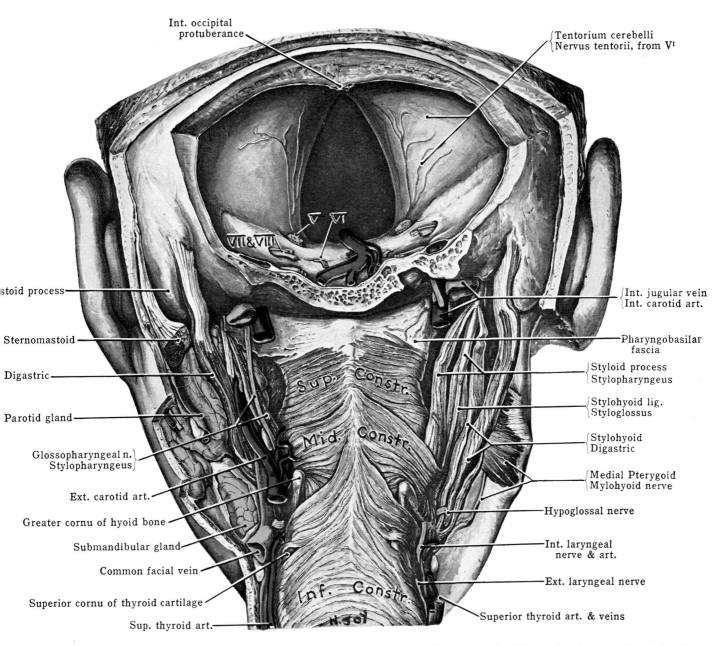

Int. occipital protuberance

Tentorium cerebelli
Nervus tentorii, from V¹

V V^{I}
VII & VIII

stoid process

Int. jugular vein
Int. carotid art.

Sternomastoid

Pharyngobasilar fascia

Digastric

Styloid process
Stylopharyngeus

Parotid gland

Stylohyoid lig.
Styloglossus

Stylohyoid
Digastric

Sup. Constr.

Glossopharyngeal n.
Stylopharyngeus

Medial Pterygoid
Mylohyoid nerve

Mid. Constr.

Ext. carotid art.

Hypoglossal nerve

Greater cornu of hyoid bone

Int. laryngeal nerve & art.

Submandibular gland

Common facial vein

Ext. laryngeal nerve

Inf. Constr.

Superior cornu of thyroid cartilage

Superior thyroid art. & veins

Sup. thyroid art.

N.501

572   Tentorium from below: Pharynx and Parotid Gland, from behind

Observe:

1. The tentorium cerebelli, forming the roof of the posterior cranial fossa, and its nerve. The basi-occipital, sawn across, and the basilar artery, formed by the union of the 2 unequal vertebral arteries, ascending on the dorsum sellae. (For bones, see fig. 497.)

2. The pharyngo-basilar fascia (i.e., the tough submucous coat) suspending the pharynx from the basi-occipital. Of the 3 Constrictors, Inferior overlapping Middle, and Middle overlapping Superior. This posterior aspect is flat or even slightly concave—not round—from side to side, being applied to the prevertebral region (fig. 561), (x-sections 579, 600).

3. The tip of the greater horn of the hyoid bone and descending from it the thyrohyoid ligament which is the posterior border of the thyrohyoid membrane, not labelled.

4. *On Right Side:* the styloid process of the temporal bone, slightly grooved on its medial side from contact with the internal jugular vein, and united to the lesser horn of the hyoid bone (not in view) by the stylohyoid ligament. Stylopharyngeus passing from the medial side of the styloid process for-

wards and medially to the interval between Superior and Middle Constrictors. Stylohyoid passing from the lateral side forwards and laterally to be split on its way to the hyoid bone by the Digastric. Styloglossus passing from the anterior aspect of the process and the ligament medially and forwards to the tongue.

5. *On Left Side:* the glossopharyngeal nerve making a spiral round Stylopharyngeus and both entering the pharyngeal wall.

6. The posterior surface of the parotid gland grooved: by the mastoid process and below this by Sternomastoid, and more medially by Digastric and by the styloid process and the 3 muscles that arise from it (see cross-sections figs. 579 and 584). The parotid gland extending from the skin almost to the pharyngeal wall and separated from the submandibular gland merely by a strong layer of fascia. From the deep fascia processes extending between the lobules of the parotid gland but the submaxillary gland free within its fascial sheath.

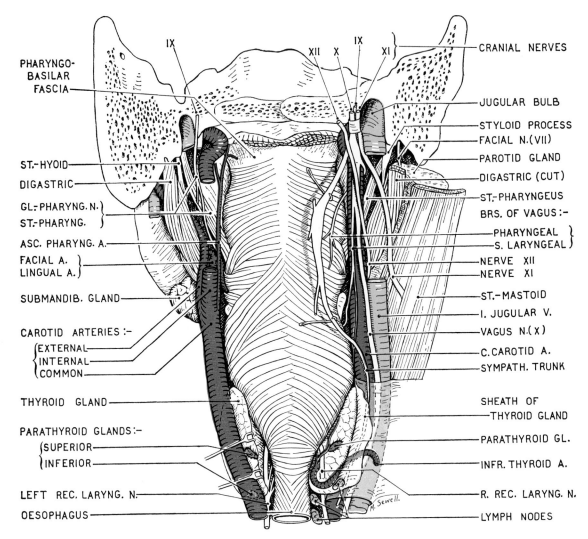

PHARYNGO-BASILAR FASCIA

IX · XII X IX XI — CRANIAL NERVES

ST.-HYOID
DIGASTRIC
GL.-PHARYNG. N.
ST.-PHARYNG.
ASC. PHARYNG. A.
FACIAL A.
LINGUAL A.
SUBMANDIB. GLAND

CAROTID ARTERIES :-
{EXTERNAL
{INTERNAL
{COMMON

THYROID GLAND

PARATHYROID GLANDS :-
{SUPERIOR
{INFERIOR

LEFT REC. LARYNG. N.
OESOPHAGUS

JUGULAR BULB
STYLOID PROCESS
FACIAL N.(VII)
PAROTID GLAND
DIGASTRIC (CUT)
ST.-PHARYNGEUS
BRS. OF VAGUS :-
PHARYNGEAL }
S. LARYNGEAL }
NERVE XII
NERVE XI
ST.-MASTOID
I. JUGULAR V.
VAGUS N.(X)
C. CAROTID A.
SYMPATH. TRUNK

SHEATH OF
THYROID GLAND
PARATHYROID GL.

INFR. THYROID A.

R. REC. LARYNG. N.
LYMPH NODES

M. Sewell.

573 Pharynx and the Last Four Cranial Nerves, from behind

Observe:

1. The narrowest and least distensible part of the alimentary canal, where the pharynx becomes the esophagus.

2. Inferior Constrictor of the pharynx overlapping Middle Constrictor, and Middle overlapping Superior.

3. Between the Superior Constrictor and the base of the skull, the semilunar area on each side where the pharyngo-basilar fascia can be seen attaching the pharynx to the basi-occipital bone.

4. The nerves and vein that emerge from the foramina on "the posterior transverse line of the skull" (fig. 571.2) and which give this line its importance. They are: (a) facial nerve, (b) internal jugular vein, and (c) last four cranial nerves. Of the 4 nerves: IX lies anterior to X and XI; and XII, which is the most medial, makes a half spiral dorsal to X as they both descend.

5. The internal carotid artery lies just behind the midpoint of the oblique line (fig. 571.1) and therefore anterior to the structures on the posterior line. Lying posterior to the artery are the sympathetic trunk and the (elongated) superior cervical ganglion from which fibers, called the int. carotid nerve, accompany the artery into the skull.

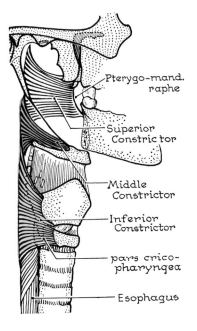

Pterygo-mand. raphe
Superior Constrictor
Middle Constrictor
Inferior Constrictor
pars crico-pharyngea
Esophagus

573.1 Diagram of the 3 constrictors of the pharynx, showing their attachments and borders.

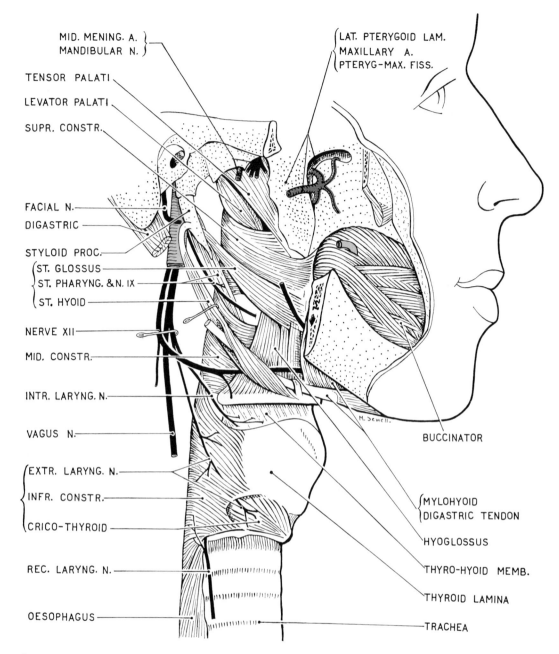

Labels on the diagram:

MID. MENING. A.
MANDIBULAR N.

LAT. PTERYGOID LAM.
MAXILLARY A.
PTERYG-MAX. FISS.

TENSOR PALATI

LEVATOR PALATI

SUPR. CONSTR.

FACIAL N.

DIGASTRIC

STYLOID PROC.

ST. GLOSSUS
ST. PHARYNG. & N. IX
ST. HYOID

NERVE XII

MID. CONSTR.

INTR. LARYNG. N.

VAGUS N.

EXTR. LARYNG. N.

INFR. CONSTR.

CRICO-THYROID

REC. LARYNG. N.

OESOPHAGUS

M. Sewell.

BUCCINATOR

MYLOHYOID
DIGASTRIC TENDON

HYOGLOSSUS

THYRO-HYOID MEMB.

THYROID LAMINA

TRACHEA

574 Pharyngeal Muscles and the Buccinator, side view

Observe:

1. Superior Constrictor and Buccinator arising from opposite sides of the pterygo-mandibular raphe.
2. Middle Constrictor overlapped by Hyoglossus, and Hyoglossus in turn overlapped by Mylohyoid.
3. Inferior Constrictor arising from the oblique line of the lamina of the thyroid cartilage (fig. 623), [from the fibrous arch that joins the tubercle on the lower border of this lamina to the inferior cornu], and, as Cricopharyngeus, from the cricoid cartilage below the cricothyroid joint (figs. 622 & 627).
4. Tensor and Levator Palati, behind the lateral pterygoid lamina or plate, helping to form the medial wall of the infratemporal region.
5. Levator Palati crossing deep to the concave upper border of

Superior Constrictor; Tensor Palati, seen better in figure 575.

6. The styloid process and the 3 muscles that arise from it—Stylo-glossus, Stylo-pharyngeus, Stylo-hyoid.
7. Styloglossus interdigitating with Hyoglossus on the side of the tongue.
   Stylopharyngeus and the glossopharyngeal nerve (IX) passing between Superior and Middle Constrictors.
   Stylohyoid split by the tendon of Digastric and attached to the hyoid bone.
8. The internal laryngeal nerve passing through the thyro-hyoid membrane between Middle and Inferior Constrictors.
9. The recurrent laryngeal nerve (via its terminal or inferior laryngeal branch) passing deep to the lower border of Inferior Constrictor.

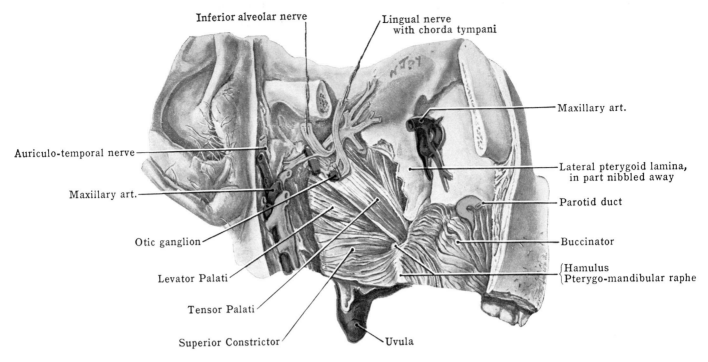

Inferior alveolar nerve

Lingual nerve with chorda tympani

Maxillary art.

Auriculo-temporal nerve

Maxillary art.

Otic ganglion

Levator Palati

Tensor Palati

Superior Constrictor

Lateral pterygoid lamina, in part nibbled away

Parotid duct

Buccinator

{Hamulus Pterygo-mandibular raphe

Uvula

575 Tensor Palati, on lateral view

Note:

1. Levator Palati crossing the upper border of Sup. Constrictor.
2. Tensor Palati forming the medial wall of the infratemporal region, and hooking round the hamulus. (For course, see fig. 619.2).
3. Otic ganglion, here retracted, lying deep to mandibular nerve and below foramen ovale. (For function, see fig. 513.2; for medial view, fig. 598.)

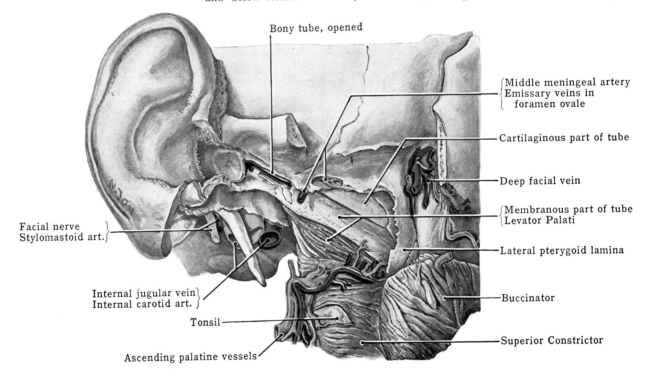

Bony tube, opened

{Middle meningeal artery Emissary veins in foramen ovale

Cartilaginous part of tube

Deep facial vein

{Membranous part of tube Levator Palati

Lateral pterygoid lamina

Buccinator

Superior Constrictor

Facial nerve Stylomastoid art.

Internal jugular vein Internal carotid art.

Tonsil

Ascending palatine vessels

576 Auditory Tube (Pharyngo-tympanic Tube), lateral view

(Tensor Palati is removed.)

Note:

1. The tonsil, here bulging through Sup. Constrictor.
2. The cartilaginous part of the tube resting on a spine on the medial pterygoid lamina; the membranous part "resting on" Levator Palati.
3. Tube, Levator, and vessels crossing the upper border of Sup. Constrictor.
4. Emissary veins from the cavernous sinus in the foramen ovale; and the deep facial vein connecting the maxillary and facial veins.

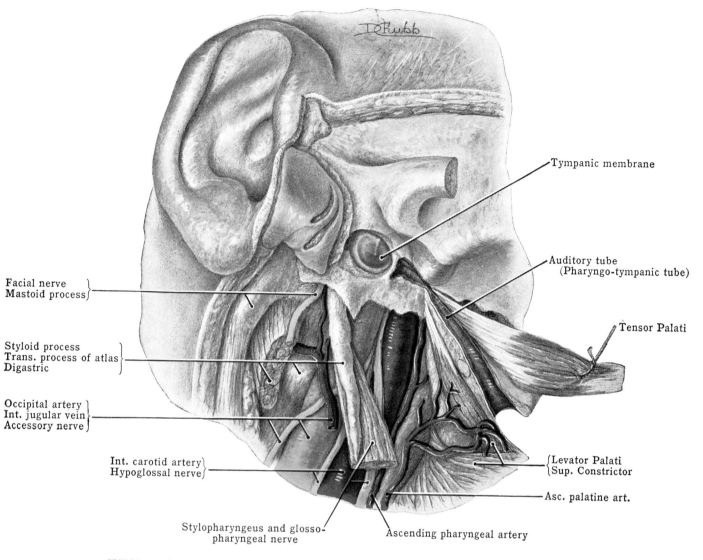

Facial nerve
Mastoid process

Styloid process
Trans. process of atlas
Digastric

Occipital artery
Int. jugular vein
Accessory nerve

Int. carotid artery
Hypoglossal nerve

Stylopharyngeus and glossopharyngeal nerve

Ascending pharyngeal artery

Tympanic membrane

Auditory tube
(Pharyngo-tympanic tube)

Tensor Palati

Levator Palati
Sup. Constrictor

Asc. palatine art.

577 Auditory Tube (Pharyngo-tympanic Tube)

Note:

1. The anterior wall of the cartilaginous part of the external acoustic meatus has two fissures—two unchondrified areas—which are closed with fibrous tissue.

2. The anterior wall of the bony part of the meatus has been ground away.

3. The tympanic membrane lies at the bottom of the meatus. It faces laterally, downwards, and forwards as though to catch sounds reflected from the ground, as one advances. The central part of the membrane is in-drawn (towards the tympanic cavity), the umbo or bottom of the concavity being at the end of the handle of the malleus. The peripheral part of the membrane is thickened at its attachment to the tympanic bone.

4. The auditory tube has been opened from pharyngeal end to tympanic end by excising its lateral membranous wall, but Tensor Palati, which arises in part from the tube, was first reflected. The tympanic segment of the tube is short and bony; the pharyngeal segment is long and cartilaginous. The two segments meet at an angle, and there the tube is narrowest. The lateral wall of the pharyngeal or cartilaginous segment of the tube is, in reality, fibrous; this wall has been excised.

5. The ascending palatine branch of the facial artery ascends on the outer surface of Superior Constrictor to its free upper border and then descends on its medial surface with Levator Palati.

6. The last 4 cranial nerves are close together between the internal jugular vein and the internal carotid artery. The vagus, however, is concealed by the hypoglossal nerve.

7. In this specimen, the stylo-mastoid artery (not labelled), which accompanies the facial nerve, springs from the occipital artery—not the posterior auricular artery as in figure 550.

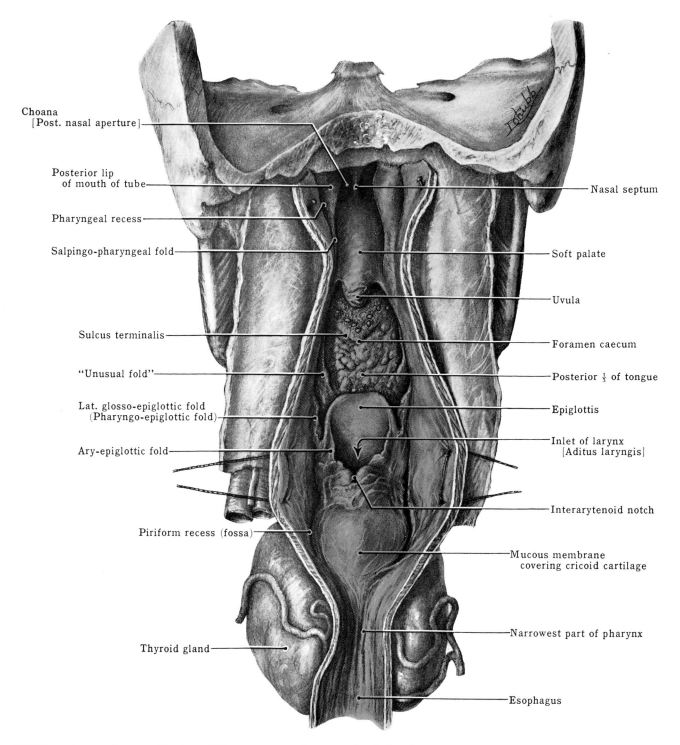

Choana
[Post. nasal aperture]

Posterior lip
of mouth of tube

Pharyngeal recess

Salpingo-pharyngeal fold

Sulcus terminalis

"Unusual fold"

Lat. glosso-epiglottic fold
(Pharyngo-epiglottic fold)

Ary-epiglottic fold

Piriform recess (fossa)

Thyroid gland

Nasal septum

Soft palate

Uvula

Foramen caecum

Posterior $\frac{1}{3}$ of tongue

Epiglottis

Inlet of larynx
[Aditus laryngis]

Interarytenoid notch

Mucous membrane
covering cricoid cartilage

Narrowest part of pharynx

Esophagus

578 Interior of the Pharynx, from behind

Observe:

1. The pharynx extending from the base of the skull to the lower border of the cricoid cartilage where it narrows to become the esophagus.

2. The soft palate ending postero-inferiorly in the uvula, and the larynx ending above at the tip of the epiglottis.

3. The 3 parts of the pharynx—nasal, oral, laryngeal.

4. The nasal part (naso-pharynx) lying above the level of the soft palate and continuous in front, through the choanae, with the nasal cavities.

5. The oral part, lying between the levels of the soft palate and

larynx, communicating in front with the oral cavity, and having the posterior $\frac{1}{3}$ of the tongue as its anterior wall. This part of the tongue is studded with lymph follicles (collectively called the lingual tonsil), and is demarcated from the anterior $\frac{2}{3}$ by the foramen caecum and the V-shaped sulcus terminalis.

6. The laryngeal part lying behind the larynx, and communicating with the cavity of the larynx through the oblique inlet or aditus. On each side of the inlet and separated from it by the ary-epiglottic fold is a piriform recess—the leader pointing to the recess is here too low.

(For side view of interior of pharynx, fig. 587.)

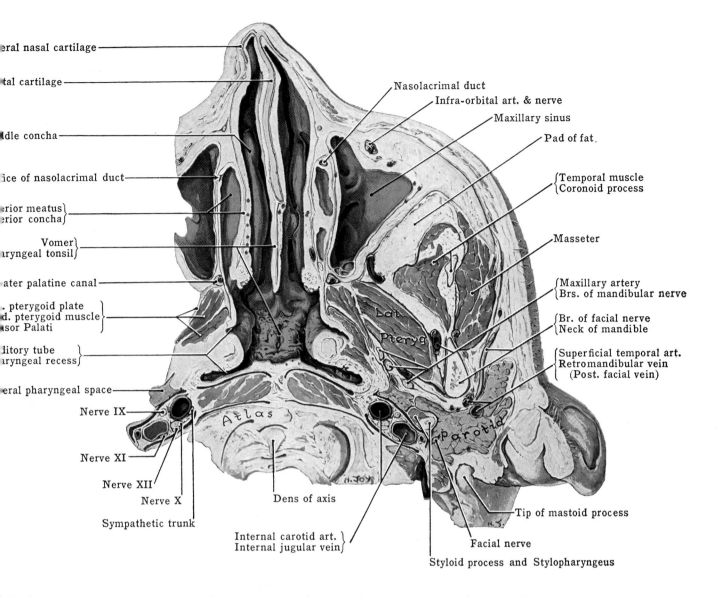

eral nasal cartilage

tal cartilage

dle concha

ice of nasolacrimal duct

rior meatus}
rior concha}

Vomer}
aryngeal tonsil}

ater palatine canal

. pterygoid plate}
d. pterygoid muscle}
sor Palati}

litory tube}
aryngeal recess}

eral pharyngeal space

Nerve IX

Nerve XI

Nerve XII

Nerve X

Sympathetic trunk

Internal carotid art.}
Internal jugular vein}

Dens of axis

Nasolacrimal duct

Infra-orbital art. & nerve

Maxillary sinus

Pad of fat

Temporal muscle}
Coronoid process}

Masseter

Maxillary artery}
Brs. of mandibular **nerve**}

Br. of facial nerve}
Neck of mandible}

Superficial temporal **art.**}
Retromandibular vein}
(Post. facial vein)}

Tip of mastoid process

Facial nerve

Styloid process and Stylopharyngeus

Lat. Pteryg.

Atlas

Parotid

579 Cross Section of Head and Neck, passing through Nasal Cavities, from below

Observe:

1. The septal cartilage continuous with the lateral nasal cartilages.
2. An unusual spur from the nasal septum pushing into the middle concha.
3. The pharyngeal tonsil somewhat overgrown (adenoids).
4. The nasolacrimal duct within the mucous membrane of the inferior meatus on one side, and its orifice on the other side.
5. The posterior ends of the inferior conchae, overgrown.
6. The pharyngeal recess spreading widely behind the mouth of the tube.
7. The mucous membrane of one maxillary sinus much thickened. The infra-orbital nerve and artery in front; the greater palatine nerve and artery behind.
8. The carotid sheath at the base of the skull, postero-lateral to the pharynx, containing the internal carotid, the internal jugular, and 5 nerves (fig. 573).
9. Around the temporal muscle, fatty tissue which is continuous with the buccal pad of fat.
10. Lateral Pterygoid passing obliquely from the medial wall (lat. pterygoid plate) of the infratemporal fossa to the lateral wall (neck of jaw).
11. The parotid gland, its deep relations, the facial nerve largely deep to it.
12. The lateral pharyngeal fatty-areolar "space" (pale green) having the pharynx medially, the carotid sheath posteriorly, the styloid process and its 3 muscles (one at this high level) laterally, branches of the mandibular nerve in a fascial septum anteriorly, and separated from the pharyngeal process of the parotid gland by the stylomandibular lig. (not labelled).

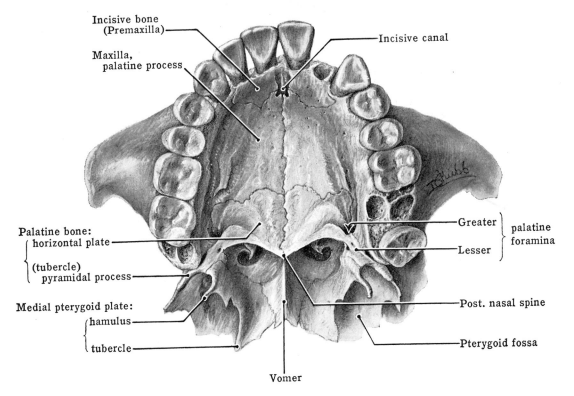

580 Bony Palate—I

(See also figure 570)

Labels for figure 580:
- Incisive bone (Premaxilla)
- Incisive canal
- Maxilla, palatine process
- Palatine bone: horizontal plate
- (tubercle) pyramidal process
- Greater } palatine foramina
- Lesser }
- Medial pterygoid plate: hamulus
- tubercle
- Post. nasal spine
- Pterygoid fossa
- Vomer

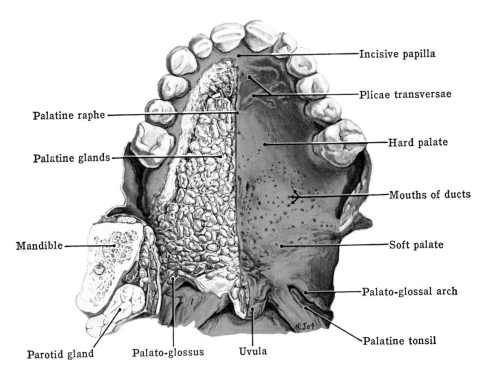

Labels for figure 581:
- Incisive papilla
- Plicae transversae
- Palatine raphe
- Palatine glands
- Hard palate
- Mouths of ducts
- Mandible
- Soft palate
- Palato-glossal arch
- Palatine tonsil
- Parotid gland
- Palato-glossus
- Uvula

581 Palate—II

Observe:

1. On the right side of the page—the transverse palatine folds, which are so conspicuous in the dog; and the orifices of the ducts of the palatine glands which give the mucous membrane an orange-skin appearance.

2. On the left side—the palatine glands, forming a very thick layer in the soft palate; a thin one in the hard palate; and absent in the region of the incisive bone and anterior part of the median raphe.

3. Posteriorly, the palate ending medianly in the uvula, and on each side in the palato-pharyngeal arch. The Palato-glossus and the palato-glossal arch extending to the under surface of the soft palate.

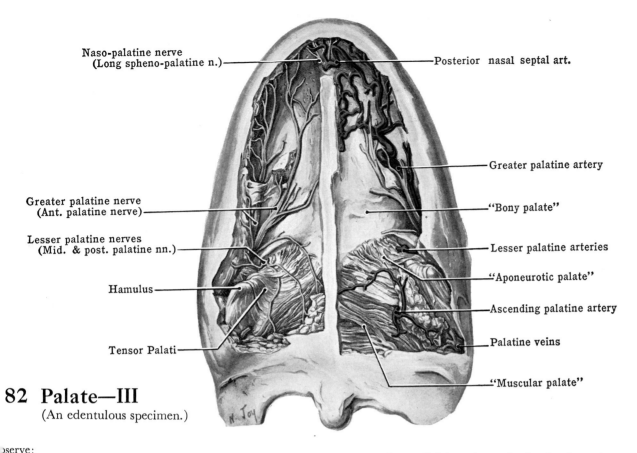

Naso-palatine nerve
(Long spheno-palatine n.)

Posterior nasal septal art.

Greater palatine artery

Greater palatine nerve
(Ant. palatine nerve)

"Bony palate"

Lesser palatine nerves
(Mid. & post. palatine nn.)

Lesser palatine arteries

Hamulus

"Aponeurotic palate"

Ascending palatine artery

Palatine veins

Tensor Palati

"Muscular palate"

N. Joy

82 Palate—III
(An edentulous specimen.)

Observe:

The palate having bony, aponeurotic, and muscular parts.
Tensor Palati hooking round the hamulus to join the palatine
aponeurosis.
Septa from the sponeurosis enclosing palatine glands.
A crest on the bony palate, having a branch of the greater
palatine nerve on each side and the artery on the lateral
side. (Commonly the artery follows the nervous pattern.)
The lateral branch of the nerve expended mainly on the

gums; the medial branch on the hard palate; the naso-
palatine nerve in the incisive region; and the lesser palatine
nerves in the soft palate.

6. Four palatine arteries, 2 being on the hard palate and 2 on
the soft:—(a) greater palatine art. which anastomoses
through the incisive canal with (b) posterior septal art.
(fig. 607), (c) lesser palatine arteries, and (d) ascending
palatine art. (fig. 577) which enters the soft palate with
Levator Palati.

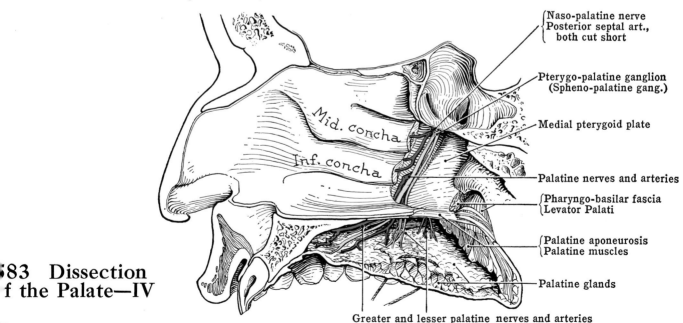

Naso-palatine nerve
Posterior septal art.,
both cut short

Pterygo-palatine ganglion
(Spheno-palatine gang.)

Medial pterygoid plate

Mid. concha

Inf. concha

Palatine nerves and arteries

Pharyngo-basilar fascia
Levator Palati

Palatine aponeurosis
Palatine muscles

Palatine glands

Greater and lesser palatine nerves and arteries

583 Dissection of the Palate—IV

Observe:

The mucous membrane, containing a layer of mucous
glands has been separated by blunt dissection. The layer of
glands is thin on the bony palate where it is part of a muco-
periosteum; it is thickest on the aponeurotic part; and is less
thick on the muscular part (fig. 587).

2. The posterior ends ($\frac{1}{3}''$) of the middle and inferior conchae
are cut through; these and the muco-periosteum are peeled
off the side wall of the nose as far as the posterior border of
the medial pterygoid plate. The papery perpendicular
plate of the palatine bone is broken through and the palatine
nerves and arteries are thereby exposed.

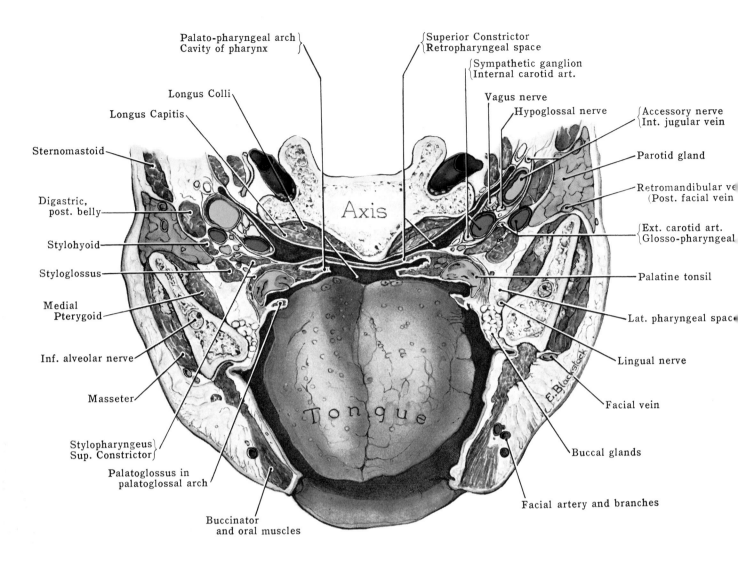

Palato-pharyngeal arch
Cavity of pharynx
Longus Colli
Longus Capitis
Sternomastoid
Digastric,
post. belly
Stylohyoid
Styloglossus
Medial
Pterygoid
Inf. alveolar nerve
Masseter
Stylopharyngeus
Sup. Constrictor
Palatoglossus in
palatoglossal arch
Buccinator
and oral muscles

Superior Constrictor
Retropharyngeal space
Sympathetic ganglion
Internal carotid art.
Vagus nerve
Hypoglossal nerve
Accessory nerve
Int. jugular vein
Parotid gland
Retromandibular ve
(Post. facial vein
Ext. carotid art.
Glosso-pharyngeal
Palatine tonsil
Lat. pharyngeal spac
Lingual nerve
Facial vein
Buccal glands
Facial artery and branches

Axis
Tongue

E. Blackstock

584 Cross Section of the Head and Neck, passing through the mouth

Observe:

1. The parotid gland filling its wedge-shaped bed or mould; the Digastric and Stylohyoid intervening between the parotid gland and the great vessels and nerves of the neck.

2. The Masseter inserted into one surface of the ramus of the jaw and the Medial Pterygoid inserted into the other.

3. The lingual nerve in contact with the ramus of the jaw.

4. Anterior to the ribbon-like Palatoglossus and its arch is the mouth; behind it is the pharynx.

5. The pharynx flattened antero-posteriorly, and the tonsil in its wall.

6. The tonsil bed formed by Superior Constrictor and Palatopharyngeus, an areolar space intervening, and limited in front and behind by the palatine arches. The carotid arteries well behind the bed.

7. The retropharyngeal space, here opened up, which allows the pharynx to contract and relax during swallowing. It is closed laterally at the carotid sheath and is limited posteriorly by the prevertebral fascia.

8. The three styloid muscles:—Stylohyoid, Styloglossus, and Stylopharyngeus. Stylopharyngeus being deepest and about to blend with Palatopharyngeus (Fig. 589).

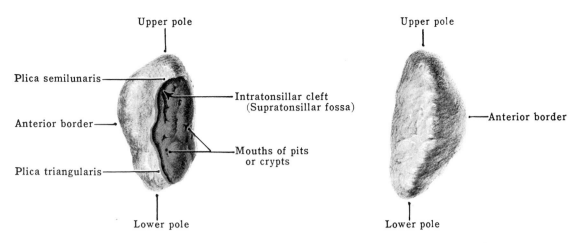

Upper pole

Plica semilunaris

Intratonsillar cleft
(Supratonsillar fossa)

Anterior border

Mouths of pits
or crypts

Plica triangularis

Lower pole

Upper pole

Anterior border

Lower pole

585 Palatine Tonsil ("The Tonsil"), medial and lateral views

Observe:

1. The long axis running vertically.
2. The fibrous capsule forming the lateral or attached surface of the tonsil. In removing the tonsil, the loose areolar tissue lying between the capsule and the thin pharyngobasilar fascia, which forms the immediate bed of the tonsil, was easily torn through.
3. The capsule extending round the anterior border and

slightly over the medial surface as a thin, free fold, covered with mucous membrane on both surfaces.

The upper part of this fold is called the plica semilunaris; the lower, the plica triangularis.

4. On the medial or free surface, the dozen stellate orifices of the testtube-like crypts, which extend right through the organ to the capsule. The intratonsillar cleft, which extends towards the upper pole.

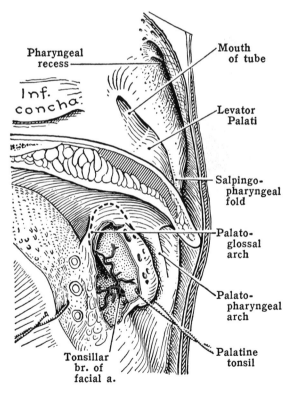

Pharyngeal recess

Inf. concha.

Mouth of tube

Levator Palati

Salpingo-pharyngeal fold

Palato-glossal arch

Palato-pharyngeal arch

Tonsillar br. of facial a.

Palatine tonsil

FIRST STAGE

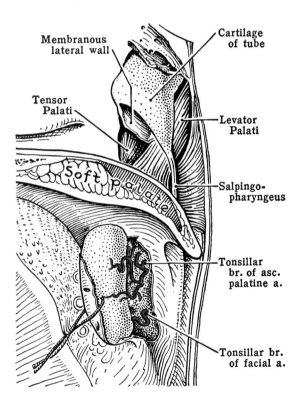

Membranous lateral wall

Cartilage of tube

Tensor Palati

Levator Palati

Soft Palate

Salpingo-pharyngeus

Tonsillar br. of asc. palatine a.

Tonsillar br. of facial a.

SECOND STAGE

586 Removal of the Tonsil. The Arterial Supply

(*Dissections by Dr. P. G. Ashmore.*)

The mucous membrane has been incised along the palatoglossal arch, and the areolar space lateral to the fibrous capsule of the tonsil has been entered.

With the point and the rounded handle of the knife, the anterior border of the tonsil has been freed and the upper part, which extends far into the soft palate, has been shelled out. The mucous membrane along the palatopharyngeal arch is now cut through.

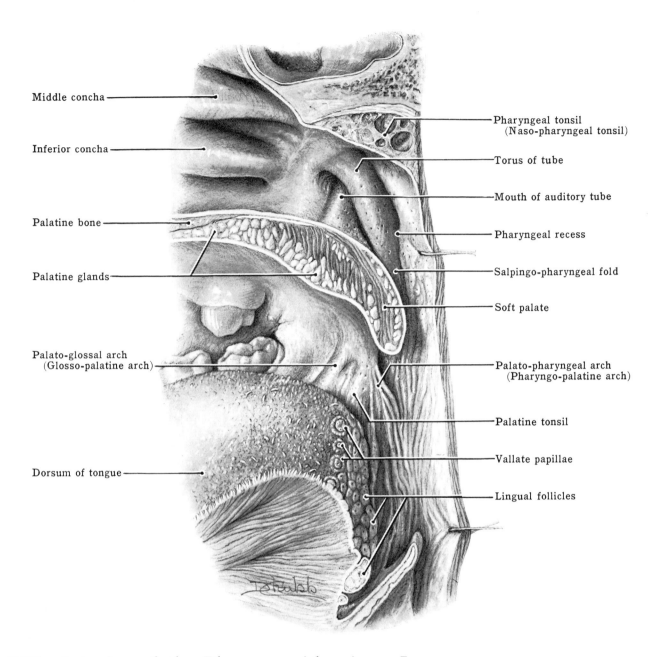

Middle concha

Inferior concha

Palatine bone

Palatine glands

Palato-glossal arch
(Glosso-palatine arch)

Dorsum of tongue

Pharyngeal tonsil
(Naso-pharyngeal tonsil)

Torus of tube

Mouth of auditory tube

Pharyngeal recess

Salpingo-pharyngeal fold

Soft palate

Palato-pharyngeal arch
(Pharyngo-palatine arch)

Palatine tonsil

Vallate papillae

Lingual follicles

587   Interior of the Pharynx, side view—I

Observe:

1. The prominent torus (superior and posterior lips) of the auditory tube and the salpingo-pharyngeal fold, which descends from the torus.

2. The location of the orifice of the tube—about ½″ behind the inferior concha.

3. The ridge, (torus levatorius) produced by Levator Palati which has the appearance of being poured out of the tube.

4. The deep pharyngeal recess behind the torus of the tube.

5. The numerous pinpoint orifices of the ducts of mucous glands about the torus and elsewhere.

6. The pharyngeal tonsil, better seen in figure 579 where deep clefts extend into the lymphoid tissue.

7. The considerable proportion of glandular tissue in the soft palate and its disposition.

8. The palato-glossal and the palato-pharyngeal arches which, in this specimen are not the sharp folds commonly seen, and the somewhat inconspicuous palatine tonsil between them.

9. The lingual follicles, each with the duct of a mucous gland opening on to its surface. Collectively, the follicles are known as the lingual tonsil.

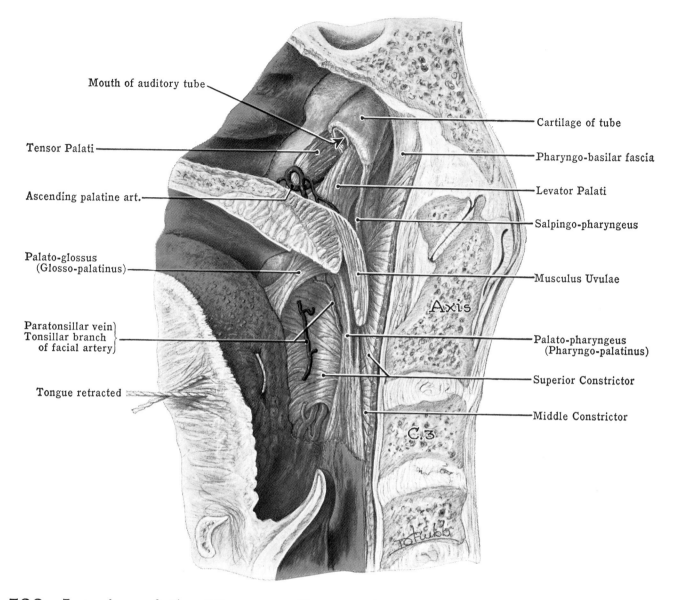

Mouth of auditory tube

Tensor Palati

Ascending palatine art.

Palato-glossus
(Glosso-palatinus)

Paratonsillar vein
Tonsillar branch
of facial artery

Tongue retracted

Cartilage of tube

Pharyngo-basilar fascia

Levator Palati

Salpingo-pharyngeus

Musculus Uvulae

Axis

Palato-pharyngeus
(Pharyngo-palatinus)

Superior Constrictor

Middle Constrictor

C.3

588   Interior of the Pharynx dissected, side view—II

The palatine and pharyngeal tonsils and the mucous membrane are removed. The submucous pharyngo-basilar fascia, which attaches the pharynx to the basilar part of the occipital bone, is thick above and thin below. It too has been removed, except at the upper arched border of Superior Constrictor.

Observe:

1. The curved cartilage of the auditory tube; its free, upper and posterior lips at the pharyngeal orifice of the tube; and Salpingo-pharyngeus descending from the posterior lip to join Palato-pharyngeus.

2. The ascending palatine branch of the facial artery descending with Levator Palati to the soft palate (fig. 577).

3. The 5 muscles of the palate (paired)—Tensor Palati (see fig. 590), Levator Palati providing most of the muscle fibres seen in the cross section of the soft palate; Musculus Uvulae, a fingerlike bundle, arising largely from the palatine

aponeurosis at the post. nasal spine (fig. 580); Palatoglossus, here a substantial band, but commonly a wisp of muscle with free anterior and posterior borders (fig. 584); and Palatopharyngeus, described with figure 589.

4. The tonsil bed from which a thin sheet of pharyngo-basilar fascia has been removed thereby exposing Palato-pharyngeus and Superior Constrictor.

Note: The bed of the palatine tonsil extends far into the soft palate; the tonsillar branch of the facial artery is here long and large; the paratonsillar vein, descending from the soft palate to join the pharyngeal plexus of veins, is a close lateral relation of the tonsil.

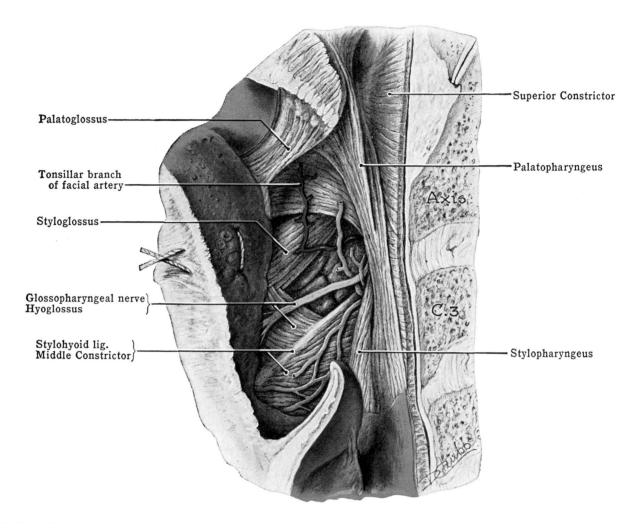

Palatoglossus

Tonsillar branch
of facial artery

Styloglossus

Glossopharyngeal nerve
Hyoglossus

Stylohyoid lig.
Middle Constrictor

Superior Constrictor

Palatopharyngeus

Axis

C.3

Stylopharyngeus

589   Deep Dissection of the Tonsil Bed—III

The tongue is pulled forward and the lower or lingual origin of Superior Constrictor is cut away.

Observe:

1. Styloglossus passing to the anterior $\frac{2}{3}$ of the tongue, where its bundles interdigitate with those of Hyoglossus, and therefore anterior to the glossopharyngeal nerve which is passing to the posterior $\frac{1}{3}$ of the tongue. This nerve, in turn lying anterior to Stylopharyngeus which descends along the anterior border of Palatopharyngeus.

2. The tonsillar branch of the facial artery, here sending a large branch (cut short) to accompany the glossopharyngeal nerve to the tongue. Lateral to the artery and the para-

tonsillar vein the submandibular salivary gland is seen.

Note: (a) In the region of the tonsil bed, Palatopharyngeus is commonly not well differentiated from Superior Constrictor, which makes it difficult or even arbitrary to decide where the lower border of Palatopharyngeus is. Elsewhere its borders are easily defined.

(b) Palatopharyngeus and Stylopharyngeus forming the longitudinal coat of the pharynx; the Constrictors form the circular coat.

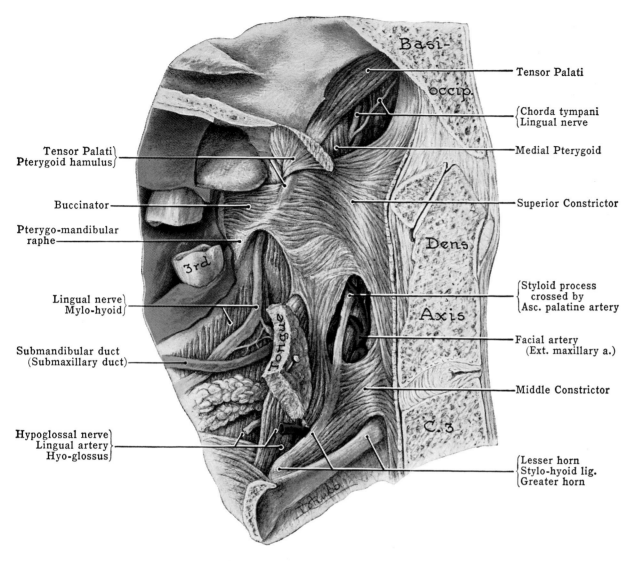

Tensor Palati

Chorda tympani
Lingual nerve

Medial Pterygoid

Superior Constrictor

Styloid process
crossed by
Asc. palatine artery

Facial artery
(Ext. maxillary a.)

Middle Constrictor

Lesser horn
Stylo-hyoid lig.
Greater horn

Tensor Palati
Pterygoid hamulus

Buccinator

Pterygo-mandibular
raphe

Lingual nerve
Mylo-hyoid

Submandibular duct
(Submaxillary duct)

Hypoglossal nerve
Lingual artery
Hyo-glossus

Basi-
occip.

Dens

Axis

C.3

3rd

Tongue

590   Superior and Middle Constrictors of the Pharynx, from within—IV

Observe:

1. Superior Constrictor arising from the pterygo-mandibular raphe which unites it to Buccinator, and from the bone at each end of the raphe (viz., the hamulus of the medial pterygoid plate superiorly and the mandible inferiorly) and also from the root of the tongue.

2. The arched upper and lower borders of Superior Constrictor extending to the median plane where the muscle meets its fellow of the opposite side.

3. Middle Constrictor arising from the angle formed by the greater and lesser horns or cornua of the hyoid bone and

from the stylohyoid lig. In this specimen, the styloid process is long (fig. 568) and is therefore a lateral relation of the tonsil.

4. The facial artery arching over the posterior belly of Digastric, and the loop of the lingual artery just below it.

5. The tendon of Tensor Palati hooking around the hamulus and then ascending to blend with the palatine aponeurosis, i.e., it takes a recurrent course.

6. The lingual nerve joined by the chorda tympani, disappearing at the posterior border of Medial Pterygoid, reappearing at the anterior border, and applied to the mandible.

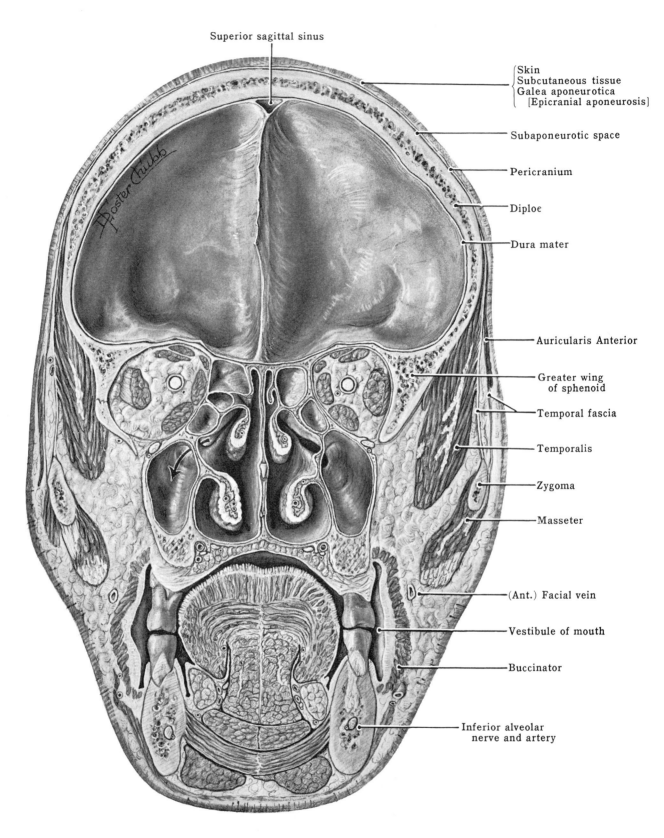

Superior sagittal sinus

Skin
Subcutaneous tissue
Galea aponeurotica
[Epicranial aponeurosis]

Subaponeurotic space

Pericranium

Diploe

Dura mater

Auricularis Anterior

Greater wing
of sphenoid

Temporal fascia

Temporalis

Zygoma

Masseter

(Ant.) Facial vein

Vestibule of mouth

Buccinator

Inferior alveolar
nerve and artery

591 Coronal Section of the Head

(For legend see figure 592.)

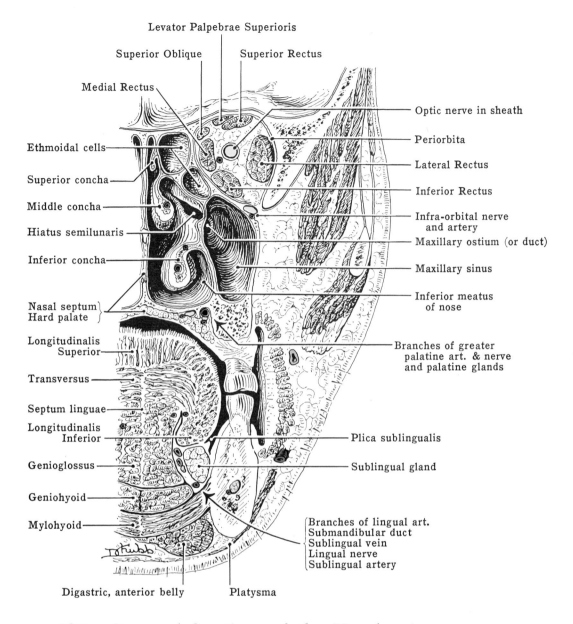

Levator Palpebrae Superioris

Superior Oblique   Superior Rectus

Medial Rectus

Optic nerve in sheath

Periorbita

Ethmoidal cells

Lateral Rectus

Superior concha

Inferior Rectus

Middle concha

Infra-orbital nerve
and artery

Hiatus semilunaris

Maxillary ostium (or duct)

Inferior concha

Maxillary sinus

Inferior meatus
of nose

Nasal septum
Hard palate

Branches of greater
palatine art. & nerve
and palatine glands

Longitudinalis
Superior

Transversus

Septum linguae

Longitudinalis
Inferior

Plica sublingualis

Genioglossus

Sublingual gland

Geniohyoid

Branches of lingual art.
Submandibular duct
Sublingual vein
Lingual nerve
Sublingual artery

Mylohyoid

Digastric, anterior belly   Platysma

592 Coronal Section of the Head
(Key to figure 591.)

Observe:

1. By reference to figure 521, that the section passes through the optic nerve and therefore through the posterior half of the orbital cavity.
2. The subarachnoid space between the optic nerve and its sheath; the orbital fat, the surrounding muscles, and the easily detachable periorbita.
3. The nasal cavity wide at the floor, but very narrow at the roof.
4. The middle concha sheltering the hiatus semilunaris into which the maxillary ostium opens.
5. The layer of glands in the mucoperiosteum of the palate; the vessels and nerves deep to the glands.
6. The median or sucking groove on the tongue which becomes deeper on forceful sucking, as may be tested with one's finger.
7. How in chewing, the tongue pushes food between the molar or millstone teeth into the vestibule and the Buccinator pushes it back again.
8. The hairs of the beard extending through the skin into the fat of the cheek and chin.

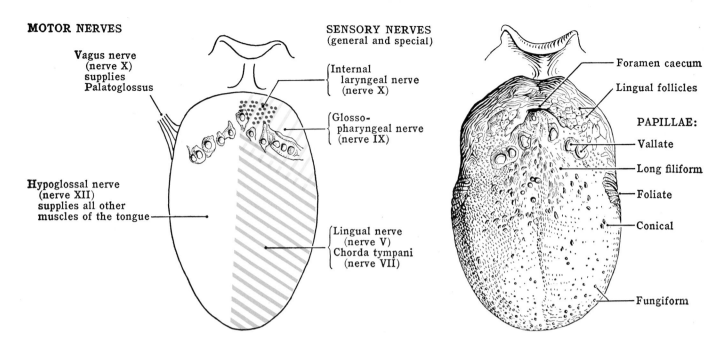

MOTOR NERVES

Vagus nerve
(nerve X)
supplies
Palatoglossus

SENSORY NERVES
(general and special)

Internal
laryngeal nerve
(nerve X)

Glosso-
pharyngeal nerve
(nerve IX)

Hypoglossal nerve
(nerve XII)
supplies all other
muscles of the tongue

Lingual nerve
(nerve V)
Chorda tympani
(nerve VII)

Foramen caecum

Lingual follicles

PAPILLAE:

Vallate

Long filiform

Foliate

Conical

Fungiform

**593 Diagram of the Nerve
Supply to the Tongue**

594 Dorsum of the Tongue

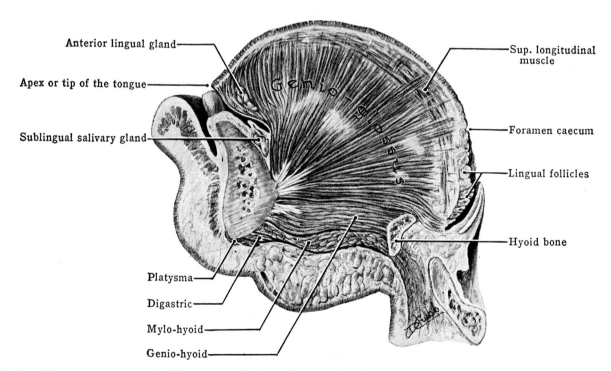

Anterior lingual gland

Apex or tip of the tongue

Sublingual salivary gland

Sup. longitudinal
muscle

Foramen caecum

Lingual follicles

Hyoid bone

Platysma

Digastric

Mylo-hyoid

Genio-hyoid

595 Tongue and Floor of the Mouth, on median section

Observe:

1. The 11 vallate papillae in figure 593 and the 7 in figure 594.

2. In figure 594, the foramen caecum, which is the patent upper end of the primitive thyro-glossal duct, and the limbs of the V-shaped sulcus terminalis, which diverge from the foramen, lie slightly behind the vallate papillae, and demarcate the developmentally different, posterior $\frac{1}{3}$ of the tongue from the anterior $\frac{2}{3}$.

3. The claw-like, conical papillae and the long filiform papillae which are directed postero-medially.

4. In figure 595 parts of the median septum of the tongue which appear as whitish areas. The anterior lingual gland, covered with a layer of muscle. The several ducts of this mixed muco-serous gland open below the tongue, but are not in view.

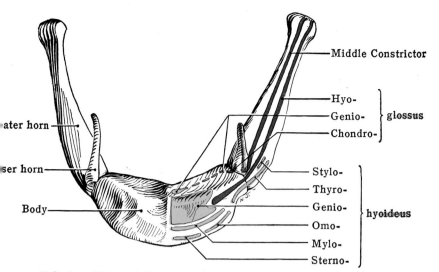

Middle Constrictor

Hyo-
Genio- } glossus
Chondro-

Stylo-
Thyro-
Genio-
Omo-
Mylo-
Sterno- } hyoideus

ater horn
ser horn
Body

596   Hyoid Bone, showing attachments of muscles

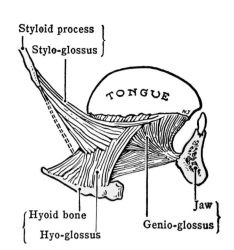

Styloid process } Stylo-glossus

TONGUE

Hyoid bone
Hyo-glossus
Genio-glossus
Jaw

596.1   Diagram of the 3 extrinsic lingual muscles to show their attachments, shapes, and directions.

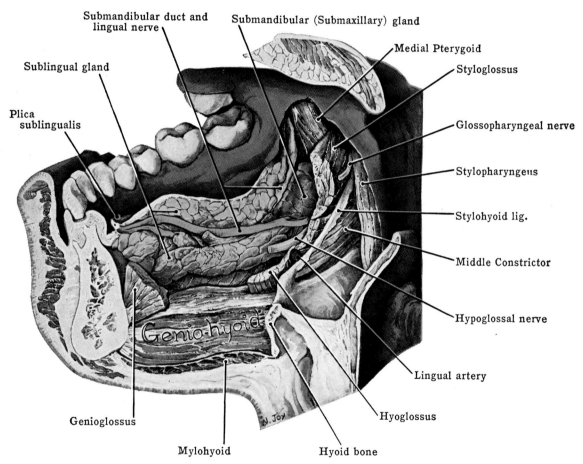

Submandibular duct and lingual nerve
Submandibular (Submaxillary) gland
Sublingual gland
Medial Pterygoid
Styloglossus
Plica sublingualis
Glossopharyngeal nerve
Stylopharyngeus
Stylohyoid lig.
Middle Constrictor
Hypoglossal nerve
Lingual artery
Genio-hyoid
Hyoglossus
Genioglossus
Mylohyoid
Hyoid bone

N. Joy

597   Floor and Side of Mouth, from which tongue is excised

Observe:

. Undisturbed:—Geniohyoid inferiorly, Middle Constrictor posteriorly, and the cut edge of the mucous membrane superiorly.

. Three divided muscles:—Genioglossus anteriorly, Hyoglossus inferiorly, and Styloglossus posteriorly.

. Other 3 divided structures:—lingual and, hypoglossal nerves, and lingual artery. The lingual nerve appearing between Medial Pterygoid and the ramus of the jaw and making three quarters of a spiral around the submandibular duct, being first superolateral, then in turn lateral, inferior,

medial, and superomedial. The hypoglossal nerve separated from the lingual artery by Hyoglossus.

4. The deep or oral part of the submandibular gland in the angle between the lingual nerve and the submandibular duct, which separate it from the sublingual gland. The orifice of the duct is seen at the anterior end of the plica sublingualis.

5. The submandibular duct adhering to the medial side of the sublingual gland, and here receiving, as it sometimes does, a large accessory duct from the lower part of the sublingual gland. For the lesser ducts see figure 547.

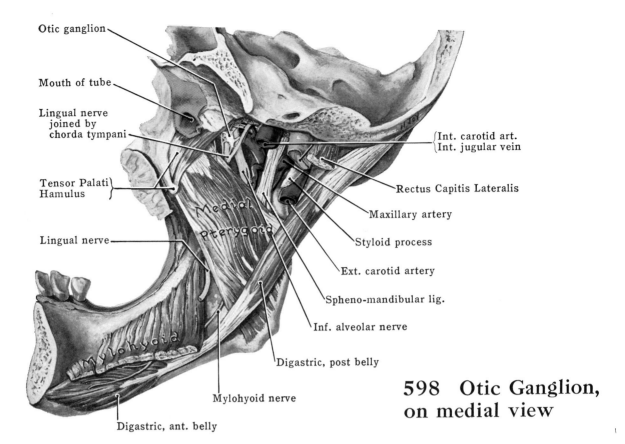

Otic ganglion

Mouth of tube

Lingual nerve
joined by
chorda tympani

Tensor Palati
Hamulus

Lingual nerve

Int. carotid art.
Int. jugular vein

Rectus Capitis Lateralis

Maxillary artery

Styloid process

Ext. carotid artery

Spheno-mandibular lig.

Inf. alveolar nerve

Digastric, post belly

Mylohyoid nerve

Digastric, ant. belly

598 Otic Ganglion, on medial view

Observe:

1. Mylohyoid with thick, free, posterior border thinning anteriorly where, below the origins of the genial muscles (see below), it must be almost functionless and may be deficient, as here, with resulting thin, free, anterior border.

2. Medial Pterygoid taking much the same direction on the medial side of the ramus as Masseter takes on the lateral.

3. Tensor Palati, here sending some fibres to the hamulus.

4. The lingual nerve, joined above Medial Pterygoid by the chorda tympani and appearing in the mouth at the anterior border of that muscle.

5. The otic ganglion lying medial to the mandibular nerve, and between foramen ovale above and Medial Pterygoid below. Tensor Palati usually covers the ganglion (fig. 659).

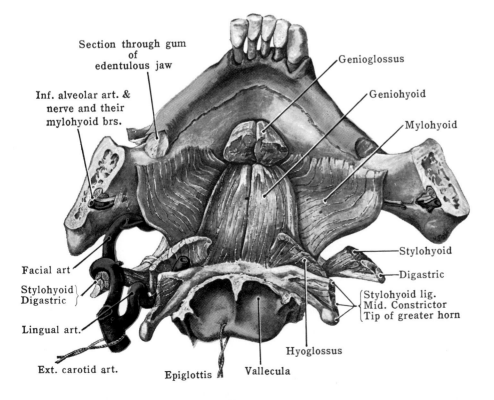

Section through gum of edentulous jaw

Inf. alveolar art. & nerve and their mylohyoid brs.

Genioglossus

Geniohyoid

Mylohyoid

Facial art

Stylohyoid
Digastric

Lingual art.

Ext. carotid art.

Epiglottis

Vallecula

Hyoglossus

Stylohyoid

Digastric

Stylohyoid lig.
Mid. Constrictor
Tip of greater horn

599 Muscles of the Floor of the Mouth

Observe:

1. Geniohyoid, paired, triangular, and occupying a horizontal plane, with apex at mental spine, base at the body of the hyoid bone, medial border in contact with its fellow, and lateral border in contact with Mylohyoid.

2. Mylohyoid arising from the mylohyoid line of the jaw (fig. 553.1); having a thick, free posterior border; thinning as it is traced forwards; and ending in a delicate, free, anterior border as it nears the origin of the genial muscles.

(Mylohyoid from below, fig. 544.)

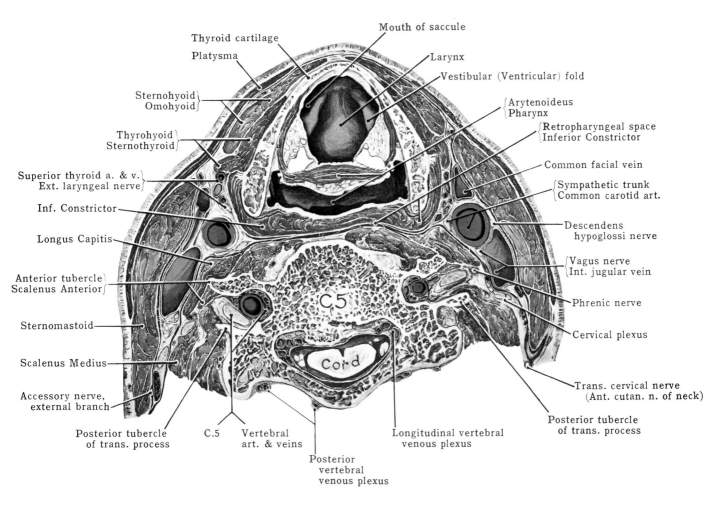

Thyroid cartilage
Platysma
Sternohyoid}
Omohyoid}
Thyrohyoid}
Sternothyroid}
Superior thyroid a. & v.}
Ext. laryngeal nerve}
Inf. Constrictor
Longus Capitis
Anterior tubercle}
Scalenus Anterior}
Sternomastoid
Scalenus Medius
Accessory nerve,
external branch
Posterior tubercle
of trans. process
C.5
Vertebral
art. & veins
Posterior
vertebral
venous plexus
Longitudinal vertebral
venous plexus
Mouth of saccule
Larynx
Vestibular (Ventricular) fold
Arytenoideus}
Pharynx}
Retropharyngeal space}
Inferior Constrictor}
Common facial vein
Sympathetic trunk}
Common carotid art.}
Descendens
hypoglossi nerve
Vagus nerve}
Int. jugular vein}
Phrenic nerve
Cervical plexus
Trans. cervical nerve
(Ant. cutan. n. of neck)
Posterior tubercle
of trans. process
C.5
Cord

600 Cross section of the Neck, passing through the middle of the Larynx, from below

Observe:

1. The thyroid cartilage shielding the larynx and the pharynx.

2. The vestibular folds, seen from below, and lateral to them the mouths of the saccules of the larynx.

3. Arytenoideus (cut obliquely, hence appearing wide) attached to the posterior surface of the arytenoid cartilage and incontinuity with Thyro-arytenoideus (not labelled).

4. Inferior Constrictor, curving round the posterior borders of the laminae of the thyroid cartilage to be attached to the oblique line (fig. 623). Sternothyroid and Thyrohyoid sharing the oblique line. (figs. 529 & 530).

5. The superior thyroid vessels and the external laryngeal nerve applied to Inferior Constrictor.

6. The 3 contents of the carotid sheath—the common carotid

artery, internal jugular vein and, in the posterior angle between them, the vagus nerve.

7. The sympathetic trunk, postero-medial to the carotid artery and medial to the vagus. The superior root of ansa cervicalis (descendens hypoglossi nerve) in front of the carotid artery.

8. The retropharyngeal space, between the pharyngeal fascia, which covers Inf. Constrictor, and the prevertebral fascia, which covers Longi Colli et Capitis. This areolar space extending laterally to the carotid sheath and readily opened up beyond it. The phrenic nerve deep to the prevertebral fascia.

9. The vertebral artery, surrounded with a plexus of veins (which inferiorly becomes the vertebral vein) and the ventral ramus of a cervical nerve (C. 5) crossing behind it.

10. Internal and external parts of the vertebral venous plexus.

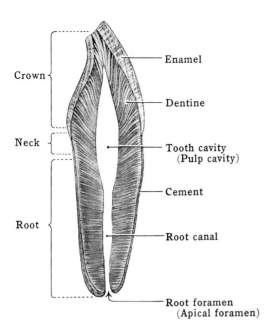

Crown
Neck
Root

Enamel

Dentine

Tooth cavity
(Pulp cavity)

Cement

Root canal

Root foramen
(Apical foramen)

601 Incisor Tooth, longitudinal section

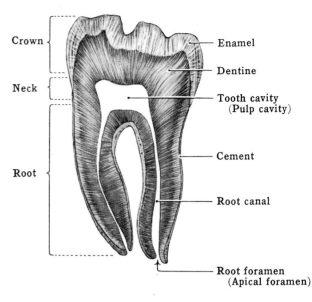

Crown
Neck
Root

Enamel

Dentine

Tooth cavity
(Pulp cavity)

Cement

Root canal

Root foramen
(Apical foramen)

601.1 Molar Tooth, longitudinal section

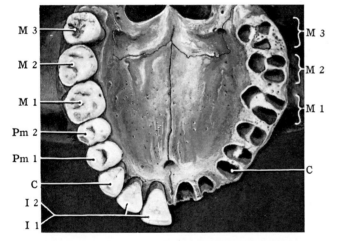

M 3
M 2
M 1
Pm 2
Pm 1
C
I 2
I 1

M 3
M 2
M 1

C

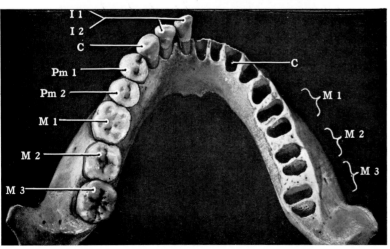

I 1
I 2
C
Pm 1
Pm 2
M 1
M 2
M 3

C

M 1
M 2
M 3

601.2 Permanent Teeth and their Sockets

Observe:

1. There are 32 permanent teeth, of which 8 are on each side of each dental arch—2 incisors, 1 canine, 2 premolars, and 3 molars. Hence the formula reads:

$$\frac{3.2.1.2.}{3.2.1.2.} \quad \frac{2.1.2.3.}{2.1.2.3.}$$

2. Upper or maxillary incisor teeth are larger than lower or mandibular incisor teeth. The upper central incisors are the largest of the incisors and the lower central are the smallest. In each dental arch the 1st molar tooth is usually the largest molar and the 3rd molar is the smallest, though the 3rd lower molar may be very large, as here.

3. Crowns: An incisor tooth has a cutting edge; a canine tooth (cuspid) has one cusp on its crown; a premolar tooth (bicuspid) has 2 (or 3) cusps; and a molar tooth has from 3 to 5 cusps. The crowns of the upper molars are either square or rhomboidal. The 1st usually has 4 cusps; the 2nd either 4 or 3; and the 3rd 3.
The crowns of the lower molars are oblong. The 1st has 5 cusps; the 2nd 4; and the 3rd from 3 to 5. The crowns are, here, well worn.

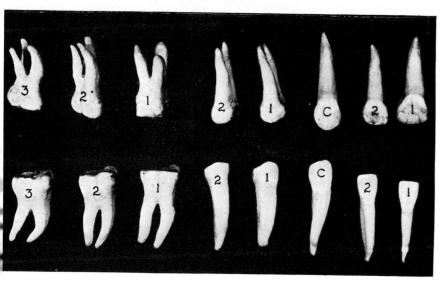

601.3 Roots of the Permanent Teeth, labial (buccal) view

Their empty sockets are shown in figure 601.2

Their empty sockets are shown in figure 601.2

Observe:

1. Lower or mandibular teeth: The incisor, canine, and premolar (bicuspid) teeth have each one root, whereas the molars have each 2 roots, a mesial (anterior) and a distal (posterior). The mesial roots generally have 2 root canals. The roots are flattened mesiodistally (i.e., from central incisor backwards to the 3rd molar).
   The sockets for the lower incisor teeth are near the labial surface of the mandible, whereas those for the lower molars are near the lingual surface.

2. Upper or maxillary teeth: The incisor and canine teeth have each one root. The premolars have each either one or 2 roots, the first premolar usually having 2, a lingual and a labial, and the second usually having one—though sometimes, as here, both premolars have 2 roots. Each of the 3 molars has 3 roots, one being lingual and 2 being labial (buccal). The roots are flattened mesio-distally, except the root of the central incisor and the lingual root of each of the 3 molars which are circular on cross section.

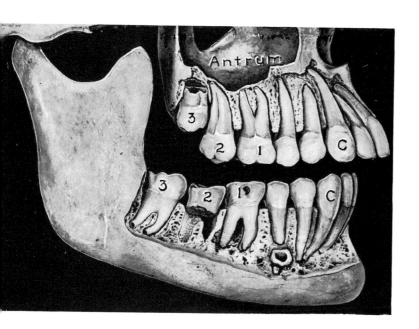

Observe:

1. The upper canine ("eye tooth") has the longest root; indeed, this is the longest tooth.
2. The roots of the upper premolars, in this specimen, are at some distance from the maxillary sinus or antrum, but the roots of the 3 molars almost penetrate into the sinus (see figs. 616 and 616.3).
3. The root of the 2nd lower premolar, very long in this specimen, does not usually extend below the level of the mental foramen.
4. The roots of the 2nd lower molar have been removed, thereby revealing the cribriform nature of the wall of a socket.
5. The upper and lower 3rd molars are not yet fully developed. The lower is more advanced than the upper—the root foramina of the lower are still large; whereas the roots of the upper have not yet formed.

601.4 Permanent Teeth, in situ, Roots exposed

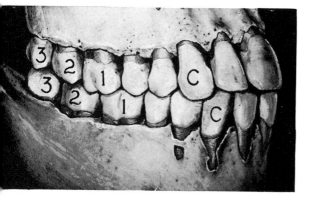

601.5 Permanent Teeth, in occlusion

Observe:

1. The upper and lower teeth begin flush, or nearly so, on one side and end flush on the other.
2. The lower central incisor is the smallest of the incisors, and the 3rd upper molar is the smallest of the molars. Except for these 2 teeth—the first in the lower row and the last in the upper—all teeth, when in occlusion, bite on two opposing teeth.
3. The upper dental arch overlaps the lower dental arch.
4. The lower incisors bite against the lingual surface of the upper incisors (fig. 458) and not edge-to-edge as in prehistoric man. As a variant there may be a considerable overbite (fig. 601.4).

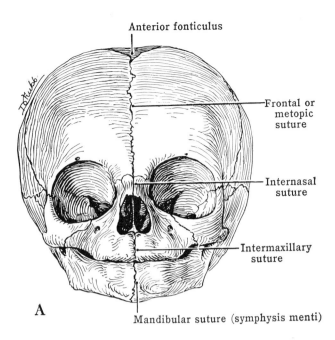

Anterior fonticulus

Frontal or metopic suture

Internasal suture

Intermaxillary suture

Mandibular suture (symphysis menti)

A

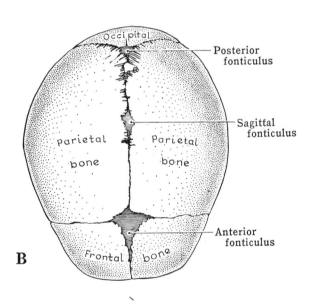

Occipital

Posterior fonticulus

parietal bone

Parietal bone

Sagittal fonticulus

Anterior fonticulus

Frontal bone

B

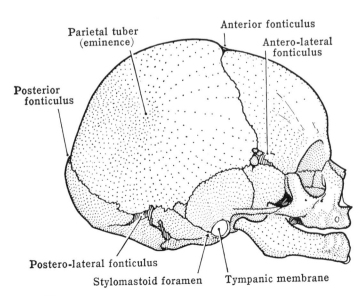

Parietal tuber (eminence)

Anterior fonticulus

Antero-lateral fonticulus

Posterior fonticulus

Postero-lateral fonticulus

Stylomastoid foramen

Tympanic membrane

C

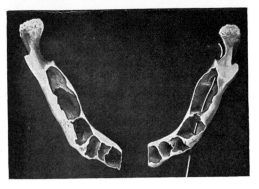

D Mandible at Birth, from above

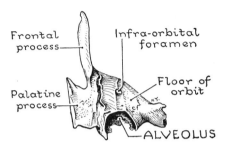

Frontal process

Infra-orbital foramen

Palatine process

Floor of orbit

ALVEOLUS

E Maxilla at Birth, posterior view
(For medial view, fig. 615.1.)

602 Skull, Mandible, and Maxilla at Birth

Note:

1. The teeth have not erupted; hence, the air sinuses are rudimentary, the maxilla and mandible are small, the angle of the mandible is obtuse and so the ramus and body of the mandible are nearly in line. The orbital cavities are large and round but the nasal cavities are not deep. The face is indeed small.

2. The mandibular suture and the frontal suture, which close during the 2nd year, are still open.

3. The tuber of the parietal bone—like that of the frontal bone—is conical. Ossification, which starts at the tubers and spreads in centrifugal waves, has not yet reached the four angles of the parietal bone. Accordingly, these are still membranous and the membrane is blended with the pericranium externally and dura mater internally to form the fonticuli. Of the fonticuli, the anterior and largest closes during the 2nd year. It is shaped like a flat kite, the long angle and tail tapering between the two halves of the frontal bone.

4. There being no mastoid process until the 2nd year, the stylomastoid foramen, which transmits the facial nerve, opens beneath the surface of the skin. The external acoustic meatus having no length, the tympanic membrane is close to the surface of the skull.

5. The maxillary antrum or sinus being very small, the floor of the orbital cavity is also the "ceiling" of the alveolus in which the rudimentary primary molar teeth lie.

6. Each half of the mandible has 5 sockets or alveoli for 5 primary teeth. The course of the inferior alveolar nerve is indicated, but the branch to the canine and incisor teeth is not shown.

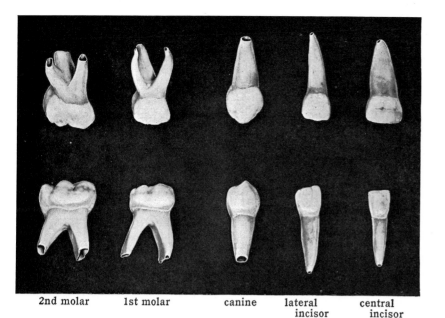

2nd molar   1st molar   canine   lateral incisor   central incisor

602.1 Primary Teeth

There are 20 primary, deciduous, temporary, or milk teeth, 5 being in each half of the mandible and 5 in each maxilla. They are named: central incisor, lateral incisor, canine, 1st molar, and 2nd molar. The formula reads

$$\frac{2.1.2. \quad 2.1.2.}{2.1.2. \quad 2.1.2.}$$

Of these 20 primary teeth the first to erupt through the gums are the lower central incisors, about the 7th month, and the last to erupt are the 2nd upper molars, about the end of the 2nd year. The 3 roots of the upper or maxillary molars and the 2 roots of the lower or mandibular molars are spread to grasp the developing Permanent Premolars (fig. 604).

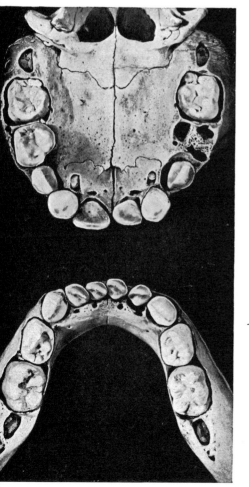

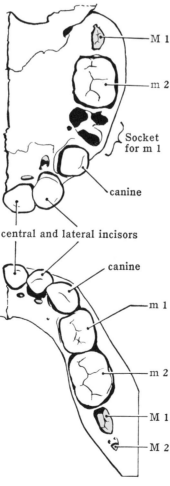

M 1
m 2
Socket for m 1
canine
central and lateral incisors
canine
m 1
m 2
M 1
M 2

602.2 Primary Dentition, aged under 2 years

The anterior fonticulus has disappeared. Only traces of the frontal and mandibular sutures remain.

(Permanent Teeth colored yellow.)

Observe:

1. The canines have not fully erupted, the 2nd molars have just started to erupt—the sequence of eruption being incisors, 1st molars, canines, 2nd molars.
2. The 2nd molars have much larger crowns than the 1st molars.
3. The socket for the 3-pronged root of the 1st upper molar is seen.
4. The foramina, seen on the lingual side of the primary incisors, lead to the alveoli for the Permanent Incisors.
5. The crowns of the unerupted 1st and 2nd Permanent Molars are partly visible.

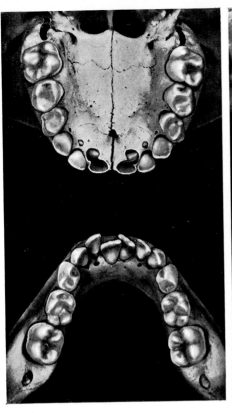

Aged 6 to 7 years

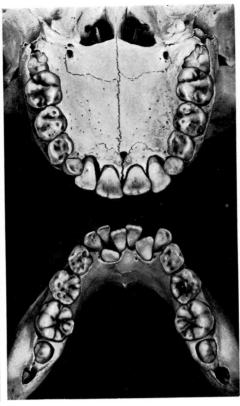

Aged 8 years

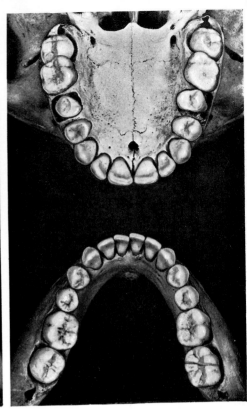

Aged 12 years

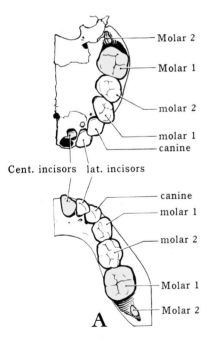

Molar 2
Molar 1
molar 2
molar 1
canine
Cent. incisors   lat. incisors
canine
molar 1
molar 2
Molar 1
Molar 2

A

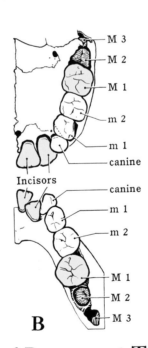

M 3
M 2
M 1
m 2
m 1
canine
Incisors
canine
m 1
m 2
M 1
M 2
M 3

B

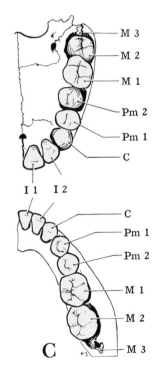

M 3
M 2
M 1
Pm 2
Pm 1
C
I 1   I 2
C
Pm 1
Pm 2
M 1
M 2
M 3

C

603 Progress in the Eruption of Permanent Teeth

Between the 6th and 12th years the primary teeth are shed and are succeeded by Permanent Teeth.

A. The 1st Molars (6th-year Molars) have fully erupted. The primary central incisors have been shed. The Lower Central Incisors have nearly fully erupted and the Upper Central Incisors are moving downwards into the empty sockets.

B. All the Permanent Incisors have erupted, the Upper and Lower Central and the Upper Lateral fully and the Lower Lateral partially. Note that the alveolus

has not yet closed around the Upper Lateral Incisors.

(Here, the root of the left lower lateral primary incisor has not been resorbed, so the tooth has not been shed. It needs the aid of a dentist.)

C. The 20 primary teeth have been replaced by 20 Permanent Teeth, and the 1st Molars and the 2nd Molars (12th-year Molars) have erupted. But, the Canines, 2nd Premolars, and 2nd Molars—especially those in the upper jaw—have not erupted fully nor have their bony sockets closed around them.

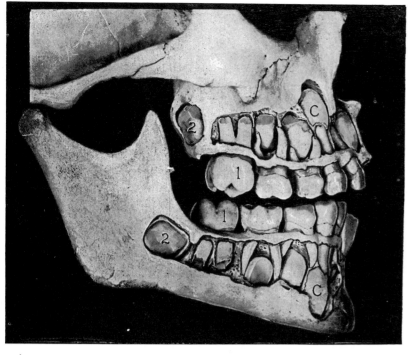

A

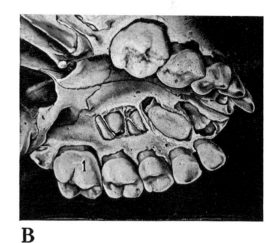

B

604 Mixed Dentition, labial and lingual views

(From the same specimen as fig. 603 A, after the removal of bone.)

The crowns of the Permanent Teeth are fully formed at the time of eruption (i.e., they grow no larger). The Permanent Incisors and Canines develop and erupt on the lingual side of the primary incisors and canines, the Lateral Incisors being the most posterior. Indeed, the Upper Lateral Incisors extend into the bony palate. The Premolar Teeth develop between the spread roots of the primary molars. The Permanent Molars have no predecessors.

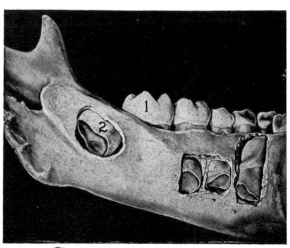

C

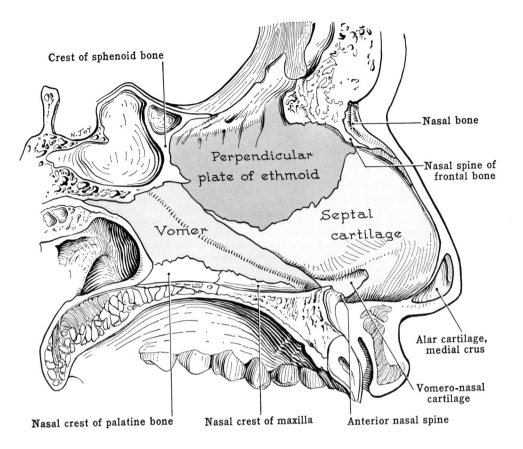

Crest of sphenoid bone

Nasal bone

Nasal spine of
frontal bone

Perpendicular
plate of ethmoid

Septal
cartilage

Vomer

Alar cartilage,
medial crus

Vomero-nasal
cartilage

Nasal crest of palatine bone   Nasal crest of maxilla   Anterior nasal spine

605   Septum of Nos

Like the palate, the septum of
the nose has a hard part and a
soft or mobile part. The skeleton
or basis of the hard septum consists of 3 parts—perpendicular
plate of ethmoid, septal cartilage,
vomer—and, around the circum-
ference of these, the adjacent bones
(frontal, nasal, maxillary, palatine, and sphenoid) make minor
contributions.

The mobile septum comprises
(a) the medial limbs (crura) of the
U-shaped alar cartilages (figs. 468
and 611), and (b) the skin and
soft tissues between the tip of the
nose and the anterior nasal spine.
Behind the vomer, an extension
of the muco-periosteum of the
septum forms a second, though
unimportant, mobile septum.

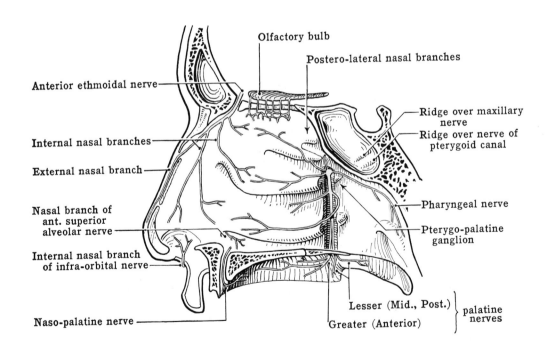

Olfactory bulb

Postero-lateral nasal branches

Anterior ethmoidal nerve

Internal nasal branches

External nasal branch

Nasal branch of
ant. superior
alveolar nerve

Internal nasal branch
of infra-orbital nerve

Naso-palatine nerve

Ridge over maxillary
nerve

Ridge over nerve of
pterygoid canal

Pharyngeal nerve

Pterygo-palatine
ganglion

Lesser (Mid., Post.)
Greater (Anterior) } palatine
nerves

Ant. ethmoidal n.   Olfactory

from
infra-orbital n.   Nasopalatin

606   Diagram of the Nerve Supply to
Lateral Wall of Nasal Cavity

(See also figures 655 and 656.)

606.1   Diagram
of the Nerves d
Nasal Septum

Observe:

Anterior ethmoidal and posterior ethmoidal branches of the ophthalmic a. entering through the cribriform plate. Only these are derived from the internal carotid, all others being from the external carotid.

The sphenopalatine a. as the main supply. Entering through the sphenopalatine foramen (fig. 608.1), it sends (a) lateral nasal branches forwards on both surfaces of the conchae, partly in bony canals, and (b) the posterior septal a. which crosses the roof of the nose below the anterior part of the floor of the sphenoidal sinus and anastomoses through the incisive foramen.

The facial a. via 3 branches: (a) the septal branch of the superior labial a.; (b) twigs from the lateral nasal a. that pierce the ala to supply the vestibular region; and (c) anastomoses from the ascending palatine a.

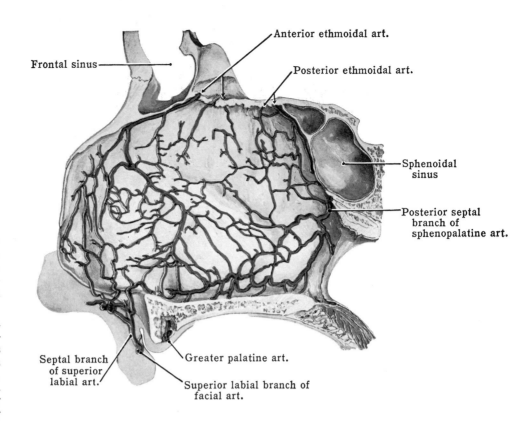

Arteries to Septum.

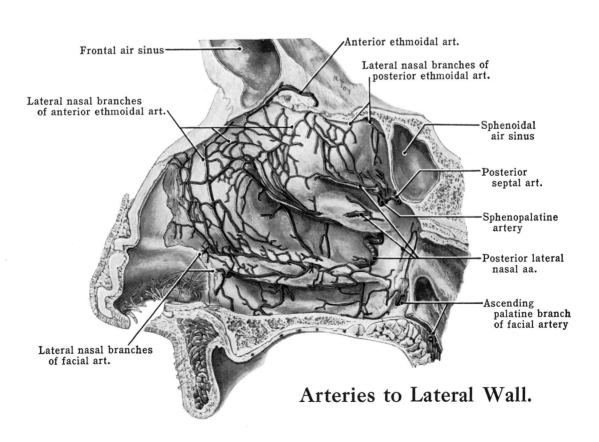

Arteries to Lateral Wall.

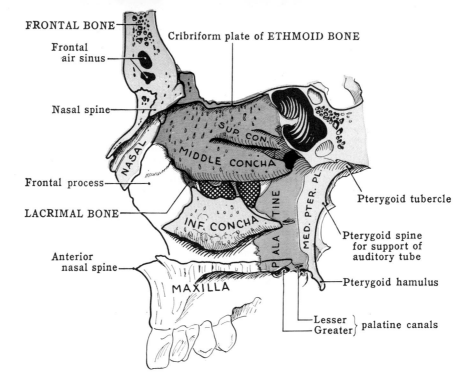

FRONTAL BONE

Frontal air sinus

Cribriform plate of ETHMOID BONE

Nasal spine

SUP. CON.

MIDDLE CONCHA

NASAL

Frontal process

LACRIMAL BONE

INF. CONCHA

PALATINE

MED. PTER. PL.

Pterygoid tubercle

Pterygoid spine for support of auditory tube

Anterior nasal spine

MAXILLA

Pterygoid hamulus

Lesser } palatine canals
Greater }

608   Bones of Lateral Wall of Nasal Cavity—I

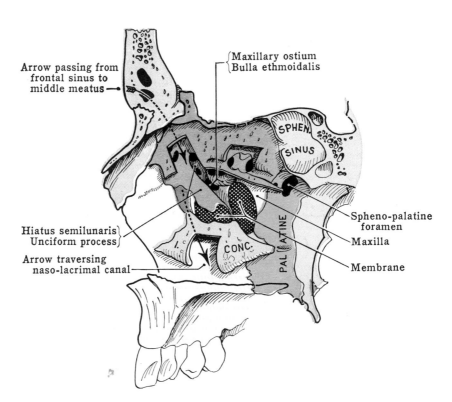

Arrow passing from frontal sinus to middle meatus →

Maxillary ostium
Bulla ethmoidalis

SPHEN.

SINUS

Hiatus semilunaris }
Unciform process }

Arrow traversing naso-lacrimal canal

I. C.

CONC.

PALATINE

Spheno-palatine foramen

Maxilla

Membrane

608.1   Bones of Lateral Wall of Nasal Cavity, dissected—II

Note:

1. The superior and middle conchae are parts of the ethmoid bone, whereas the inferior concha is a bone of itself.

2. The pterygoid process is part of the sphenoid bone (fig. 619.1). Its medial plate forms the posterior part of the lateral wall of the bony nasal cavity.

3. The fragile, perpendicular plate of the palatine bone has a notch at its upper border, which, when in articulation with the body of the sphenoid bone, forms the spheno-palatine foramen (fig. 615.3).

4. The groove on the nasal bone is for the external nasal branch of the anterior ethmoidal nerve (fig. 606).

5. The hiatus semilunaris is bounded below by the unciform process of the ethmoid bone. The maxillary ostium opens on to the hiatus. Accessory maxillary ostia may occur in the membrane that closes the maxillary hiatus.

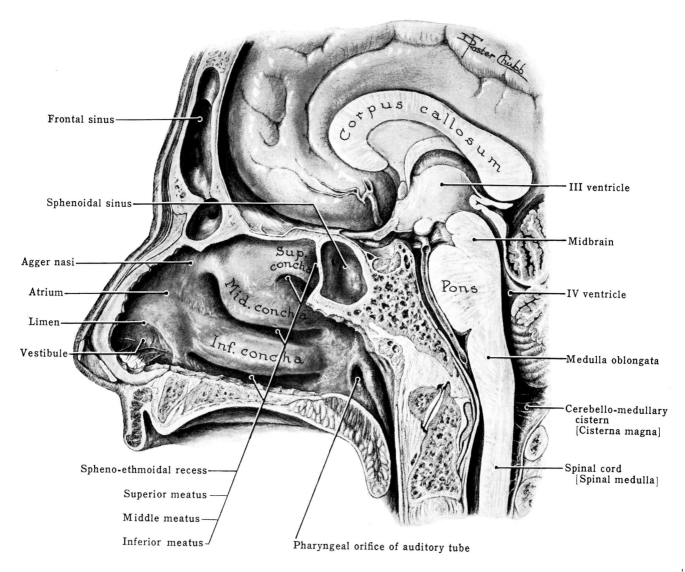

Frontal sinus

Sphenoidal sinus

Agger nasi

Atrium

Limen

Vestibule

Corpus callosum

III ventricle

Midbrain

Pons

IV ventricle

Medulla oblongata

Cerebello-medullary cistern [Cisterna magna]

Spinal cord [Spinal medulla]

Sup. concha

Mid. concha

Inf. concha

Spheno-ethmoidal recess

Superior meatus

Middle meatus

Inferior meatus

Pharyngeal orifice of auditory tube

609   Lateral Wall of Nasal Cavity—I

Observe:

1. The vestibule, above the nostril or naris and in front of the inferior meatus. The hairs growing from its skin-lined surface, spreading in all directions.

2. The atrium, above the vestibule and in front of the middle meatus.

3. The inferior and middle conchae, curving downwards and medially from the lateral wall, dividing it into 3 nearly equal parts, and covering the inferior and middle meatuses respectively.

4. The superior concha, small and in front of the sphenoidal sinus. The middle concha, with an angled lower border, ending below the sphenoidal sinus. The inferior concha, with a slightly curved lower border, ending below the middle concha, $\frac{1}{3}''$ to $\frac{1}{2}''$ in front of the orifice of the tube—i.e., about the width of the medial pterygoid plate (fig. 608).

5. The floor of the nose, inclined slightly downwards and backwards, at the level of the atlas.

6. The roof comprising:— (a) an anterior sloping part, corresponding to the bridge of the nose; (b) an intermediate horizontal part, formed by the delicate cribriform plate; (c) a perpendicular part in front of the sphenoidal sinus and, (d) a curved part, below the sinus, which is confluent with the roof of the naso-pharynx.

7. The pons and the fourth ventricle at the level of the sphenodial sinus.

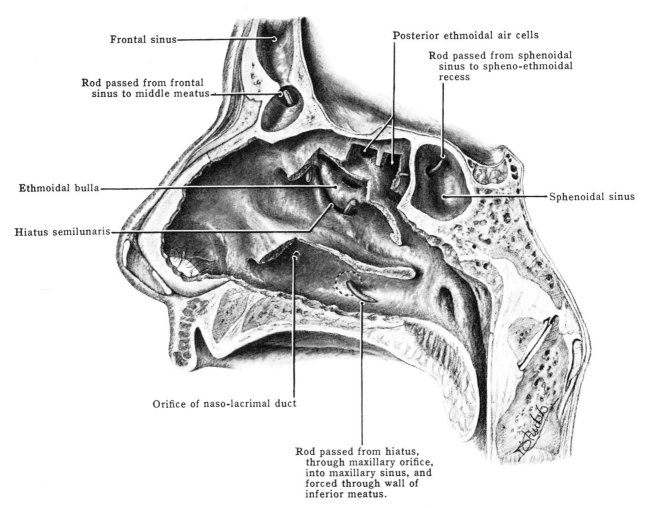

Frontal sinus

Rod passed from frontal sinus to middle meatus

Ethmoidal bulla

Hiatus semilunaris

Orifice of naso-lacrimal duct

Posterior ethmoidal air cells

Rod passed from sphenoidal sinus to spheno-ethmoidal recess

Sphenoidal sinus

Rod passed from hiatus, through maxillary orifice, into maxillary sinus, and forced through wall of inferior meatus.

610   Lateral Wall of Nasal Cavity, dissected—II

Parts of the superior, middle, and inferior conchae are cut away.

Observe:

1. The sphenoidal sinus, in the body of the sphenoid bone; its orifice, above the middle of its anterior wall, opening into the spheno-ethmoidal recess.

2. The orifices of posterior ethmoidal cells opening into the superior meatus.

3. A cell, in this specimen, opening on to the upper surface of the ethmoidal bulla.

4. The attachment of the inferior concha, steep in its anterior $\frac{1}{3}$, but gently sloping in its posterior $\frac{2}{3}$. The orifice of the naso-lacrimal duct, a short (variable) distance below the angle of union of the anterior $\frac{1}{3}$ and posterior $\frac{2}{3}$.

5. The sharp probe forced through the thinnest portion of the medial wall of the maxillary sinus, well above the level of the floor of the nasal cavity.

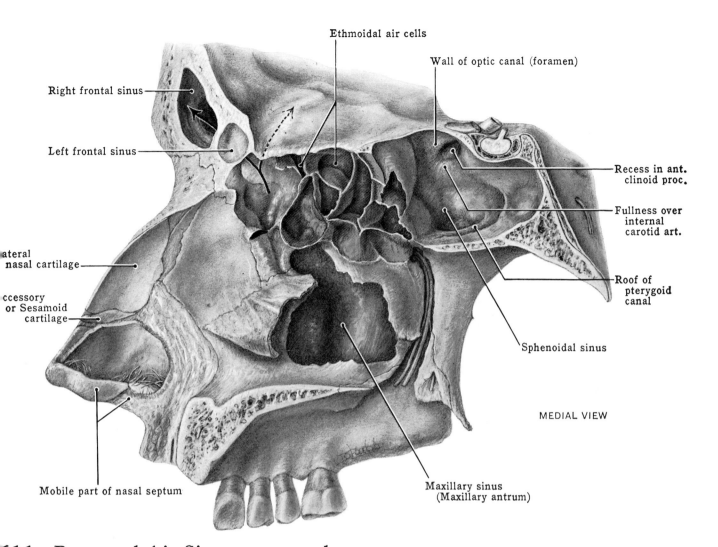

Ethmoidal air cells

Wall of optic canal (foramen)

Right frontal sinus

Left frontal sinus

Recess in ant. clinoid proc.

Fullness over internal carotid art.

ateral nasal cartilage

ccessory or Sesamoid cartilage

Roof of pterygoid canal

Sphenoidal sinus

MEDIAL VIEW

Mobile part of nasal septum

Maxillary sinus (Maxillary antrum)

611 Paranasal Air Sinuses, opened

Observe:

. The ethmoidal cells (pink), collectively called a sinus, like a honey-comb, and having the thin orbital plate of the frontal bone for a roof (figs. 520 & 617).

2. An anterior ethmoidal cell (blue) invading the diploe of the squama of the frontal bone to become a frontal sinus. It is ethmoidal in origin, but frontal in location. An offshoot (broken arrow) invades the orbital plate of the frontal bone.

3. The sphenoidal sinus (blue) here, very extensive—compare with figure 610—extending (a) backwards below the hypophysis cerebri to the dorsum sellae, (b) laterally, below the optic nerve, into the anterior clinoid process, and (c) downwards to the pterygoid process, but leaving the pterygoid canal rising as a ridge on the floor of the sinus.

4. The maxillary sinus (yellow) pyramidal in shape; its base (largely nibbled away), contributing to the lateral wall of the nasal cavity; its apex being in the zygomatic process; and its orifice being at its highest point.

611.1

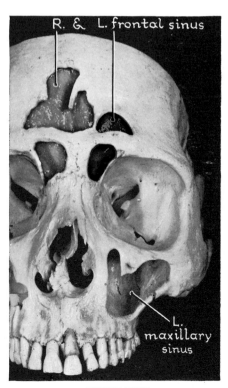

R. & L. frontal sinus

L. maxillary sinus

FRONT VIEW

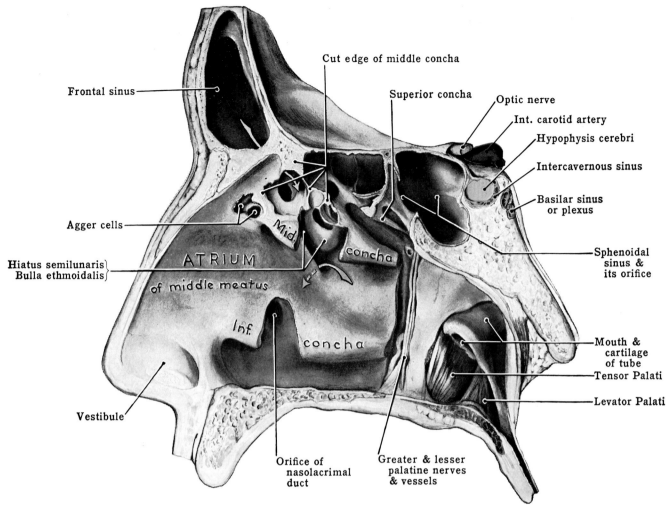

Frontal sinus

Cut edge of middle concha

Superior concha

Optic nerve

Int. carotid artery

Hypophysis cerebri

Intercavernous sinus

Basilar sinus or plexus

Agger cells

Mid. concha

Sphenoidal sinus & its orifice

Hiatus semilunaris
Bulla ethmoidalis

ATRIUM
of middle meatus

Inf. concha

Mouth & cartilage of tube

Tensor Palati

Levator Palati

Vestibule

Orifice of nasolacrimal duct

Greater & lesser palatine nerves & vessels

612   Paranasal Air Sinuses

Note:

1. The frontal sinus with its outlet at its lowest point, leading into the middle meatus medial to the hiatus semilunaris. The hiatus ends blindly in front as an anterior ethmoidal cell, and posteriorly as the maxillary orifice, indicated by an arrow.

2. Lateral to the agger nasi, there are 2 agger cells: one is a diverticulum from the frontal sinus; the other from the hiatus.

3. The sphenoidal sinus of average size, and with a very large orifice.

4. A bullar cell with its orifice above.

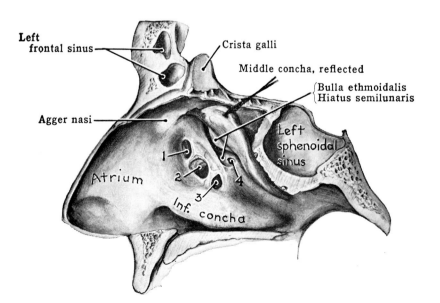

Left frontal sinus

Crista galli

Middle concha, reflected

Bulla ethmoidalis
Hiatus semilunaris

Agger nasi

Atrium

Left sphenoidal sinus

Inf. concha

613   Accessory Maxillary Orifices

Note:

1. In addition to the primary or normal ostium (not in view), there are here present 4 secondary or acquired ostia resulting from the breaking down of the membrane shown in cross-hatching in figure 608.1.

2. The septum between the right and the left sphenoidal sinus, here occupies the median plane—it is usually deflected to one side or other.

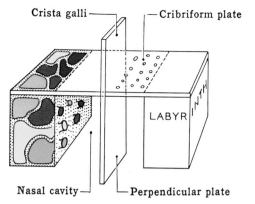

Crista galli — — Cribriform plate

Nasal cavity — — Perpendicular plate

LABYRINTH

614 Scheme of the Ethmoidal Air Cells, collectively called a sinus

The ethmoidal air cells may be likened to a number of rubber balloons projecting into an oblong box and variously inflated to the full capacity of the box. Indeed, one (occasionally more) of the anterior balloons bursts through the lid of the box (i.e., the roof of the ethmoidal labyrinth) and invades the neighbouring territory (i.e., the frontal bone) to a variable extent and acquires the name "frontal air sinus".

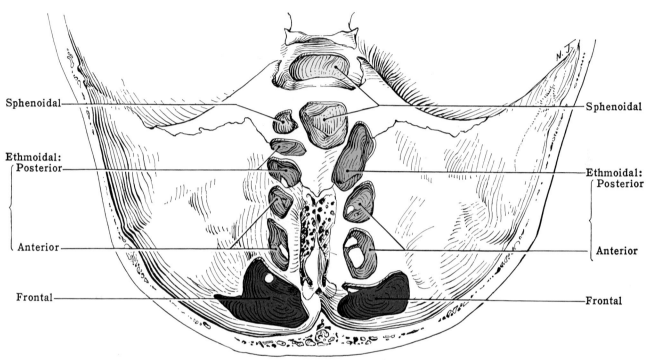

Sphenoidal

Ethmoidal:
Posterior

Anterior

Frontal

Sphenoidal

Ethmoidal:
Posterior

Anterior

Frontal

614.1 Air Sinuses Surrounding the Cribriform Plate, from above

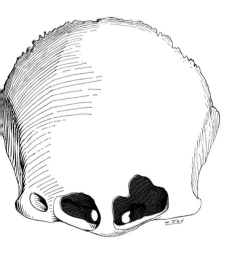

614.2 Frontal Air Sinuses, from the front

The orifices of the sinuses are at the lowest points of the sinuses.

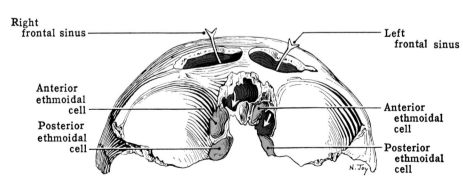

Right frontal sinus

Left frontal sinus

Anterior ethmoidal cell

Posterior ethmoidal cell

Anterior ethmoidal cell

Posterior ethmoidal cell

614.3 Frontal Air Sinuses, from below

The right frontal air sinus is here, as usual, an extension of an anterior ethmoidal cell. The corresponding left cell (blue) is small, but the next cell behind it has invaded the diploe of the frontal bone and so become a frontal sinus.

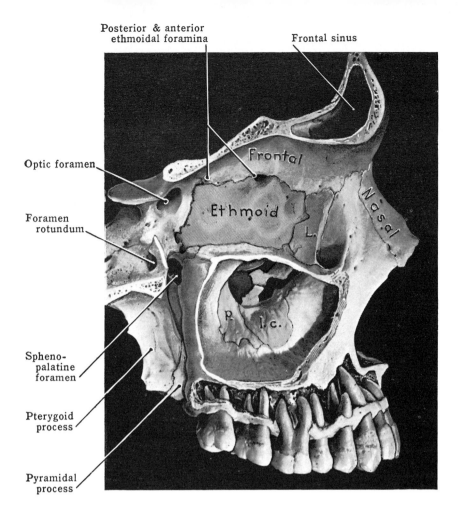

Posterior & anterior ethmoidal foramina

Frontal sinus

Optic foramen

Foramen rotundum

Spheno-palatine foramen

Pterygoid process

Pyramidal process

Frontal *Ethmoid* *L.* *Nasal*

p. *l.c.*

615   Medial Wall of Orbital Cavity and of Maxillary Sinus

Ic.—inferior concha (green)
L.—lacrimal bone (blue)
P.—palatine bone (yellow)

Note:

1. The site of the hiatus semilunaris betwee[n]
   bulla of the ethmoid bone above and the un[c]
   (= hook-like) process below.
2. The pterygo-palatine fossa between ptery[goid]
   process, maxilla, palatine bone, and sph[e]
   bone. The foramen rotundum opens into the [...]
   from the middle cranial fossa and the sph[eno-]
   palatine foramen opens into the nasal cavity.

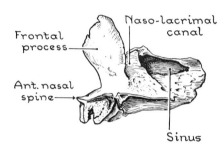

Frontal process

Naso-lacrimal canal

Ant. nasal spine

Sinus

615.1   Maxilla at birth, medial view

(For posterior view, fig. 602E.)

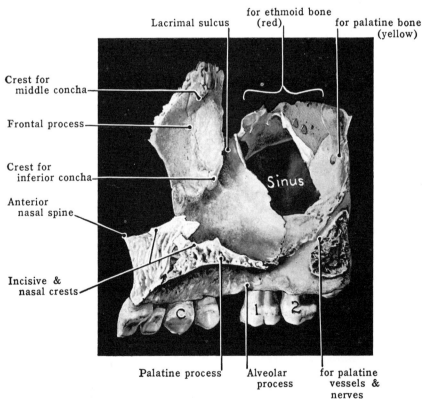

Crest for middle concha

Frontal process

Crest for inferior concha

Anterior nasal spine

Incisive & nasal crests

Lacrimal sulcus

for ethmoid bone (red)

for palatine bone (yellow)

Sinus

C *1* *2*

Palatine process

Alveolar process

for palatine vessels & nerves

615.2   Medial Aspect of Maxilla

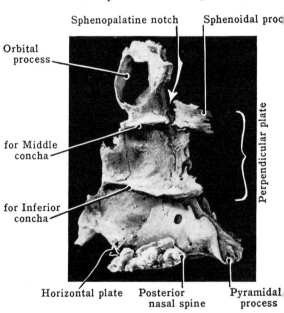

Orbital process

Sphenopalatine notch

Sphenoidal proc[ess]

for Middle concha

for Inferior concha

Perpendicular plate

Horizontal plate

Posterior nasal spine

Pyramidal process

615.3   Medial Aspect of Palatine Bone

Note:

1. The pyramidal process has 2 grooves for the pyteryg[oid]
   process.
2. The cell in the orbital process is an extension of eith[er]
   the maxillary sinus, an ethmoidal cell, or the sphenoi[d]
   sinus.

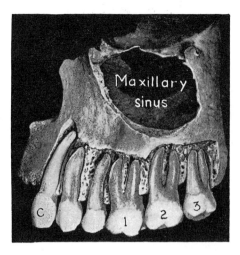

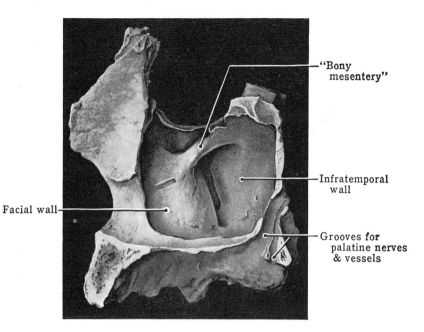

16 Maxillary Sinus, left side, lateral view

Note:

The roots of the teeth are, here, at some distance from the sinus.

Contrast this figure with figures 601.4 and 615 where the roots of the teeth come closer to the floor of the bony sinus, and with figure 616.3 where they penetrate it.

616.1 Maxillary Sinus, medial view

Note:

1. The "bony mesentery" for the infra-orbital nerve and vessels, here, projecting, not from the roof, but from the lateral wall.
2. The anterior or facial wall pushing far into the sinus.
3. The grooves for the greater and lesser palatine nerves.

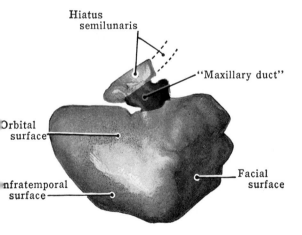

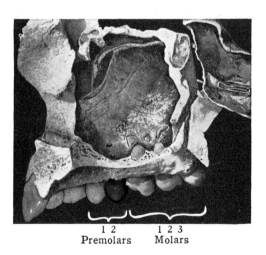

616.2 Cast of the right Maxillary Sinus, lateral view

Note:

The so-called orifice or ostium, which opens into the hiatus semilunaris, is usually a duct, in shape flattened oval or slit-like, and of the following average dimensions: Length of the duct along its anterior wall, 6.0 mm, and along its posterior wall, 5 mm; similarly, the long diameter of the oval, 6.0 mm, and the short diameter, 3.5 mm. J.C.B.G.

616.3 Maxillary Sinus, medial view

Note:

The roots of 3 teeth, here, penetrate the bony floor.

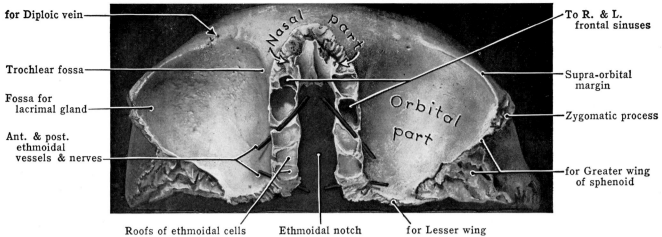

for Diploic vein

Trochlear fossa

Fossa for lacrimal gland

Ant. & post. ethmoidal vessels & nerves

Nasal part

Orbital part

To R. & L. frontal sinuses

Supra-orbital margin

Zygomatic process

for Greater wing of sphenoid

Roofs of ethmoidal cells   Ethmoidal notch   for Lesser wing

617   Frontal Bone, inferior aspect

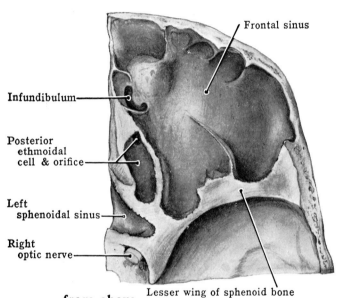

Frontal sinus

Infundibulum

Posterior ethmoidal cell & orifice

Left sphenoidal sinus

Right optic nerve

Lesser wing of sphenoid bone

from above

617.1   Extensive Frontal Sinus

This sinus occupies the entire orbital part of the frontal bone.

An anterior ethmoidal cell bulges dome-like into the floor, of the frontal sinus.

The left sphenoidal sinus crosses the median plane and helps to form the roof of the right optic canal.

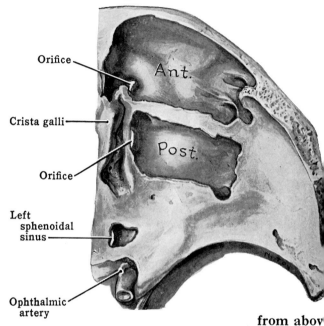

Orifice

Ant.

Crista galli

Post.

Orifice

Left sphenoidal sinus

Ophthalmic artery

from abov

617.2   Extensive Ethmoidal Cel

This cell occupies the hinder half of the orbital part of the frontal bone, behind an average sized frontal sin

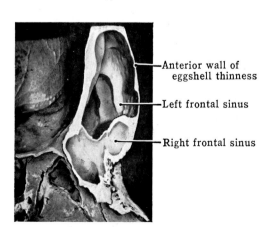

Anterior wall of eggshell thinness

Left frontal sinus

Right frontal sinus

617.3   Frontal Sinus, with thin anterior wall

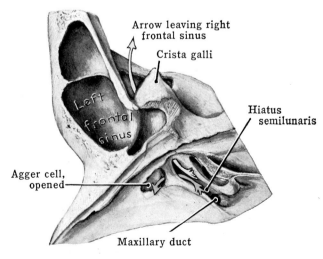

Arrow leaving right frontal sinus

Crista galli

Left frontal sinus

Hiatus semilunaris

Agger cell, opened

Maxillary duct

617.4   Frontal Sinus in the Crista Galli

The left sinus here extends far across the median plane. The right sinus opens at the summit of the hiatus. The agger cell is here a diverticulum from the hiatus.

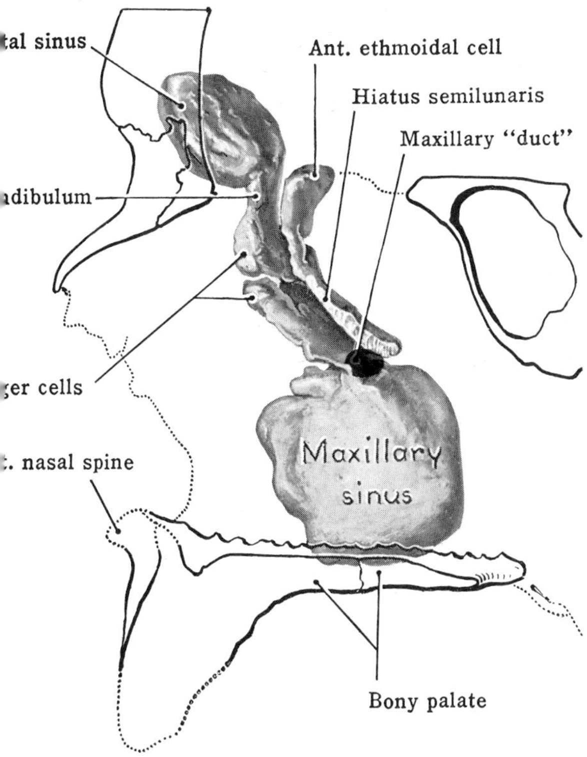
tal sinus
Ant. ethmoidal cell
Hiatus semilunaris
Maxillary "duct"
idibulum
ger cells
Maxillary sinus
. nasal spine
Bony palate

8 Cast of the Frontal and Maxillary uses, medial view

e frontal sinus lies above the orbital cavity and has its opening at its vest point, whereas the maxillary sinus lies below the orbital cavity d has its opening on a level with its highest point.

d this frontal sinus failed to develop, the anterior ethmoidal cell own) would have taken its place in default.

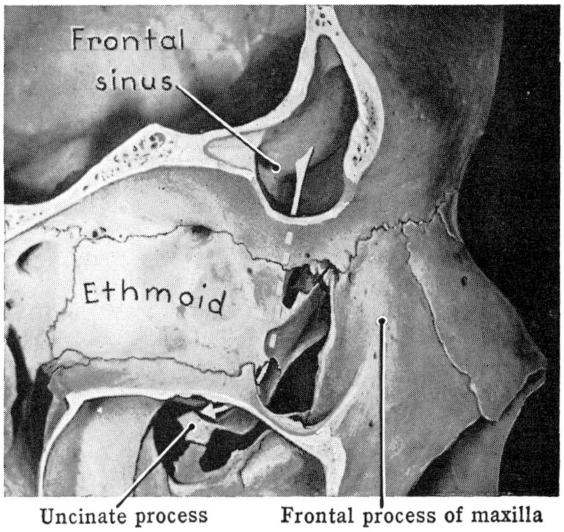
Frontal sinus
Ethmoid
Uncinate process
Frontal process of maxilla

618.1 Frontonasal Duct

From figure 615 after removal of the lacrimal bone.

The golden arrow suggests that, if there were fluid in the frontal sinus, it would drain through the infundibulum ethmoidale, (situated at the lowest point of the sinus) into the hiatus semilunaris and thence into the maxillary sinus via its orifice or duct (618), situated on a level with its highest point.

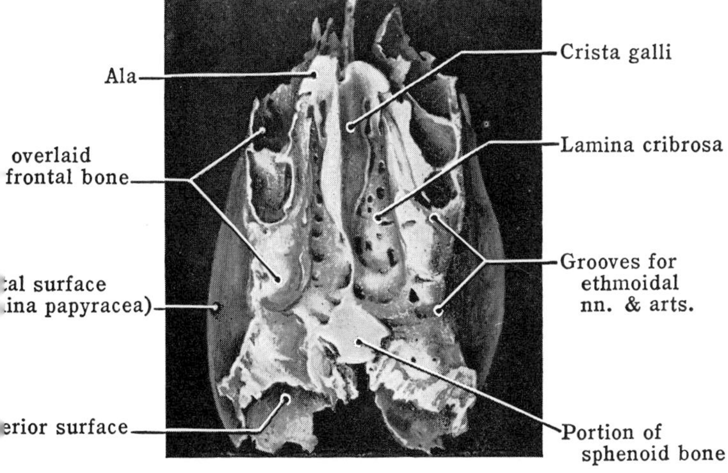
Ala
overlaid
frontal bone
al surface
ina papyracea)
erior surface
Crista galli
Lamina cribrosa
Grooves for ethmoidal nn. & arts.
Portion of sphenoid bone

8.2 Ethmoid Bone, superior aspect

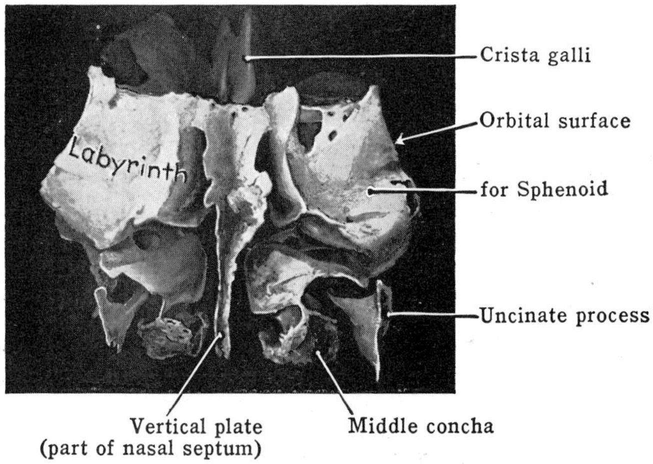
Labyrinth
Crista galli
Orbital surface
for Sphenoid
Uncinate process
Vertical plate
(part of nasal septum)
Middle concha

618.3 Ethmoid Bone, posterior aspect

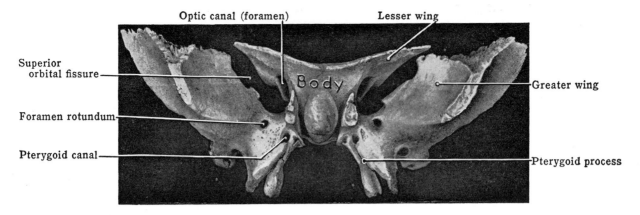

Optic canal (foramen) Lesser wing

Superior
orbital fissure

Body

Greater wing

Foramen rotundum

Pterygoid canal

Pterygoid process

619   Sphenoid Bone of a Child

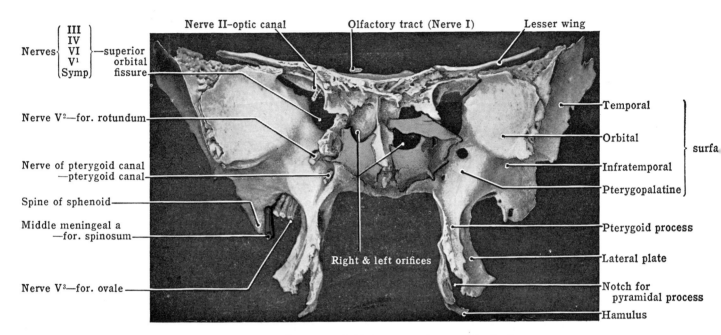

Nerves { III IV VI V¹ Symp } —superior orbital fissure

Nerve II–optic canal   Olfactory tract (Nerve I)   Lesser wing

Nerve V²—for. rotundum

Nerve of pterygoid canal —pterygoid canal

Spine of sphenoid

Middle meningeal a —for. spinosum

Nerve V³—for. ovale

Right & left orifices

Temporal

Orbital

Infratemporal

Pterygopalatine

surfa

Pterygoid process

Lateral plate

Notch for pyramidal process

Hamulus

619.1   Sphenoid Bone of an Adult

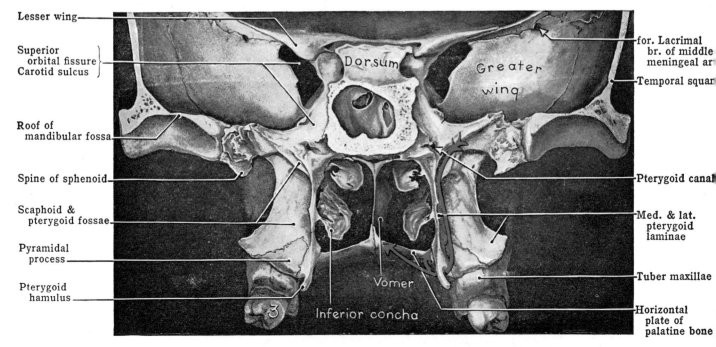

Lesser wing

Superior orbital fissure
Carotid sulcus

Roof of mandibular fossa

Spine of sphenoid

Scaphoid & pterygoid fossae

Pyramidal process

Pterygoid hamulus

Dorsum

Greater wing

Vomer

Inferior concha

for. Lacrimal br. of middle meningeal ar

Temporal squar

Pterygoid canal

Med. & lat. pterygoid laminae

Tuber maxillae

Horizontal plate of palatine bone

619.2   A Coronal Section of the Skull

619 Sphenoid Bone of a Young Child, front view

The right and left sphenoidal sinuses do not invade the body until about the 4th year. (For enlarging sinus, figs. 511, 610 & 611.)

619.1 Sphenoid Bone of an Adult, front view

Note:

On each side 6, or 50%, of the 12 cranial nerves are closely related to the sphenoid, nerve V piercing it in 3 divisions. The nerve of the pterygoid canal and the middle meningeal artery pierce the bone.

The parts coloured pink are the sphenoidal conchae.

619.2 A Coronal Section of the Skull, showing the sphenoid bone and surroundings, posterior view

Note:

1. The 2 posterior nasal apertures [choanae] separated from each other by the vomer, and each bounded below by the horizontal plate of the palatine bone, laterally by the medial pterygoid lamina, and above by the ala of the vomer and the vaginal process of the medial pterygoid lamina (not labelled). The inferior and middle conchae are visible within.

2. The pterygoid fossa, bounded medially by the medial pterygoid lamina, which extends upwards to the pterygoid canal and which ends below the level of the palate, as the hamulus (i.e. the pulley of the Tensor Palati). The Tensor (scarlet arrow) arises from the canoe-shaped scaphoid fossa.

3. The very thin (even translucent) roof of the mandibular fossa.

4. The occasional foramen through which the middle meningeal and lacrimal arteries anastomose.

620.1 Extensive Sphenoidal Sinus, left side ⟶

Note:

1. This very extensive sinus extends laterally between the maxillary nerve and the nerve of the pterygoid canal, inflating the greater wing of the sphenoid bone and the pterygoid process. It extends forwards into the lateral wall of the orbital cavity, backwards to the mandibular nerve which passes through the foramen ovale, laterally to the temporal fossa, and downwards to the roof and medial walls of the infratemporal fossa.

2. The greater (superficial) petrosal nerve is seen leaving the hiatus facialis, running above the carotid canal, descending through the foramen lacerum, and, when joined by sympathetic fibres (not shown), it becomes the nerve of the pterygoid canal (fig. 657).

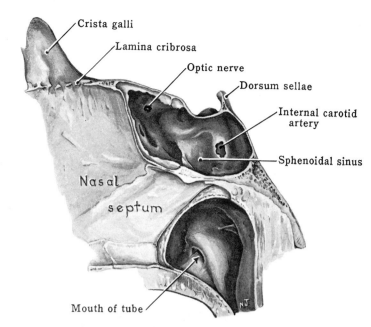

Crista galli
Lamina cribrosa
Optic nerve
Dorsum sellae
Internal carotid artery
Sphenoidal sinus
Nasal septum
Mouth of tube

620 Right Sphenoidal Sinus, very large and thin walled

Note:

1. The sinus extends from an average-sized orifice placed half way down the anterior wall, to the dorsum sellae and basi-occipital. It passes below the chiasmatic sulcus and the hypophyseal fossa (fig. 612).

2. The internal carotid artery and the optic nerve have a papery covering of bone and project in relief from the lateral wall.

3. Between nerve and artery a diverticulum leads into the anterior clinoid process.

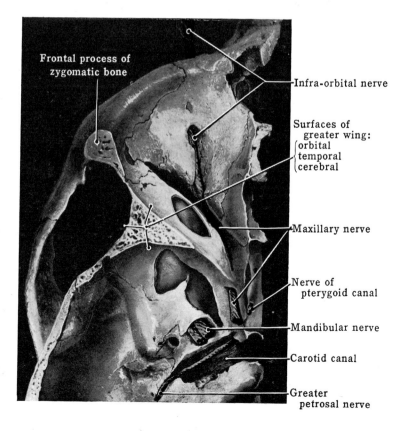

Frontal process of zygomatic bone
Infra-orbital nerve
Surfaces of greater wing: orbital temporal cerebral
Maxillary nerve
Nerve of pterygoid canal
Mandibular nerve
Carotid canal
Greater petrosal nerve

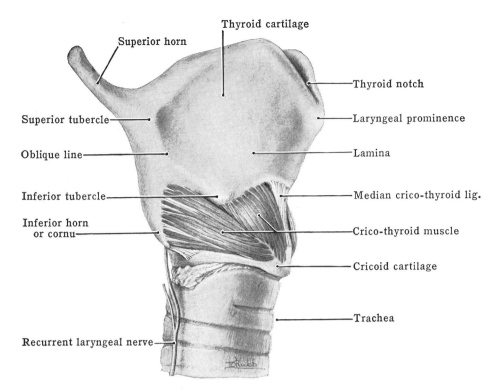

Superior horn

Thyroid cartilage

Thyroid notch

Superior tubercle

Laryngeal prominence

Oblique line

Lamina

Inferior tubercle

Median crico-thyroid lig.

Inferior horn
or cornu

Crico-thyroid muscle

Cricoid cartilage

Trachea

Recurrent laryngeal nerve

621 Thyroid Cartilage: Crico-thyroideus, side view.

Observe:

The Cricothyroid arising from the outer surface of the arch of the cricoid cartilage and having 2 parts—
(a) a straight, which is inserted into the lower border of

the lamina of the thyroid cartilage, and (b) an oblique, which is inserted into the anterior border of the inferior horn.

(For nerve supply, see below & fig. 530.)

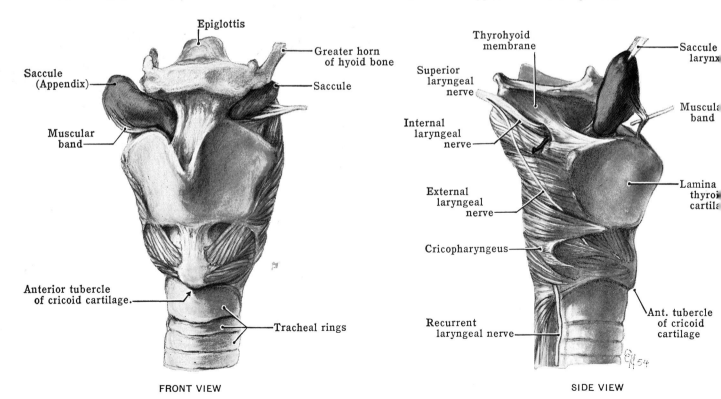

Epiglottis

Greater horn
of hyoid bone

Saccule
(Appendix)

Saccule

Muscular
band

Anterior tubercle
of cricoid cartilage.

Tracheal rings

FRONT VIEW

Thyrohyoid
membrane

Saccule
larynx

Superior
laryngeal
nerve

Muscula
band

Internal
laryngeal
nerve

External
laryngeal
nerve

Lamina
thyroi
cartila

Cricopharyngeus

Recurrent
laryngeal nerve

Ant. tubercle
of cricoid
cartilage

SIDE VIEW

622 Large Laryngeal Saccules (Appendices)

The saccule shown in fig. 628 may be very large, as here. In certain apes it is enormous. Although the sac is applied to the internal laryngeal nerve, these 2 structures, — sac and nerve — perforate the thyrohyoid membrane separately

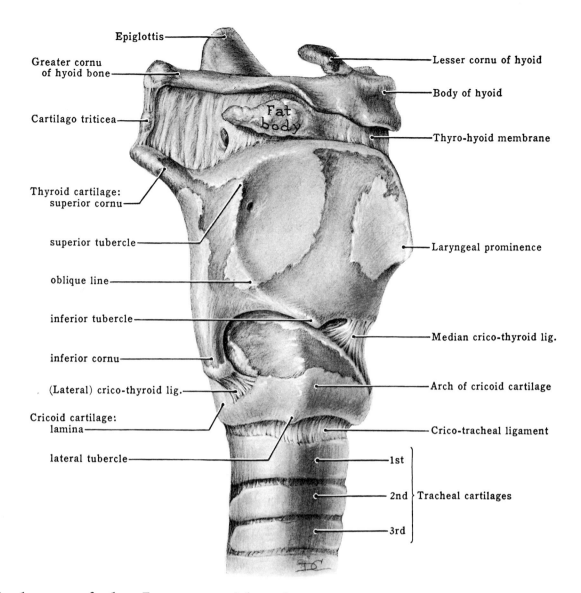

Epiglottis

Greater cornu of hyoid bone

Cartilago triticea

Fat body

Lesser cornu of hyoid

Body of hyoid

Thyro-hyoid membrane

Thyroid cartilage: superior cornu

superior tubercle

oblique line

inferior tubercle

inferior cornu

(Lateral) crico-thyroid lig.

Cricoid cartilage: lamina

lateral tubercle

Laryngeal prominence

Median crico-thyroid lig.

Arch of cricoid cartilage

Crico-tracheal ligament

1st

2nd ⎱ Tracheal cartilages

3rd ⎰

23 Skeleton of the Larynx, side view

The larynx extends vertically from the tip of the epiglottis to the lower border of cricoid cartilage. The hyoid bone or tongue bone is not regarded as part of the larynx.

Serve:

The lesser cornu of the hyoid bone, still partly cartilaginous, and not yet fused with the body. The thyroid and cricoid cartilages, on the other hand, partly ossified.

The right lamina of the thyroid cartilage, projecting anteriorly above the point of union with its fellow to form the laryngeal prominence. Its posterior border, prolonged into a superior and an inferior cornu; of these, the inferior articulates with the cricoid cartilage. The oblique line (for the attachment of 3 muscles—Inferior Constrictor, Sterno-thyroid, Thyrohyoid) curving from the superior tubercle to the inferior tubercle.

The cricoid cartilage, having 2 parts—an arch anteriorly, and a lamina posteriorly.

The thyro-hyoid membrane:— (a) attaching the whole length of the upper border of the thyroid lamina to the upper border (not lower, see fig. 629) of the body and greater cornu of the hyoid bone; (b) thickened posteriorly to form the thyro-hyoid ligament which contains a nodule of cartilage; (c) pierced by the internal laryngeal nerve and companion vessels; and (d) evaginated by a fat body.

The median cricothyroid ligament, uniting the median parts of the adjacent borders of the cricoid and thyroid cartilages. The remainder of the lower border of the thyroid cartilage gives attachment to the Cricothyroid (fig. 621); whereas, the remainder of the upper border of the arch of the cricoid cartilage gives attachment to the Lateral Crico-arytenoid (fig. 628) and the cricothyroid ligament (fig. 629).

The upper border of the arch of the cricoid, inclined; the lower border, resembling that of the thyroid cartilage and projecting anteriorly beyond the trachea. By this projecting feature the cricoid cartilage can be identified in life.

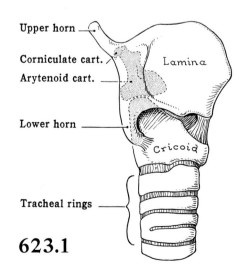

Upper horn

Corniculate cart.

Arytenoid cart.

Lamina

Lower horn

Cricoid

Tracheal rings

623.1

Diagram:

The thyroid cartilage shields the arytenoid cartilage and the upper part of the cricoid cartilage on which the arytenoid rests.

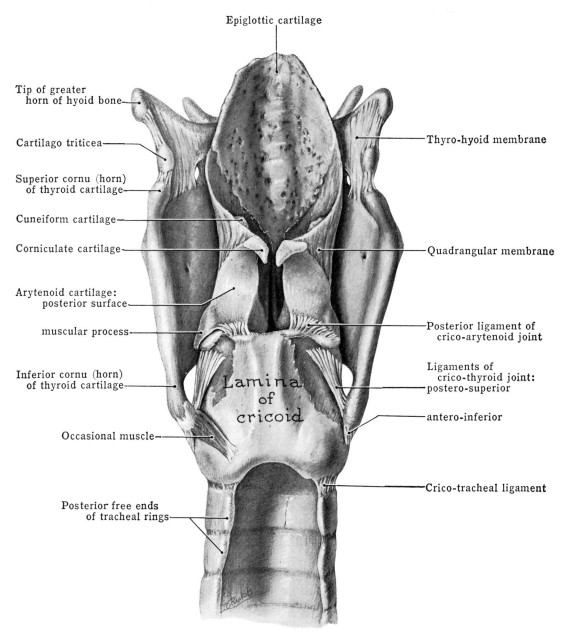

Epiglottic cartilage

Tip of greater horn of hyoid bone

Cartilago triticea

Superior cornu (horn) of thyroid cartilage

Cuneiform cartilage

Corniculate cartilage

Arytenoid cartilage: posterior surface

muscular process

Inferior cornu (horn) of thyroid cartilage

Occasional muscle

Posterior free ends of tracheal rings

Thyro-hyoid membrane

Quadrangular membrane

Posterior ligament of crico-arytenoid joint

Ligaments of crico-thyroid joint: postero-superior

antero-inferior

Crico-tracheal ligament

Lamina of cricoid

624 Skeleton of the Larynx, from behind (Cartilages, membranes, and ligaments)

Observe

1. The thyroid cartilage, shielding the smaller cartilages of the larynx (epiglottic, arytenoid, corniculate, and cuneiform): The hyoid bone—though not a part of the larynx—likewise shields the upper part of the epiglottic cartilage.

   The rounded posterior border of the thyroid cartilage, prolonged into an upper and a lower cornu: The lower cornu articulating with the cricoid cartilage at a synovial joint (figs. 628 & 629), the capsule of which is reinforced by 2 distinct mooring bands (postero-superior and antero-inferior) and not uncommonly by a muscle, the Kerato-cricoid, as shown.

2. The quadrangular membrane, connecting the border of the epiglottic cartilage to the arytenoid and corniculate cartilages, having a free upper border, and ending below as the vestibular ligament (fig. 632).

3. The posterior, concave surface of the 3-sided, pyramidal arytenoid cartilage.

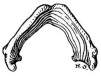

Female

625.1

Compare the angles formed by the thyroid cartilages—male & female—with those of the pubic arches in figures 218 and 220.

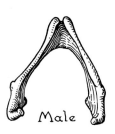

Male

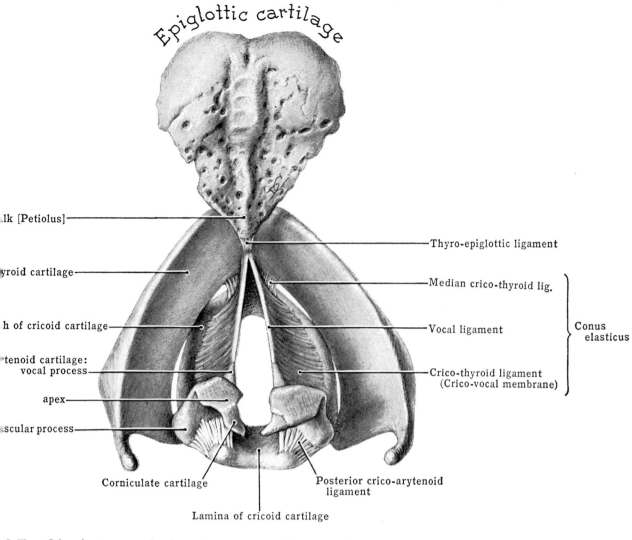

Epiglottic cartilage

...lk [Petiolus]

...yroid cartilage

...h of cricoid cartilage

...tenoid cartilage:
vocal process

apex

...scular process

Corniculate cartilage

Lamina of cricoid cartilage

Thyro-epiglottic ligament

Median crico-thyroid lig.

Vocal ligament

Crico-thyroid ligament
(Crico-vocal membrane)

Conus
elasticus

Posterior crico-arytenoid
ligament

25   Skeleton of the Larynx, from above

...bserve

The right and the left lamina of the thyroid cartilage, united anteriorly at an "angle" of
about 60° in the male and 90° in the female (cf. the subpubic angle, figs. 218 & 220).

The epiglottic cartilage, shaped like a bicycle saddle, pitted for mucous glands, and attached
at its apex by ligamentous fibres to the angle of the thyroid cartilage above the vocal ligaments.

The arytenoid cartilage (paired), having a blunt apex prolonged as the corniculate cartilage;
a rounded, lateral, basal angle called the muscular process; and a sharp, anterior basal
angle, called the vocal process, for the attachment of the vocal ligament.

The strong posterior crico-arytenoid ligament, which prevents the arytenoid cartilage from
falling into the larynx.

The vocal ligament, which forms the skeleton of the vocal fold, extending from the vocal
process to the "angle" of the thyroid cartilage, and there joining its fellow below the thyro-
epiglottic ligament.

The crico-thyroid ligament blending in front with the median crico-thyroid ligament (fig.
623), and sweeping upwards from the upper border of the arch of the cricoid cartilage to
the vocal ligament. Hence, when the vocal ligaments are in apposition, the membranes of
opposite sides form a roof for the infraglottic section of the larynx below them. The 3 ligaments—median cricothyroid lig., cricothyroid lig., and vocal lig.—are sometimes referred
to bilaterally as the *conus elasticus*, but the term is indefinite.

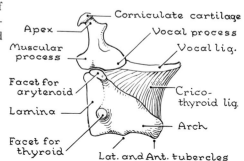

Apex

Muscular
process

Facet for
arytenoid

Lamina

Facet for
thyroid

Corniculate cartilage

Vocal process

Vocal lig.

Crico-
thyroid lig.

Arch

Lat. and Ant. tubercles

625.2

Diagram: Crico-thyroid and Vocal ligaments, side view.

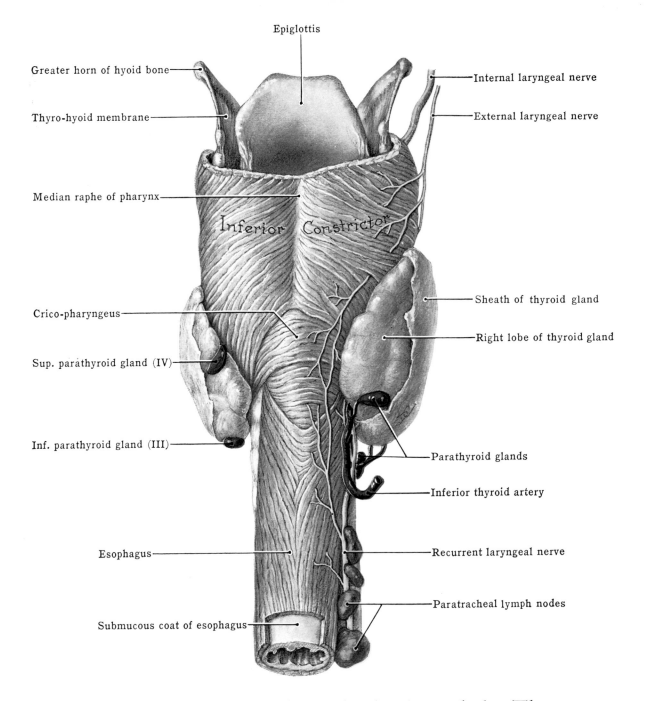

Epiglottis

Greater horn of hyoid bone

Thyro-hyoid membrane

Median raphe of pharynx

Inferior Constrictor

Crico-pharyngeus

Sup. parathyroid gland (IV)

Inf. parathyroid gland (III)

Esophagus

Submucous coat of esophagus

Internal laryngeal nerve

External laryngeal nerve

Sheath of thyroid gland

Right lobe of thyroid gland

Parathyroid glands

Inferior thyroid artery

Recurrent laryngeal nerve

Paratracheal lymph nodes

626 Thyroid Gland, the Parathyroid Glands, and the Three Laryngeal Nerves, from behind

Observe:

1. The right and left lobes of the thyroid gland, unequal in size, applied to the Inferior Constrictor of the pharynx, the trachea, and the esophagus. (For X-section, see fig. 535.)

2. The superior parathyroid gland, here, as usual, fusiform in shape and lying in a crevice on the posterior border of the lateral lobe of the thyroid gland. The inferior gland, more circular and applied to the lower pole of the thyroid gland. On the right side, both parathyroid glands are rather low, the inferior gland (verified histologically) being altogether below the thyroid gland.

3. The internal laryngeal nerve, which is sensory (see fig. 627). The external laryngeal nerve, supplying Inferior Constrictor and Crico-thyroid (see figs. 530 & 532). The recurrent laryngeal nerve, which is mixed, supplying esophagus, trachea (fig. 534), and Inferior Constrictor, dividing into 2 branches which ascend variously related to the branches of the inferior thyroid artery.

Terminology: The end branch of the recurrent laryngeal nerve is officially named "inferior laryngeal nerve" and it accompanies the inferior laryngeal artery (fig. 628.1) into the larynx.

(For Interior of Pharynx, undisturbed, see fig. 578.)

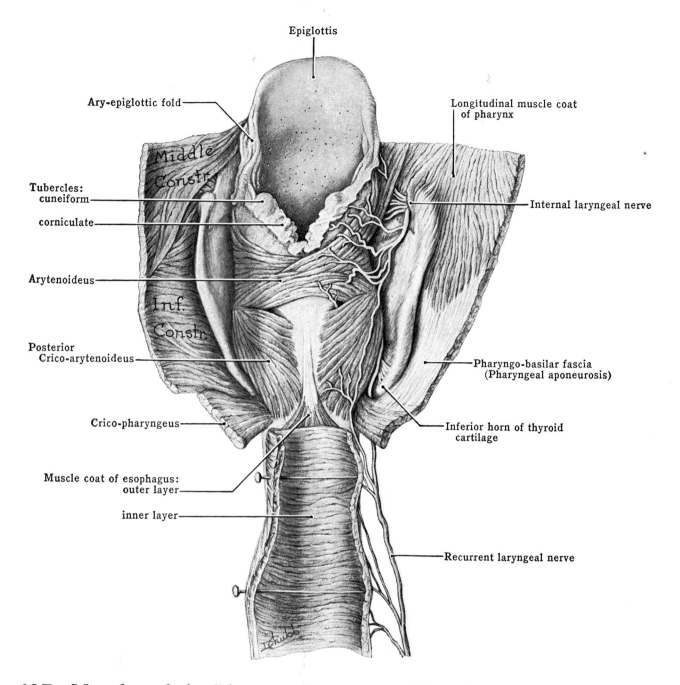

Epiglottis

Ary-epiglottic fold

Longitudinal muscle coat
of pharynx

Middle Constr.

Tubercles:
cuneiform

corniculate

Internal laryngeal nerve

Arytenoideus

Inf. Constr.

Posterior
Crico-arytenoideus

Pharyngo-basilar fascia
(Pharyngeal aponeurosis)

Crico-pharyngeus

Inferior horn of thyroid
cartilage

Muscle coat of esophagus:
outer layer

inner layer

Recurrent laryngeal nerve

627 Muscles of the Pharynx, Larynx, and Esophagus, posterior view

The mucous membrane of the pharynx and esophagus is removed; the left Palato-pharyngeus also is removed and the Constrictors are thereby uncovered.

Observe:

1. On the epiglottis, the pinpoint orifices of the glands that occupy the pits on the epiglottic cartilage (fig. 625).

2. Palato-pharyngeus and Stylo-pharyngeus together constituting the inner or longitudinal muscle coat of the pharynx (figs. 588 & 589), inserted into the pharyngo-basilar fascia and thyroid cartilage.

3. The esophagus, having inner or circularly arranged muscle fibres and outer or longitudinally arranged fibres; the latter suspending the esophagus from the cricoid cartilage.

4. Inferior Constrictor, attached not to the posterior border of the thyroid cartilage (but to the oblique line and the tubercles, fig. 623). Its lowest fibres, called Crico-pharyngeus, which act as a sphincter, attached to the cricoid cartilage.

5. The fan-shape of Crico-arytenoideus Posterior. Its upper fibres rotate the arytenoid cartilage laterally; its lower fibres pull the cartilage downwards.

6. Arytenoideus (Interarytenoideus), having transverse fibres; and also oblique fibres which are continued into the ary-epiglottic fold as Ary-epiglotticus.

7. The recurrent laryngeal nerve (mixed—motor and sensory), entering the larynx as two branches of which the anterior runs immediately behind the crico-thyroid joint.

8. The internal laryngeal nerve (sensory) piercing the thyrohyoid membrane as several diverging branches.

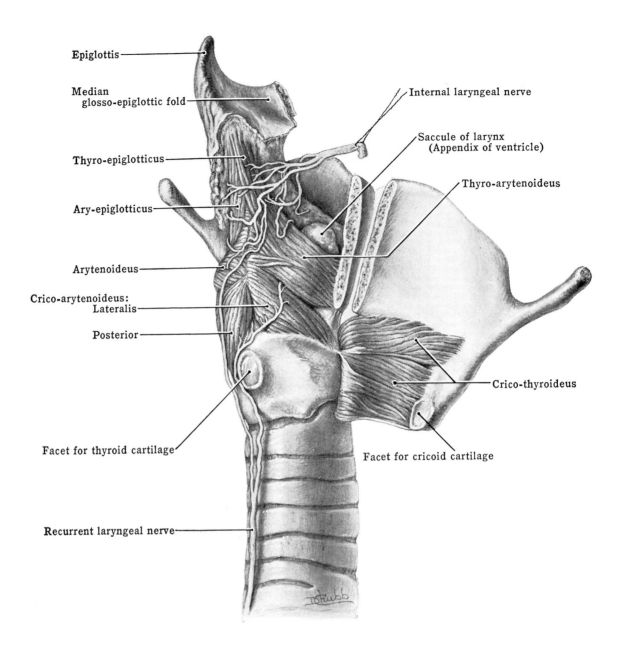

Epiglottis

Median glosso-epiglottic fold

Thyro-epiglotticus

Ary-epiglotticus

Arytenoideus

Crico-arytenoideus:
Lateralis

Posterior

Facet for thyroid cartilage

Recurrent laryngeal nerve

Internal laryngeal nerve

Saccule of larynx
(Appendix of ventricle)

Thyro-arytenoideus

Crico-thyroideus

Facet for cricoid cartilage

628 and 628.1 Muscles, Nerves and Arteries of the Larynx: Cricothyroid Joint, side view

The thyroid cartilage is sawn through on the right of the median plane; the crico-thyroid joint is laid open; the right lamina of the thyroid cartilage is turned forwards, stripping Crico-thyroideus off the arch of the cricoid cartilage.

Observe:

1. Crico-arytenoideus Lateralis, arising from the upper border of the arch of the cricoid carti-lage, and inserted with Crico-arytenoideus Posterior into the muscular process of the arytenoid cartilage.

2. Thyro-arytenoideus, inserted with Arytenoideus into the lateral border of the arytenoid cartilage; and its uppermost fibres continued to (or towards) the epiglottis as Thyro-epi-glotticus.

3. The blind upper end of the laryngeal saccule, see also figure 622.

4. The internal and recurrent laryngeal nerves, described with figure 627.

5. In figure 628.1, note the anastomoses between superior and inferior laryngeal arteries (being branches of sup. and inf. thyroid arts. respectively). Arterial twigs piercing the epiglottic cartilage at the sites of the pits for glands.

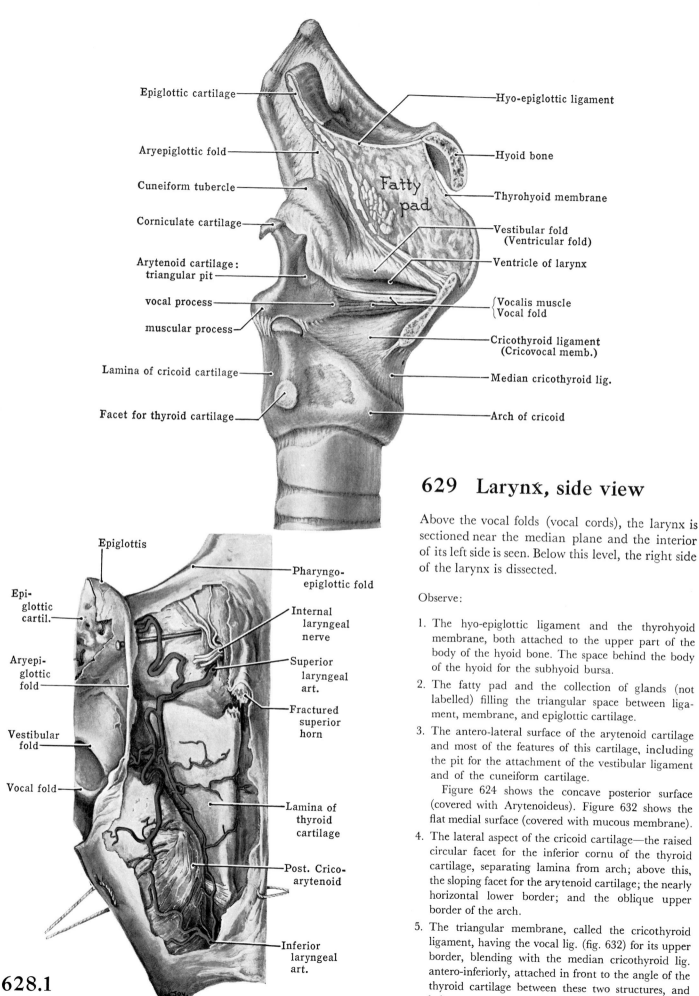

Epiglottic cartilage

Aryepiglottic fold

Cuneiform tubercle

Corniculate cartilage

Arytenoid cartilage: triangular pit

vocal process

muscular process

Lamina of cricoid cartilage

Facet for thyroid cartilage

Hyo-epiglottic ligament

Hyoid bone

Thyrohyoid membrane

Fatty pad

Vestibular fold (Ventricular fold)

Ventricle of larynx

{ Vocalis muscle
{ Vocal fold

Cricothyroid ligament (Cricovocal memb.)

Median cricothyroid lig.

Arch of cricoid

Epiglottis

Epi-glottic cartil.

Aryepi-glottic fold

Vestibular fold

Vocal fold

Pharyngo-epiglottic fold

Internal laryngeal nerve

Superior laryngeal art.

Fractured superior horn

Lamina of thyroid cartilage

Post. Crico-arytenoid

Inferior laryngeal art.

628.1

629 Larynx, side view

Above the vocal folds (vocal cords), the larynx is sectioned near the median plane and the interior of its left side is seen. Below this level, the right side of the larynx is dissected.

Observe:

1. The hyo-epiglottic ligament and the thyrohyoid membrane, both attached to the upper part of the body of the hyoid bone. The space behind the body of the hyoid for the subhyoid bursa.

2. The fatty pad and the collection of glands (not labelled) filling the triangular space between ligament, membrane, and epiglottic cartilage.

3. The antero-lateral surface of the arytenoid cartilage and most of the features of this cartilage, including the pit for the attachment of the vestibular ligament and of the cuneiform cartilage.

   Figure 624 shows the concave posterior surface (covered with Arytenoideus). Figure 632 shows the flat medial surface (covered with mucous membrane).

4. The lateral aspect of the cricoid cartilage—the raised circular facet for the inferior cornu of the thyroid cartilage, separating lamina from arch; above this, the sloping facet for the arytenoid cartilage; the nearly horizontal lower border; and the oblique upper border of the arch.

5. The triangular membrane, called the cricothyroid ligament, having the vocal lig. (fig. 632) for its upper border, blending with the median cricothyroid lig. antero-inferiorly, attached in front to the angle of the thyroid cartilage between these two structures, and below to the cricoid cartilage.

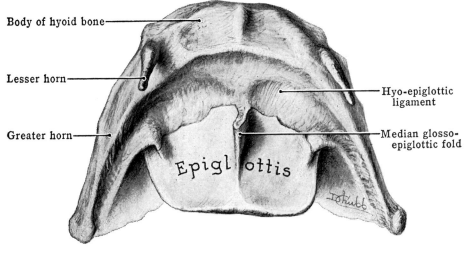

Body of hyoid bone

Lesser horn

Greater horn

Epiglottis

Hyo-epiglottic ligament

Median glosso-epiglottic fold

630 Hyo-epiglottic Ligament, from above

Observe:

1. The hyo-epiglottic ligament, uniting the ⊙ glottic cartilage to the hyoid bone.

2. The three parts of the hyoid bone, and the asy⊙ metry of the greater and lesser horns or cor⊙ of opposite sides. (Hyoid bone, see fig. 596.)

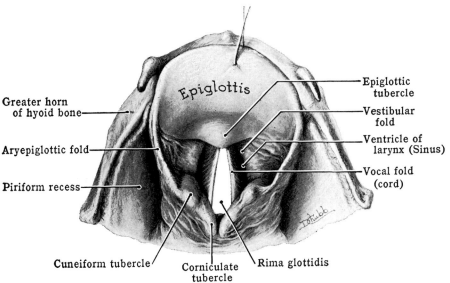

Greater horn of hyoid bone

Aryepiglottic fold

Piriform recess

Cuneiform tubercle

Corniculate tubercle

Rima glottidis

Epiglottis

Epiglottic tubercle

Vestibular fold

Ventricle of larynx (Sinus)

Vocal fold (cord)

631 Larynx, from abov⊙

Observe:

1. The inlet or aditus to the larynx, bounde⊙ front by the free, curved edge of the epiglo⊙ behind, by the arytenoid cartilages, the cor⊙ late cartilages, which cap them, and the in⊙ arytenoid fold which unites them; and, on e⊙ side, by the aryepiglottic fold, which con⊙ the upper end of the cuneiform cartilage.

2. The vocal folds, closer together than the ves⊙ ular folds (false cords) and, therefore, vis⊙ below them. The sharpness of the vocal fo⊙ the fullness of the vestibular folds.

3. The mucous membrane, smooth and adhe⊙ in the epiglottic region and over the v⊙ folds, but loose and even wrinkled posterio⊙ where movement is free.

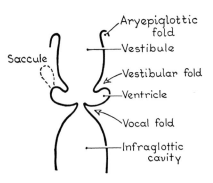

Aryepiglottic fold

Vestibule

Saccule

Vestibular fold

Ventricle

Vocal fold

Infraglottic cavity

631.1 Diagram of the 3 compartments of the larynx, on coronal section

These are—a vestibule, a middle compartment having a right and a left ventricle, and an infraglottic cavity.

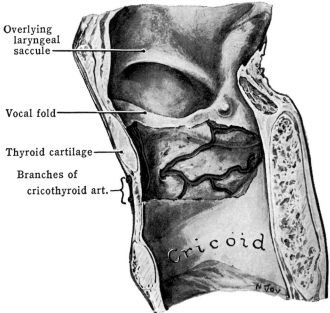

Overlying laryngeal saccule

Vocal fold

Thyroid cartilage

Branches of cricothyroid art.

Cricoid

631.2 Distribution of Cricothyroid Arter⊙

This branch of the superior thyroid art. anastomoses with its fellow i⊙ front of the median cricothyroid lig., as shown in figure 528. Lymp⊙ vessels accompany it.

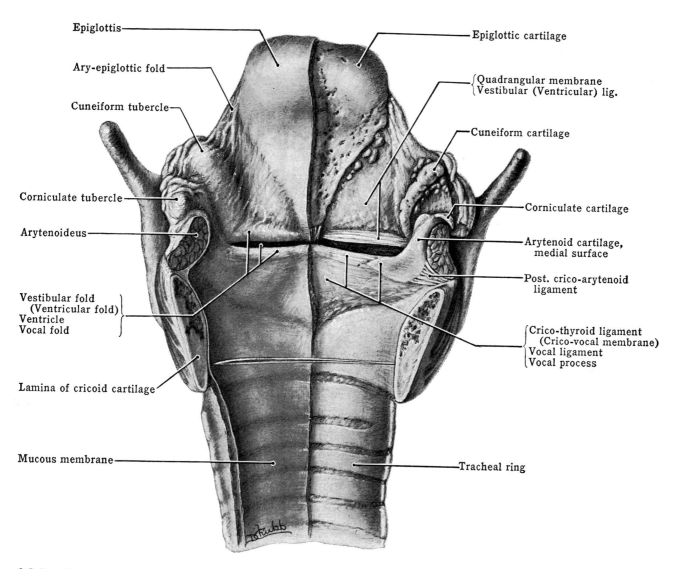

Epiglottis

Ary-epiglottic fold

Cuneiform tubercle

Corniculate tubercle

Arytenoideus

Vestibular fold
  (Ventricular fold)
Ventricle
Vocal fold

Lamina of cricoid cartilage

Mucous membrane

Epiglottic cartilage

Quadrangular membrane
Vestibular (Ventricular) lig.

Cuneiform cartilage

Corniculate cartilage

Arytenoid cartilage,
  medial surface

Post. crico-arytenoid
  ligament

Crico-thyroid ligament
  (Crico-vocal membrane)
Vocal ligament
Vocal process

Tracheal ring

632   Interior of the Larynx, posterior view

The posterior wall of the larynx is split medianly, and the two sides are held apart. On the left side, the mucous membrane, which is the innermost coat of the larynx, is intact; on the right side, the mucous and submucous coats are peeled off and the next coat, consisting of cartilages, ligaments and a fibro-elastic membrane, is thereby laid bare.

Observe:

1. Arytenoideus and the lamina of the cricoid cartilage, divided posteriorly.
2. The entrance to the larynx to be oblique; the lower limit, at the lower border of the cricoid cartilage where the trachea begins, to be horizontal.
3. The 3 compartments of the larynx—(a) the uppermost compartment or vestibule, above the level of the vestibular folds; (b) the middle, between the levels of the vestibular and vocal folds, and having a right and a left canoe-shaped depression, the ventricles; and (c) the lowest or infraglottic cavity, below the level of the vocal folds.

4. The mucous membrane, particularly smooth and adherent over the epiglottic cartilage and vocal ligaments; and particularly loose and wrinkled about the arytenoid cartilages, where movement is free.
5. The two parts of the fibro-elastic membrane—(a) an upper quadrangular, and (b) a lower triangular. The upper part, the quadrangular membrane, which is thickened below to form the vestibular ligament. The lower part, the crico-thyroid ligament (conus elasticus), which begins below as the strong median cricothyroid ligament and ends above as the vocal ligament. Between the vocal and the vestibular ligament, the membrane, lined with mucous membrane, is evaginated to form the wall of the ventricle.
6. The cuneiform cartilage; (a) more club-shaped than wedge-shaped, (b) composed of elastic cartilage and pitted for, and surrounded with, glands, like the epiglottic cartilage of which it is a detached part, and (c) attached to the arytenoid cartilage beside the posterior end of the vestibular ligament.
7. The posterior ligament of the crico-arytenoid joint, anchoring the arytenoid cartilage. The flat, medial, submucous surface of the arytenoid cartilage.

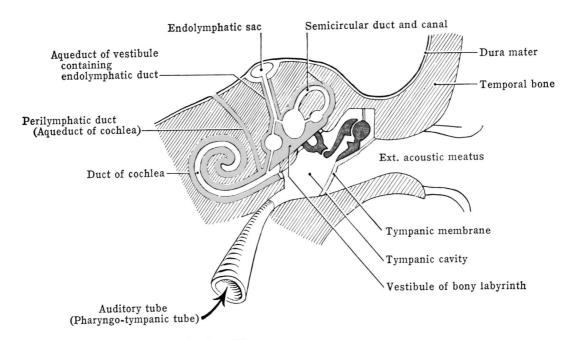

Aqueduct of vestibule containing endolymphatic duct

Endolymphatic sac

Semicircular duct and canal

Dura mater

Temporal bone

Perilymphatic duct (Aqueduct of cochlea)

Duct of cochlea

Ext. acoustic meatus

Tympanic membrane

Tympanic cavity

Vestibule of bony labyrinth

Auditory tube (Pharyngo-tympanic tube)

633 General Scheme of the Ear

The ear is divisible into 3 parts—external, middle, internal.

The external ear comprises (a) the auricle and (b) the external acoustic meatus, the medial end of which is closed by the tympanic membrane.

The tympanic membrane is set obliquely and is slightly conical, its most in-drawn point or umbo being at the lower end of the handle of the malleus which is attached to the membrane.

The middle ear or tympanum lies between the tympanic membrane and the internal ear.

Three ossicles (red)—malleus, incus, stapes—stretch from the lateral to the medial wall of the tympanum. Of these, the malleus is attached to the tympanic membrane; the stapes is attached by an annular ligament to the oval opening, called the fenestra vestibuli; and the incus connects these two ossicles.

The part of the tympanic cavity that lies above the level of the external acoustic meatus is the epitympanic recess (not labelled). It contains the upper ends of the malleus and incus.

The auditory tube opens into the anterior wall of the tympanic cavity; the aditus ad antrum opens from the epitympanic recess backwards to the mastoid antrum (fig. 639).

The internal ear comprises a closed system of membranous tubes and bulbs, called the membranous labyrinth, which are filled with fluid, called endolymph, and are bathed in surrounding fluid called perilymph (blue). The perilymph is contained within the bony labyrinth, but this system is not a closed one, for, as represented in fig. 633, perilymph and cerebrospinal fluid are confluent in the posterior cranial fossa. There is, however, good evidence that this system also is closed, the perilymphatic duct ending as a perilymphatic sac. (Wharton Young.)

When the tympanic membrane vibrates, the malleus vibrates with it and transmits the vibrations via the incus to the stapes. The stapes, being attached to the margins of the fenestra vestibuli (oval window) by an annular ligament, transmits the vibrations to the perilymph within the vestibule.

A secondary tympanic membrane which closes the fenestra cochleae (round window), receiving the vibrations transmitted to the incompressible perilymph, is itself made to vibrate in turn.

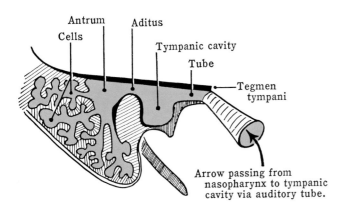

Antrum

Cells

Aditus

Tympanic cavity

Tube

Tegmen tympani

Arrow passing from nasopharynx to tympanic cavity via auditory tube.

633.1 Diagram of Tegmen Tympani

The mastoid air cells are in communication with the outside air via the mastoid antrum, aditus ad antrum, tympanic cavity, and bony and cartilaginous parts of the auditory tube.

A thin plate of bone, called the tegmen tympani, forms a roof for these.

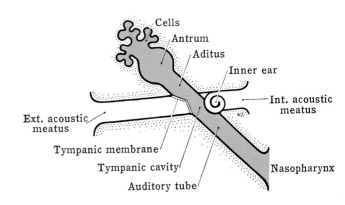

Cells

Antrum

Aditus

Inner ear

Int. acoustic meatus

Ext. acoustic meatus

Tympanic membrane

Tympanic cavity

Auditory tube

Nasopharynx

633.2 Scheme of Meatuses and Airway

showing the line of the meatuses and the line of the airway (from nasopharynx to mastoid cells) intersecting at the tympanic cavity.

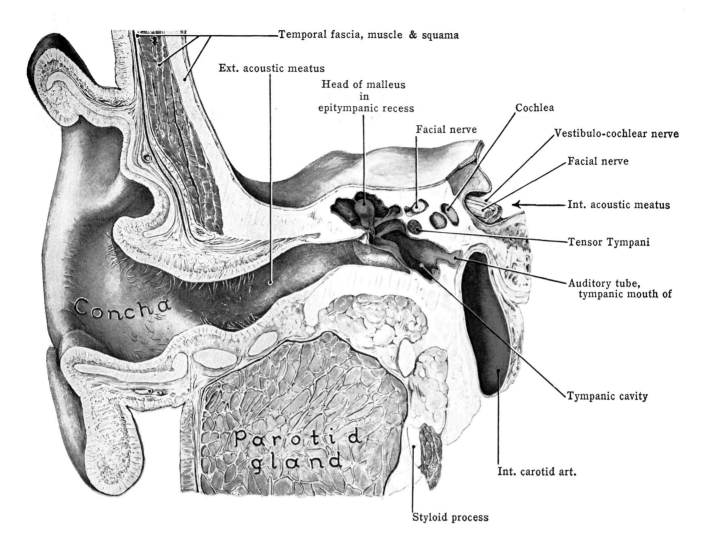

Temporal fascia, muscle & squama

Ext. acoustic meatus

Head of malleus in epitympanic recess

Facial nerve

Cochlea

Vestibulo-cochlear nerve

Facial nerve

Int. acoustic meatus

Tensor Tympani

Auditory tube, tympanic mouth of

Tympanic cavity

Int. carotid art.

Styloid process

Concha

Parotid gland

634 Ear on Coronal Section, anterior view

(Inner ear tinted blue; mucous membrane of the middle ear pink.)

Observe:

1. The external acoustic (auditory) meatus which from tragus to ear drum is 1¼″ long, half the length being cartilaginous and half bony. Narrowest near the drum due to the rise on the floor, hence the "well" where fluid might collect at the medial end of the meatus.

2. The cartilaginous or mobile part of the external meatus, lined with thick skin and having hairs and the mouths of many glands; the bony part lined with a thin epithelium which adheres to the periosteum and also forms the outermost layer of the tympanic membrane.

3. The obliquity of the tympanic membrane which meets the roof of the meatus at an obtuse angle and the floor at an acute one.

4. The middle ear or tympanic cavity, extending above the level of the drum as the epitympanic recess, and the recess extending laterally above the bony meatus.

5. The tympanic cavity widest above, narrow below, and narrowest at the level of the umbo where the membrane is indrawn and faces the promontory of the cochlea.

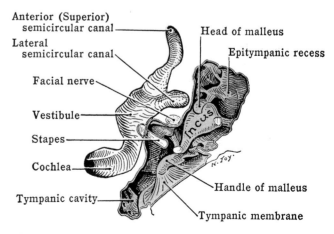

Anterior (Superior) semicircular canal

Lateral semicircular canal

Facial nerve

Vestibule

Stapes

Cochlea

Tympanic cavity

Head of malleus

Epitympanic recess

Incus

Handle of malleus

Tympanic membrane

(Inset from another specimen, posterior view.)

6. The thin shell of bone covering the facial nerve. The grooved anterior crus of the stapes and the anterior half of its base closing the fenestra vestibuli. The long axis of the stapes inclined upwards and medially—not lying horizontally.

7. The lateral canal, above facial nerve (fig. 637).

635 Tympanic Membrane, on lateral view

(Exposed by grinding away the bony exterior meatus.)

Observe:

1. The tympanic membrane, oval rather than round, and shaped like a funnel with rolled rim and a depressed part, called the umbo, at the tip of the handle of the malleus which is situated antero-inferior to the centre of the membrane.

2. The stria mallearis, which overlies the handle of the malleus, extending upwards to the prominentia, which overlies the lateral process of the malleus.

3. Above the prominentia the membrane is thin and is called the pars flaccida. The pars flaccida lacks the radial and circular fibres present in the remainder of the membrane (pars tensa). The junction between the two parts, flaccid and tense, is marked by an anterior and a posterior line which run from the prominentia to the free ends of the horseshoe-shaped tympanic ring (fig. 646).

4. The pars flaccida forms the lateral wall of the superior recess (fig. 641) of the tympanic cavity.

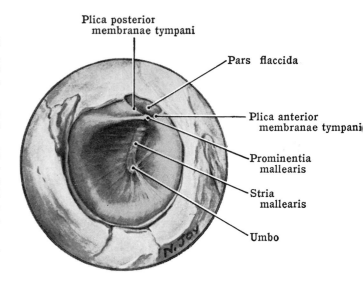

Plica posterior membranae tympani
Pars flaccida
Plica anterior membranae tympani
Prominentia mallearis
Stria mallearis
Umbo

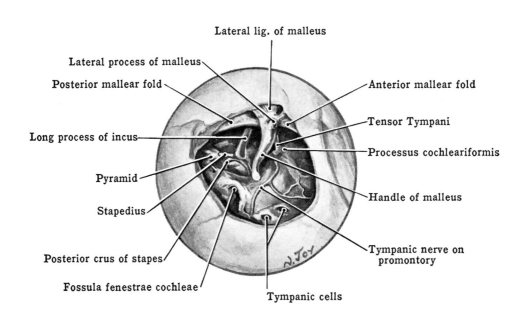

Lateral lig. of malleus
Lateral process of malleus
Posterior mallear fold
Long process of incus
Pyramid
Stapedius
Posterior crus of stapes
Fossula fenestrae cochleae
Tympanic cells
Anterior mallear fold
Tensor Tympani
Processus cochleariformis
Handle of malleus
Tympanic nerve on promontory

636 Tympanic Cavity, infero-lateral view, after removal of the tympanic membrane

Observe:

1. The direction of the handle of the malleus and of the long process of the incus which lies behind it; also the posterior and anterior mallear folds of mucous membrane in which the chorda tympani passes between the two bones (fig. 641).

2. The fulness of the promontory with grooves for the tympanic nerve (a branch of the glossopharyngeal nerve) and its connections.

3. The end of a fossula at the deep end of which is the fenestra cochleae or round window, closed by the secondary tympanic membrane (not in view).

4. The tendon of Stapedius passing forwards to the neck of the stapes; the tendon of Tensor Tympani passing laterally to the neck of the malleus.

5. The lateral ligament of the malleus and the neck of the malleus forming the medial wall of the superior recess of the tympanic membrane (fig. 641).

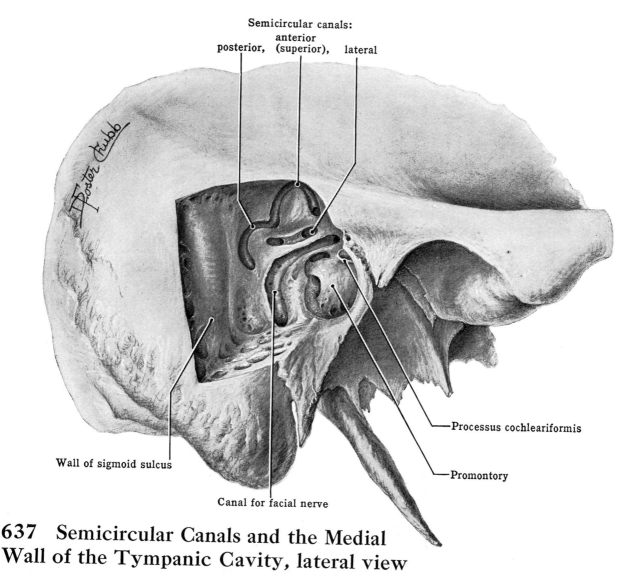

Semicircular canals:
anterior
posterior, (superior), lateral

Processus cochleariformis

Promontory

Wall of sigmoid sulcus

Canal for facial nerve

637 Semicircular Canals and the Medial Wall of the Tympanic Cavity, lateral view

The mastoid cells, seen in coronal section in figure 643, are largely removed and the inner table of the skull, here forming the semi-tubular wall of the sigmoid sulcus, is exposed. The posterior wall of the external acoustic meatus and the mastoid antrum are removed.

Observe:

1. The 3 semicircular canals, lying in the 3 planes of space, are opened.

2. The anterior and posterior canals, placed vertically and at right angles to each other. The lateral canal, placed horizontally and at right angles to the anterior and posterior canals.

3. The medial end of the anterior canal and the upper end of the posterior canal, uniting to form the crus commune. The lateral canal lying in the medial wall of the aditus ad antrum.

4. The features of the medial or labyrinthine wall of the tympanic cavity:
   (a) The promontory, lying 2 mm deep to the umbo, and overlying the basal turn of the cochlea.
   (b) The processus cochleariformis, at the end of the canal for Tensor Tympani. It acts as a pulley for the Tensor.
   (c) The fenestra vestibuli, close behind the pulley and medial to it. It is closed by the foot-plate of the stapes, which is bound to its margin by an annular ligament.
   (d) The fossula leading to the fenestra cochleae, below the vestibular window and separated from it by a rounded bar which projects backwards from the promontory.
   (e) The facial canal (opened) running horizontally backwards, between the vestibular window and the lateral semicircular canal, to the junction of the medial and posterior walls, then descending in the posterior wall to its orifice, the stylomastoid foramen.

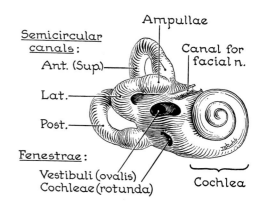

Semicircular canals:
Ant. (Sup.)
Lat.
Post.

Ampullae
Canal for facial n.

Fenestrae:
Vestibuli (ovalis)
Cochleae (rotunda)

Cochlea

637.1 Bony Inner Ear, lateral view

To aid in orientation of fig. 637.

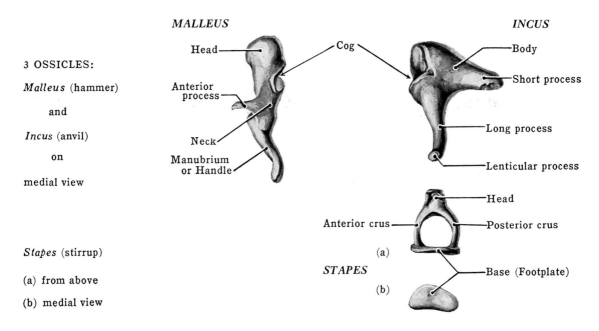

3 OSSICLES:

Malleus (hammer)

and

Incus (anvil)

on

medial view

Stapes (stirrup)

(a) from above

(b) medial view

3 Ossicles of the middle ear in their relative positions.

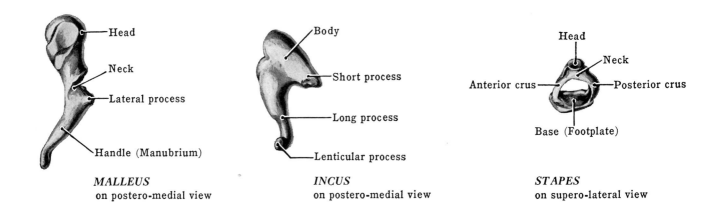

MALLEUS
on postero-medial view

INCUS
on postero-medial view

STAPES
on supero-lateral view

638 Ossicles of the Middle Ear

(Malleus, Incus, and Stapes)

The head of the malleus and the body and short process of the incus lie in the epitympanic recess.

The saddle-shaped articular surface of the head of the malleus and the reciprocally saddle-shaped articular surface of the body of the incus form the incudo-mallear synovial joint.

The anterior process of the malleus and the short process of the incus (it might better have been called the posterior process) are in line and are moored fore and aft by ligaments.

The handle of the malleus, from lateral process to tip, is imbedded in the tympanic membrane.

The end of the long (vertical) process of the incus has a convex articular facet for articulation with the head of the stapes, at the incudo-stapedial synovial joint.

The hole in the stapes in the embryo transmits an artery, the stapedial artery. It is now closed by an obturator. The upper border of the footplate is convex; and it is deeper anteriorly than posteriorly. The two crura are grooved. The anterior crus is the more slender and straighter and it is fixed to a small area on the plate; the posterior crus is attached to the whole depth of the plate.

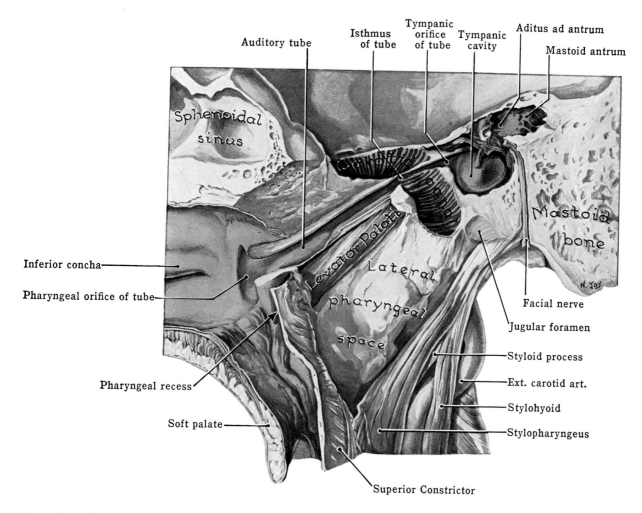

Labels on upper figure:
- Auditory tube
- Isthmus of tube
- Tympanic orifice of tube
- Tympanic cavity
- Aditus ad antrum
- Mastoid antrum
- Sphenoidal sinus
- Mastoid bone
- Inferior concha
- Pharyngeal orifice of tube
- Levator Palati
- Lateral pharyngeal space
- Facial nerve
- Jugular foramen
- Pharyngeal recess
- Styloid process
- Ext. carotid art.
- Stylohyoid
- Stylopharyngeus
- Soft palate
- Superior Constrictor

639 Auditory Tube (Pharyngo-tympanic Tube), exposed from the medial or pharyngeal aspect.

Observe:

1. The general direction of the tube—upwards, backwards, and laterally from nasopharynx to tympanic cavity.

2. The funnel-shaped pharyngeal orifice of the tube, situated $\frac{1}{2}''$ behind the inferior concha of the nose.

3. The cartilaginous part of the tube, $1''$ long, resting throughout its length on Levator Palati, but affording it almost no origin.

4. The bony part of the tube passing lateral to the carotid canal, $\frac{1}{2}''$ long, narrow at the isthmus where it joins the cartilaginous part, wider at its tympanic orifice, and less steep than the cartilaginous part.

5. Tensor Tympani, lying above a bony ledge, called the processus cochleariformis, and inserted into the neck of the malleus.

6. The chorda tympani lying in a "mesentery", the anterior and posterior mallear folds, and the anterior and posterior recesses of the tympanic membrane lateral to the respective folds.

7. The anterior mallear fold acting as a mesentery for Tensor Tympani also, and continuous with a fold that passes forwards from the head of the malleus.

8. The upper half of the lateral pharyngeal space, seen on cross section in figures 579 & 584.

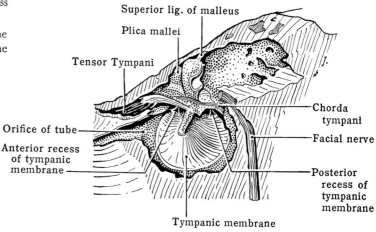

Labels on lower figure:
- Superior lig. of malleus
- Plica mallei
- Tensor Tympani
- Chorda tympani
- Facial nerve
- Orifice of tube
- Anterior recess of tympanic membrane
- Posterior recess of tympanic membrane
- Tympanic membrane

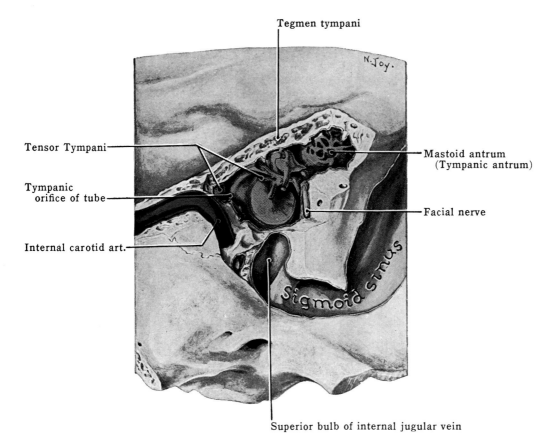

Tegmen tympani

Tensor Tympani

Tympanic
orifice of tube

Internal carotid art.

Mastoid antrum
(Tympanic antrum)

Facial nerve

Sigmoid sinus

Superior bulb of internal jugular vein

640 Walls of the Tympanic Cavity or Middle Ear

(Exposed with a drill, from the medial aspect.)

Observe:

1. The tegmen tympani forming the roof of the tube, tympanic cavity, and antrum, here fairly thick but commonly papery in thinness.

2. The int. carotid artery as the main feature of the anterior wall; the int. jugular vein the main feature of the floor; and the facial nerve the main feature of the posterior wall.

3. The supero-lateral part of the anterior wall leading to the auditory tube and Tensor Tympani; the supero-lateral part

of the posterior wall leading to the mastoid antrum.

4. The tympanic membrane forming much of the lateral wall. Above it is the epitympanic recess in which are housed the greater parts of the malleus and incus.

5. A ligament suspending the malleus from the tegmen tympani; the short process of the incus moored by ligaments to the fossa incudis in the floor of the aditus to the antrum.

6. The chorda tympani passing between incus and malleus.

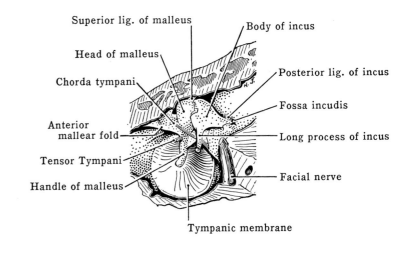

Epitympanic recess   Aditus

Tube

Facial n. (VII)

ANTERIOR   POSTERIOR

Int. carotid art.

Carotid sheath

Superior jugular bulb

Superior lig. of malleus   Body of incus

Head of malleus   Posterior lig. of incus

Chorda tympani   Fossa incudis

Anterior mallear fold   Long process of incus

Tensor Tympani   Facial nerve

Handle of malleus

Tympanic membrane

640.1

Diagram: Features of Walls of Tympanic Cavity.

ANTERIOR → POSTERIOR →

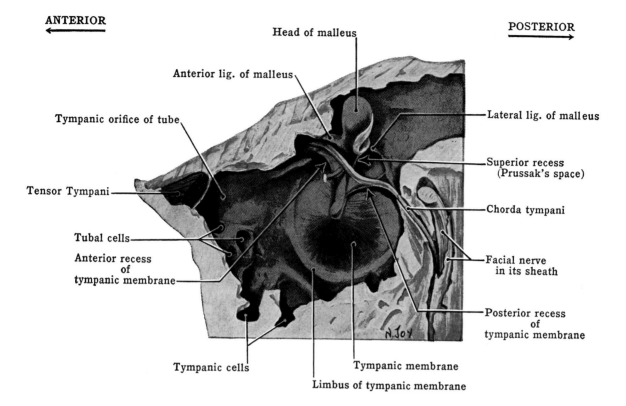

Head of malleus — Anterior lig. of malleus — Tympanic orifice of tube — Tensor Tympani — Tubal cells — Anterior recess of tympanic membrane — Lateral lig. of malleus — Superior recess (Prussak's space) — Chorda tympani — Facial nerve in its sheath — Posterior recess of tympanic membrane — Tympanic cells — Tympanic membrane — Limbus of tympanic membrane

641 Lateral Wall of the Tympanic Cavity, medial view

Observe:

1. The oval tympanic membrane, with a greater vertical than horizontal diameter (9 mm. x 8 mm.).

2. The handle of the malleus incorporated in the membrane, its end being at the umbo.

3. The anterior process of the malleus anchored forwards by the anterior lig. This lig. is almost continuous through the petro-tympanic fissure with the spheno-mandibular lig.

4. The facial nerve within its tough periosteal tube. The chorda tympani leaving the facial nerve, and as it goes to the front wall (a) lying within 2 crescentic folds of mucous membrane, the anterior and posterior mallear folds, which, so to speak, suspend it from the tympanic membrane at the junction of its flaccid and tense parts, (b) crossing the neck of the malleus above the tendon of Tensor, and (c) following the anterior process and anterior lig.

5. The 3 recesses of the membrane—the anterior and the posterior recess, which extend upwards between the mallear folds and the pars tensa of the membrane, and thirdly the superior recess. The superior recess extends forwards (see arrow) between the neck of the malleus and the pars flaccida, and it is limited below by the short process of the malleus and above by the lateral lig. (fig. 636). This space may open posteriorly, lateral to the incus, as here, or it may open downwards into the posterior recess.

6. The fibro-cartilaginous margin or limbus of the membrane which fastens it to the sulcus in the tympanic bone.

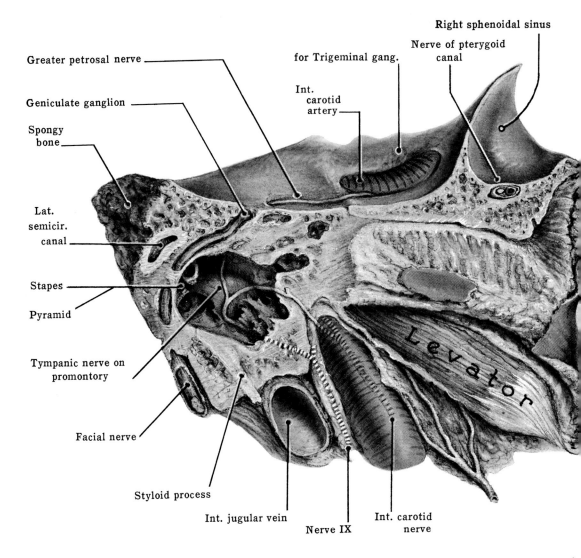

Greater petrosal nerve

Geniculate ganglion

Spongy bone

Lat. semicir. canal

Stapes

Pyramid

Tympanic nerve on promontory

Facial nerve

Styloid process

Int. jugular vein

Nerve IX

Int. carotid nerve

for Trigeminal gang.

Int. carotid artery

Nerve of pterygoid canal

Right sphenoidal sinus

Levator

641.1   Auditory Tube and Tympanic Cavity, right side

The Lateral Wall of the cavity is dominated by the tympanic membrane, handle of malleus and chorda tympani nerve (fig. 641).

The Medial Wall has a broad bulging, the promontory, which overlies the 1st turn of the cochlea (figs. 637 and 649). On it the tympanic nerve (fig. 659) and carotico-tympanic branches of the int. carotid nerve (fig. 514.1) form a plexus, the tympanic plexus, which supplies the neighbourhood and gives off the lesser petrosal nerve (fig. 659).

Procedure (modified, after R. D. Laurenson). Using dissecting room material, collected at the end of a session, and aided by a short hack saw, the squamous and mastoid parts of the temporal bone are sawn across coronally from suprameatal spine (fig. 462), through the mastoid antrum, into the posterior cranial fossa. The posterior part of the bone is then discarded.

The thin roof (tegmen) of the antrum and aditus (fig. 633.1) is nibbled away until the incus comes into view (fig. 648). The *incus* is now picked from its articulation with *malleus* laterally, and *stapes* medially.

A probe, passed from the pharynx up the auditory tube, until arrested at the isthmus, will serve as a directional guide.

Identify the *int. carotid artery* medially, beneath the

trigeminal ganglion (figs. 513 and 514) at the foramen lacerum, and the *middle meningeal artery* laterally, at the foramen spinosum (fig. 512).

A saw cut from the gap left by the incus to the space between the two arteries (carotid & meningeal) will pass between the *greater and lesser petrosal nerves*, being parallel, and continue into the tube.

The incus having been removed, the only structure that crosses the path of the saw is *Tensor Tympani tendon*, which passes from medial to lateral wall. Unintentionally, but fortunately, in this specimen a shaving of the medial wall (containing the fleshy Tensor in its semicanal and the processus cochleariformis) were included with the lateral part, leaving the tendon intact.

Structures, divided and seen on both medial and lateral parts.
a) Levator Palati, supporting the tube.
b) Auditory tube, cartilaginous above & medially; membranous below & laterally (fig. 639).
c) Right sphenoidal sinus, having the pterygoid canal below.
d) Internal carotid artery.
e) Internal jugular vein.
f) Facial nerve.
g) A petrosal nerve, either greater or lesser.

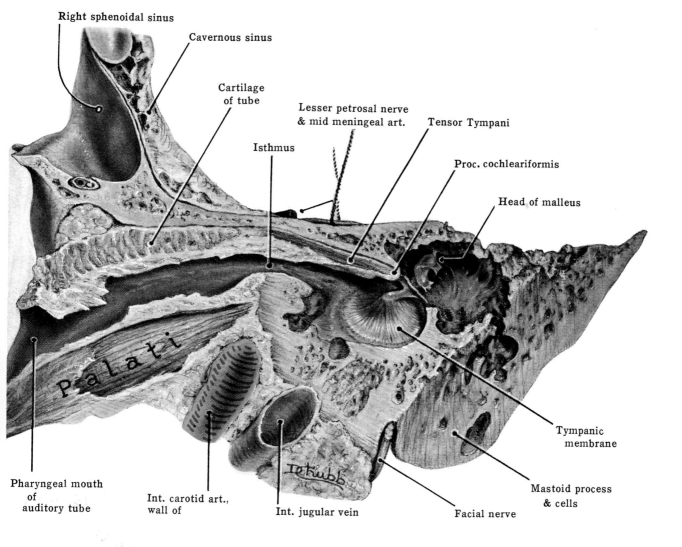

Right sphenoidal sinus

Cavernous sinus

Cartilage of tube

Lesser petrosal nerve & mid meningeal art.

Tensor Tympani

Isthmus

Proc. cochleariformis

Head of malleus

Palati

Tympanic membrane

Pharyngeal mouth of auditory tube

Int. carotid art., wall of

Int. jugular vein

Facial nerve

Mastoid process & cells

split longitudinally into lateral and medial parts.

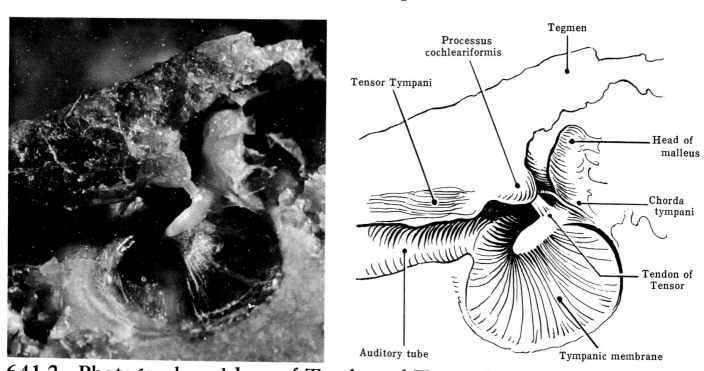

Processus cochleariformis

Tegmen

Tensor Tympani

Head of malleus

Chorda tympani

Tendon of Tensor

Auditory tube

Tympanic membrane

641.2   Photograph and key of Tendon of Tensor Tympani passing from medial to lateral wall (Courtesy of Frank Humelbaugh.)

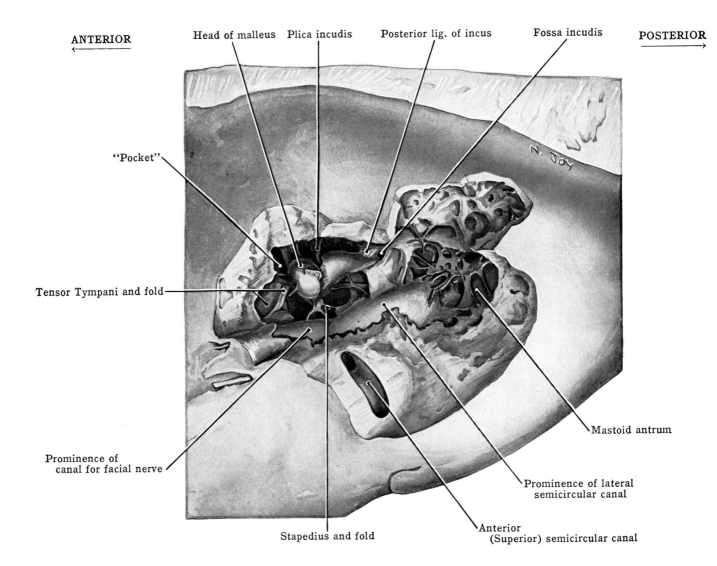

Head of malleus   Plica incudis   Posterior lig. of incus   Fossa incudis

"Pocket"

Tensor Tympani and fold

Prominence of
canal for facial nerve

Mastoid antrum

Prominence of lateral
semicircular canal

Stapedius and fold

Anterior
(Superior) semicircular canal

642 Tympanic Cavity and Mastoid Antrum, from above

The bony roof, or tegmen tympani, has been removed with the aid of an
electric drill.

Observe:

1. Extensive folds, strands, "mesenteries", and pockets of mucous membrane.
2. The mesentery for Tensor Tympani (commonly perforated) and the mesentery for Stapedius and stapes.
3. The head of the malleus and the body and short crus of the incus in the epitympanic recess. The short process of the incus moored by two ligamentous bands to the sides of the fossa incudis on the floor of the aditus ad antrum.
4. The strand from the body of the incus to the lateral wall is commonly an extensive fold as in fig. 648 and the result is a pocket. The superior ligament of the malleus (not labelled) is cut short.

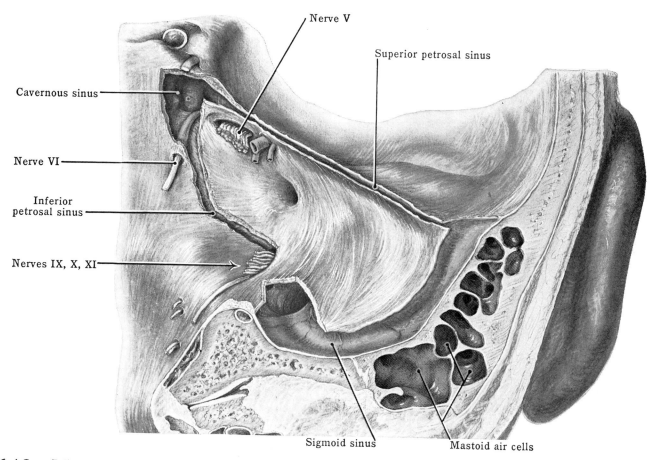

Nerve V

Superior petrosal sinus

Cavernous sinus

Nerve VI

Inferior
petrosal sinus

Nerves IX, X, XI

Sigmoid sinus

Mastoid air cells

643 Mastoid Air Cells—Dural Sinuses

Observe:

1. Mastoid cells (pink), lined with mucous membrane, and occupying the diploe (fig. 633.1). The branching ducts through which these cells communicate with the antrum. The two lowest cells almost bursting through the outer table of the skull.

2. The posterior surface of the petrous bone encircled with 3 sinuses—sigmoid, superior petrosal, and inferior petrosal.

The two petrosal sinuses draining the cavernous sinus.

3. The sup. petrosal sinus, at the attached margin of the tentorium, bridging nerve V. The sigmoid sinus, nerves IX, X, and XI, and the inf. petrosal sinus disappearing into the jugular foramen.

4. Nerve VI, passing through the inf. petrosal sinus and bending forwards to enter the cavernous sinus. (Fig. 514.)

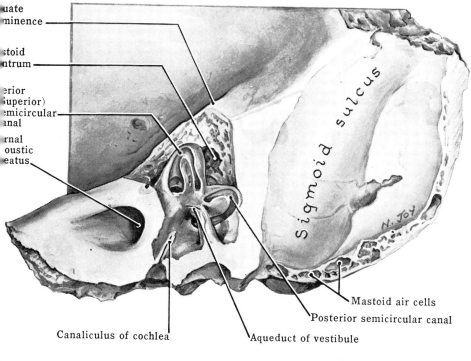

uate
minence

stoid
ntrum

erior
Superior)
emicircular
anal

rnal
oustic
eatus

Sigmoid sulcus

N. Joy

Mastoid air cells

Posterior semicircular canal

Canaliculus of cochlea

Aqueduct of vestibule

644 Semicircular Canals and the Aqueducts, postero-superior view

Observe:

1. The anterior semicircular canal, set vertically, below the arcuate eminence, and making a right angle with the posterior surface of the petrous bone.

2. The posterior semicircular canal, nearly parallel to the posterior surface of the bone, close to that surface, and only 5 mm. from the sigmoid sulcus.

3. The aqueduct of the vestibule, which contains the ductus endolymphaticus and opens medial to the posterior canal.

4. The canaliculus of the cochlea, which contains the perilymphatic duct (aqueduct of cochlea) and opens at the apex of the depression for the ganglion of nerve IX.

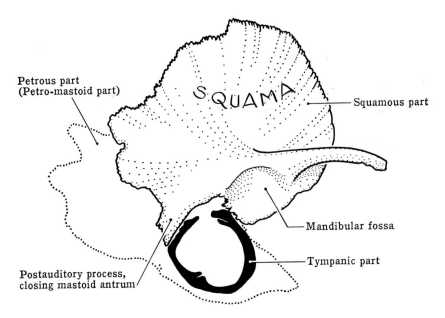

Petrous part
(Petro-mastoid part)

SQUAMA

Squamous part

Mandibular fossa

Tympanic part

Postauditory process,
closing mastoid antrum

645   Temporal Bone at Birth, lateral view

Note:

1. The 3 parts of the temporal bone—squamous, petrous, tympanic—separable at birth.
2. The mandibular fossa is shallow. The postauditory process, descending from the squamous part, closes the mastoid antrum laterally.
3. No mastoid process has yet appeared on the petrous part, there being as yet no mastoid cells.
4. The tympanic part is a ring that is incomplete above; no tympanic plate has yet grown to give length to the external acoustic meatus; hence the tympanic membrane is close to the surface of the skull.

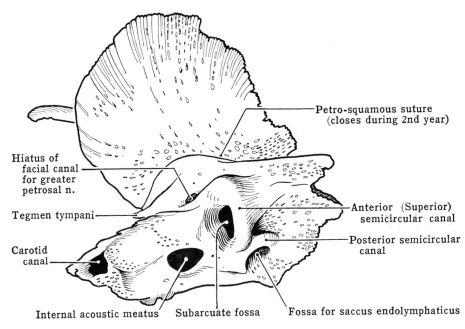

Petro-squamous suture
(closes during 2nd year)

Hiatus of
facial canal
for greater
petrosal n.

Tegmen tympani

Anterior (Superior)
semicircular canal

Posterior semicircular
canal

Carotid
canal

Internal acoustic meatus   Subarcuate fossa   Fossa for saccus endolymphaticus

645.1   Temporal Bone at Birth, posterior view

Note:

1. The hollows round about the anterior and posterior semicircular canals are not yet filled in with bone; hence, these canals project as bony rims.
2. The subarcuate fossa, within the arc of the anterior semicircular canal, is large and looks medially. The fossa within the arc of the posterior canal is likewise large; it looks downwards and laterally and lodges the endolymphatic sac, shown in figure 650.

46 Temporal Bone during the first year of life, lateral view

(The mastoid antrum has been opened.)

Note:

There is a mastoid antrum, but no mastoid process, and accordingly no mastoid cells.

The tympanic bone is a ring, incomplete above. It has no length, but sprouting from its lateral border are two spines.

The stylo-mastoid foramen, from which the facial nerve emerges, is near the skin surface.

The tympanic cavity is large.

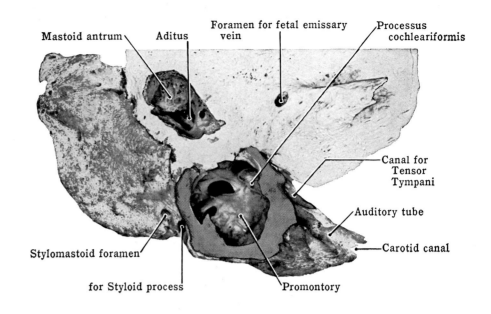

47 Temporal Bone during the third or fourth year, lateral view

(The mastoid antrum and the epitympanic recess have been opened.)

Note:

The mastoid process is appearing. The walls of the antrum are like a honeycomb.

The enlarging spines on the tympanic ring are nearer to meeting and so to enclosing a temporary foramen (closed by membrane) in what is becoming the tympanic plate. This plate will form the anterior, the inferior, and part of the posterior, wall of the external acoustic meatus (fig. 558).

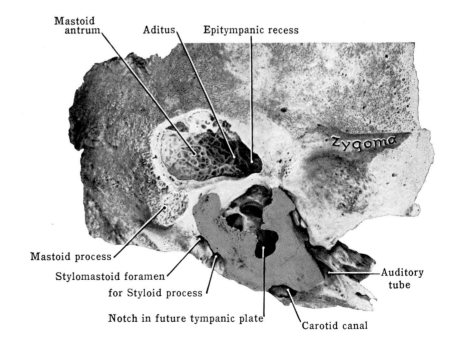

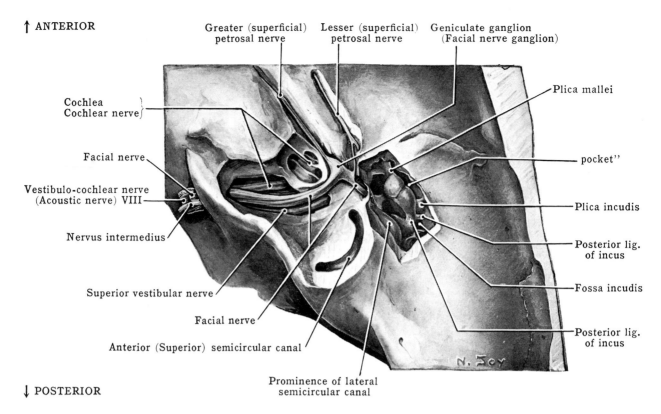

↑ ANTERIOR

Greater (superficial) petrosal nerve

Lesser (superficial) petrosal nerve

Geniculate ganglion (Facial nerve ganglion)

Cochlea
Cochlear nerve

Facial nerve

Vestibulo-cochlear nerve (Acoustic nerve) VIII

Nervus intermedius

Superior vestibular nerve

Facial nerve

Anterior (Superior) semicircular canal

Plica mallei

pocket"

Plica incudis

Posterior lig. of incus

Fossa incudis

Posterior lig. of incus

↓ POSTERIOR

Prominence of lateral semicircular canal

648   Geniculate Ganglion, from above

(The Ganglion of the Facial Nerve.)

Observe:

1. The facial nerve, the nervus intermedius, and the vestibulo-cochlear nerve, entering and traversing the internal acoustic meatus. The facial nerve, joined by the nervus intermedius, running close behind the cochlea and, therefore, across the roof of the vestibule (fig. 649) to the geniculate ganglion and at the ganglion making a right angle bend, called the genu, and then curving downwards and backwards within its bony canal, called the facial canal, whose papery lateral wall separates it from the tympanic cavity.

2. The petrosal branch of the middle meningeal artery, which

enters the canal at the hiatus (fig. 513), running with the nerve.

3. The geniculate ganglion, which is the cell station of fibers of general sensation and of taste (fig. 657), situated at the genu and in line with the internal acoustic meatus. Through the ganglion run forward fibers of the greater (superficial) petrosal nerve on their way to the pterygopalatine ganglion; from the facial nerve, beyond the ganglion, goes a communicating branch to the lesser (superficial) petrosal nerve on its way to the otic ganglion. Further on, but not in view, the chorda tympani leaves the facial nerve and joins the lingual which conducts it to the submandibular ganglion.

MEDIAL

LATERAL

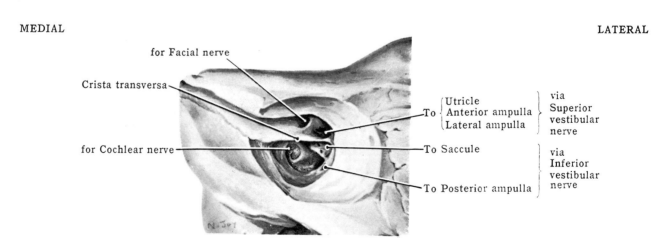

for Facial nerve

Crista transversa

for Cochlear nerve

To Utricle
Anterior ampulla
Lateral ampulla — via Superior vestibular nerve

To Saccule

To Posterior ampulla — via Inferior vestibular nerve

648.1   Fundus of the Internal Acoustic Meatus

(The walls of the meatus have been ground away.)

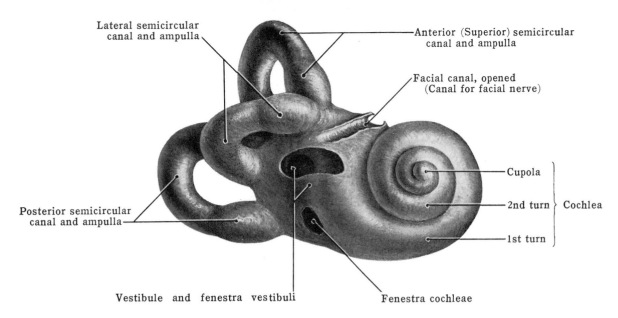

Lateral semicircular canal and ampulla

Anterior (Superior) semicircular canal and ampulla

Facial canal, opened (Canal for facial nerve)

Cupola ⎤

2nd turn ⎬ Cochlea

1st turn ⎦

Posterior semicircular canal and ampulla

Vestibule and fenestra vestibuli

Fenestra cochleae

649 Bony Labyrinth, lateral view, right side

Observe.

1. The 3 parts of the bony internal ear or bony labyrinth-cochlea, in front; vestibule in the middle; semicircular canals, behind.

2. The 2½ turns or coils of the cochlea; the first or basal coil, which lies deep to the medial wall of the tympanic cavity, communicating with the tympanic cavity through the fenestra cochleae (round window). In life this fenestra is closed by the secondary tympanic membrane.

3 The vestibule, crossed above by the facial canal and com-

municating with the tympanic cavity through the fenestra vestibuli (oval window). In life this window is closed by the base or foot-piece of the stapes.

4. The 3 semicircular canals—anterior, posterior, lateral. The anterior and posterior canals set vertically at a right angle to each other; the lateral canal set horizontally and at a right angle to the two others. Each canal, forming about ⅔ of a circle, and each having an ampulla at one end. The lateral canal is the shortest; the posterior canal is the longest. (See figs. 637 & 644.)

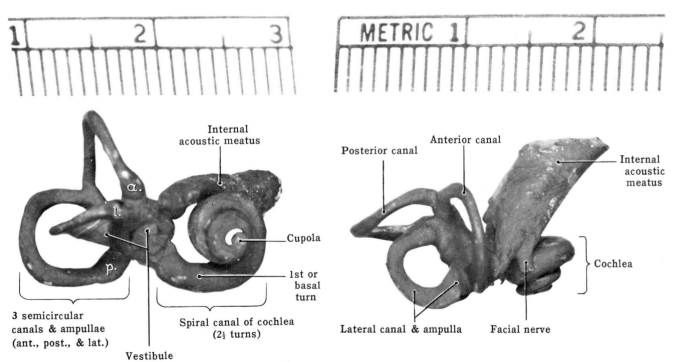

Internal acoustic meatus

Cupola

1st or basal turn

Posterior canal

Anterior canal

Internal acoustic meatus

Cochlea

3 semicircular canals & ampullae (ant., post., & lat.)

Spiral canal of cochlea (2½ turns)

Vestibule

Lateral canal & ampulla

Facial nerve

649.1-649.2 Plastic Cast of Interior of Bony Labyrinth, lateral view and from above, photographs

Observe:

1. As can be seen, the length of this cast—from the anterior end of the cochlea to the posterior end of the posterior semicircular canal-is 18 mm to 19 mm.

2. The casts of the semicircular canals are flattened, or compressed, from side to side.

3. Each of the three canals has two ends—a simple and an ampullary (or dilated). These open into the vestibule by 5 openings, the simple ends of the two vertical canals having a common crus.

650 Membranous Labyrinth, lateral view, right side

From a reconstruction made by Dr. Milne Dickie and Dr. J. S. Fraser.

Note:

The membranous labyrinth or membranous internal ear is contained within the bony labyrinth or bony internal ear.

It is a closed system of ducts and chambers, filled with endolymph and surrounded with, or bathed in, perilymph.

It has 3 parts—the duct of the cochlea, within the cochlea; the saccule and the utricle, within the vestibule; the 3 semicircular ducts, within the 3 semicircular canals.

One end of the duct of the cochlea is closed; the other end communicates with the saccule through the ductus reuniens.

The saccule in turn communicates with the utricle through the utriculo-saccular duct (not labelled). From this duct springs the endolymphatic duct, which occupies the aqueduct of the vestibule and ends in the endolymphatic sac (fig. 633). Into the utricle the 3 semicircular ducts open by 5 openings.

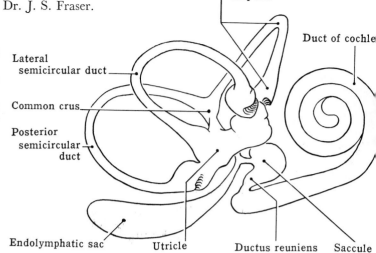

Anterior (Superior) semicircular duct and membranous ampulla

Duct of cochlea

Lateral semicircular duct

Common crus

Posterior semicircular duct

Endolymphatic sac   Utricle   Ductus reuniens   Saccule

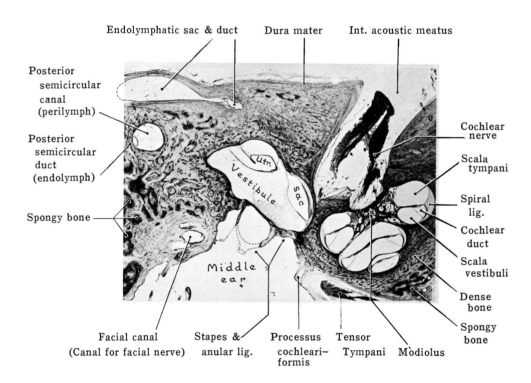

Endolymphatic sac & duct   Dura mater   Int. acoustic meatus

Posterior semicircular canal (perilymph)

Posterior semicircular duct (endolymph)

Spongy bone

Cochlear nerve

Scala tympani

Spiral lig.

Cochlear duct

Scala vestibuli

Dense bone

Spongy bone

Facial canal (Canal for facial nerve)   Stapes & anular lig.   Processus cochleariformis   Tensor Tympani   Modiolus

650.1 Labyrinth, or Inner Ear, on cross section

(Photograph by courtesy of Sylvia Bensley.)

Observe:

1. At the top, the endolymphatic sac lying extradurally.

2. The stapes to be broken. Its anular ligament, extending from its basis (foot-plate) to the fenestra vestibuli, is short behind and long in front, so it moves more like a door than a piston.

3. The utricle, pulled away from its recess in the vestibule; likewise the saccule, but to a milder extent.

4. The modiolus, which is the central bony core of the cochlea, resembles a screw-nail, its spiral bony lamina (or thread, fig. 648) is attached by the spiral membrane (basilar membrane) to the peripherally placed spiral ligament.

5. The cochlear duct, triangular on cross-section, has for its sides (a) spiral membrane, (b) spiral ligament, and (c) vestibular ligament which is delicate.

6. Above the cochlear duct (scala media) is the scala vestibuli, which leads off the vestibule; below it is the scala tympani, which leads to the fenestra cochleae which is closed by the secondary tympanic membrane.

7. The cochlear duct and 3 semicircular ducts are attached to the convex sides of their respective bony canals; that is, they are not completely surrounded with perilymph, as commonly represented in diagram.

8. The bony labyrinth to be composed of dense bone largely embedded in spongy bone. This makes it possible to define it.

*The Cranial Nerves
and the Dermatomes*

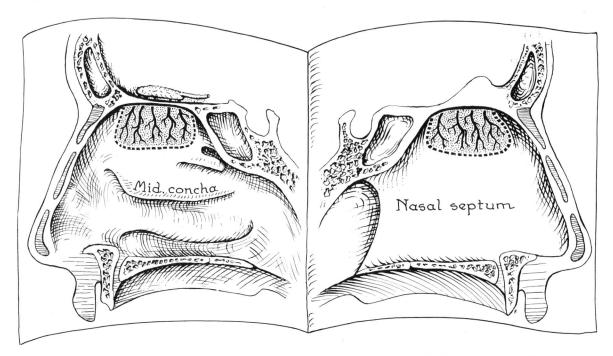

651   Scheme of the Distribution of the Olfactory Nerve

(Cranial Nerve I)

The olfactory area is usually much smaller than that shown here, and it is irregular in outline due to streamer-like invasion by non-olfactory, ciliated, columnar epithelium. The decrease in size is believed to result mainly from the destruction of the sensory olfactory neurons in the course of recurring infections of the nasal mucosa.

A study of the olfactory nerves in 143 adults (over 21 years of age) revealed that only 12% had a full complement of olfactory nerve fibres, that 8% had lost all fibres on one side, and that 5% had lost all fibres on both sides.

There is considerable variation in the number of olfactory nerve fibres in individuals of a given age, but on the average there is a loss of 1% of fibres per year during postnatal life, i.e., at the age of 50 years the average person has lost 50% of fibres and at the age of 75 years, 75% of fibres. (*C. G. Smith.*)

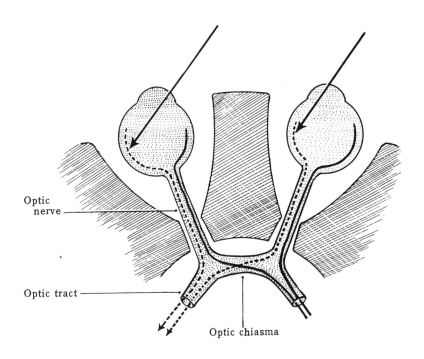

652   Scheme of the Distribution of the Optic Nerve

(Cranial Nerve II)

Rays of light from the right half of the visual field impinge on the left half of each retina, and impulses set up there travel along nerve fibres that pass to the left optic tract. Similarly, rays of light from the left half of the visual field set up impulses that reach the right optic tract. Thus, the nerve fibres from the nasal half of each retina are the ones that cross in the optic chiasma; those from the temporal half of each retina remain uncrossed.

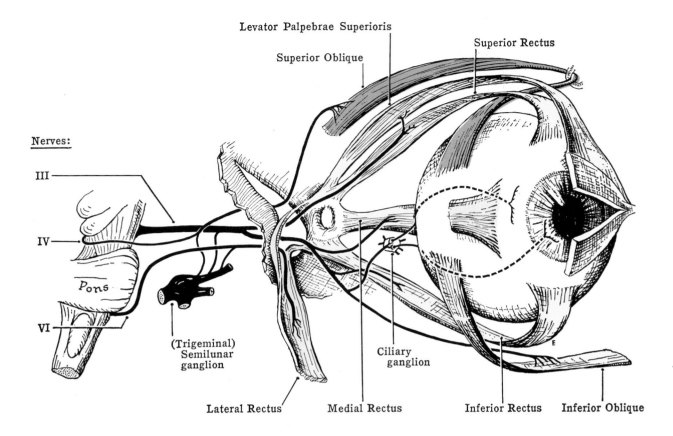

Nerves:

III

IV

Pons

VI

Levator Palpebrae Superioris

Superior Oblique

Superior Rectus

(Trigeminal)
Semilunar
ganglion

Ciliary
ganglion

Lateral Rectus   Medial Rectus   Inferior Rectus   Inferior Oblique

653   Scheme of the Distribution of the Oculomotor, Trochlear, and Abducent Nerves

(Cranial Nerves III, IV, and VI)

These 3 motor nerves, after receiving proprioceptive fibers from the trigeminal nerve, supply the orbital muscles. Nerves IV and VI each supply one muscle and nerve III supplies the remaining five muscles.

The trochlear nerve supplies Superior Oblique—the muscle that passes through a trochlea or pulley; the abducent nerve supplies Lateral Rectus—the muscle that abducts; and the oculomotor nerve supplies Levator Palpebrae Superioris, Superior Rectus, Medial Rectus, Inferior Rectus, and Inferior Oblique and, via the ciliary ganglion, it supplies the ciliary muscle and the Sphincter Pupillae.

Sympathetic fibres (not shown) from segments T.1 and 2, via the superior cervical sympathetic ganglion, supply the Dilator Pupillae and also involuntary muscle fibres (a) in the upper lid, (b) in the lower lid, and (c) bridging the inferior orbital fissure.

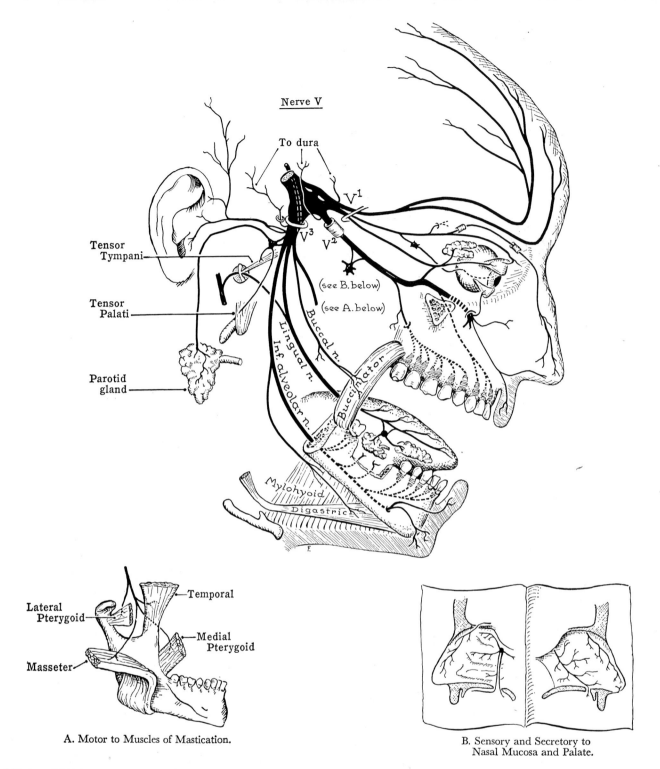

Nerve V

To dura

V¹

V³

V²

Tensor
Tympani

Tensor
Palati

Parotid
gland

(see B. below)

(see A. below)

Buccal n.

Lingual n.

Inf. alveolar n.

Buccinator

Mylohyoid

Digastric

f.

Lateral
Pterygoid

Temporal

Medial
Pterygoid

Masseter

A. Motor to Muscles of Mastication.

B. Sensory and Secretory to
Nasal Mucosa and Palate.

654, 655, 656   Scheme of the Distribution of the Trigeminal Nerve

(Cranial Nerve V)

The cutaneous distribution of the 3 divisions of nerve V is shown in figure 470.1. Each division supplies not the skin surface only but also the whole thickness of tissue from skin surface to mucous surface.

Each of the 3 divisions sends a twig to the dura mater—V¹ to the tentorium cerebelli; V² & V³ to the floor and side wall of the middle cranial fossa.

Each of the 3 divisions is connected with a parasympathetic ganglion—V¹ with the ciliary, V² with the

pterygopalatine, and V³ with the submandibular and otic. These ganglia are excitor cell stations whose preganglionic fibres travel with nerves III, VII, and IX. The postganglionic fibres are distributed with the branches of nerve V to smooth muscles of the eyeball and to glands.

The ophthalmic nerve (V¹) is sensory: (a) to the eyeball and cornea via the ciliary nerves (fig. 520); hence, if paralysed, the ocular conjunctiva is insensitive to touch; (b) to the frontal, ethmoidal, and sphenoidal

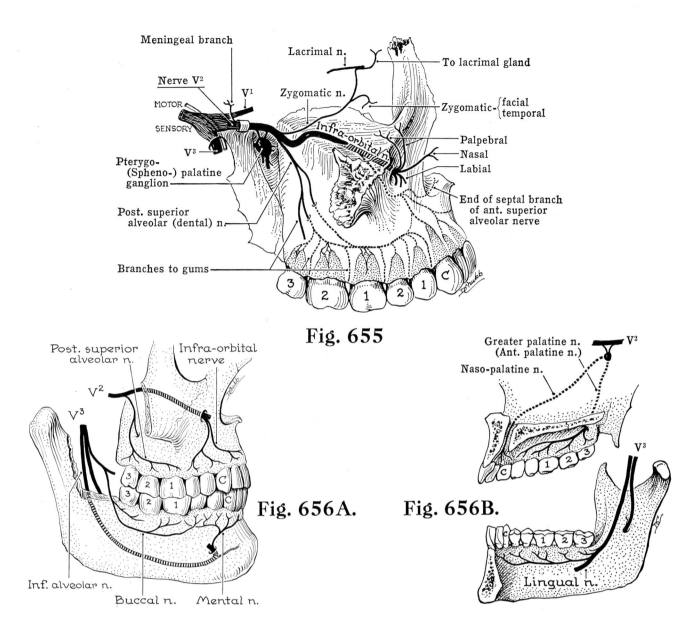

Fig. 655

Fig. 656A.   Fig. 656B.

air sinuses via the supra-orbital and ethmoidal nerves; and (c) to the skin and conjunctival surfaces of the upper eyelid and to the skin and mucous surfaces of the external nose (fig. 606).

The maxillary nerve (V^2) is sensory: (a) to the upper teeth and gums (see below); (b) to the face, both surfaces of the lower lid, the skin of the side and vestibule of the nose, and both surfaces of the upper lip (fig. 470); (c) via the pterygopalatine ganglion (fig. 606) to the mucoperiosteum of the nasal cavity, palate, and roof of the pharynx; and (d) to the maxillary, ethmoidal, and sphenoidal air sinuses; (e) secretory fibres from this ganglion pass with the zygomatic and then with the lacrimal nerve to the lacrimal gland (fig. 655).

The mandibular nerve (V^3) is motor: (a) to the 4 muscles of mastication—but not to Buccinator; (b) to the 2 Tensores (Tympani and Palati) via the otic ganglion; and (c) to Mylohyoid and anterior belly of Digastric. It is sensory: (a) to the lower teeth and gums (see below); (b) to both surfaces of the lower lip by the mental nerve; (c) to the auricle and temporal region by the auriculotemporal nerve which also sends twigs

to the external meatus and outer surface of the ear drum, and conveys secretory fibres from the otic ganglion to the parotid gland; (d) to the mucous membrane of the cheek by the buccal nerve (fig. 559); and (e) to the anterior two-thirds of the tongue, floor of the mouth, and gums by the lingual nerve which also distributes the chorda tympani.

The gums and teeth—Nerve V^2 subserves sensation to the upper gums by 4 branches (fig. 656) and to the upper teeth by 2 branches, viz., the posterior and anterior superior alveolar (dental) nerves (fig. 655). Nerve V^3 subserves the lower gums by 3 branches and the lower teeth by one branch, viz., inferior alveolar. The gums are also supplied by twigs that perforate the alveoli (fig. 655). The territory of any of these gingival and dental nerves may either be extended or contracted, e.g., twigs of the mental and lingual nerves may cross the median plane to supply the gums of the opposite side, and the inferior alveolar nerves may decussate in the mandibular canal to supply the incisors of the opposite side.

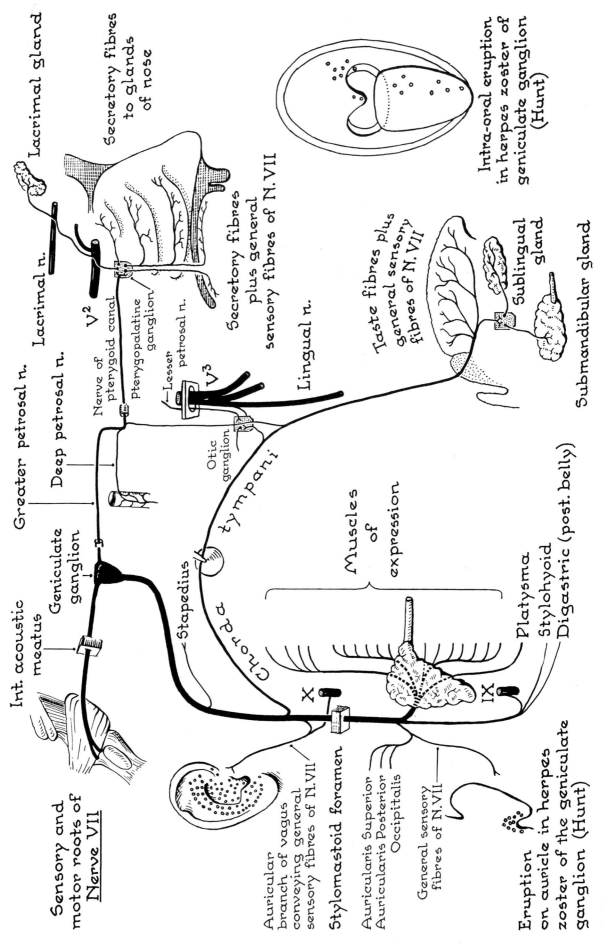

Lacrimal gland

Secretory fibres to glands of nose

Secretory fibres plus general sensory fibres of N. VII

Lacrimal n.

V²

Nerve of pterygoid canal

Pterygopalatine ganglion

Lesser petrosal n.

V³

Lingual n.

Otic ganglion

Greater petrosal n.

Deep petrosal n.

Int. acoustic meatus

Geniculate ganglion

Sensory and motor roots of Nerve VII

Stapedius

Chorda tympani

Muscles of expression

Platysma
Stylohyoid
Digastric (post. belly)

X

IX

Stylomastoid foramen

Auricular branch of vagus conveying general sensory fibres of N. VII

Auricularis Superior
Auricularis Posterior
Occipitalis

General sensory fibres of N. VII

Eruption on auricle in herpes zoster of the geniculate ganglion (Hunt)

Taste fibres plus general sensory fibres of N. VII

Sublingual gland

Submandibular gland

Intra-oral eruption in herpes zoster of geniculate ganglion (Hunt)

657 Scheme of the Distribution of the Facial Nerve

(Cranial Nerve VII)

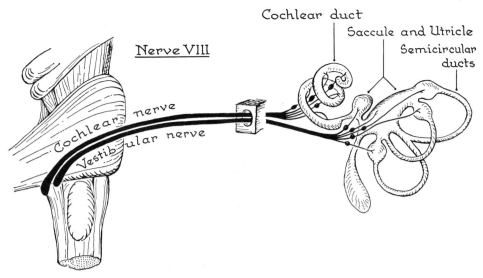

Cochlear duct

Nerve VIII

Saccule and Utricle

Semicircular ducts

Cochlear nerve

Vestibular nerve

658 Scheme of the Distribution of the Vestibulo-cochlear Nerve

(Auditory or acoustic nerve. Cranial Nerve VIII)

This nerve has two parts: (a) the cochlear nerve, or nerve of hearing, whose fibres transmit impulses from the spiral organ of Corti in the cochlear duct; and (b) the vestibular nerve, or nerve of balancing, whose fibres transmit impulses from the maculae of the saccule and utricle and in the ampullae of the three semicircular ducts.

657 Scheme of the Distribution of the Facial Nerve

Motor to the muscles of expression—i.e., muscles around the eye, nose, mouth, and ear; of the scalp above and the platysma below. It also supplies Stapedius, Stylohyoid, and Digastric (post. belly). Levator Palpebrae is not of this group, but Buccinator is. Hence, if the facial nerve is paralysed (a) the "eye" remains open and cannot close, and (b) food collects in the vestibule of the mouth, pushed there by the tongue, and the Buccinator cannot return it (fig. 591).

Secretory (1) via the greater superficial petrosal nerve and nerve of the pterygoid canal to the pterygopalatine ganglion, thence by relay to the glands of the nose and palate and to the lacrimal gland; (2) via the chorda tympani (a) to the submandibular (submaxillary) ganglion whence fibres are relayed to the submandibular and sublingual salivary glands; and, (b) via its connection with the otic ganglion, it activates the parotid gland.

Sensory fibres, with cell stations in the geniculate ganglion, carry impulses (a) from the deep tissues of the face, (b) from the external meatus, the auricle, and, (c) via the chorda tympani and greater petrosal nerve, from the tongue and palate.

Taste fibres, with cell stations in the geniculate ganglion, pass (a) from the palate non-stop through the pterygopalatine ganglion, nerve of the pterygoid canal, and greater petrosal nerve to the geniculate ganglion; and (b) from the anterior two-thirds of the tongue two routes are followed: (1) via the chorda tympani to the facial nerve and so to the geniculate ganglion, and (2) by a branch of the chorda that traverses the otic ganglion to join the greater petrosal nerve and so to the geniculate ganglion. As evidence of this double route is the fact that the chorda tympani may be cut without any loss of taste, whereas cutting the greater petrosal nerve may result in loss of taste. (Schwartz, H. G., and Weddell, G., 1938.)

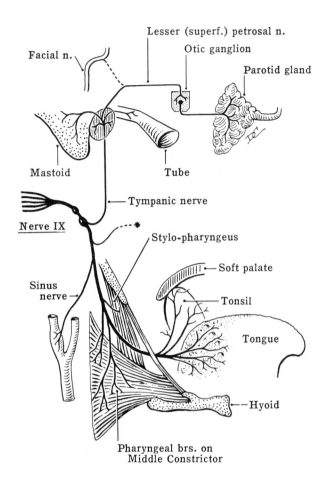

Facial n.

Lesser (superf.) petrosal n.

Otic ganglion

Parotid gland

Mastoid

Tube

Tympanic nerve

Nerve IX

Stylo-pharyngeus

Sinus nerve

Soft palate

Tonsil

Tongue

Hyoid

Pharyngeal brs. on Middle Constrictor

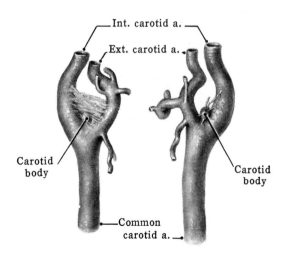

Int. carotid a.

Ext. carotid a.

Carotid body

Carotid body

Common carotid a.

659.1

Carotid Body, viewed from behind in two stages. This particular body appeared black from engorged surface veins and, so, was easily recognized.

659 Scheme of the Distribution of the Glossopharyngeal Nerve

(Cranial Nerve IX)

Motor fibres supply one muscle—Stylopharyngeus.

Secretory fibres travel via the tympanic and lesser petrosal nerves to the otic ganglion, there to be relayed via the auriculotemporal nerve to the parotid gland. It has been observed that cutting the chorda tympani reduces permanently the secretion not only of the submandibular gland but also of the parotid. Cutting the glossopharyngeal nerve above the connecting branch it sends to the nerve to Digastric (post. belly) also reduces secretion in the three large salivary glands. Hence, it is surmised that secretory fibres travel down nerve IX, through the connecting branch to the nerve to Digastric (indicated by a star in fig. 659 and shown in fig. 657), thence up the stem of nerve VII and along the chorda (a) to the submandibular ganglion where the impulses are relayed to the submandibular and sublingual glands, and (b) to the otic ganglion where the impulses are relayed to the parotid gland. (Reichert, F. L., and Poth, E. J.)

General sensory fibres supply almost the entire one half of the pharyngeal wall, including the oro-pharyngeal isthmus (i.e., under surface of the soft palate, tonsil, pharyngeal arches, and posterior third of the tongue). They also supply the dorsum of the soft palate, the auditory tube, tympanum, medial surface of the ear drum, mastoid antrum, and mastoid air cells. The pharyngeal branch of the maxillary nerve (fig. 606) attends to the roof of the pharynx; the lesser palatine nerves (fig. 582) to the anterior parts of the soft palate; and the internal laryngeal nerve to the lowest part of the pharynx (fig. 627) and somewhat to the surroundings of the laryngeal orifice (fig. 593).

Taste fibres supply the posterior third of the tongue including the vallate papillae (fig. 593).

The sinus nerve is afferent from the carotid sinus and carotid body.

The carotid sinus responds to pressure changes within the artery: the carotid body is believed to respond to chemical changes (concentration of carbon dioxide) in the blood.

Note: (1) The glossopharyngeal nerve, like the facial nerve, activates each of the three large salivary glands. (2) Clinical evidence is undecided as to the share taken by nerves VII, IX, and X in conveying sensation from the auricle and external meatus and in supplying the muscles of the palate.

660 Scheme of the Distribution of the Vagus Nerve

(Cranial Nerve X)

Motor: (a) The fibres received from the cranial root of the accessory nerve (fig. 661) supply the muscles of the pharynx (Stylopharyngeus excepted), of the palate (Tensor Palati excepted, but including Palatoglossus), and of the larynx (without exception). The foregoing are skeletal muscles.
> (b) Inhibitory to the cardiac muscle.

Motor to all smooth muscle, secretory to all glands, and afferent from all mucous surfaces in the following parts—pharynx (lowest part), larynx, trachea, bronchi and lungs; esophagus (entire), stomach, and gut down to the left colic flexure; liver, gall gladder and bile passages; pancreas and pancreatic ducts; and perhaps spleen and kidney.

Taste: from the few taste buds about the epiglottis.

Branches arise from the vagus thus:

In the jugular fossa—(a) a meningeal branch to the dura of the posterior cranial fossa; and (b) an auricular branch to the outer surface of the ear drum, the external acoustic meatus, and the back of the auricle (figs. 551 & 552).

In the neck—(a) the pharyngeal branch is motor to Superior and Middle Constrictors and muscles of the soft palate; (b) the superior laryngeal nerve, via the internal laryngeal nerve, is sensory to the larynx above the vocal cords and to the lowest part of the pharynx (fig. 627) and, via the external laryngeal nerve, motor to Inferior Constrictor and Cricothyroid (figs. 532 & 626), (c) a twig (sinus nerve) to the carotid sinus, and (d) two cardiac branches.

In the thorax—(a) the recurrent nerve sends a motor branch to Inferior Constrictor, is motor to all the laryngeal muscles (excepting Cricothyroid), and is both afferent and efferent to the larynx below the level of the cords, as well as to the upper part of the esophagus; (b, c, and d) cardiac and pulmonary branches and the esophageal plexus.

In the abdomen—see figure 133.

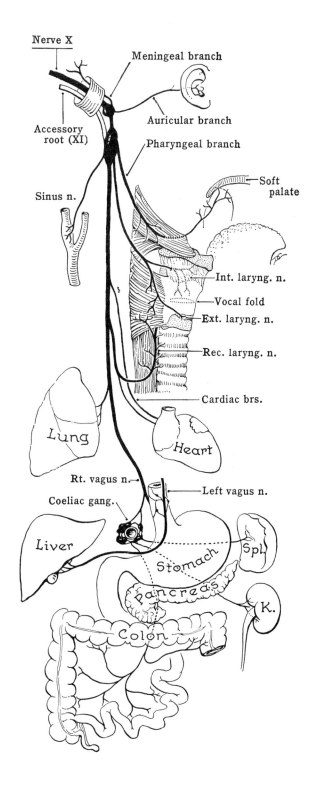

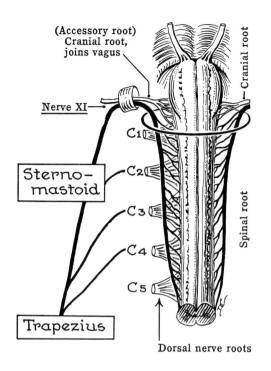

(Accessory root) Cranial root, joins vagus

Cranial root

Nerve XI

C1

Sterno-mastoid

C2

C3

Spinal root

C4

C5

Trapezius

Dorsal nerve roots

661 Scheme of the Distribution of the Spinal Part of the Accessory Nerve

(Cervical Nerve XI)

The spinal root of the accessory nerve, joined by fibres from the ventral ramus of C.2, supplies Sternomastoid and, joined by fibres from the ventral rami of C.3 & 4, supplies Trapezius. Experiments on lower animals (cat, rabbit and monkey) give evidence that the ventral rami fibres of cervical nerves 2, 3, & 4 are proprioceptive, that is, sensory only. (*K. B. Corbin and F. Harrison.*) In man, however, there is clinical evidence (both surgical and medical) that these contributions from C.2, 3, & 4 convey motor as well as sensory fibres. (*H. W. Wookey; K. G. McKenzie; W. Haymaker and B. Woodhall.*) The spinal root of the accessory nerve usually passes through the dorsal root ganglion of C.1 and may receive sensory fibres from it (*A. A. Pearson*).

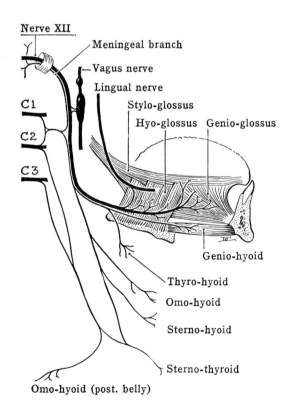

Nerve XII

Meningeal branch

Vagus nerve

Lingual nerve

Stylo-glossus

C1

Hyo-glossus   Genio-glossus

C2

C3

Genio-hyoid

Thyro-hyoid

Omo-hyoid

Sterno-hyoid

Sterno-thyroid

Omo-hyoid (post. belly)

662 Scheme of the Distribution of the Hypoglossal Nerve

(Cranial Nerve XII)

This efferent nerve supplies all the intrinsic (longitudinal, transverse, and vertical) and extrinsic (Styloglossus, Hyoglossus, and Genioglossus) muscles of the tongue, Palatoglossus excepted.

It receives a mixed (motor and sensory) branch from the loop between the ventral rami of C.1 and 2. The sensory or afferent fibres in part take a recurrent course and end in the dura mater of the posterior cranial fossa. The motor or efferent branch supplies Geniohyoid and Thyrohyoid, and it provides a descending branch which unites with a descending branch of C.2 and 3 to form a loop, the ansa cervicalis. This and the ansa supply the remaining depressor muscles of the hyoid bone.

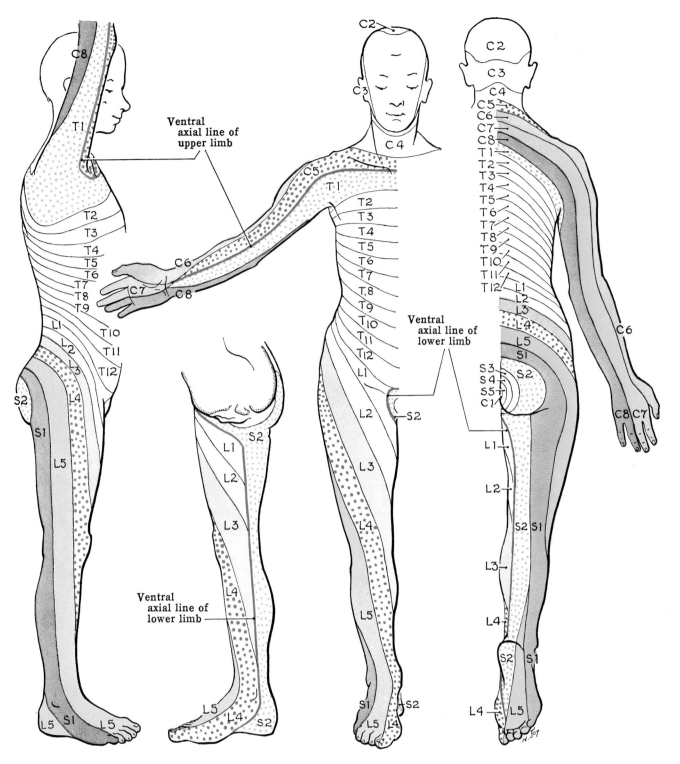

663 Dermatomes of the Upper and Lower Limbs

(Modified, after Keegan, J. J., and Garrett, F. D.)

According to the clinical, surgical, and experimental findings of Keegan and Garrett, the dermatomes of the limbs from the 5th cervical to the 1st thoracic, and from the 3rd lumbar to the 2nd sacral extend as a series of bands from the mid-dorsal line of the trunk into the limbs, as illustrated. When the function of even a single dorsal nerve root is interrupted, faint but definite diminution of sensitivity can be demonstrated in the dermatome. The best method to detect and plot the area of diminished sensitivity is by the use of light pin scratch for pain sensation, although it can be found for temperature and for tactile sensation also.

Note: Pearson, A. A. and Bass, J. J. find that in the human embryo it is unusual for the dorsal rami of C. 6, 7 and 8 to possess cutaneous branches, for only about 10% do; and that C.5 and T.1 possess them in only 67% and 82% respectively. In contrast, they do find that in rabbit embryos each of these dorsal rami (C.5—T.1) possesses a cutaneous branch.

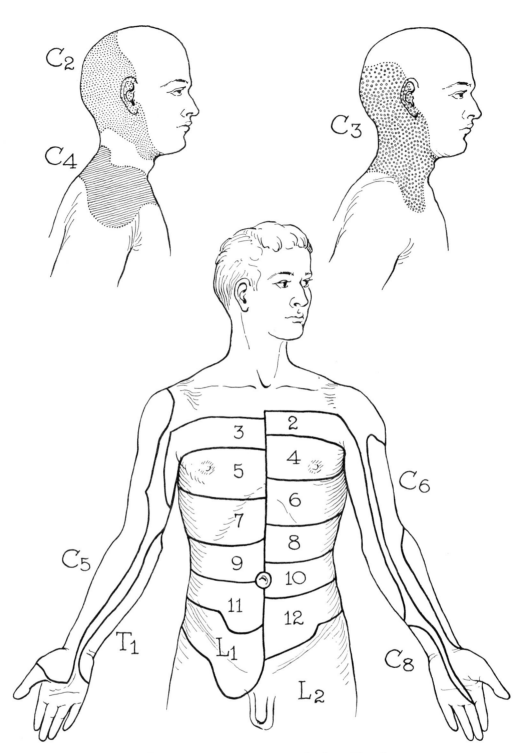

664   Dermatomes of the Upper Parts of the Body

(Modified, from Fender, after Foerster)

A dermatome is an area of skin supplied by the dorsal (sensory) root of a spinal nerve.

The dermatomes were determined by plotting (a) the areas of vasodilation that resulted on stimulation of individual dorsal nerve roots, and (b) the areas of "remaining sensibility" after cutting three roots above and three roots below a given nerve root. The areas plotted represent the average .finding for each dorsal root based on pain sensation. Areas determined for temperature sensation have similar limits, but those for touch are more extensive.

Note that there is considerable overlapping of contiguous dermatomes; that is to say, each segmental nerve overlaps the territories of its neighbours. As a result, no anesthesia results unless two or more consecutive dorsal roots have lost their functions.

The 7th cervical dermatome (not depicted) begins lower on the upper arm than the 6th and includes most, or all, of the hand.

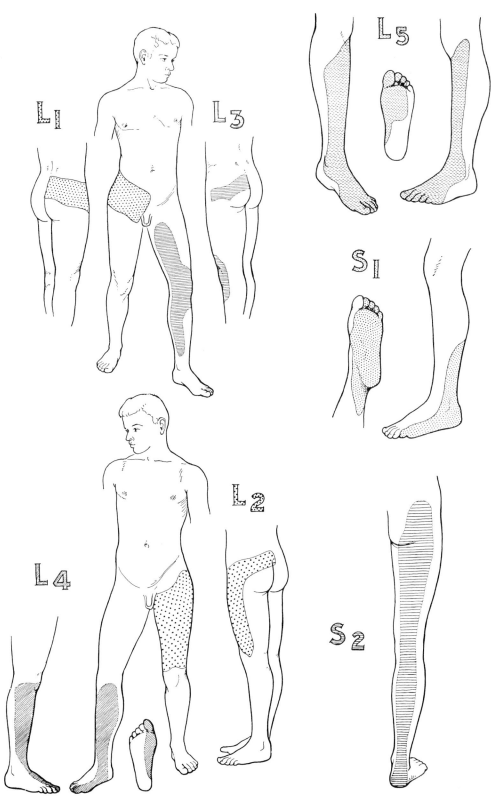

665 Dermatomes of the Lower Limb
(Modified, from Fender, after Foerster)

References

Figure

27 BARLOW, R. N. The sternalis muscle in American whites and Negroes. Anat. Rec., *61:* 413, 1935.

27 SEIB, G. A. The musculus pectoralis minor in American whites and American Negroes. Am. J. Phys. Anthropol., *23:* 389, 1938.

28 J. C. B. G. Data collected by the author.

42 C. G. S. Data collected by Carleton G. Smith.

47 TERRY, R. J. A study of the supracondyloid process in the living. Am. J. Phys. Anthropol., *4:* 129, 1921.

47 TERRY, R. J. On the racial distribution of the supracondyloid variation. Am. J. Phys. Anthropol., *14:* 459, 1930.

48 TROTTER, M. Septal apertures in the humerus of American whites and Negroes. Am. J. Phys. Anthropol., *19:* 213, 1934.

48.1 HAZLETT, J. W. The superficial ulnar artery with references to accidental intra-arterial injection. Canad. M. A. J., *61:* 289, 1949.

85 APPLETON, A. B. A case of abnormal distribution of the musculocutaneous nerve. J. Anat. & Physiol., *46:* 89, 1911.

85 HUTTON, W. K. Remarks on the innervation of the dorsus manus with special reference to certain rare abnormalities. J. Anat. & Physiol., *40:* 326, 1906.

85 LEARMONTH, J. R. A variation in the distribution of the "radial nerve." J. Anat., *53:* 371, 1919.

85 STOPFORD, J. S. B. The variation in distribution of the cutaneous nerves of the hand and digits. J. Anat., *53:* 14, 1918.

89 LANDSMEER, J. M. F. The anatomy of the dorsal aponeurosis of the human finger and its functional significance. Anat. Rec., *104:* 31, 1949.

97-D R. K. G. Data collected by R. K. George.

98 McKERN, T. W., AND STEWART, T. D. Skeletal age changes in young American males. Quartermaster Research & Development Center, Natick, Mass., U. S. A., 1957.

98 FRANCIS, C. C., AND WERLE, P. P. The appearance of centers of ossification from birth to 5 years. Anat. Rec., *24:* 273, 1939.

98 FRANCIS, C. C. The appearance of centers of ossification from 6 to 15 years. Anat. Rec., *27:* 127, 1940.

98 PRYOR, J. W. Differences in the time of development of centers of ossification in the male and female skeleton. Anat. Rec., *8:* 252, 1922.

104 PRYOR, J. W. Time of ossification of the bones of the hand of the male and female. Am. J. Phys. Anthropol., *8:* 401, 1925.

Figure

104 GREULICH, W. W., AND PYLE, S. I. Radiographic Atlas of Skeletal Development of the Hand and Wrist, 2nd ed. Stanford University Press, 1959.

104.2,1 GEORGE, R. Topography of the unpaired visceral branches of the abdominal aorta. J. Anat., *69:* 196, 1935.

119 HARRISON, R. G. The distribution of the vasal and cremasteric arteries to the testis, etc. J. Anat., *83:* 267, 1949.

132 MICHELS, N. A. Blood Supply and Anatomy of the Upper Abdominal Organs. J. B. Lippincott Company, Philadelphia, 1955.

133 McCREA, E. A. The abdominal distribution of the vagus. J. Anat., *59:* 18, 1924.

133 MITCHELL, G. A. G. Innervation of the stomach. *In* Anatomy of the Autonomic Nervous System, p. 281. E. & S. Livingstone, Ltd., Edinburgh, 1953.

135 FALCONER, C. W. A., AND GRIFFITHS, E. The anatomy of the blood vessels in the region of the pancreas. Brit. J. Surg., *37:* 334, 1950.

135 MICHELS, N. A. *et al.* The superior mesenteric vein—an anatomic and surgical study of eighty-one subjects. J. Internat. Coll. Surgeons, *41:* 339, 1964.

137–140 HJORTSJO, C. H. The topography of the intrahepatic duct systems (and of the portal vein). Acta anat., *11:* 599, 1951.

137–140 HJORTSJO, C. H. The intrahepatic ramifications of the portal vein. Lunds Universitets Arsskrift, *52:* 20, 1956.

137–140 HEALEY, J. E., SCHROY, P. C., AND SORENSEN, R. J. The intrahepatic artery in man. J. Internat. Coll. Surgeons, *20:* 133, 1953.

137–140 HEALEY, J. E., AND SCHROY, P. C. Anatomy of the biliary ducts within the human liver. A. M. A. Arch. Surg., *66:* 599, 1953.

137–140 SCHMIDT, H., AND GUTTMAN, E. Systematische Anatomie der Gallengange des Menschen. Acta anat. *28:* 1, 1956.

137–140 ELIAS, H., AND PETTY, D. Gross anatomy of the blood vessels and ducts within the human liver. Am. J. Anat., *90:* 59, 1952.

137–140 ELIAS, H. Nomenklatur der intrahepatischen Gefasse. Anat. Anzeiger, *102:* 1/4, 73, 1955.

143 DASELER, E. H., ANSON, B. J., HAMBLEY, W. C., AND REIMANN, A. F. The cystic artery and constituents of the hepatic pedicle. Surg. Gynec. & Obst., *85:* 47, 1947.

143–145 VANDAMME, J. P. J. *et al.* A re-evaluation of the hepatic and cystic arteries—the importance of the aberrant hepatic branches. Acta anat. *73:* 192, 1969.

Figure

144 J. C. B. G. From data collected by the author.

145 MICHELS, N. A. Blood Supply and Anatomy of the Upper Abdominal Organs. J. B. Lippincott Company, Philadelphia, 1955.

145 PARKE, W. W., MICHELS, N. A., AND GHOSH, C. M. Blood supply of the common bile duct. Surg. Gynec. & Obst., *117:* 47, 1963.

152 CURTIS, G. M., AND MOVITZ, D. The surgical significance of the accessory spleen. Ann. Surg., *123:* 276, 1946.

152 HALPERT, B., AND GYORKEY, F. Accessory spleen in the tail of the pancreas. A. M. A. Arch. Path., *64:* 266, 1957.

152 HALPERT, B., AND GYORKEY, F. Lesions observed in accessory spleens of 311 patients. Am. J. Clin. Path., *32:* 165, 1959.

157 MILLBOURN, E. On the excretory ducts of the pancreas in man, with special reference to their relations to each other, to the common bile duct and to the duodenum: radiological and anatomical study. Acta anat., *9:* 1, 1950.

157 DAWSON, W., AND LANGMAN, J. An anatomical-radiological study on the pancreatic duct pattern in man. Anat. Rec., *139:* 59, 1961.

157 HORSEY, W. J., AND PAUL, W. Personal observations.

158 WOODBURNE, R. T., AND OLSEN, L. L. The arteries of the pancreas. Anat. Rec., *111:* 255, 1951.

158 PIERSON, J. M. The arterial blood supply of the pancreas. Surg. Gynec. & Obst., *77:* 426, 1943.

158 MICHELS, N. A. The anatomic variations of the arterial pancreaticoduodenal arcades etc. J. Internat. Coll. Surgeons, *37:* 13, 1962.

160.1 EDWARDS, E. A. Functional anatomy of the porta-systemic (porta-caval) communications. Arch. Int. Med., *88:* 137, 1951.

160.1 MICHELS, N. A. Newer anatomy of the liver and its variant blood supply and collateral circulation. Am. J. Surg., *112:* 337, 1966.

161 BOYDEN, E. A. The "Phrygian cap" in cholecystography; congenital anomaly of the gall-bladder. Am. J. Roentgenol., *33:* 589, 1935.

161 BOYDEN, E. A. The accessory gall-bladder. Am. J. Anat., *38:* 177, 1926.

162 BASMAJIAN, J. V. The marginal anastomoses of the arteries to the large intestine. Surg. Gynec. & Obst., *99:* 614, 1954.

162 BASMAJIAN, J. V. The main arteries of the large intestine. Surg. Gynec. & Obst., *101:* 585, 1955.

162 MICHELS, N. A., SIDDHARTH, P., KORNBLITH, P. L. AND PARKE, W. W. The variant blood supply to the small and large intestines—based on four hundred dissections etc. J. Internat. Coll. Surgeons *39:* 127, 1963. *Also* The variant blood supply to the descending colon, rectosigmoid and rectum. Dis. Colon Rectum, *8:* 251, 1965.

163.2 GOLIGHER, J. C. The blood supply to the sigmoid colon and rectum. Brit. J. Surg., *37:* 157, 1949.

167 ROSS, J. A. Vascular patterns of small and large intestine compared. Brit. J. Surg., *39:* 330, 1952.

170.1 JAY, G. D., III, MARGULIS, R. R., McGRAW, A. B., AND NORTHRIP, R. R. Meckel's diverticulum: survey of 103 cases. Arch. Surg., *61:* 158, 1950.

172 WAKELEY, C. P. G. The position of the vermiform appendix as ascertained by the analysis of 10,000 cases. J. Anat., *67:* 277, 1933.

Figure

172 MAISEL, H. The position of the human vermiform appendix in fetal and adult age groups. (About 55% are pelvic and 26% retrocecal or retrocolic.) Anat. Rec., *136:* 385, 1960.

180 CLARK, K. The blood vessels of the adrenal gland. J. Roy. Coll. Surgeons, Edin., *4:* 257, 1959.

183.1 GRAVES, F. T. The Arterial Anatomy of the Kidney. John Wright & Sons, Ltd., Bristol, 1971.

183.1 GRAVES, F. T. The anatomy of the intrarenal arteries and its application to segmental resection of the kidney. Brit. J. Surg., *42:* 132, 1954.

183.1 GRAVES, F. T. The anatomy of the intrarenal arteries in health and disease. Brit. J. Surg., *43:* 605, 1956.

183.1 RICHES, E. W. The present status of renal angiography. Brit. J. Surg., *42:* 462, 1955.

183.1 ROBERTS, J. B. M. Conservative renal surgery—an anatomical basis. Brit. J. Surg., *48:* 1, 1960.

183.1 FINE, H. AND KEEN, E. N. The arteries of the human kidney. J. Anat., *100:* 881, 1966.

184.2 LOFGREN, F. An attempt at homologizing different types of pyelus (renal pelvis). Urol. Internat., *5:* No. 1, 1956.

184.2 LOFGREN, F. Some Features in the Renal Morphogenesis and Anatomy with Practical Considerations. Institute of Anatomy, University of Lund, Lund, Sweden, 1956.

186 LOWSLEY, O. S. Postcaval ureter—operation for its correction. Surg. Gynec. & Obst., *82:* 549, 1946.

186 PICK, J. W., AND ANSON, B. J. Retrocaval ureter. J. Urol., *43:* 672, 1940.

187 BELL, E. T. Anomalies. *In* Renal Diseases, p. 55. Lea & Febiger, Philadelphia, 1946.

187 LLOYD, L. W. The renal artery in whites and American Negroes. Am. J. Phys. Anthropol., *20:* 153, 1935.

187 MERKLIN, R. J., AND MICHELS, N. A. The variant renal and suprarenal blood supply with data on the inferior phrenic, ureteral and gonadal arteries. J. Internat. Coll. Surgeons, *29:* 41, 1958.

187 ADACHI, B. Multiple renal arteries. *In* Das Arteriensystem der Japaner. Kyoto, 1928.

187 CAMPBELL, M. Ureteral reduplication (double ureter). *In* Urology, vol. 1, p. 309. W. B. Saunders Company, Philadelphia, 1954.

187 ANDERSON, G. A., RICE, G. G., AND HARRIS, B. A. Pregnancy and labor complicated by pelvic ectopic kidney anomalies; a review. Obst. & Gynec. Surv., *4:* 737, 1949.

187 GRAVES, F. T. The arterial anatomy of the congenitally abnormal kidney. Brit. J. Surg., *56:* 533, 1969.

188.3 SEIB, G. A. The azygos system of veins in American whites and American Negroes, including observations on inferior caval venous system. Am. J. Phys. Anthropol., *19:* 39, 1934.

191.1 THORNTON, M. W. AND SCHWEISTHAL, M. R. The phrenic nerve: its terminal divisions and supply to the crura of the diaphragm. Anat. Rec., *164:* 283, 1969.

191.1 BOTHA, G. S. M. The anatomy of phrenic nerve termination and the motor innervation of the diaphragm. Thorax, *12:* 50, 1957.

196 WILDE, F. R. The anal intermuscular septum. Brit. J. Surg., *36:* 279, 1949.

206 NILSSON, S. The human seminal vesicle. Acta chir. Scandinav. (Suppl. 269), Stockholm, 1962.

207.1 LOWSLEY, O. S. The development of the human prostate gland. Am. J. Anat. *13:* 299, 1912.

Figure

214 LEARMONTH, J. E. A contribution to the neurophysiology of the urinary bladder in man. Brain, *54:* 147, 1931.

214 LANGWORTHY, O. R., KOLB, L. C., AND LEWIS, L. G. *In* Physiology of Micturition. The Williams & Wilkins Company, Baltimore, 1940.

255 BASMAJIAN, J. V. The distribution of valves in the femoral, external iliac and common iliac veins and their relationship to varicose veins. Surg. Gynec. & Obst., *95:* 537, 1952.

257 FLEMING, J. F. R., AND LEVY, L. F. Personal observations.

279 WOLCOTT, W. E. The evolution of the circulation in the developing femoral head and neck. Surg. Gynec. & Obst., *77:* 61, 1943.

279 TRUETA, J., AND HARRISON, M. H. M. Normal vascular anatomy of the femoral head in adult man. J. Bone & Joint Surg., *35B:* 442, 1953.

309 R. K. G. Data collected by R. K. George.

323 J. C. B. G. Data collected by the author.

324 SENIOR, H. D. An interpretation of the recorded arterial anomalies of the human leg and foot. J. Anat., *53:* 130, 1919.

324 QUAIN, R. The Anatomy of the Arteries of the Human Body. Taylor and Walton, London, 1844.

350 FRANCIS, C. C., AND WERLE, P. P. See reference for Figure 98.

350 McKERN, T. W., AND STEWART, T. D. See reference for Figure 98.

356 C. E. S. Data collected by Charles E. Storton.

356 HARRIS, R. I., AND BEATH, T. Army Foot Survey, vol. 1, p. 52. National Research Council of Canada, Ottawa, 1947.

373.1 McKERN, T. W., AND STEWART, T. D. See reference for Figure 98.

378 Ho, G. T. Personal observations.

382 ROWE, G. G., AND ROCHE, M. B. The etiology of separate neural arch. J. Bone & Joint Surg., *35A:* 102, 1953.

382 STEWART, T. D. The age incidence of neural-arch defects in Alaskan natives considered from the standpoint of etiology. J. Bone & Joint Surg., *35A:* 937, 1953.

386 RISSANEN, P. M. The surgical anatomy and pathology of the supraspinous and interspinous ligaments etc. Acta orthop. Scandinav. (Suppl. 46), Copenhagen, 1960.

390 BATSON, O. V. The function of the vertebral veins and their role in the spread of metastases. Ann. Surg., *112:* 138, 1940.

390 BATSON, O. V. The vertebral vein system. Am. J. Roentgenol., *78:* 195, 1957.

394 TROTTER, M. Synostosis between manubrium and body of the sternum in whites and Negroes. Am. J. Phys. Anthropol., *18:* 439, 1934.

394 McKERN, T. W., AND STEWART, T. D. See reference for Figure 98.

400 ADSON, A. W. Cervical ribs: symptoms, differential diagnosis and indications for section of insertion of scalenus anticus muscle. J. Internat. Coll. Surgeons, *16:* 546, 1951.

403 KROPP, B. N. The lateral costal branch of the internal mammary artery. J. Thoracic Surg., *21:* 421, 1951.

Figure

413.2 WOODBURNE, R. T. The costo-mediastinal border of the left pleura in the precordial area. Anat. Rec., *97:* 197, 1947.

413.2 CUNNINGHAM, D. J. Text-Book of Anatomy, 9th ed., Figures 597–600, Oxford University Press, New York, 1951.

413.2 LACHMAN, E. A comparison of the posterior boundaries of lungs and pleura as demonstrated on the cadaver and on the roentgenogram of the living. Anat. Rec., *83:* 521, 1942.

424 JACKSON, C. L., AND HUBER, J. F. Correlated applied anatomy of the bronchial tree and lungs with a system of nomenclature. Dis. Chest, *9:* 319, 1943.

425 BOYDEN, E. A. Segmental Anatomy of the Lungs. McGraw-Hill Book Company, New York, 1954.

425 BOYDEN, E. A. The nomenclature of the bronchopulmonary segments and their blood supply. Dis. Chest, *39:* 1, 1961.

437 JAMES, T. N. Anatomy of the Coronary Arteries, Hoeber, New York, 1961.

437 JAMES, T. N. Anatomy of the coronary arteries in health and disease. Circulation, *32:* 1020, 1965.

437 WINTERSCHEID, L. C. Collateral circulation of the heart. *In* Collateral Circulation in Clinical Surgery, edited by Strandness, D. E., W. B. Saunders Company, Philadelphia, 1969.

445.1 WALLS, E. W. Dissection of the atrioventricular node and bundle in the human heart. J. Anat., *79:* 45, 1945.

446.4 ADACHI, B. Das Arteriensystem der Japaner. Kyoto, 1928.

446.4 QUAIN, R. The Anatomy of the Arteries of the Human Body. Taylor and Walton, London, 1844.

446.4 THOMSON, A. Third Annual Report of the Committee of Collective Investigation of the Anatomical Society of Great Britain and Ireland for the Year 1891–1892. J. Anat. & Physiol., *27:* 191, 1893.

446.4 LOTH, E. Anatomie des Partes Molles. Masson et Cie, Paris, 1931.

447.1 McDONALD, J. J., AND ANSON, B. J. Variations in origin of arteries derived from the aortic arch in American whites and Negroes. Am. J. Phys. Anthropol., *27:* 91, 1940.

447.1 ANSON, B. J. *In* Callander's Surgical Anatomy, 4th ed., p. 318. W. B. Saunders Company, Philadelphia, 1957.

447.1 STEWART, J. R., KINCAID, O. W., AND EDWARDS, J. E. An atlas of vascular rings and related malformations of the aortic arch system. Charles C Thomas, Publisher, Springfield, Ill., 1964.

447.2 HILEL, N., AND GERSHON, G. Thoracic duct terminating on the right side associated with aberrant retroesophageal right subclavian artery. Thorax, *23:* 266, 1968.

453 ROSS, J. K. A review of the surgery of the thoracic duct. Thorax, *16:* 12, 1961.

454 SWIGART, L. V. L., SIEKERT, R. G., HAMBLEY, W. C., AND ANSON, B. J. The esophageal arteries, an anatomic study of 150 specimens. Surg. Gynec. & Obst., *90:* 234, 1950.

455 SEIB, G. A. See reference for Figure 188.3.

457.1 CAULDWELL, E. W., SIEKERT, R. G., LININGER, R. E., AND ANSON, B. J. The bronchial arteries. (Data on origin, number and course in 300 specimens.) Surg. Gynec. & Obst., *86:* 395, 1948.

Figure

471 WHITNALL, S. E. *In* Anatomy of the Human Orbit. Oxford Medical Publications, London, 1921.

471.5 HUELKE, D. F. A study of the transverse cervical and dorsal scapular arteries. Anat. Rec., *132:* 233, 1958.

471.5 ADACHI, B. A. transversa scapulae and a. transversa colli. *In* Das Arteriensystem der Japaner, vol. 1, pp. 147 and 182. Kyoto, 1928.

471.5 READ, W. T., AND TROTTER, M. The origins of transverse cervical and of transverse scapular arteries in American whites and Negroes. Am. J. Phys. Anthropol., *28:* 239, 1941.

471.5 MacINTOSH, D., AND SMITH, G. G. Personal observations.

483 KIMMEL, D. L. Innervation of spinal dura mater and dura mater of the posterior cranial fossa. Neurology, *11:* 800, 1961.

484 SUH, T. H., AND ALEXANDER, L. Vascular system of the human spinal cord (radicular vessels). Arch. Neurol. & Psychiat., *41:* 659, 1939.

484 MacDONALD, I. B., McKENZIE, K. G., AND BOTTERELL, E. H. Anterior rhizotomy. J. Neurosurg., *3:* 421, 1946.

484 SMITH, C. G. Changes in length and position of the segments of the spinal cord with changes in posture in the monkey. Radiology, *66:* 259, 1956.

484.1 JIT, I., AND CHARNAKIA, V. M. The vertebral level of the termination of the spinal cord. J. Anat. Soc. India, *8:* 93, 1959.

484.1 REIMANN, A. F., AND ANSON, B. J. Vertebral level of termination of the spinal cord with a report of a case of a sacral cord. Anat. Rec. 88: 127, 1944. *Also in* Callander's Surgical Anatomy, 4th ed., p. 771. W. B. Saunders Company, Philadelphia, 1958.

486 HAWKINS, T. D., AND MARTIN, L. Incidence of hyperostosis frontalis interna. J. Neurol. Neurosurg. & Psychiat., *28:* 171, 1965.

499 STILES, H. J. *In* Cunningham's Textbook of Anatomy, 4th ed., p. 1359. Oxford Medical Press, London, 1913.

502 KIMMEL, D. L. The nerves of the cranial dura mater etc. Chicago M. School Quart., *22:* 16, 1961.

504.2 BROWNING, H. The confluence of dural venous sinuses. Am. J. Anat., *93:* 307, 1953.

505 ALKSNE, J. F. Circle of Willis [Cerebral arterial circle], variations in. *In* Strandness, D. E.: Collateral circulation in clinical surgery, edited by Strandness, D. E., p. 596, W. B. Saunders Company, Philadelphia, 1969.

505.2 JONES, T., AND SHEPARD, W. C. A Manual of Surgical Anatomy. W. B. Saunders Company, Philadelphia, 1945.

511 McKERN, T. W., AND STEWART, T. D. See reference for Figure 98.

511 POWELL, T. V., AND BRODIE, A. G.: Closure of sphenooccipital synchondrosis. (In general, male closure age starts between 13–16 years and is completed by 20; female between 11–14 years and is completed by 17.) Anat. Rec., *147:* 15, 1963.

523.1 McCULLOCH, C. The zonule of Zinn: its origin, course, and insertion and its relation to neighboring structures. Tr. Ophth. Soc., *52:* 525, 1954.

555 HJORTSJO, C-H. The mechanism in the temporomandibular joint (Excerptum). Acta odont. Scandinav. *XI:* fasc. 1, 1953.

Figure

560.3 PEARSON, B. W., MacKENZIE, R. G., AND GOODMAN, W. S. The anatomical basis of transantral ligation of the maxillary artery in severe epistaxis. Laryngoscope, *79:* 969, 1969.

566.1 LEWIS, G. F. Personal observations.

566.2 MacINTOSH, D., AND SMITH, C. G. Personal observations.

567 ADACHI, B. Arteria vertebralis. *In* Das Arteriensystem der Japaner, vol. 1, p. 138. Kyoto, 1928.

567 BELL, R. H., SWIGART, L. L., AND ANSON, B. J. The relation of the vertebral artery to the cervical vertebrae. Quart. Bull. Northwestern Univ. M. School, *24:* no. 3, 184, 1950.

567 COBB, W. M. The ossa suprasternalia in whites and American Negroes and the form of the superior border of the manubrium. J. Anat., Pt 2, *71:* 245, 1937.

624 HETHERINGTON, J. The kerato-cricoid muscle in the American white and Negro. Am. J. Phys. Anthropol., *19:* 209, 1934.

633 YOUNG, M. W. The termination of the perilymphatic duct. Anat. Rec., *112:* 404, 1952.

639 GRAVES, G. O., AND EDWARDS, L. F. The Eustachian tube. (A review of its descriptive, microscopic, topographic and clinical anatomy.) Arch. Otolaryg., *39:* 359, 1944.

641.1 LAURENSON, R. D. A rapid method of dissecting the middle ear. Anat. Rec., *151:* 503, 1965.

651 SMITH, C. G. Incidence of atrophy of the olfactory nerves in man. Arch. Otolaryng., *34:* 533, 1941.

657 SCHWARTZ, H. G., AND WEDELL, G. Observations on the pathways transmitting the sensation of taste. Brain, *61:* 99, 1938.

657 HUNT, J. R. Geniculate neuralgia. Arch. Neurol. & Psychiat., *37:* 253, 1937.

659 REICHERT, F. L., AND POTH, E. J. Recent knowledge regarding the physiology of the glossopharyngeal nerve in man with analysis of its sensory, motor, gustatory and secretory functions. Bull. Johns Hopkins Hosp., *53:* 131, 1933.

659.1 ADAMS, W. E. The Comparative Anatomy of the Carotid Body and Carotid Sinus. Charles C Thomas, Publisher, Springfield, Ill., 1958.

659.1 BOYD, J. D. Observations on the human carotid sinus and its nerve supply (with illustration). Anat. Anz., *84:* 386, 1937.

661 CORBIN, K. B., AND HARRISON, F. The sensory innervation of the spinal accessory and tongue musculature in the rhesus monkey. Brain, *62:* 191, 1939.

661 HAYMAKER, W., AND WOODHALL, B. Peripheral Nerve Injuries, 2nd ed. W. B. Saunders Company, Philadelphia, 1953.

661 PEARSON, A. A. The spinal accessory nerve in human embryos. J. Comp. Neurol., *68:* 243, 1938.

663 FENDER, F. A. Foerster's scheme of the dermatomes. Arch. Neurol. & Psychiat., *41:* 688, 1939.

665 KEEGAN, J. J., AND GARRETT, F. D. The segmental distribution of the cutaneous nerves in the limbs of man. Anat. Rec., *102:* 409, 1948.

665 PEARSON, A. A., AND BASS, J. J. Cutaneous branches of the posterior primary rami of the cervical nerves. Anat. Rec., *139:* 263, 1961.

665 PEARSON, A. A., AND BASS, J. J. Further observations on the cutaneous branches of the posterior primary rami of the cervical nerves in embryos. Anat. Rec., *142:* 266, 1962.

Index

References are to Figure Numbers

The chief references to any item are printed in bold type

Abdomen, cross section of, 178
  preview of, 104.2
  skeleton of, 104.2
Acetabulum, 276–278, 282–284
Acromion, 1, 25, 26
  unfused epiphysis, 40
Aditus; to larynx, 578
  ad antrum, 555, 633.1, 639
Agger nasi, 609, **613**
Air cells—
  agger cells, 612, 618
  of ethmoid. See "Sinus, ethmoidal"
  mastoid, 633.1, 641.1, **643**
  tubal, 641
  tympanic, 641
Ala; of ethmoid, 508
  of sacrum, 219, **373**
Ampulla—
  of deferent duct, 206
  of semicircular canals, 649
  of semicircular ducts, 650
  of uterine tube, 232
Anastomoses around knee, 289–291
  porta-caval, 160.1
Angle—
  acromial, 2, **26**
  calcanean, of cuboid, 345
  of clitoris, 224
  of mandible **460**, 461, **553**, 557
  of rib, 392, **398**, 409
  of sacrum, infero-lateral, 373, 374
  of scapula, **1, 2,** 25
  sternal, 11, **393**, 394, 397, See also "Joints, sterno-manubrial"
Annulus. See "Anulus" & "Ring"
  fibrosus, 384–387
  ovalis. See "Limbus"

ANOMALIES—
  Appendix, vermiform, 172
  Arch, axillary, 27
    aortic arch, 446.4, 447
  Arteries—
    brachial, 28
    brachiocephalic trunk (innominate), 446, 447
    carotid, internal, 567.1

ANOMALIES, Arteries (*cont.*)
  coronary, 439
  circumflex humeral, 41
  cystic, 143
  dorsalis pedis, 324
  hepatic, 144, 135 & 148 (see text)
  innominate, 446, 447
  lateral costal, 403
  lingual, 566.1
  median, persisting, 97
  obturator, 212
  popliteal, high division, 324
  profunda brachii, 41
  renal, 151, 184, 187
  subclavian, right, 447.2
  suprascapular, 471.5 (see text)
  tibial, 324
  transverse cervical, 471.5
  ulnar, superficial, 48.1
  vertebral, 446.4, 567
  of bile passages, 161
  Bones—
    acromion, epiphysis, 40
    atlas, occipitalization of, 489
    carpals, 97
    cuneiform, bipartite, 356
    fabella, 323
    foramen, supratrochlear, 48
    frontalis, hyperostosis of, 486
    humerus, 47, 48
    interparietal, 488
    mandible, 553.2
    metacarpals, 97
    metatarsals, 349
    navicular, accessory, 356
    occipital, 487–489
    os; acromiale, 40
      incae, 488
      japonicum, 557.1
      trigonum, 356
    ossicles, suprasternal, 567
    paramastoid, 487
    patella, bipartite, 323
    process; paramastoid, 487
      styloid, 568, 568.1
      supracondylar, 47
    ribs, 400–402

ANOMALIES, Bones (*cont.*)
  sacrum, 380, 381
  sesamoid, gastrocnemius, 323
    peroneus longus, 356
    tibialis posterior, 356
  sternum, 396, 397
  talus, 356
  tibiale externum, 356
  vertebral column, 375–383, 489
  wrist, 97
Diverticulum; duodenal, 171
  ilei (Meckel's), 170.1
Ducts; biliary, 161
  pancreatic, 155–157
Gall bladder, 161
Gland, thyroid, 539
  of Joint; shoulder, 42, 43
  sacro-iliac (synostosis), 223.1
Kidney, 187
Larynx, saccule of, 622
Ligament, stylohyoid, 568
Lung, azygos lobe, 457
Muscles—
  axillary arch, 27
  biceps brachii, 28
  coraco-brachialis, 28
  extensor digitorum brevis, 97
  levator glandulae thyroideae, 539
  palmaris longus, 97
  pectorales, 27
  piriformis and sciatic nerve, 323
  scalenus minimus, 537, **567**
  sternalis, 27
Nerves—
  accessory and jugular vein, **566.2**
  ansa cervicalis and jugular vein, **566.2**
  of hand, cutaneous, 85, 97
  laryngeal, recurrent, 532
  median, 97
  phrenic and great veins, **566.2**
  sciatic and piriformis, 323
  ulnar, 85, 97
Sinuses, air, 610–620
Spleen, accessory, 152
Sacro-iliac synostosis, 223.1
Sacrum, 380, 381
Spondylolisthesis, 383

Anomalies (*cont.*)

ANOMALIES (*cont.*)

stylohyoid ligament, 568, **568.1**

ureter, 186, 187

vena cava; inferior, 185–186

superior, 456

fold of, 440, 456

Ansa; cervicalis (hypoglossi), 542

superior root (desc. hypoglossi n.), **541, 542,** 551

inferior root (desc. cervicalis n.), **541,** 542, 566.2

subclavia, 430, 537, **561**

Antihelix, 469

Antitragus, 469

Antrum—

of Highmore. See "Sinus, maxillary"

mastoid (tympanic), 633.1, **639, 642, 646,** 647

pyloric, 127, 128

Anulus; fibrosis, 384–387

ovalis. See "Limbus"

Aorta—

complete, 189.1, 457.2

diagram of, 413

thoracic, 429, **452**

ascending, **433, 434, 440, 441**

arch, 414, **433–435, 449–**452

anomalies, 446.4, 447

descending, **429, 431, 442, 450**

branches, 454, 457.1

abdominal, 164, 165, **179**

branches, 188, 188.1

Aperture. See also "Hiatus; Opening; Orifice."

nasal, anterior. See "Aper. piriform"

nasal, posterior. See "Choana"

piriform, 461, 464A (see text)

Apex—

of coccyx, 373, 374

of head of fibula, 242, 243

of heart, 434

of lung, 414.1–416

of sacrum, 373

Aponeurosis—

bicipital, 44, **45**

dorsal, of toes. See "Expansion"

epicranial, **490,** 498.1

of obliquus abdominis externus, 105, **109**

palatine, 582, 583

palmar, 59, 70, 72

pharyngeal. See "Fascia, pharyngobasilar"

plantar, 325, 327

bony attachments, 314

lateral cord of, 331

of transversus abdominis, **174, 190,** 478, 479

tricipital; See "Fascia on anconeus"

Appendix—

of epididymis, 116

epiploica, 162, **164, 165**

of larynx. See "Saccule"

testis, 116

vermiform, 162, **169,** 170

in female, 235–237

veriations, **172,** 235

Aqueduct—

of cochlea. See "Duct, perilymphatic", 633, 644 (see text)

of vestibule, 497, **633, 644**

Arachnoid mater. See "Mater"

Arc of Riolan, 158, 165

Arch—

of aorta. See "Aorta"

of atlas, 562, 563

axillary, 27

of azygos vein, 435, 450–452, **457**

carpal, dorsal, 78, 79

palmar, 71

coraco-acromial, 36, 38 (text)

costal. See "Ribs"

of cricoid cartilage, **623,** 629

jugular venous, 527

lumbo-costal. See "Lig. arcuate"

neural, 359, 365

palatine, 584, 587

palato-glossal (glosso-palatine), 584, 587

palato-pharyngeal (pharyngo-palatine), 584, 587

palmar; deep, 71

superficial, 67

pubic, 242

superciliary, 459

tendinous (of levator ani), 209

vertebral, 357, 358

cervical, 367

thoracic, 370

lumbar, 371

anomalies, 376, 382

zygomatic, 459, 461

Area, dangerous, (scalp), **458,** 498.1

ARTERIES—

acromio-thoracic. See "A. thoraco-acromial"

alveolar, 559

aorta. See "Aorta"

appendicular, 162, **169**

arcuate, 306

auricular, posterior, **467,** 550, **551**

diagrams of, 500, 543.2

axillary, 15–17, 474, 475

basilar, 503

of bile passages, 145, 146

brachial, 20

section at midarm, 15, **34**

section at elbow, 55

lower part of, 45, 46

high division, 28

brachio-cephalic (innominate). See "Trunk, brachio-cephalic"

bronchial, 451, **454**

buccal, 559

of bulb, penis, **201,** 205

caecal, 169

calcanean, 319.1, 321, 325

cardiac. See "A. coronary"

carotid;

common, in neck, **471.4,** 530, **534**

in thorax, left, **429, 432–435, 449, 452**

external, 542, 549, **552**

diagram of, 471.4, **543.2**

internal; in skull, 505, **513, 514,** 520

in neck, **542, 543.2,** 551, **552,** 584

at base of skull, **573, 577,** 579

in temporal bone, 514.1, 639, 640

tortuous, 567.1

carpal; dorsal, 67, **78,** 79, **81**

palmar, 60, 71

cecal, 169

celiac, (trunk), **132.1,** 153, 154, **179,** 188

Arteries (*cont.*)

cerebellar, superior, 503, **505**

cerebral; anterior, 503, 505, **520**

middle, 505, 520

posterior, 503, 505, **513**

cervical; ascending, **471.4, 531,** 536

deep [profunda], 457.1, 491

transverse [colli], 471.4, 471.5, **473–475, 531,** 536, 561

circle, cerebral (of Willis), 505, 513 (not labelled)

circumflex; femoral, 279

lateral, 263

medial, 263, 270

humeral; anterior, 17

posterior, 17, **32, 33,** 39

variations, 41

iliac; deep, **112,** 258

superficial, **105,** 252–254

scapular, 15, **17, 32**

coeliac, **132.1,** 153, 154, **179,** 188

colic; left, 163

middle, **135,** 162–165

right, 135, 153, **162**

communicating, of brain; anterior, 520

posterior, **505,** 513

coronary, **433, 437, 440, 446.1**

varieties of, 439

costal, lateral, 403

cremasteric, 111, **112, 119,** 256

cricothyroid, 549, 631.2

to crus penis. See "deep of penis"

cystic, 132.1, 142, **145, 160**

variations, 143

deep; circumflex iliac, **112,** 202, 258

end branches of, 111

of penis, 200, 201

deferential (of vas deferens), 119, 202

dental. See "A. alveolar"

digital; of foot, 306, 325–327

of hand, 67, 70, 71, 78

dorsal carpal of ulnar, 67, 81

dorsal scapular, *25.1,* 26.1, 471.5 (see text), 531

dorsalis; indices, 74, **78,** 79

linguae, 549

nasi, 524

pedis, **306,** 307, 324

penis, 199–201

pollicis, 74, **78,** 79

scapulae, *25.1,* 26.1, 471.5 (see text), **531**

of duodenum, 132, **135, 158, 159**

epigastric; inferior, **106, 112,** 205, 216

in female, 233, 235

superficial, 105, **252**

superior, **106**

epiploic, 132

esophageal, 132, 135, 454

ethmoidal, 520, 524, 607

of face, 466

facial (ext. maxillary)—

diagram of, 543.2

in neck, 542, 546, **599**

in face, 466, 467

branches; ascending palatine, 577, 588, 590

tonsillar, 543.2, **548,** 586, **589**

submental, 527, **546**

labial, sup. & inf., **458** (not labelled), **607**

ARTERIES, facial (ext. maxillary, branches) (*cont.*)
lateral nasal, 466, 607
facial, transverse, 466, **467, 543.2,** 550
femoral, 257–259, 263, 264
at adductor hiatus, 263.1
cross section; 256.1, 264
to head of femur, 279, 283
gastric; left, **132, 134,** 153
right, 132, 135, 145
short, 132
gastro-duodenal, **132,** 145, 148 **153**
gastro-epiploic; left, **132,** 135, 149
right, **132,** 135, 153
genicular, 287, **289–291,** 296, 298
descending (genus suprema), 290
gluteal—
in buttock, 270, 271
in pelvis, 210, 211, 213
hemorrhoidal. See "A., rectal"
hepatic, 132.1, 135, **142,** 146, 148
intrahepatic course, 140, 141
variations, 144
hypogastric. See "A., iliac, internal"
umbilical branch, **205, 210,** 211
ilial, **162,** 167, 169
ileo-colic, 153, **162,** 164, **165,** 169
iliac; common, **165,** 179, 188
external, **112,** 179, **202, 210,** 216
internal, **210,** 211, 235
branches of, 210, 213
ilio-lumbar, 211, 213
infra-orbital, 556, 560
inguinal, superficial, **105,** 252–254
innominate. See "Trunk, brachiocephalic", 432–435, 448–450, **452,** 531, **536**
anomalies, 446.1–447.2
intercostal; scheme, 405
anterior, 406, 407 (not labelled)
posterior, 409, **410, 428,** 429, 457.1
supreme (superior), 429, **430,** 454, **457.1**
interosseous; anterior, 52
common, 52
posterior, 52, 79
recurrent, 57, 79
of intestine, 162–167
jejunal, 162, 167
labial, posterior, (of perineum), 226
labyrinthine (int. auditory), 505
lacrimal, 520, 524
laryngeal; superior, 530, 628.1
inferior, 535 (see text), 628.1
of round ligament, 122
limb, lower (diagram), 244
upper (diagram), 3
lingual, 543.2, 548, **549, 551,** 599
variations in origin, 566.1
lumbar, 188–190
malleolar, 306
mammary, internal. See "A., thoracic, internal"
marginal, of Drummond, 163
to masseter, 551, 559
maxillary (internal); 559, **560**
diagram of, 543.2, **556**
3rd part, 560.3
external. See "A., facial"
median, 60, 97
meningeal; middle, 502, 513, 560
surface anatomy, 499
accessory, 556, 560 (see text)

ARTERIES, meningeal (*cont.*)
mesenteric; inferior, **163**–165, 179, 235
superior, 135, 153, 158, 162, 179
metacarpal; dorsal, 78
palmar, 71
metatarsal; dorsal, 306
plantar, 326
mylohyoid, 546, 599
of nasal cavities, 607
nasal posterior, lateral, & septal, 560.3, 607
nasopalatine. See "A., septal, posterior"
obturator, 210, 211
accessory (abnormal), 212
occipital, 491, 542, 543.2, 551, **552**
in posterior triangle, 472, **473,** 477
in scalp, 24, **500**
oesophageal, 132, 135, **454**
ophthalmic, 516, 520, **524**
ovarian, 232, **233,** 235
palatine
ascending, 543.2, 577, **582, 588, 590,** 607
descending, 556, **560.3**
greater, 556, **560,** 582, **583,** 592
lesser, 582, **583**
palmar superficial, 59
of pancreas, 153, 154, **158,** 159
pancreatica magna, 154
pancreatico-duodenal; inferior and superior, 153, 154, 158, 159
of pelvis, 210, 211, 213, 216
of penis, **199**–201, 216
perforating; of foot, 306, 326
of hand, 72, 78
of thigh, **244,** 258, 270
pericardiaco-phrenic, 428
perineal, 216
peroneal, **310,** 319, **320**
perforating branch, 306
pharyngeal br. of maxillary a., 560.3
pharyngeal, ascending, 471.4, **573, 577**
phrenic, inferior, **179,** 180, 188
plantar, 319, **321, 326,** 330
popliteal, 285, **287, 289,** 320
high division of, 324
princeps pollicis, 65, **71.1**
profunda; brachii, 32, 33
variations, 41
cervicis. See "A., cervical, deep"
femoris, 257–259, 263, 264
linguae, 549 (see text)
of pterygoid canal, 560.3
pudendal; external, **105,** 252–254
internal; in buttock, 270, 271
in pelvis, 195, 210, 213
pulmonary—
See "Trunk, pulmonary," **433,** 434, 436
right and left, 433–435, **450**
in root of lungs, 415, 416, 428, 429
in lung, **419, 422,** 423, 451
radial—
in forearm, 59–61
in palm, 71, 72
recurrent branch of, 46
in "snuff-box," 74, 78, **79**
at wrist, 66, 67, 71
radialis indicis (palmar digital), 67, **71,** 79
rectal (hemorrhoidal)—
inferior, **192,** 195, 216
middle, 195, 210, 211

ARTERIES, rectal (*cont.*)
superior, 163, 195
renal, 177, **179,** 183.1, 188
accessory, 151, **184,** 187
segmental, 183.1, 183.2, 184.1
retro-duodenal, 135 (unlabelled), 158
sacral, lateral, 211, 213
saphenous, 263
of scalp, 500
scapular, dorsal, 471.5 (see text), 531
alternative origin, **25.1**
of sciatic nerve, 280
scrotal, posterior, 192, 201
septal, posterior, 560.3, 607
sigmoid, (inf. left colic), 163, 163.2, 165
of sole, diagram, 326
spermatic; external. See "A., cremasteric"
internal. See "A., testicular"
spheno-palatine, 556, 560.3, **607**
splenic, 132, **135,** 149, 154, 158, 159
sternomastoid, 541, **542**
scheme of, 543.2
of stomach, 132
stylomastoid, 550, 577 (see text)
subclavian—
anomalies, 446.4, 447, **532**
right and left, 434, 435, 448–452, **536**
right only, 430, 475, 531, 537
left only, **429, 536 B**
subcostal, 179, **190**
sublingual, **548,** 592
submental, 527, 542, **546**
subscapular, 15, **17**
supraduodenal, 132, **153**
supra-orbital, 500, **520,** 524
suprascapular, 25, **32, 531,** 533, 536
supratrochlear; of arm, "See ulnar collateral inferior"
of head, 500, **524**
tarsal, 306
temporal—
deep, 559
middle, 543.2
groove for, 557
superficial, **466, 467,** 550
origin of, 559
in scalp, 500
testicular, 165, **179**
in iliac fossa, 202, 210
near testis, 119
at origin, 177, **188**
thoracic—
internal (mammary), 405–407, 430, 432
origin of, 449, **561**
lateral, 3, 15, **16**
supreme (superior), 17
thoraco-acromial, 14, 16
of thymus, 448
thyroid; inferior, **531, 534, 536,** 561
superior, **529,** 530, 532, 534, **542,** 548
tibial; anterior, 305, **306,** 320
posterior, 310, 319–322
absence of, 324
tonsillar, **548, 586,** 588, 589
transverse—
cervical [colli], 473–**475, 531,** 536
abnormal, 25.1, **471.5,** 536, 567
scapular. See "Art. suprascapular"
ulnar—
in forearm, 59–61, 63
in palm, 67, 71

Arteries (*cont.*)

ARTERIES, ulnar (*cont.*)
    recurrent branch of, 56, 57, **61**
    superficial, 48.1
    variation, 48.1
    at wrist, 66, 67
  ulnar collateral, 20, 45–47
  umbilical, obliterated, **205, 210, 211**
  of ureter, 189
  uterine, 232.1, 234
  vaginal, 232.1, 234
  of vas deferens. See "A. deferential"
  vertebral—
    anomalous, 446.4, 567
    at origin, 452, 536, 537, **561**
    in skull, 503, **564**, 565
    in suboccipital region, 493–495
  vesical, **210**, 211, 234, **238**
Articulation. See "Joint"
Asterion, 461
Atlas, **367, 368,** 495, 563
  occipitalization of, 489
  relations of transverse process, 552, 561
Atrium; of heart, 433–436, 443
  of middle meatus of nasal cavity, 609, **612**
  of nose, 609
Auricle—
  of ear, 469
    vessels and nerves of, 551
  of heart, 434, **436**
Axilla, 13–23
  cross-section of, 22
Axis vertebra (Epistropheus), **367, 368,** 563

Back, 24, 173–175
Band; ilio-tibial. See "Tract"
  moderator. See "Trabecula, septomarginal" 444, 445.1
Bar, costo-transverse, 367, 368
Base of mandible, 460, 461
Basi-occipital bone (Basi-occiput), **507,** 510, **511,** 565, 571.2
Bed; of parotid, 465, **551, 552**
  of stomach, 134, **149**
  of tonsil, 584, 588–590
Bile passages, **142,** 145, **148,** 153, 154, **156**
  intrahepatic course, 140, 141, 160
  arteries of, 142–146, 159
  and right hepatic artery, 135, **144,** 148
Bladder, gall. See "Gall bladder"
  urinary, 197
    blood supply, 210
    from above, 202, 233
    from behind, 205, 207
    interior, 208
    cross section; female, 191.6
      male, 191.6
    median section; female, 236
      male, 203, 204
    nerve supply, 214
    trigone; female, 232.1, 235
      male, 208
Body—
  ano-coccygeal. See "Lig." 236
  of hyoid bone, 596, 623
  mammillary, 506
  of mandible, 462
  Pacchionian. See "Granulations, arachnoid"
  perineal. See "tendon, central"

Body (*cont.*)
  of sphenoid, 507, 511
  of sternum, 393
  of vertebra, 357–360
Bones. See also individual bones
  lower limb, ossification of, 350–355
  upper limb, ossification of, **98–104**
Brain; base, 506
  median section, 609
  stem, dorsal view, 495
Breast, 12
Bregma, 461
Brim, pelvic, 221
Bronchial tree, 417, 420
Broncho-pulmonary segments, 425–427
Bronchus, 415–429, **451,** 458
Bulb and **Bulbus—**
  jugular; superior, 573, **640**
    inferior & superior, 543.3
  oculi [eyeball], 471.2, 519–522
  olfactory, **506,** 606
  of penis (urethral), 193, 198
    on section, 200, 201
  of vestibule, of vagina, 228, 229
Bulla ethmoidalis, 608.1, 610
Bundle; atrioventricular, 445
  neurovascular, 15
Bursa—
  omental (Sac, lesser); 134, 135, 149
    diagram, 130.1, 130.2, 176
  synovial—
    of tendo calcaneus, 315, 333, **339**
    of biceps brachii, 51, **62.1**
    calcanean, subcutaneous, 333
    of gastrocnemius, 302
    of gluteus maximus, 270
    interspinous, 386
    of medial ligament of knee, 294
    of obturator externus, 275
    of obturator internus, 275, **281**
    of olecranon, 51, **55**
    of popliteus, 288, **302**
    of psoas, 281
    of quadriceps femoris [suprapatellar], 301
    of semimembranosus, 287, 302
    subacromial, **35,** 39
    subdeltoid, 22, **35,** 38.1
    subhyoid (text), 629
    subscapular, 22, **36,** 39
    of tendo calcaneus, 315, 333, 339
    trochanteric, 270
    of vastus lateralis, 270
Buttresses—
  of face, 463
  of nose, 464

Caecum. See Cecum
Calcaneus (Calcaneum), **311–316,** 336, 337, 344
Calyx [Calix], renal, 183
Canal—
  adductor, 259 (see text), 263
    on cross-section, 264 (see text)
  anal, 193–196
    median section, female, 236
      male, 203
  carotid, 569, 571.1
  condylar, 496, **512, 569**

Canal, condylar (*cont.*)
  anterior. See "C. hypoglossal"
  posterior. See "C, condylar"
  for facial nerve, **637, 639,** 642, 648-**649**
  femoral, 254, 281 (on section)
  hypoglossal, 508, **512, 569, 571.2**
  infra-orbital, 518
  inguinal;
    female, 120–122
    male, 109–112
    schematic, 113
  innominatus. See "Canaliculus"
  naso-lacrimal, 464, 579
  optic (Foramen, optic), 508, **512, 518**
    and sphenoidal sinus, 611, 620
  palatine, 608
  palato-vaginal or pharyngeal, 560.1
  pterygoid, **611,** 619–619.2
  pudendal, 192, 215
  pyloric, 127, 128
  sacral, 219, 373, **374**
  semicircular, 637, 644, 645.1, **649**
  vertebral, 357 (see text). See also "Foramen, vertebral"
  Vidian. See "C., pterygoid"
Canaliculus; of cochlea, 497, **644**
  innominatus, 509
  lacrimal, 519
Capitate bone. See "Carpus"
Capitulum, 1, 51, **55**
Capsule. See "Joint"
  renal; fatty, 175, 178
    fibrous, 178, 183
  Tenon's. See "Fascia bulbi"
Carpus; anterior aspect, 62
  facets, 95
  posterior aspect, 86
Cartilage—
  alar. See "C., nasal"
  arytenoid, **624,** 625, **629, 632**
  of auricle, 469
  corniculate, **624,** 625, 629, 632
  costal, 391, 393 (see text).
  cricoid, 528, **621–625,** 628, 629
  cuneiform, 624, **632**
  of epiglottis. See "Epiglottis"
  nasal, **468,** 579, 605, **611**
  semilunar. See "Meniscus of knee"
  septal, **468,** 579, **605**
  sesamoid, of nose, **468,** 611
  subvomerine. See "C. vomeronasal"
  thyroid, 528, **621–625,** 627, 628
    male & female, 625.1
  triticea, **623,** 624
  vomero-nasal, 605
Cauda equina, 484
Cave, trigeminal (of Meckel), 514, **554,** 565
Cavity—
  glenoid, 38
  infraglottic, 631.1
  nasal, 459, **605–612**
    coronal section, 517, 591
  orbital, 459, **518–521,** 524, 525
    coronal section, 517, 592
    sagittal section, 471.2
  pericardial. See "Pericardium"
  pleural, 412
  tympanic, 633–642
Cecum, **162,** 164, 169, 170
Cells, air. See "Air cells, Sinus, Antrum"
Centrum of vertebra, 359, **360, 365**

Cerebellum, 506
Cervix uteri, **232–234**
Chiasma, optic, 506, 521
Choana (aperture, nasal, post.), 569, **578**
Chorda tympani. See "Nerve, ch. tympani"
Chordae tendineae, **445,** 446
Cistern; cerebello-medullary, 609
  chyli, 452
Clavicle, 1, **11, 19,** 391, 529, **534**
Cleft, intratonsillar, 585
Clitoris, **224,** 225, **228,** 229
Clivus, 497, 508
  definition, 496 (in text)
Coccyx; anterior aspect, 364, 373
  lateral aspect, 222
    median section, 217, 236
    posterior aspect, 374
Cochlea, 633, 634, 648, **649**
Colliculus; seminalis (prostatic), 208
  of midbrain, 513
Colon—
  ascending, 162, 164, 165
  descending, 163–165
  pelvic. See "Colon, sigmoid"
  succulation of, 162
  sigmoid (pelvic), 163–165
  tenia of, 162, **164, 169**
  transverse, 149, **162–165**
Column; anal, 196, **203**
  renal, 183
  vertebral, 363, 364
    anomalies of, 375–383, 489
    See also "Vertebra"
Conchae; nasal, 592, 608, **609**
  sphenoidal, 619.1 (see text)
Condyle—
  of femur, 242, 243, 300
  of mandible. See "Head of mandible"
  occipital, 569
  of tibia, **242,** 243, **294**
Cone of muscles, space, 471.2, 517 (see text)
Conjunctiva, 519
Conus arteriosus. See "Infundibulum of
    right ventricle"
  elasticus, **625,** 632 (see text)
Coracoid process, 1, **16,** 26
Cord—
  of brachial plexus, 16–20
  lateral, of plantar aponeurosis, 331
  oblique, of forearm, 49
  spermatic, 105, 111
    coverings of, 106, 113, 117
  spinal, **482, 484,** 494, 495, 506
  vocal. See "Fold, vocal"
Cornea, **522**
Cornu; of coccyx, 222, **374**
  of hyoid bone, 541.1
  of sacrum, 222, **374**
Corona of glans penis, 198, 199
Corpus—
  callosum, 458, 609
  cavernosum penis, 197, **198,** 200
  spongiosum penis (cavernosum ure-
    thrae), 197, **198,** 200
Cortex of kidney, 183
Costa. See "Rib"
Crescent of foramina, (in sphenoid), 509
Crest—
  falciform, of ischium, 222
  frontal, 508
  iliac, 222, **242, 273**

Crest (cont.)
  infratemporal, **558,** 569
  intertrochanteric, 243
  lacrimal; (of lacrimal bone), 462, **518**
    of maxilla, 518 (see text)
  nasal; of maxilla, 605
    of palatine bone, 605
  obturator, 284
  occipital; external, 485, **569**
    internal, 508
  "pronator," of ulna, 52
  pubic, 109, 221
  of rib head, 398
  of rib neck, 398
  of sacrum, 374
  of scapular spine, 25
  sphenoidal, 605
  supinator, 51
  supramastoid, 462, 499, **557**
  of trapezium. See "Tubercle of trape-
    zium"
  of ulna, pronator, 52
  urethral, 208
Crista; galli, 503, **508,** 614
  terminalis, (of heart), 443
Cross sections. See "Sections"
Crus—
  antihelicis, 469
  clitoridis, 224
  of diaphragm, 191
  helicis, 469
  of inguinal ring, 110
  penis, 193, **198,** 200
Cuboid bone, **312–314,** 345–347
Cuneiform bones, **311–314,** 343, 346–347
  bipartite, 356
Cupola; of cochlea, 649
  of diaphragm, 432
  of pleura (cervical pleura), 448–**451**
Curvature of stomach, 127
Cusp. See "Valve"

Dartos, 199 (see text)
Dens of axis, 367, 368, 562, 563
Dentine, 601
Dentition, 601–604
Dermatomes, 663–665
Diaphragm—
  the diaphragm:
    abdominal aspect, 190, 191, 407
    from above, 431
    nerve supply, 191.1
    side view, 428, 429
  oral, 544 (in text)
  pelvic; 191.6 (diagram)
    from above, 209, 231
    from below, 194
  urogenital; female, 228, **229**
    male, **201**
Diaphragma sellae, 503
Digestive system—
  diagram of, 124
Diploe, 591
Disc, articular—
  inferior radio-ulnar, **52,** 90, 91, **94**
  intervertebral, 384–390
  of knee. See "Meniscus"
  sterno-clavicular, 19 (see text), **534**
  temporo-mandibular, 552, **554, 555**
Diverticulum; of duodenum, 171
  of ileum (Meckel's), 170.1

Door. See "Porta"
Dorsum—
  ilii, 243
  ischii, 243
  sellae, 508, 511, 512
Duct and **Ductus—**
  bile, 142, 147, **148, 154,** 156, 159
    and right hepatic artery, 144, 148
    arteries of, 145
  of cochlea, 633, **650,** 650.1
  cystic, 142, 144–**147**
    abnormal, 161
    opened, 156
  deferens (Vas deferens), 115, **210**
    near bladder, 205–208
    at pelvic brim, **202,** 216
    near testis, 114, **118,** 119
  ejaculatory, 115, 206, **207,** 207.1
  endolymphatic, 497, 633, 644 (see text)
  fronto-nasal, 618.1
  hepatic, 142, 145–**147,** 156
    accessory, 161
  lacrimal. See "Canaliculus"
  lactiferous, 12
  lymphatic, right, 453
  maxillary, **616.2,** 618
  naso-lacrimal, 471.1, **519,** 579, **610**
  pancreatic, 156, 157
  para-urethral (Skene's), 227 (see text)
  parotid (Stensen's), 466, **467,** 550, **559**
  perilymphatic, 633, 644 (see text)
  prostatic ductules, 207.1
  reuniens, 650
  semicircular, 633, **650**
  submandibular (submaxillary), 546–549,
    592
    medial view, 590, **597**
  tear. See "Canaliculus, lacrimal"
  of testis, 113–119
  thoracic, **451–454**
    in cross-section of thorax, 431
    on esophagus, 429, 451
    in root of neck, 533, 534, **536**
  of vestibular gland, 228, 229
Duodenum, 124, **153, 154, 156**
  1st part, **126** (see text), 134
  2nd part, **147,** 156, **178**
  3rd part, 164, 165
  arteries of, **153,** 154, 158, **159**
  diverticula, 171
  interior, 168
  relations of, **126,** 153, **176–178**
Dura mater. See "Mater"

Ear—
  of child, 645–647
  coronal section, **634**
  external; auricle, **469, 634**
    cartilage of, 469, 577
    meatus, **461,** 552, **634**
    vessels and nerves, **467,** 550, **551,** 552
  internal, 633, 648, **649, 650**
    cast of, 649.1
  middle [tympanic cavity], 633, 634, 636–
    642
    ossicles, 633, 638
  scheme of, 633
  section through, 634
  tympanic membrane, 633–**635,** 639–**641,**
    641.1

Eminence—
 arcuate, 512, 644
 articular. See "Tubercle, articular"
 frontal. See "Tuber, frontal"
 ilio-pubic (-pectineal), 219, 222
 parietal. See "Tuber, parietal"
Enamel of tooth, 601
Epicondyle—
 of femur, 242, **293**
 of humerus, 1, 2, **49**, 56
Epididymis, 116–119
 cross-section, 114
Epiglottis, **578**, 623–632
Epiphyses. See also "Ossification"—
 bones of lower limb, 351–355
  acetabulum, 277, 278
  femur, upper end, 282
 bones of upper limb, 99–104
  acromion, 40
 vertebra, 359–361
Epistropheus. See "Axis vertebra"
Esophagus—
 arterial supply, 454
 hiatus, 191
 in neck, 532–536
 in thorax, 450–452
  cross-section, 430, 431
  behind pericardium, 442
  pleural aspect, 428, 429
 in abdomen, 124, 126, **128**, 134, **135**
Ethmoid bone—
 from above and behind, 618.2, 618.3
 from the front, 464
 cribrosa (cribriform) plate, 458, 464, 508,
  618.2
 orbital plate, **615**, 618.1
 perpendicular plate, 460, **605**
 scheme of, 614
Excavation. See "Pouch"
Expansion, extensor [dorsal]—
 of toes, 307
 of fingers, 87–89
  bony attachments, 77
Eyeball [Bulbus oculi], 519–523.6
 general structure, 523.1
 dissection of ox's eye, 523.2
 microscope sections, 523.3, 523.4
 in situ, 471.2, 517
Eyelids, 470, 471

Face, 466, 467, 470
 buttresses of, 463
 sensory nerves of, 470.1
Falx; cerebelli, 458, **503**
 cerebri, 458, **503**
 inguinalis, [conjoint tendon], **110–112**,
  abdominal view, 216
 female, 123
Fascia—
 of abdomen, 105
 on anconeus, 31, **56**
 of back. See "F., lumbar"
 Buck's, deep of penis, 199
 bulbi, 471.2
 Camper's, 105 (see text)
 clavipectoral, 14
 Colles'. See "Fascia of perineum, superficial," 192
 cremasteric, 117
  section, 191.6B

Fascia (cont.)
 dorsal. See "F., lumbar"
 of foot. See "Aponeurosis, plantar"
 of gluteus medius, 24, **271**, 272.1
 hypothenar, 70
 iliaca, 190, 205, **256**, 258
 ilio-psoas. See "F., psoas"
 lata, 256
 of leg, 304, **305**, 319
 lumbar, **173–175**, 478–**481**
 of neck; of anterior triangle, 527, 533,
  535
  of posterior triangle, 472–**474**, 542
 obturator, **193**, 209, 217, **241** (see text)
 omohyoid, 474, **542**
 palmar. See "Aponeurosis, palmar"
 palpebral. See "Septum, orbital," 470
 of pectineus, **254**, 258, 274, **281**
 of pelvis; female, 237–241
  male, 203, 205, 207
 of penis, 199
 of perineum, 192, 194
 pharyngo-basilar, 573, **588**, 627
 plantar. See "Aponeurosis, plantar"
 of popliteus, **287**, 319
 pretracheal, 527
 prevertebral, 531, 533, 535 (not labelled)
 prostatic, 194, **207**, 208 (see text)
 of psoas, 256, 481
 of quadratus lumborum, 481
 recto-vesical, 203, 207
 renal, 175, 178
 Scarpa's, 105 (see text)
 of sole. See "Aponeurosis, plantar"
 spermatic; external, 117
  internal, 117
 of submandibular gland, 542
 temporal, **465**, 466, **591**
 thenar, 70
 of thigh, 256, 264
 thoracolumbar (lumbodorsal), **173**, 478
 transversalis, 112, 113
 of urogenital diaphragm. See "Membrane, perineal"
 of vagina, 229, 241 (see text)
Fat. See also "Pad of fat"
 digital process of, 225–227
 extraperitoneal [subperitoneal], 190, 205
 labial process of, 225–227
 perinephric. See "Capsule, renal, fatty,"
  175, 178
Femur, 242, 243
 muscle attachments, **265, 266**, 276.1, **288,
  295, 297**
 upper epiphyses, 282
Fenestra; cochleae, 636, 637.1, **649**
 vestibuli, 637, 637.1, **649**
Fibres, intercrural, 105, 108, **109**
Fibula, 303, 310, 315
 muscle attachments, 303
Filum; terminale, 484
 of spinal dura mater (terminale externum), 203, **484**
Fimbria of uterine tube, 232
Fissure—See also "Sulcus"
 cerebral, lateral, 506
 of lung (interlobar), 414, **415, 416**
 orbital; inferior, 518, **558**
  superior, 509, **518, 619.1**
 petro-occipital, 497
 petro-squamous, 510

Fissure (cont.)
 pterygo-maxillary, 558 (see text), 574
 squamo-tympani, 558 & 569 (not labelled)
 tympano-mastoid, **557**, 569, 671.2
Fold—See also "Plica"
 alar, of knee, 299
 ary-epiglottic, **578, 627, 631**, 632
 glosso-epiglottic; lateral, 578
  median, 628, **630**
 ileo-cecal, **169**, 235
 infrapatellar, 299
 interureteric, 208
 mallear, 636, 641 (see text)
 mucous, of tympanum, **642, 648**
 pharyngo-epiglottic. See "F., lateral
  glosso-epiglottic"
 recto-uterine, **233**, 236, **237**
 sacro-genital [recto-vesical], 202
 salpingo-pharyngeal, 578, **587**
 spiral in cystic duct, 156
 synovial. See "Pad of fat"
 transverse vesical, 233
 vena cava, left, 440, 456
 vestibular (ventricular), 629, 631, 632
 vocal (cord), 535, 629, **631, 632**
Follicle, lingual, **587**, 594, 595
Fonticulus (Fontanelle), 602
Foramen—
 alveolar (dental), 558
 "anastomatic" (lacrimal), 509, 518, 619.2
 cecum; of skull, 508
  of tongue, 578, 594
 condylar, posterior. See "Canal"
 costo-transverse. See "F., transversarium"
 "crescent of," in sphenoid, 509
 for dens, 563
 dental. See "For., alveolar"
 epiploic, **126**, 135, 148
  diagram, 130.2
 ethmoidal, 508, **518**, 607, **615**, 617
 incisive, 569, 580
 infra-oribital, **459**, 518
 intervertebral, 387
 jugular, 512, **569**, 571.2
 lacerum, **512, 569**, 571.2
 lacrimal. See "For., anastomatic"
 magnum, **507**, 510, 564, **570**
 mandibular, 553.1
 mastoid, 485, **512, 569**
 mental, 459, **553**
 obturator, 222, **242**
 optic. See "Canal, optic"
 ovale; inside skull, **508**, 509, **512**, 620.1
  outside skull, 558, **569**, 571.2, **619.1**
 palatine, 569, **580**
 parietal, 485
 rotundum, 509, **512**, 615, **619.1**
 sciatic; greater, **217, 272**, 273
  lesser, **217**, 273
 spheno-palatine, 558, **608.1, 615**
 spinosum; inside skull, **508**, 509, 512
  outside skull, 558, **569**, 571.1, **619.1**
 sternal, **396**, 404
 stylo-mastoid, **569**, 571.2
  at birth, 646, 647
 supra-orbital, 459, or notch, 518
 supratrochlear, of humerus, 48
 transversarium (transverse), 365–367
 transverse; of atlas, 367, **563**
  of axis, 367, **563**

Foramen (*cont.*)
   vertebral, **358**, 360
   zygomatico-facial, 459
Fornix of vagina, 236 (see text)
Fossa—See also **"Pouch and Recess"**
   acetabular, **276**, 282–284
   articular. See "F., mandibular"
   canine, 459, 462
   cerebellar, 508
   coronoid, 51
   cranial; anterior, 507, **508**, 591
      middle, 509–516
         posterior, 507, 508, **510–512**
         from behind, 495–**497**, 643
   cubital, 44–46
   digastric, 553.1
   duodenal [recesses], 163.1
   for gall-bladder, 146
   hypophyseal, 508, **512**
   iliac, 219, **222**, 242
   incisive, 459, 462
   incudis, 642
   infraspinous, 2
   infratemporal, 554–556, **557–560**
   intersigmoid, 202 (see text)
   intrabulbar, 203
   ischio-rectal, 193, 205, **241**
      cross section, 191.6 (female)
   for lacrimal sac, 518
   malleolar, fibula, 303, 335
   mandibular (temporo-mandibular), **558**, 569, 570, 571.1, 619.2
      at birth, 645
   navicular, of urethra, 199.1, 203
   olecranon, 51
   ovalis; of heart, 443
      of thigh. See "Opening, saphenous"
   pararectal, 202
   paravesical, **202**, 233
   piriform. See "Recess, piriform"
   pituitary. See "F., hypophyseal"
   popliteal, 285–289
   pterygoid, 580, **619.2**
   pterygo-palatine (maxillary), 558, 560.1
      definition, 615 (see text)
   radial, 51
   for saccus endolymphaticus, 645.1
   scaphoid; of auricle. See "Scapha"
      of sphenoid bone, 569, **619.2**
   subarcuate, 497, **645.1**
   sublingual, 553.1
   submandibular, 553.1
   supinator, 51
   supra-tonsillar. See "Cleft, intratonsillar"
   temporal, 460
   temporo-mandibular. See "F., mandibular"
   terminal (of urethra), See "F., navicular"
   Vermian, **508**, 564
Frenulum clitoridis, 227
   of prepuce, 199
Frontal bone—
   cerebral surface, 507, 614.1
   from below, 617
   front and side, 459–462
   hyperostosis, 486
   median section, 608
   showing frontal sinuses, 611–614.3, 617–617.4
Fundus of gall bladder, 156

Fundus (*cont.*)
   of stomach, 124, 127
   of uterus, 233.1

Galea aponeurotica. See "Aponeurosis epicranial"
Gall-bladder; 147, 156
   arteries of, 142, **143, 145, 146**
   parts and interior, 156
   relations, 125, **126, 134,** 136
   variations, 161
   veins, 146.1
Ganglion—
   celiac, 179, **180,** 191.3, 660
   cervical. See "G., sympathetic," 561
   ciliary, 520, 521, 523.6
      scheme of, 653
   geneculate (of facial nerve), 648, 657
      distribution of, 657
   otic, 598
      scheme of, 513.2, 657, **659**
   pelvic (of Frankenhaeuser), 240
   posterior root. See "G., spinal"
   pterygopalatine, **560.2,** 583, 606
      scheme of, **547.1,** 657
   semilunar (trigeminal), 513
   sphenopalatine. **See** 'G., pterygopalatine"
   spinal, 19, 410, **483, 538**
   stellate, 537
   submandibular (submaxillary), 547, 548
      scheme of, **547.1,** 657
   sympathetic; cervical, 561
      cervicothoracic [stellate], 537
      lumbar, 189, 190
      sacral, 213
      thoracic, 428, 429
      vertebral, 534, 537 (see text), **561**
   trigeminal. **See** "G., semilunar"
Glabella, 460, 461
Gland—
   adrenal. See "Gl. suprarenal"
   buccal, 584
   bulbo-urethral (Cowper's), 115, 205
   ciliary, 471
   Haversian. See "Pad of fat, synovial"
   labial, 547 (see text)
   lacrimal, 470, 517, 519–521, **523.6**
      nerve supply, **560.2,** 655, **657**
   lingual, anterior, 595
   lymphatic. See "Nodes, lymph"
   mammary, 12
   molar, 559
   nasal, nerve supply, 657
   paired, three, 210.1
   palatine, **581,** 583, **587**
      nerve supply, 657
   parathyroid, 573, **626**
   parotid, 466, **467, 550,** 572
      bed, 465, **550–552**
      on cross-section, 579, 584
      nerve supply, 657, 659
   pituitary. See "Hypophysis cerebri"
   prostate. **See** "Prostate"
   salivary, 547
   sublingual, 597
      inferior view, 545
      lateral view, 547
      medial view, 597
      nerve supply, 547, **657**

Gland (*cont.*)
   submandibular (submaxillary), 465
      inferior view, 544
      lateral view, **541,** 547
      medial view, 589 (see text), 597
      nerve supply, 657
   suprarenal, 151, **177,** 179, **180,** 185
   tarsal, 471
   thymus, **448,** 528
   thyroid, 539
      cross-section, 535, 536
      front and side views, 528–534
      posterior view, 573, **626**
      variations, 539
   of tongue, anterior, 595
   unpaired, three (liver, pancreas, spleen), 104.2F
   vestibular, greater (of Bartholin), 228, 229
Glans clitoridis, **224,** 227, **228**
   penis, 197–**199, 203**
Granulations, arachnoid, 502, 503
Groove—See also **"Sulcus"**
   for arch of aorta, (on lung), 416
   atrio-ventricular. See "Sulcus, coronary"
      for azygos arch, (on lung), 415
   bicipital, 1
   carotid, 508, 512
   chiasmatic (optic), 505, 508, **512**
   coronary (atrio-ventricular), 434, 435
   costal, 398
   for digastric muscle, 569
   for esophagus, 415, 416
   for first rib, 415, 416
   for inferior petrosal sinus, 508, 512
   for inferior vena cava, 415
   infra-orbital, 518
   for innominate vein, 415
   intertubercular (bicipital), 1
   interventricular (longitudinal), 434, 435
   for middle meningeal artery, 512
   for middle temporal artery, 557
   mylo-hyoid, 533.1
   for occipital artery, 485, **569**
   for esophagus, 415, 416
   optic. See "Gr., chiasmatic"
   for petrosal sinus, 497, 512
   for radial nerve (spiral), 2
   for sagittal sinus, 508
   for sigmoid sinus, 508, **512**
   spiral, for radial nerve, 2
   for subclavian vessels, 399, 416
   subcostal. See "G., costal"
   for superior vena cava, 415
   for transverse sinus, 508
   for trigeminal nerve, 497
   for vertebral artery, 367
Gums, nerve supply, 655, 656
Gutter for cervical nerves, 366–368, 538 (in text)
   for lumbricals of hand, 70

Hamate bone. See "Carpus"
Hamulus, pterygoid, 569, 580, 608, **619.2**
   with attachments, 575, 582, **590**
Hand—
   bones; dorsal aspect, 86
      palmar aspect, 62
      epiphyses, 104
   cross-section, **65,** 71.1

Hand (*cont.*)

Hand (cont.)
  muscle attachments; dorsal aspect, 77
    palmar, **58,** 82
  nerves; motor, 68.1
    sensory, 83–85
Head, "The";
  coronal section, 517, 554, **591**
  median section, **458,** 503, 595, 609
  transverse section, 579, 584
Head—
  of femur, 276.1–282
  of fibula, 242, 293, **295, 301–303**
  of humerus, 2
  of mandible, **462,** 507, **553,** 557
  of metacarpal, 62
  of metatarsal, 312
  of phalanx of finger, 62
  of radius, **1,** 51, 55
  of rib, 398
  of talus, 312
  of ulna, **1, 2,** 52
Heart; exterior of, 433–436, 440
  interior of, 443–446
Helix, 469
Hernia of intervertebral disc, 386
Hiatus—See also "Opening and Orifice"
  in adductor magnus, 263.1
  in diaphragm, 191, 191.2
  for greater (superficial) petrosal nerve (of
    facial canal), 512
  sacral, 374
  saphenous (fossa ovalis), 106, **110,** 253–
    256
  semilunaris, **592, 608.1, 610,** 612
Hip bone [Os coxae], 222, **242, 243**
  ligamentous attachments, 217, 273–275
  muscle attachments, 265, 266, 276
  orientation, 221.1
  in youth, 277
Hook of hamate bone, 62, 72, **93,** 95
Horn. See "Cornu"
Humerus, 1, 2
  anomalies of, 47, 48
  cross-sections, 104.1
  lower end, 49, 50, 55
  muscle attachments, 11, **29, 30**
Hyoid bone, 596, 623
  with larynx, **623,** 624, **629,** 630
  in median section, 595, 597
  in midline of neck, 527, 540–542
  as reference point, 541.1
  within pharynx, 590
Hyperostosis frontalis, 486
Hypophysis cerebri, **505,** 612

Ileum, **162, 166,** 168–170
Ilium, 277, 276, & see Hip bone
  muscle attachments, 265, 266
  in youth, 277, 278, **351**
Impression, cardiac, of lung, 415, 416
  trigeminal, 512
Incisive bone (Premaxilla), 580
Incisura. See also "Notch"
  intertragica, 469
  semilunaris. See "Notch, trochlear"
Incus, 638
Infundibulum—
  ethmoidal, **517,** 618
  of hypophysis, 506
  of right ventricle, **444**
  of uterine tube, 232

Inion. See "Protuberance, occipital, ext."
Inlet of larynx. See "Aditus"
Innominate bone. See "Hip bone"
Interparietal bones, 488
Intersection, tendinous, 105
Intestines, **124,** 162, 163
  interior of, 168, 170
  large, 164, 165
Iris, 522
Ischium, 222, 242, 243
  ligamentous attachments, 217, 273
  muscle attachments, 276
  in youth, 277
Isthmus; of auditory tube, 639
  of thyroid gland, 539
  of uterine tube, 232

Jaw—See "Mandible"
Jejunum, 162
  interior of, 168
  upper end, **153, 158,** 176
Joint—
  acromio-clavicular, 36
  ankle, 322, 332–340
  of atlas, 495, 562, **563, 565**
  calcaneo-cuboid, 308, 337, **338, 342**
  carpal, 90, 93, 95
  carpo-metacarpal, 95
  costo-transverse, 398.1, 410, 411
  cranio-vertebral, 565
  of cricoid, 623, **624,** 628
  elbow, **49, 50,** 54, 57
    cross-section of, 55
  foot; bones, 311–314, 343–348
    ligaments, 332, 337–342
  hip, 274–284
    cross-section of, 281
  intercarpal, 90
  interchondral, 404
  intermetacarpal, 95
  intermetatarsal, 347, 348
  interphalangeal, of fingers, 96
  intervertebral, 384–389
  inversion and eversion, 336–338
  knee, 292–302
  manubrio-sternal, 404, 432
  metacarpo-phalangeal, 96
    of hallux, 329.2
  radio-carpal, 90–95
  radio-ulnar; inferior, 90–95
    middle, 52
    superior, 49–55
  sacro-iliac, 221–223
    synostosis of, 223.1
  shoulder, 36–39
    cross-section, 22
    variations, 42, 43
  sterno-clavicular, 533, 534
  sterno-costal, 404
  sterno-manubrial, 404
  symphysis pubis, 203, 209
  talo-calcanean, 334, 336–340
  talo-navicular, 336, **337,** 338–342
  tarso-metatarsal, 332, 342, 343
  temporo-mandibular, **551–555,** 557, 558
  tibio-fibular; inferior, **322,** 332, **338**
    contact surfaces, 303, 333, 334
    superior, 293, 301 (not labelled)
  vertebral. See "J., intervertebral"
  wrist, 90–95
  xiphi-sternal. See "Junction"

Jugum sphenoidale, 507, **507.1,** 512
Junction—
  costo-chondral, 391
  neuro-central, **359,** 365
  xiphi-sternal, 393

Kidney, **179,** 181–183.2
  anomalies of, 185–187
  anterior aspect, 147–151, 176–178
  peritoneal relations, 176, 177
  posterior approach, 175, 189
  pyramids, numbers of, 184.2
  segments, 184
  segmental arteries, 183.1, 183.2

Labium; majus, **225,** 226, **236**
  minus, **225,** 229, **236**
Labrum; acetabular, 282, 284
  glenoid, 38
Labyrinth; ethmoidal, 614, 618.3
  of internal ear, 649, 650
Lacertus fibrosus. See "Aponeurosis, bicipi-
  tal"
Lacrimal bone, 461, **518, 608,** 615
Lacuna lateralis, (of dura) 502
Lambda, 461, **485**
Lamina—See also "**Plate**"
  cribosa [cribriform], 464
  of cricoid, 623, **624,** 629
  pterygoid, 619.1, 619.2
    from below, 569, **580**
    lateral, **558,** 574
    medial, 583, **608**
  of vertebra, **358,** 388
Larynx, 621–632
Leg, cross-section of, 310

LIGAMENTS—
  accessory plantar. See "Lig., plantar
    (plate)"
    volar. See "Lig. palmar (plate)"
  acetabular, transverse, 284
  acromio-clavicular, 36
  alar (check) of dens, 565
  anular (annular); of radius, 49–54, 57
    of stapes, 650.1
  ano-coccygeal (body), 236
  apicis dentis, 562 (see text)
  arcuate; of diaphragm, (lateral, medial
    & median) 191, 191.3
    pubic, 217, **236**
  arteriosum, 429, 433–435, **449–451**
  atlanto-axial, accessory, 565
  atlantis; cruciform, 562, 565 (see text)
    transverse, 562, **563, 565**
  bifurcated, 332, 337, **338**
  broad, of uterus, **232,** 233–235, **236**
  calcaneo-cuboid; dorsal, 338
    plantar (short plantar), 342
  calcaneo-fibular, 322, 337, **338**
  calcaneo-navicular; lateral, 338
    plantar (spring lig.), **337,** 339, 341, **342**
  calcaneo-tibial. See "L., tibiocalcanean
  cardinal, 241
  carpal, transverse. See "Retinaculum,
    flexor or wrist"
  cervical, lateral. See "L. cardinal"
  check, of levator palpebrae, **517,** 520,
    521

LIGAMENTS (*cont.*)

collateral (medial & lateral)—
  of elbow, 49, 50, 53
  of finger, 96
  of knee, **293,** 295–298, **300**–302
conoid, 36
of Cooper; in breast, 12
  of pelvis (pectineal), 108, 274
coraco-acromial, 26, 36
coraco-clavicular, 25, **36**
coraco-humeral, 26, 38
coronary, of knee, **294,** 298, **300**
  of liver, **131,** 177
costo-clavicular, 19 (not labelled)
costo-transverse, 409, **410, 411, 431**
costo-vertebral, 410
costo-xiphoid, 404
crico-arytenoid, 624, 625, 632
crico-thyroid (crico-vocal memb.), 625, **629,** 632
  median, 528, **623,** 625, **629**
crico-tracheal (membrane), 623, 624
cruciate of knee, **292**–**294, 300,** 302
cruciform of atlas, 562, 565 (see text)
crural, cruciate and transverse. See "Retinacula, extensor, of ankle"
cubo-navicular, 342
cuneo-cuboid, 342
cuneo-navicular, 332, 342
cutaneous, of fingers, 68, 71.1
deltoid, **322,** 332–334, **339** (see text)
denticulate, **482,** 484, 564
falciform, of liver, **125,** 131, 134
flavum, **385**–**388,** 458, 538
  fundiform of penis, 110
gastro-lienal (-splenic), 150
gleno-humeral, **37,** 39
of head of femur, 281–284
hyo-epiglottic, 629, 630
ilio-femoral, **274,** 281, 284
ilio-lumbar, 190
of incus, **642,** 648
infundibulo-pelvic. See "Lig. suspensory of ovary"
inguinal, 108, **109,** 258
interchondral, 404
intermetatarsal, **332,** 341, **342**
interosseous; sacro-iliac, 223
  talo-calcanean, 337, **338,** 340
  tibio-fibular, 303 (see text), **334**
interspinous, 385, 386
intra-articular. See also "Disc"
  sternocostal, 404
ischio-femoral, 275
laciniate. See "Retinaculum, flexor of ankle"
lacunar, **108, 254,** 258
lateral; of ankle, **380,** 322, **338**
  of elbow, 50, 53
  of knee, **293,** 296, 300–**302**
latum uteri, See "Lig. broad"
lieno-renal, **134,** 135, 150, **151,** 177
of liver, **125,** 131, **136,** 142, 177
longitudinal of vertebral bodies—
  anterior, **386, 388,** 410, 562
  posterior, 386, 388, **389, 411,** 562
lumbo-costal, 480
of malleolus, lateral, **308, 322,** 338
of malleus, anterior, 641
  lateral, 636, 641
    superior, 639, 640 (insets)

LIGAMENTS (*cont.*)

medial, of ankle. See "Lig., deltoid"
  of elbow, **49**
  of knee, **293, 294, 298,** 299
metacarpal, transverse; deep, 72
  superficial, 59 (not labelled)
metatarsal, tranverse; deep, 330
  superficial, 325
of neck of rib. See "L., costo-transverse," 431
oblique, posterior, of knee. See "L., popliteal, oblique"
of ovary, **232,** 233, 237.1
  suspensory, 232, **233, 236,** 237
of palm, superficial transverse, 59
palmar (plate; accessory), 72, 96
patellar, 295, **300, 301**
pectineal (Cooper's), 108, **274**
of penis; fundiform, 110
  suspensory, 198.1
perineal, transverse, 201
phrenico-colic, 149
piso-hamate, 71, 72
piso-metacarpal, 72
plantar; (plate; accessory), 330, 331
  calcaneo-navicular, **337,** 339, 341, **342**
  long, 331, **341**
  short [calcaneo-cuboid], 341, **342**
popliteal, oblique, 269
Poupart's. See "Lig., inguinal"
pterygo-mandibular. See "Raphe"
pubic, arcuate (inferior), 217, 236
pubo-prostatic, 194, 203
pubo-vesical, 236 (not labelled)
pulmonary, 415, 416
radiate; sterno-costal, 404
  of head of rib, 410
radio-carpal, palmar, 60, **90**
recto-uterine, 237
reflex inguinal, 109, 110
retinacular (link), 89
round; of head of femur, 281–284
  of liver, **136,** 139, 142
  of uterus—
    inguinal canal, 121, 122
    in labium, 225, 227
    in pelvis, **232, 233**–**238**
sacro-iliac; ventral (anterior), 217
  dorsal (posterior), 273
sacro-spinous, 217, 273
sacro-tuberous, 217, 271, **273**
of skin of fingers, 68, 71.1
spheno-mandibular, **560,** 598
spring. See "Lig., plantar calcaneo-navicular".
sterno-clavicular, 533, 534
sterno-costal, 404
stylo-hyoid, 549, **589, 590,** 597
  ossified, 568
suprascapular [trans. scapular], 25, 26
supraspinous, 385, 386
suspensory of clitoris, 227
  of ovary, 232–237
  of penis, 198.1
talo-calcanean, lateral, 340
  interosseous, 337, **338,** 340
talo-fibular; anterior, 332, **338**
  posterior, 322
talo-navicular (dorsal), 332, 338
tarso-metatarsal, **332,** 339, 341, **342**
temporo-mandibular, 551

LIGAMENTS (*cont.*)

teres; femoris, 281–284
  hepatis, **136,** 139, 142
  uteri. See "Lig., round"
thyro-arytenoid. See "Lig., vocal"
thyro-epiglottic, 625
thyro-hyoid. See "Membrane"
tibio-calcanean, 339
tibio-fibular; anterior inferior, 308, 332, **338**
  inferior transverse, 322
  interosseous, 303 (see text), **334**
  posterior inferior, 322
  superior, 293
tibio-navicular (of deltoid), 339
tibio-talar (of deltoid), 333, 334, 339
transverse; of acetabulum, 284
  of atlas, 562, 563, 565
  of humerus, 36
  metacarpal; deep, 72
    superficial, 59 (not labelled)
  perineal, 201
  metatarsal; deep, 330
    superficial, 325
  of scapula, 25, 26
tibio-fibular, inferior, 322
trapezoid, 36
triangular, of liver, 131, 136, **177**
of tubercle of rib. See "L., costotransverse"
utero-sacral [recto-uterine], 237
of vena cava, left. See "Fold"
venosum, 142
  fissure for, 130, 131.1
vertebral, **385**–**389,** 410, 411
vestibular (ventricular), 632
vocal, **625,** 632
Ligamentum nuchae, **491,** 494
Limbus of fossa ovalis, 443
  of tympanic membrane, 641
Limen nasi, 609
Line or **Linea**—
  alba, 106, 178
  arcuate; of ilium, 221
    of rectus sheath, 106
  aspera, 243
  epiphyseal, of upper end of femur, 282
  gluteal, 273
  intercondylar, of femur, 243
  intertrochanteric, 242, **274**
  myo-hyoid, 553.1
  nuchal; inferior, **485,** 569
    superior, 462, **485**
    supreme, 485, **490**
  oblique; of base of skull, 571.1
    of mandible, 459, **462,** 553.1
    of radius, 1, 2
  pectineal [pecten pubis], 219, **221,** 242
  popliteal. See "Linea, soleal"
  soleal, 243, **315**
  spiral, of femur, 243
  supracondylar; of femur, 243
    of humerus, **1,** 51
  temporal, **462,** 485
  transverse, of base of skull, 571.2
  trochanteric. See "L., intertrochanteric"
Lingula; of lung, **416,** 425
  of mandible, 553.1
Lip of vertebra, cervical, 367
Liver, 125, 134, 136
  bare area, **130.3,** 131

Liver (*cont.*)

Liver (*cont.*)
  corrosion preparations, 137–141
  fissures, sulci, lobes, 125.1, 136, 136.1
  caudate lobe, 125.1, **126** (text), 135, **136**
  peritoneal attachments, 130–131
  porta, **125.1**, 142, 145–148
  sections, 126, 160
  segments, 137, 141
  veins, portal intrahepatic, 138
    hepatic, 137.1, 188.2
Lobule of external ear, 469
Lunate bone. See "Carpus"
  fused with triquetrum, 97
Lung, 414–416
  azygos, lobe of, 457
  broncho-pulmonary segments, 424–427
  hilus, dissection of, 423–423.3
  intrapulmonary bronchi, 417, 420
    vessels, 418, 419, 421, 422
  root of, 428, 429, **450**, 451
Lunule of aortic cusp, 446.2
Lymph Nodes (Glands)—
  abdominal, 165, 189
  auricular; preauricular, 550
    retroauricular (posterior), 467
  axillary, lateral, 22 (not labelled)
  cervical, deep, 494, 533, 535
  colic, epicolic, paracolic, 165
  (of Cloquet) deep inguinal, 254, 281
  cubital (supratrochlear), 44
  cystic, 145
  iliac external, 112 (not labelled), 241
  inguinal; deep, 112, 251
    superficial, 251
  lumbar (lateral aortic), 191.3
  occipital, 24, 477
  pancreatic, 148, **153**, 154
  paracolic, 165
  parasternal, 406 (see text)
  paratracheal, 626
  parotid; deep, 554
    superficial, 467, 554
      (preauricular), 550 (see text)
  submandmibular, 541 (see text)
  submental, 527 (see text)
  tracheobronchial, 450, 452
Lymph vessels inguinal, **251**, 256

Malleolus, 315, 333, 334
Malleus, 635, **638**, 641, **641.1**, 642
Mandible, 459–462, **553**
  at birth, 602
Manubrium sterni, 11, 393
Margin, orbital, 459
Mass, lateral; of atlas, 367, **563**
    of sacrum. See "Sacrum, pars lateralis"
Mastoid bone. See "Temporal bone"
Mater—
  cranial dura, 502, 503, 504
  spinal arachnoid, 482, **484**, 538
  spinal dura, 482–484.1, 538
Maxilla—
  at birth, 602.E, 615.1
  front and side views, 459–462
  in infratemporal fossa, 558
  in palate, **569**, 570
  in walls of nose, 608, 615.2
Meatus—
  acoustic (auditory)—
    external, **461**, 552, 633, **634**
    internal, 497, 512, **644, 648, 648.1**

Meatus (*cont.*)
  of nose, 592, 608–**609**
Mediastinum of thorax—
  diagrams, 412, 413.1
  posterior, 431, 442
  side views, 428, 429
  superior, 448–451
  superior and posterior, 452–455, 457.1
Medulla; of kidney, 183
  oblongata, 609
  spinal. See "Cord, spinal"
Membrane—
  atlanto-occipital—
    anterior, 562
    posterior, 492 (see text)
  costo-coracoid, 14.1
  crico-thyroid. See "Ligament"
  crico-tracheal. See "Ligament"
  crico-vocal, 625, 629, 632
  hyo-epiglottic. See "Ligament"
  intercostal, 405, 409, 410
  interosseous; of forearm, 49, **52**
    of leg, **306, 310**, 332
  obturator, 217, **284**
  perineal; female, 227, **228**
    male, 192, **193, 201**
      on section, 203
  quadrangular, 624, **632**
  tectorial, 562, 565
  thyro-hyoid, **623**, 624, **629**
    at front of neck, 528, 574
  tympanic, 633, **634, 635**, 641
Meninges. See "Mater"
Meniscus of knee, from above, 294
  back, front & sides, 293, 296, 298–302
Mesentery, 162
  root of, cut, 164
  of vermiform appendix, **169**, 235, 237
Meso-appendix, **169**, 235, 137
Mesocolon; sigmond (pelvic), **165**, 202
    root of (female), 233, **235**
  transverse, 134, 164, **165, 176**
Meso-esophagus, 431 (see text)
Mesometrium, 233.1
Mesosalpinx, 232
Mesotendon, 69.1
Mesovarium, 232
Metacarpal bones—
  anterior aspect, 62
  bases, 95
  muscle attachments, 58, 77
  posterior aspect, 86
  separate styloid process, 97
Metatarsal bones, 311–314, **343, 348**
  variations, 349
Midbrain, **506**, 609
Modiolus, 648, 650.1
Mons pubis, 225, 227
Mouth, coronal section of, 591
  floor of, 584, 595
  roof of, 580–582
  side of, 597
Multangular bone. See "Carpus"
  greater. See "Trapezium" 62, 86, 95
  lesser. See "Trapezoid" 62, 86, 95

MUSCLES—
  abductor digiti minimi (quinti) pedis,
    327, **330, 331**
    bony attachments, 314

MUSCLE, abductor (*cont.*)
  digiti minimi (hand), 67, 68, 81
    bony attachments, 58
  hallucis, 327, **330, 331**
    bony attachments, **311**, 314
    posterior part, 321, 322
  pollicis brevis, 61, 67, 68
    bony attachments, 58
  pollicis longus, 78, 79
    insertion, 58, **72**
    near wrist, **66,** 67, 75
    origin, 77
    synovial sheath, 86.1
  adductor brevis (thigh), 261–264
    bony attachments, 265, 266
  hallucis, 314, **330**
  longus, **257–263**, 264
    bony attachments, 265, 266
  magnus, 262–264, **269**, 271
    bony attachments, **266, 276**, 297
    tendinous hiatus, 263.1
  pollicis, **67**, 70, **71**, 74
    bony attachments, 58
  anconeus, 56, **57**, 78
    bony attachments, 77
    fascia on, 31, **56**
    nerve supply, 56.1
  articular, of knee (genus), 298.1
  aryepiglotticus, 628
  arytenoideus, **627**, 628, 632
  auricularis; posterior, 467, 472
    anterior and superior, 467
  axillary arch, 27
  of back, 477–481
    suboccipital region, 490–494
  biceps brachii, 18, 20
    attrition, 28
    bony attachments, 29, 38
    long head, 38, 39, 42
    lower end, **45**, 46, **49**
    short head, 15, 16
    third head, 28
    upper end, 18
  femoris, 267–269, 271
    bony attachments, 265, **266, 295**
    insertion, 300, 302
    lower part, 285, **287**
  brachialis, 20, 34
    bony attachments, 29, 30
    lower end, 45, **46**, 61, 62.1
    upper end, 18, **31**, 33
  brachio-radialis, 59–61, 78
    bony attachments, 58
    at elbow, 45, 46
    lower end, 66
    upper end, 31
  broncho-oesophageal, 451 (see text)
  buccinator, **465**, 467, **559, 574**, 590
    coronal-section, 591
  bulbo-spongiosus (-cavernosus), **192**, 203,
    204
    in female, 227, 228
  caninus. See "M., levator anguli oris"
  chondroglossus, orgin of, 596
  compressor naris, 466
  constrictors of pharynx, 572–574
    inferior, 600, **626**, 627
    middle and superior, 584, 589, **590**
  coraco-brachialis, 15, 16, 18, **20**
    anomaly, 28

MUSCLE, coraco-brachialis (*cont.*)
  bony attachments, 11
  corrugator supercilii, 466, **470**
  cremaster, 110, **111**, 117
    nerve to, 256
    section, 191.6B
    female, 121
  crico-arytenoideus, **627, 628**
  crico-pharyngeus, 622, 626, **627**
  crico-thyroid, **621,** 628
    at front of neck, 528–530
  deltoid, 14, **31,** 474
    anterior aspect, 13, 14
    bony attachments, **11, 30**
    deep relations, 26, **32**
    posterior aspect, 24
    structure, 31.1
  depressor anguli oris, 466, 467, 470
    labii inferioris, 466, 526
    of larynx, **527–529, 542**
  diaphragm, The. See "Diaphragm"
  digastric, 540, **598**
    anterior belly, **527,** 541, **546**
    posterior belly, 540.2, 546, **550–552**
  erector spinae (sacrospinalis), **479,** 480
    cross-section, 178, **481**
  of expression, 466
  extensor carpi radialis brevis, 46, **61, 78**
    bony attachments, 77
    insertion, 78, **87**
    synovial sheath, 86.1
    carpi radialis longus, 61, **78**
    bony attachments, **58,** 77
    insertion, 87
    synovial sheath, 86.1
    upper end, **31,** 46
    carpi ulnaris, **78,** 79
    bony attachments, **58,** 77
    insertion, **71,** 81
    synovial sheath, 86.1
    digiti minimi (V), (hand), 78, 86.1, 87
    digitorum (communis), 78, 79
    bony attachments, 77
    insertion, 88
    near wrist, 86.1, 87
    digitorum brevis, 307–309
    bony origin, 313
    digitorum longus, 304, 305, **307, 310**
    bony origin, 303
    hallucis longus, **305, 307,** 310
    bony attachments, 303, 313
    synovial sheath, 309
    hallucis brevis, **307,** 313
    iliocostalis, 479
    indicis, 77–**79,** 86, **87**
    pollicis brevis, 78, 79
    bony attachments, **76,** 77
    tendon of insertion, **75,** 86.1, 87
    pollicis longus, 78, 79
    bony attachments, 76, 77
    tendon of insertion, 75
  of eyeball, extrinsic, 519–523
  flexor; accessorius [quadratus plantae], 322, **328, 329,** 330
    bony origin, **311,** 314
    carpi radialis, 59
    bony attachments, 58
    at wrist, 66, 72
    carpi ulnaris, 56, 57, **60, 61,** 63
    bony attachments, 58, 77, **82**
    at wrist, **66, 67, 72,** 81

MUSCLES, flexor (*cont.*)
  digiti minimi (foot) V., 314, 327, **331**
  digiti minimi (hand) V., 58, **68,** 71
  digitorum accessorius. See "M., quad-ratus plantae"
  digitorum brevis, 314, **327, 331**
  digitorum longus—
    at ankle, 321, 322
    bony attachments, 314, 316
    in foot, **328,** 329, **331**
    in leg, **310,** 319, **320**
  digitorum profundus, 61, 62.1
    bony attachments, **58, 77**
    insertion, **72,** 88
    synovial sheath, 69
    near wrist, 71
  digitorum superficialis (sublimis), 59, 60
    bony attachments, 58, 62
    insertion, **72,** 88
    synovial sheath, 69
    near wrist, 66, 71
  hallucis brevis, 314, 330, **331**
  hallucis longus—
    at ankle, 321, 322
    bony attachments, **314, 316**
    in foot, 325–331
    in leg, **310, 319,** 320
  pollicis brevis, 61, **67, 68**
    bony attachments, 58
  pollicis longus, 61, 62.1
    bony attachments, 58
    synovial sheath, 69
    in wrist and hand, 60, 66, **71**
  frontalis, **466,** 470, 498.1
  gastrocnemius, 310, **317**
    bony attachments, 288, 295, **316**
    upper end, 285–287, 302
  gemelli, 271, 272
    bony attachments, 266, 276.1
  genio-glossus, 548, 592, **595,** 597
  genio-hyoid, **545,** 548, 592, 595, **599**
  glosso-palatinus. See "M., palatoglossus"
  gluteus; maximus, 264, **267**
    bony attachments, 266
    bounding perineum, 192
    deep relations, 270, 271
    pelvic aspect, 217
    medius, 267–271
    aponeurotic origin, 272.1
    bony attachments, 266
    insertion, 276.1
    minimus, **271,** 284
    bony attachments, 265, **266, 276.1**
  gracilis, **262,** 263, 264
    bony attachments, 276, 297
    lower part, 285, **298,** 320
    upper part, 258, 259
  hyo-glossus, 546–548, 574, 589, 590
  hypothenar, 67, **68,** 70, **71**
  iliacus, 261
    bony attachments, 265
    in femoral triangle, 258, 259
    in iliac fossa, 190
  ilio-coccygeus, 194, 209, 230.1
  ilio-costalis, 479, 481
  incisive, 470
  infraspinatus, **32,** 33, 39
    bony attachments, 30
  intercostalis; externus, 405, 406, **408, 409**
    innermost, 405, 410

MUSCLES, intercostalis (*cont.*)
  internus, 405–409
  interossei; of foot, 307, **331**
    of hand, **72,** 87
    bony attachments, **58,** 76, **77**
    insertion, 88
    1st dorsal, see also **67,** 70, 75, **79**
  interspinales, **481, 493,** 538
  intertransverse, **480,** 481, **538,** 561
  ischio-cavernosus, 192
    in female, 227
  kerato-cricoid (text), 624
  latissimus dorsi, **24**
    in axilla, 15, 17, 18
    on cross-section, 431, 481
    insertion, 11
    in lumbar region, 107, 173
  levator; anguli oris, 470
    ani—
      from above, 209
      from below, 192, **194**
      coronal section, 205
      in female, 230, 231, 241
      median section, 203, 204
    costae, 409, **411,** 479
    glandulae thyroideae, 539
    labii superioris, **466,** 470 (see text)
    labii superioris alaeque nasi, **466,** 470
    palati, **574–577, 586–588, 639,** 641.1
    palpebrae, 470, **471.2,** 517, **520**
    prostatae, 194, 209
    scapulae, 24, 25, 477, **478,** 561
    nerve supply, 473, 474
    scapular attachment, 30
  of limbs—
    lower, list of, 251
    upper, list of, 10
  longissimus, **479,** 491
    cross-section, 481
  longus; capitis, 561
    colli (cervicis), 428, 561
  lumbricales; of foot, 327, **328**
    of hand, **61,** 68
    insertion, 88
  masseter, 465–467
    cross-section, 551, 579, **591**
  of mastication, nerves, 654
  mentalis, 466, **470**
  multifidus, **480,** 481, 493
  mylohyoid—
    front of neck, **544,** 545, **546,** 547
    from within mouth, 590, 598, **599**
    on section, **547, 591,** 595
  obliquus; abdominis externus, **105–109, 173,** 174, 406
    abdominis internus, **106,** 110, 125, 173
    capitis, inferior, 490, **492,** 494
    superior, 490, **492**
    oculi inferior, **519,** 522.1, 525
    superior, **519–**522.1, 525
  obturator externus, 271, **272, 274**
    bony origin, 276
    grooving femur, 276.1
    internus, **272, 281**
    in pelvis, **216**
    in buttock, 268–271, 275
    insertion, 276.1
  occipitalis, 477, **490**
  occipito-frontalis, 458
  omohyoid, 542
    inferior belly, 25, **474,** 533

Muscles (*cont.*)

MUSCLES, omohyoid (*cont.*)
    superior belly, 527, **528,** 541
  opponens digiti minimi, 58, **61,** 68, 81
    pollicis, 58, 61, **68**
  orbicularis; oculi, 466, 467
    pars lacrimalis, 471.1
    oris, 470
  palato-glossus, 588, 589
  palato-pharyngeus, 588, 589
  palmaris brevis, 59, **67**
    longus, **59,** 66, 67
  papillary, 444–446
  pectinati, 443
  pectineus, 258–260, 263, **274**
    bony attachments, 276, 276.1
  pectoralis major, **13, 14,** 107
    abdominal part, 105, 106
    anomaly, 27
    in axilla, 15, 16
    bony attachments, 11
    insertion, 16, 17
    minor, **14–16, 406**
    anomaly, 27
    bony attachments, 11
    insertion, 19
  perineal, deep transverse. See "Dia-
    phragm, urogenital"
    superficial, **192,** 227
  peroneus brevis, **304, 306**
    at ankle, **308,** 322
    bony attachments, **303, 313, 316**
    on cross-section, 310
    synovial sheath, 309
    digiti quinti, 306
    longus, **304,** 306, **310**
    bony attachments, 303, 314
    on side of foot, **308,** 322
    in sole, 308, **341**
    synovial sheath, 309
    tertius, 304, **305,** 310
    bony attachments, 303, 313
    on foot, 308, 309
  pharyngeal, 573, **574, 588–590,** 627
  pharyngo-palatinus. See "M., palato-
    pharyngeus"
  piriformis—
    bony insertion, 276.1
    in buttock, 268–271, **273**
    in pelvis, 209, 213, **216**
  plantaris, 286–288, **310**
  platysma, 13, 467, **470,** 472, **526**
  popliteus, 287, **302,** 320
    bony attachments, 288, 295
    tendon of, 294, 296, 301
  prevertebral, 561
  procerus, 466, **470**
  pronator quadratus, 59, **72**
    bony attachments, 58
    teres, 46, **59**
    bony attachments, **58,** 77
    deep relations, 60
    insertion, **62.1,** 79
  psoas major—
    in abdomen, 179, **190,** 256
    on cross-section, **178,** 481
    insertion, 275, 276.1
    in thigh, 259–261
    minor, 260
  pterygoid; lateral, 559, 579
    medial, 547, 559, **560,** 584, **598**
  pubo-coccygeus, 209, 216

MUSCLES, pubo-coccygeus (*cont.*)
  from below, 193
  medial aspect, 204
  female, 230, 231
  pubo-rectalis, **194,** 196, 203, **204**
    female, 230
  pubo-vaginalis, 229, 230
  quadratus femoris, 268–271, **273**
    bony attachments, 276, 276.1
    labii inferioris. See "M., depressor
     labii inferioris"
    labii superioris. See "M., levator labii
     superioris"
    lumborum, 175, 179, **190, 480,** 481
    plantae, 311, 314, 322, **328,** 329
  quadriceps femoris, 261, 301
    See also "M., rectus femoris & vasti"
  rectus abdominis, **105,** 406
    lower end of, 125
    sheath of, 105, 106, 178
    capitis anterior, 561
    capitis lateralis, **495,** 561
    capitis posterior, 490, **492,** 494
    of eyeball, 517–523
    femoris, **260,** 263
    bony origin, 276
    upper part, 259, 274, **284**
    on section, 264, 281
  rhomboid major, 24, **478**
    scapular insertion, 30
    minor, 24, **478**
  rotatores, 411, 493
  sacro-spinalis. See "M., Erector Spinae"
  salpingo-pharyngeus, 588
  sartorius, 256–259, **260,** 263, 264
    bony attachments, 265, 297
    insertion, 298, 320
  scalenus—
    anterior, **531,** 535, **536,** 561
    in posterior triangle, 473–475
    medius, 473–475, **536,** 561
    minimus, 537, **567**
    posterior, 406, 474, **475**
  semimembranosus, 264, 267, **268**
    bony attachments, **266, 288,** 297
    in thigh, 270, 271
    insertion, **262,** 298, **302**
    in popliteal region, 285–287
  semitendinosus, 264, 267, **268**
    bony attachments, **266,** 276, 297
    in thigh, 270, 271
    insertion, **262,** 298
    popliteal region, 285–287
  serratus anterior, 13, **22, 23, 478**
    in axilla, 15–18, 107
    in posterior triangle, 474
    bony attachments, **11, 29**
    posterior inferior, 173, 478
    posterior superior, 478
  soleus, 310, 317, **318,** 319
    bony attachments, **288,** 316
    insertion, 329
    upper end, 286, **287**
    cross section, 310
  sphincter ani externus, **192, 193, 194,** 196
    median section, 203, **204**
    ani internus, 193, **194, 196**

MUSCLES, sphincter (*cont.*)
  pyloric, 128
  urethrae, 203
    female, 230, 230.1
  spinalis, 479
  splenius capitis, 473, **479,** 494
    cervicis, **479**
  stapedius, 636
  sternalis, 27
  sterno-hyoid, **528, 529,** 542
    origin of, 406, **407**
  sterno-mastoid, **473,** 527, 541, **542**
    origin of, 11, 406
  sterno-thyroid, 528, **529,** 542
    origin of, 406, **407**
  stylo-glossus, **548,** 572, 584, **589**
  stylo-hyoid, 542, **551, 552,** 574, 584
  stylo-pharyngeus, 549, **572,** 577, 584, **589**
  subclavius, **16,** 406, 474, **475**
  subcostal, 410
  subscapularis, 15, 17, **18,** 33
    bony attachments, 11, 29
    on cross-section, 22
  supinator, 46, 61, **62.1**
    bony insertion, 58, 77
    posterior aspect, 57, **79**
  supraspinatus, 25, **26**
    attrition, 42
    bony attachments, 29, 30
  synergist, 86.3
  tarsal, 471.2
  temporalis, **465, 551,** 559
    on section, 560, 579, 591
  tensor fasciae latae, **259,** 261
    palati, 575, 577, 588, **590**
    course, 619.2 (see text)
    tympani, 641, 641.1, 641.2
    veli palantini. See "M., tensor palati"
  teres major, **32,** 33
    anterior aspect, 15, 17, **18,** 20
    bony attachments, 29, 30
    minor, 32, 33
    bony attachments, 30
    at shoulder joint, 39
  thenar, 68–70
  of thumb, "outcropping," 78, 79
  thyro-arytenoid, 628
  thyro-epiglottic, 628
  thyro-hyroid, **529,** 541, **542**
  tibialis anterior, 304, **305**
    at ankle, **307, 309,** 332
    bony attachments, **303,** 311, **314**
    insertion, **329, 341**
    section at midleg, 310
    posterior, 310, 320
    bony insertion, 311, 314
    bony origin, 303
    tendon of, **321,** 322, 329, **341**
    section at midleg, 310
  of tongue, intrinsic, 592, 595
  transversus abdominis, **106,** 111, 407, **408**
    posterior part, 174, 190
    on section, 125
    thoracis, 406, 407
    perinei profundus. See "Diaphragm
     urogenital"
    perinei superficialis, 192, 227
  trapezius, 24, 25, **472**
    bony insertion, **11,** 30
  triangularis. See "M., depressor anguli
    oris"

MUSCLES (*cont.*)

triceps brachii, 20, **31–33**
  bony attachments, **30, 38**
  lower end, 56
  section at midarm, 34
vastus intermedius, **261,** 263, 264
  bony attachments, 265, 266
  lateralis, 260, **261,** 263, **264**
    bony attachments, **265, 266,** 276.1
    insertion, 296
  medialis, 260, **261,** 263, **264**
    bony attachments, **265, 266,** 276.1
    insertion, 298
vocalis, 629
zygomaticus major, **466,** 467, **470**
  minor, 470 (see text)

Naris. See "Nostril"
Nasal bones, 459, 461, **464,** 605, **608**
Nasion, 460, 461
Navicular bone, 311–314
  facets, 343, 345, 346
Neck—"the";
  front of, 526–530, 543
  landmarks, 540.1
  parotid region, 550, 551
  deep to parotid region, 552, 577
    root of, **449,** 531–537, **561**
  sections, cross-, 494, 535, 584, 600
    median, 458
  triangles of, 540
    anterior, 541, 542
    posterior, 472–476
Neck—
  of femur, **243,** 275, 279
  of fibula, 242, **315**
  of humerus, 1
  of mandible, 462, **553,** 557
  of radius, 51
  of rib, **398,** 411
  of tooth, 601

NERVES

of abdominal wall; anterior, 105–107
  posterior, 24, 173–175
abducent (*VI*)—
  in post. fossa, **506,** 565, **643**
  in mid fossa & orbit, 513, **514,** 516, 521
to abductor hallucis, 321
accessory (*XI*)—
  in anterior triangle, **541, 542, 550,** 551
  at base of skull, 561, **573**
  deep to parotid bed, **552,** 577
  distribution of, 660, **661**
  piercing dura, 564, 565
  and jugular vein, 566.2
  in posterior triangle, **472–474,** 540
  superficial origin, 495, 506
  supply trapezius, 24, **25**
acoustic (auditory). See "N. vestibulo-
    cochlear," 495, 506, 565, 648
  scheme of, 658
to adductor magnus, 270, 271
alveolar (dental) **559, 560, 655, 656**
to anconeus, 56.1
auricular; great **467, 472,** 541
  posterior, **467,** 550
auriculo-temporal—
  in infratemporal fossa, 560
  in parotid region, 550, 552
  in temporal region, 466, **467, 470.1,** 500

NERVES (*cont.*)

axillary (circumflex), **17–19, 32,** 33, 39
of back, 24
to biceps femoris, 270, 271
buccal; of facial, 467
  of mandibular, 470, 470.1, 559, **560**
to bulbo-spongiosus, 205
calcanean, medial, 249, **325**
cardiac, 449, 450
carotid, internal, 514.1, 641.1
carotid sinus, 659, 660
caudal, anterior, 213
cervical—
  roots and rami, 476, **538**
    dorsal rami, 480, 483
    ventral rami, 454, **561**
  1st nerve, 564, 565
    (cutaneous br.), 491, 492
  1st and 2nd nerves, **495,** 564
  of facial nerve, 467, **472**
  cervical plexus, 561
  in anterior triangle, 526
  in posterior triangle, 472–476
  in suboccipital region, 490–492, 495
  in upper limb, 7, 8, **13**
chorda tympani—
  distribution of, 593, **657**
  in neck, **560,** 590, 598
  in tympanum, **641**
ciliary, 520, 523.6
circumflex. See "N., axillary"
to clitoris, 228
to coccygeus, 213
to coraco-brachialis, 16
cranial—
  piercing dura mater, 495, 505, **565**
  schemes of, 651–662
  superficial origins, 506
  see also individual nerves
to cremaster, 256
cutaneous—
  of abdomen, 105–107, 173–175
  of arm, **7, 8,** 32
  of back, 24
  of face, 470
  of foot, 248, 325
  of forearm, **7, 8,** 44
  of hand, 7, 8, **68,** 70, **83–85**
    variations, **85,** 97
  of lower limbs, 248, 249, 325
  of neck, 472, 477, 526
  palmar, 7, 84
  of scalp, 500
  of thigh (femoral cutaneous), **248,** 249
    intermediate, 258
    lateral, 190, **256,** 258
    medial, 258
    posterior, 270, 271
      perineal branch of, **192,** 205, **226**
  of thorax, 13, 107
  of trunk, 13, 15, **24,** 105, **107**
  of upper limb, 7, 8
dental. See "N. alveolar"
descendens; cervicalis. See "Ansa cervi-
    calis, inf, root"
  hypoglossi. See "Ansa cervicalis, sup.
    root"
to digastric, 552
digital; of foot, 325, 327
  of hand, 67, **68,** 70, 83
dorsal; of penis, **199–201, 215,** 216

NERVES, dorsal (*cont.*)

scapular. See "N. to rhomboids"
erigentes. See "N. splanchnic, pelvic"
ethmoidal; anterior, 520, **521,** 606
  posterior, 521
to extensor digitorum brevis, 305
of face; motor, 467
  sensory, 470
facial (*VII*)—
  scheme of, 657
  in cranial cavity, 495, **506, 565**
  in temporal bone, **637,** 639, **641, 648**
  in parotid region, **550,** 552, **577**
  on face, 467
  cervical branch, 467, **472,** 541
  secretomotor fibers, 547.1
femoral; in iliac fossa, 179, **190, 256**
  in thigh, 263
to flexor carpi ulnaris, **57,** 61
to flexor digitorum profundus, 61
to flexor pollicis brevis, 68
frontal, **513,** 516, 520
gastric, 133
to gastrocnemius, 286
genito-femoral; in abdomen, 190, 202
  genital & femoral brs., 248, 256
gingival, 559, 560
  diagram of, 655, 656
glosso-pharyngeal (*IX*)—
  scheme of, 659
  superficial origin, 506
  piercing dura, 564, **565**
  pit for ganglion, 497
  in the neck, **552,** 572–574
  at bed of tonsil, 589
  to tongue, 593
gluteal; inferior, 213, **270**
  superior, 213, **271**
to glutei, 213, 270, 271
to gums. See "N., gingival"
hemorrhoidal, inferior. See "N. rectal
    inferior," 192, 215, 216
hypoglossal (*XII*)—
  scheme of, 662
  superficial origin, 506
  in cranial cavity, 564, 565
  at base of skull, 561, 573
  deep to parotid bed, 552
  in triangles of neck, **542,** 550–552
  in floor of mouth, 547, **548,** 590, 597
iliohypogastric; ventral br., **106,** 110, **111**
  lateral cutaneous br., 107, **173,** 249
  dorsal part, **174,** 190
ilio-inguinal; ventral branch, 105, **110,
    111,** 253
  dorsal part, 179, **190**
infra-orbital, **470,** 560, 560.2, 655
infratrochlear, **470,** 470.1, 520, **521**
intercostal, 405–410, 428–430
  cutaneous branches, 13, 24, **105, 107**
intercosto-brachial, **7, 8,** 13, **15,** 107
internal carotid, 514.1, 641.1
interosseous of forearm; anterior, 61,
    62.1, 63
  posterior, **46,** 61, **79**
labial, posterior, 226
lacrimal, 470, **513,** 516, 520, 560.2
laryngeal; external, 529, **530,** 532, 542
  branches to inferior constrictor, 626
  internal, **542,** 574, 626–**628**
  recurrent—

NERVES, laryngeal, recurrent (*cont.*)
    anomalous right nerve, 532
    left nerve in thorax, 433, 449–**451**
    in neck; left, 530, **534**
        right, 531, 626
        within larynx, 627, 628
    superior, **622**, 660 (see text)
  to latissimus dorsi, 15, 17, 18
  to levator ani, 204–**209**, 213
  to levator scapulae, 473, 474
  lingual—
    in infratemporal fossa, 559, **560**
    viewed from neck, 544, **547, 548**
    viewed from mouth, **590, 593, 597**
  lower limb—
    cutaneous distribution, 248, 249, 325
    motor distribution, 250
  lumbar, 190
    dorsal rami, 24
  lumbo-inguinal. See "N. genitofemoral, femoral br."
  to lumbricals of hand, 68, 72
  mandibular (V³), 513, 560, 620.1
    scheme of, 654, 656
  to masseter, **551**, 559, **560**
  maxillary (V²)—
    scheme of, 654–656
    at origin, 513
    in pterygo-palatine fossa, 560.2, 620.1
    branches, superficial, 470, 470.1
    nasal and palatine, 582, 583, **606**
  median, 9, 19
    in arm, 20
    in axilla, 16, 19
    at elbow, 45, **46**, 55
    in forearm, 60, 61
    in hand, 67, 68
    at wrist, 66
      variation, 28, 47, 97
  mental, **470**, 470.1, 656
  musculo-cutaneous, of arm, 9, 19
    in arm, **18**, 20
      variation, 28
    in axilla, 16, 18
    near elbow, 44–**46**
  musculo-cutaneous, of leg. See "N. peroneal, superficial"
  mylo-hyoid, 542, **546**, 560, 598
  nasal; external, **470**, 470.1, **606**
    internal, 606
  naso-ciliary, **514**, 516, **521**
  naso-palatine, 582, 583, **606.1**
  to obliquus abdominis externus, 13, **107**
  obturator; in abdomen, 190
    accessory, 190
    cutaneous branches, 248, 249
    in pelvis, **210, 213**, 216
    in thigh, 258, **263**, 264, 274
  to obturator internus, **213, 270**
  occipital—
    greater, 24, 472, 477, **490–492**, 500
    lesser, **472**, 477, 500
    third, **477**, 500
  oculo-motor (III)—
    at base of brain, 505, **506**
    leaving dura, 565
    in middle fossa, 513, **514**
    in orbital cavity, 520, **521**, 525
    distribution, 653
  olfactory (I), 606
    distribution, 651

NERVES (*cont.*)
  ophthalmic (V¹), 513–516
    cutaneous branches, 470, **470.1**, 500
  optic (II), 520, 521
    in cranial cavity, **506**, 513, 516
    in orbital cavity, 471.2, 522.1, 525
    of orbit, motor, 525
  palatine, 582, 583, 592, 606
  to palato-glossus, 593
  to pectorales, 14, 16
  to penis, 199, 201
  perineal, **192, 215**
    branch of fourth sacral, 192, (213)
    branch of post. cutan. of thigh, **192, 226**, 249, **271**
  peroneal; common (popliteal, lateral), **285–287, 303, 304**
    deep & superficial, 303–306, 310
    cutaneous branches, 248, 249, 285
  petrosal; greater (superf), **513**, 514, 620.1
    hiatus and canal for, 512, 648
    distribution, 547.1, 657
    lesser (superficial), 513, 648
    distribution, 513.2, 659
  pharyngeal, of maxillary n., 560.2
    distribution, 606
  phrenic—
  in neck, **473–475, 531**, 533, 536, **561**
    at root of neck, 449
    in thorax, **428, 429**, 431, 432
  to piriformis, 213
  plantar, 321, 325, 327
  to platysma, 467
  popliteal—
    lateral. See "N., peroneal, common"
    medial. See "N., tibial"
  to popliteus, 286, 287, **320**
  presacral. See "Plexus, hypogastric inferior"
  of pterygoid canal (Vidian), **560.2**
    cross section, 641.1
    scheme, 657
  to pterygoid, lateral, 560
  pudendal, 213, 241, 270
    diagram of, 215
  to quadratus femoris, 213
  to quadratus plantae, 330
  radial; in axilla, 17, **18**, (see text), 19
    in arm, 32, 33
    deep branch. See "N., inteross. of forearm, posterior"
    at elbow, 46, 55
    in forearm, 60, **61**
    in hand, cutaneous, 7, 8, **83**
    superficial branch, 46, 59, 61, 66, 73
    at wrist, 59, 73
  rami—
    ventral (anterior); spinal—
      cervical, 476, **495, 538, 561**
      lumbar, 483
      scheme of, 405
    communicantes (sympathetic);
      neck, 561
      abdomen, 189, 190
      pelvis, 213
      thorax, 428, 429
    dorsal (posterior); spinal—
      cervical, 476, 495, **538**
      cutaneous branches, 477
      lumbar and sacral, 480, 483
      thoracic, 409, **411**

NERVES (*cont.*)
  rectal, inferior, **192**, 215, 216
  to rectus femoris, 263
  recurrent. See "N., laryngeal, recurrent"
  to rhomboids, 25.2, **473**, 474
  sacral, 204, **213**, 216
    perineal branch of fourth, **192**, 230.1
    dorsal rami, 249
  saphenous, **248**, 249, **263, 321**
  to sartorius, 263
  of scalp, 500
  sciatic—
    arterial supply, 280
    in buttock, 273
    in pelvis, 213
    and piriformis, 323
    in thigh, 264, 270, 271
  scrotal, posterior, 192
  segmental (spinal)—
    cervical, 538, 538.1
    thorax & abdomen, 13.1, 405
    lower limb, 663, 665
    upper limb, 663, 664
  to semimembranosus, 270
  to semitendinosus, 270
  sensory. See "N., cutaneous"
  to serratus anterior, in neck, 473, **475**
    in axilla, 15, 17, 18, **23**, 107
  sinus, carotid, 659, 660
  to soleus, 286
  spermatic, external. See "N., genitofemoral, genital br."
  spheno-palatine, long. See "N., nasopalatine"
  spinal, 13.1, 538.1
  spinal accessory. See "N., accessory"
  splanchnic; in thorax 410, **428, 429**
    in abdomen, 190, 191.3
    in pelvis, 204, 210, **213**, 214
  to sternomastoid. See "N., accessory"
  to stylo-hyoid, 552
  subcostal, 107, **173–175, 190**
  to subscapularis, 15, 18
  suboccipital (dorsal br. of C.1) 490–492
  supraclavicular, 7, 8, **13, 472**, 526
  supra-orbital, **470**, 513, 520
    diagrams of, 470.1, 500
  suprascapular, 17, 25, 32, **475**
  supratrochlear, 470, 470.1
  sural, 249
    near ankle, 246, 247
    in popliteal fossa, 285, 286
  sympathetic trunk. See "Tr. sympathetic"
  to temporalis, 559, 560
  tentorii, 572
  to teres major, 15, 17, 18
    minor, 32
  to thenar muscles, 66
  thoracic; diagram of, 405. See also "Nn. intercosal & subcostal"
    long. See "N. to serratus anterior"
  thoracodorsal. See "N. to latissimus dorsi"
  to thyro-hyoid, **542, 546**
  tibial; (medial popliteal), 285–287
    (posterior tibial), 310, 319–322
    cutaneous branches, **249**, 285, 321
  of tongue, 593
  to trapezius, **24**, 25, 473 (see text)
  to triceps brachii, **15**, 17, 18, 20, **33**

NERVES (*cont.*)
  trigeminal (V)—
    cutaneous branches, **470,** 470.1, 500
    distribution, 654–656
    groove for, 497, 565, 643
    in middle cranial fossa, 513, 514
    in post. cranial fossa, 495, 565, **643**
    superficial origin, 506
  trochlear (IV), 513, 514–516
    at base of brain, 505, 506
    distribution, 653
    leaving dura, 565
    in orbital cavity, **520,** 521
    superficial origin, 495
  tympanic, 636, 641.1
    distribution, 659
  ulnar, 9, 19
    in arm, 20
    in axilla, 16, 19
    at elbow, 46, 55–**57**
    in forearm, 60, 61, 63
    in hand, 66–68, 72
      dorsal branch, 80, 83
    at wrist, 64, 67
      variation, 97
  upper limb—
    motor distribution, 9, 10
    cutaneous distribution, 7, 8
  vagus (X)—
    distribution, 660
    superficial origin, 495, 506
    piercing dura, 565
    in neck—
      at base of skull, 561, 573
      deep to parotid bed, 552
      in anterior triangle, **530, 531, 550–**
        552
    in thorax—
      left, 429
      right, 428
      in superior mediastinum, 433, 449,
        450
      in posterior mediastinum, 442
    in abdomen, 133, 180
    to vasti, 263
  vestibulocochlear, VIII (acoustic), 495,
    506, 565, 648
    scheme of, 658
  zygomatic, 560.2
    zygomatico-facial, 470, 560.2
    zygomatico-temporal, 470.1, **551,** 560.2
Nipple, 12, 107
Node—
  lymph. See "Lymph nodes"
  atrioventricular [a.v.], 445.1
  sinu-atrial, 445.1
Nose—
  anterior [piriform] aperture, 461, 464A
  buttresses of, 464
  nasal cartilages, 468, 605
  nasal cavity, 459, 605–612
  posterior aperture [choana], 569, 578
Nostril, 468, 609–611 (not labelled)
Notch. See also "Incisura"
  acetabular, 276
  angular, of stomach, 127
  cardiac; of lung, 414, **414.1,** 416
    of stomach, 127
  clavicular, of sternum, 393
  costal, 393
  fibular, of tibia, 303

Notch (*cont.*)
  interarytenoid, 578
  intercondylar, of femur, 243, 293
  jugular (suprasternal), **11, 393,** 528
  mandibular, 553, 557
  mastoid, 485
  radial, of ulna, 51, **53**
  sacro-coccygeal, 374
  sciatic, greater & lesser, 222, 243
  semilunar, of ulna. See "N., trochlear"
  of stomach, 127
  supra-orbital. See "Foramen"
  suprasternal, **11, 393,** 528
  thyroid, 621
  trochlear; of frontal, 518
    of ulna, 51, **52,** 53
  ulnar, of radius, 52
  vertebral, 358
Nucleus pulposus, 384, 386

Occipital bone—
  anomalies, 487–489
  at birth, 485.1
  inner surface, 507, **508,** 512
  outer surface, 462, **485, 569**
Oesophagus, Esophagus—
  arterial supply, 454
  in neck; right and left sides, 532, 534
    cross-section, 535, 536
  in thorax, 450–452
    cross-section, 430, 431
    behind pericardium, 442
    pleural aspect, 428, 429
  in abdomen, 125, 126, 134, 135
    hiatus, 179, 191
Olecranon, 2, 49–56
Olive, 506
Omentum, greater, **125,** 126, 164
  lesser, **126,** 136
    diagram of, 130
Opening. See also "**Orifice, Foramen,** and
    Hiatus"
  in diaphragm, 191
  saphenous, 106, **110,** 253–256
  tendinous (in adductor magnus), 263.1
Orbit (orbital cavity)—
  bony, 459, 518
  contents, 519–525
  cone of muscles, 471.2, 517 (see **text**)
  section; coronal, 516, 517
    sagittal, 471.2
Orifice—
  aortic, **436, 445,** 446.1, .2, .3
  of appendix, 170
  atrio-ventricular, 443–445 (see **text**)
  cardiac, of stomach, 128, 129
  ileo-cecal, 170
  of naso-lacrimal duct, 610, 612
  of pharyngeal tube, 609, **639**
  of pulmonary trunk, **436, 444,** 446.3
  pyloric, 128
  urethral, female, 227, **228, 236**
    male—
      external, 199.1, 203
      internal, 203, 208
  of uterus (external), 232, 236
  of vagina, 227, **230**
Os; acetabuli, 278
  acromiale, 40
  coxae. See "Hip bone"
  Incae, 488

Os (*cont.*)
  Japonicum, 557.1
  trigonum, 356
Ossicles of ear, 633, 636, **638,** 642
  suprasternal, 567
Ossification. See also "Epiphyses"—
  acetabulum, 278
  acromion, 40, 100
  hip bone, in youth, 277, 278
  jugum sphenoidale, 507.1
  limb, lower, 350–355
    upper, 98–104
  mandible, at birth, 602
  maxilla, at birth, 602
  occipital bone, at birth, 485.1
  sacrum, in youth, 373.1
  skull, at birth, 602
  sphenoid, lesser wings, 507.1
  spheno-occipital synostosis, 511
  sternum, in youth, 394
  temporal bone, in childhood, 645–647
  vertebra, in childhood, 359, 360
Ostium; maxillary, **608.1,** 612, 616.2, **618**
  pelvic, of uterine tube, 232
Ovary, **232,** 235, **236,** 237.1

Pacchionian bodies. See "Granulations,
    arachnoid"
Pad of fat; buccal (sucking), 470
  "pericardiaco-phrenic," 428, 429, 431
  synovial—
    at ankle & foot, 337, 338
    at elbow, 53, 55
    at hip, 282
    at knee, 299
    at shoulder, 37, 39
    at vertebrae, **385,** 538
    at wrist & hand, 91, 93
Palate, 458, 581–583
  bony, 580
    hard, 581
    coronal section, 591, 592
  soft, 578
    median section, 586, **587–590**
Palatine bone; from behind, 619.2
  from below, 570, **580**
  nasal aspect, 605, **608,** 615.3
Palm, 59, 61, 65–72
Palpebrae. See "Eyelids"
Pancreas, 134, 135, **153, 154**
  arteries, 158, 159
  ducts, 156, 157
  relations, 147–151, 176, 177
Papilla; duodenal, 168
  renal, 183
  of tongue, 587, **594**
Parathyroid. See "Gland, parathyroid"
Parietal bone, 461, 485, 507
Passages, bile. See "Bile passages"
Patella, **242,** 260, 299, **300**
  bipartite, 323
Pecten pubis, 219, **221**
  of anal canal, 196.1
Pedicle of vertebra, 358, 388
Peduncle, middle cerebellar, 506
Pelvis—
  false (greater), 218–221
  female; bones, 220–221
    floor of, 231
    from above, 233
    from in front, 234, 235, 241

Pelvis, *female (cont.)*
cross-section, 191.6
median section, 236–240
vessels on side wall, 238
walls, 217
male; bones, 218, 219
coronal section, 205
cross-section, 191.6
from above, 202
floor, 209
median section, 203, 204
orientation, 221.1
of kidney, 182, 183
varieties of, 187
Penis, 197–201, 203
ligaments; fundiform, 110
suspensory, 198.1
Perforation, sternal, 396, 404
Pericardium—
diaphragmatic surface, 431
front view, 414, **432,** 448
interior of, 434, 435, **441**
posterior relations, 442
side view, 428, 429
Perichondrium, costal, 404, 406 (text)
Perineum, female, 224–230
male, 192–201
Peritoneum—
diagrams of, 130–131
of hepato-renal pouch, 130.3, 147
of lesser sac. See "Bursa, omental"
of pelvis; female, 233–236
male, 202–204
of posterior abdominal wall, 176, 177
Petrous bone. See "Temporal bone"
Phalanges; of foot, 311–314
of hand, **62, 86,** 96
Pharynx—
interior of, **578,** 587, 627
posterior view, **572,** 573, 626
section, cross-, 579, 584, 600
side view, 574
tonsil & bed, 585–590
Pinna. See "Auricle of ear"
Pisiform bone. See "Carpus"
Plane, transpyloric, 104.2
Plate. See also "**Lamina**"
cribrosa (cribriform), **458,** 464, 508, **618.2**
horizontal, of palatine bone, 570, **580**
hyaline, of vertebra, **385,** 386
orbital, of frontal bone, 507, 617
palmar. See "Lig. palmar", 72, 96
perpendicular; of ethmoid, **605,** 614
of palatine bone, **608,** 615.3
pterygoid. See "Lamina"
tympanic, **558,** 569
vertical. See "P., perpendicular"
Platysma, 13, 467, **470,** 472, **526**
Pleura—
abdominal relations, 149
apical relations, 430
cervical relations, 450, 451, 561
diaphragmatic relations, 431
mediastinal relations, 428, 429
reflexions, 413.2
scheme of, 412.1
Plexus—
nerve; brachial, 16–**19,** 473–**476,** 561
cardiac. See "Nerve, cardiac"
celiac (ganglion), 179, **180,** 191.3
cervical, 561. See also "Nerve, cervical"

Plexus, nerve *(cont.)*
coccygeal, 213
esophageal, **428,** 442 (see text)
hypogastric, superior (presacral nerve), 165, 235
inferior (pelvic plexus), 240
lumbar, 190
phrenic, 179, 180
pulmonary; anterior, 433, **449,** 450,
posterior, 428 (not labelled)
renal, 180
sacral, 213
venous; prostatic, 208
vertebral, 390, 491–**494** (see text), 600
vesical, 208, 241 (see text)
Plica. See also "**Fold**"
semilunaris of tonsil, 585
sublingualis, 592, **597**
triangularis of tonsil, 585
Pocket. See "Pouch"
Pole of skull, posterior, 485
Pons, 506, 609
Porta hepatis, 126, **136, 142,** 145–148
pedis, 322 (see text)
Pouch. See also "Fossa & Recess"—
hepato-renal (of Morison), 147
mucous of tympanum, 641, **642,** 648
perineal; deep, 205 (see text)
superficial (Colles), 192
recto-uterine (Douglas), 233, 236
recto-vesical (in male), 202, 203
subphrenic, 130.3
vesico-uterine, 233, 236
Prepuce; of clitoris, 227
of penis, 199, 203
Premaxilla, 580
Process—
accessory, of vertebra, **366,** 369, 371
alveolar, 459
of calcaneum. See "Tubercle"
clinoid; anterior, **508, 513–515**
posterior, **512–514**
cochleariformis, **637,** 641.2, 646, 650.1
coracoid, 1, 16, 26
coronoid; of mandible, 462, **553,** 557
of ulna, 1, 49, **51–53,** 55
"digital of fat", 225–227
frontal; of maxilla, 459, **462,** 464A, **608**
of zygoma, 459, 462
jugular, 495, 561, **570**
mammillary, **366,** 369, 371
mastoid—
from behind, 485
from below, 569
side view, 461, 551
odontoid, of axis. See "Dens"
olecranon, 49–56
palatine, of maxilla, 569, **570**
paramastoid, 487
post-auditory, 645
pterygoid, 619.1
function of, 463
pyramidal, of palatine bone, **558,** 580, **619.2**
spinous. See "Vertebra"
styloid—
of fibula. See "Head, apex of"
of radius, 1, **52,** 90–94
of temporal bone—
from below, **570,** 571.1
with relations, **552,** 572, 577, 579

Process, *styloid,* of temporal bone *(cont.)*
side view, 461, 557
at tonsil bed, 590
anomaly, 568
of ulna, 1, **52,** 90–94
supracondylar, of humerus, 47
transverse—
of atlas, 540.1, 552, 561, **563**
of coccyx, **222, 373**
of vertebra. See "Vertebra"
(uncinate), unciform, 608.1, **618.1,** 618.3
vaginal, of temporal bone, 557
vaginalis peritonei, 233
vermiform, 162, **169,** 170
in female, 235, 236
vocal, **629,** 632
xiphoid, 11, 393
zygomatic, of frontal bone, 459, **462,** 463
of temporal bone. See "Zygoma"
Prominence, laryngeal, **527,** 621, 623
Promontory of sacrum, **221,** 373
of tympanic cavity, 636, **637,** 646
Prostate, 197
from behind, 205, 207
from below, 193, **194**
on section, 203, 208
Protuberance—
mental, 460, 553
occipital; external [inion], 461, **485**
internal, 508
Pterion, 461
Pubis, 219, **222, 242**
muscle attachments, 216, **265, 276**
in youth, 277
Pupil, 522
Pylorus, **127,** 149, 153
interior of, 128, 168
Pyramid; of medulla, 506
renal, 183
of tympanic cavity, 636

Radius, 1, 2, 52
cross-sections, 104.1
lower end, 90–94
muscle attachments, 58, 77
upper end, 49–52
Ramus—
of ischium, 222
of mandible, 462, 557
of nerve. See "Nerve, rami"
of pubis, **222,** 284
Raphe—
of palate, 581
of pharynx, 626
pterygo-mandibular, **574, 575, 590**
Ray, medullary, 183
Recess. See also "Pouch & Sinus"—
apical of nasal cavity, 458
costo-diaphragmatic, pleural, 431, 455
costo-mediastinal, pleural, 431
duodenal, 163.1
epitympanic, **634,** 647
hepato-renal, 130.3, 147
ileocecal, 169
intersigmoid, 202
lateral, of fourth ventricle, 506
pharyngeal, **578, 579,** 587
phrenico-costal. See "R. costodiaphragmatic"
piriform, 578, 631

Recess (*cont.*)
  pleural—
    costodiaphragmatic, **126, 179,** 431, **455**
    costo-mediastinal, 431
  sacciform; of elbow, 54
    of wrist, 90
  of sigmoid mesocolon, 202 (see text)
  spheno-ethmoidal, 609, 610
  subphrenic, 130.3
  of tympanic membrane, 641
  upper. See under "Bursa, omental"
Rectum—
  arteries of, 195
  female—
    from above, 233
    median section, 236
    from perineum, 241
    piercing levator ani, 231
  male—
    from above, 202
    median section, 203
    from perineum, 194
    piercing levator ani, 209
    relations, anterior, 205
Region—
  anal, 192
  inguinal; female, 120–123
    male, 109–112
  nuchal, cross-section, 494
  parotid, 467, 550–552
  prevertebral, 561
  suboccipital, 490–493
    cross-section, 494
  suprahyoid, 546–549
  urogenital, 192
  Rete; carpal, dorsal, 78
  testis, 114
Retinaculum—
  extensor; of ankle, 306–309
    of wrist, 78, 81, **87**
  flexor; of ankle, 319–321
    of wrist, 61, **68,** 69, **72,** 90.1
  peroneal, 306, **308**
Ribs, 2, 11, 398, 399
  anomalies of, 400–402
  articulated, 391, 392, 410, 411
  eleventh, 174
  lumbar rib, 480
  morphology, 365
  twelfth, 173–175, 190, 191
Ridge. See also "Line"
  longitudinal, of stomach, 128
  supracondylar; of femur, 243
    of humerus, 1, 2, **51**
  Rima glottidis, 631
Ring; aortic, 447.1
  femoral, 254 (see text), **258**
  inguinal, deep, 111
    superficial, **108**–110, 120
Root—
  of lung, **415, 416,** 432, 450
  of nerve, **482,** 538, 564
  of tooth, 601, 601.1, 601.3, 602.1
  of vertebra. See "Pedicle"

S

Sac—
  conjunctival, 471.2
  dural, 483
  endolymphatic, 633, 650
  lacrimal, 471.1, **519**

Sac (*cont.*)
  lesser. See "Bursa, omental," **134, 135,**
    149, 176
    diagrams of, 130
    mouth of. See "Foramen, epiploic,"
      126
    pericardial. See "Pericardium"
Sacculation of colon, 162, 170
Saccule; of labyrinth of ear, 650, 650.1
  of larynx, 622, 628
Sacrum—
  base of, 219, 221
  dorsal aspect, 374
  lateral aspect, **222,** 363
  median section, 203, 236
  pelvic aspect, 364, 373
Scala; tympani, 650.1
  vestibuli, 650.1
Scalp—
  arteries & nerves of, 500
  dangerous area, 458, 498.1
Scapha (scaphoid fossa), 469
Scaphoid bone. See "Carpus"
Scapula, **1, 2,** 391, 392
  muscle attachments, 29, 30
  orientation, 38
Sclera, 522
Scrotum, schematic, 113
Sections—
  coronal sections—
    ankle joint, 334
    cavernous sinus, 515
    head, 554, **591**
    heel, 334
    hip joint, 282
    nasal cavity, 591
    orbital cavity, 516, 517, 592
    talo-calcanean joint, 334
    temporomandibular joint, 554
    tongue, 591
    uterus, 233.1
  cross-sections—
    abdomen, 178
    ankle joint, 333
    arm, 15, 34
    axilla, 22
    elbow joint, 55
    eyeball, 523.1
    femoral sheath, 281
    finger, 71.1
    forearm, 63
    hand, 65
    head, 579, 584
    hip joint, 281
    humerus, 104.1
    leg, 310
    liver, 160
    lumbar region, 481
    neck, 494, 535, 600
    parotid gland, 579, 584
    pelvis; female, 191.6
      male, 191.6
    radius and ulna, 104.1
    sacro-iliac joint, 223
    shoulder joint, 22
    testis, 114
    thigh, 264
    tongue, 591
    tonsil, 584
    wrist, 64
  median sections—

Sections, median sections (*cont.*)
  head, 458, 503
  neck, 458
  pelvis, male, 203, 204
    female, 236
  tongue, 595
  sagittal sections—
    broad ligament, 233.2
    eyelid, 471
    orbital cavity, 471.2
    temporomandibular joint, 555
Segments; broncho-pulmonary, 424–427
  hepatic, 137
  renal, 184
Septum—
  intermuscular; of arm, lateral, 57
    medial, 20, 46, **57**
    of leg, 310, 319–321
    of thigh, lateral, 271, 287, 296
  interventricular, 444, 445
  linguae, **592,** 595 (text)
  nasal, 458, 464 (text), **605**
  orbital (palpebral fascial), 470, 471.1
  peroneal [crural], 310, 320
  rectovaginal, 241
  rectovesical, 194, 203
  vesico-vaginal, 241
Sesamoid bones—
  of hallux, 311, **329,** 329.1, 329.2
  of hand, 65, 72 (not labelled)
  in gastrocnemius, 323
  in peroneus longus, 356
  in tibialis posterior, 356
Seamoid cartilages, nasal, 468
Sheath—
  axillary, 15
  carotid, **534,** (in text) 535, 579, **584,** 600
  of facial nerve, 641
  femoral, 253, **254,** 256, **281**
  fibrous digital; in foot, 325, 330
    in hand, 67, 69, **72**
    bony attachments, 62, **71.1**
  of optic nerve, 592
  of rectus abdominis, 105, 106
  synovial; diagram, 69.1
    of biceps brachii, 36
    in foot, 309
    in hand, 69, 86.1
Sinus—
  aortic, 445, 446.2
  carotid, nerve of, 659, 660
  cavernous, 515, 643
  coronary, 438, **440, 443,** 456
  of epididymis, 114, 116
  ethmoidal (cells), **610, 611, 612**
    from above, **520,** 614.1, 617
    scheme of, 614
  frontal, **609–615,** 617–**618.1**
  of larynx. See "Ventricle"
  mastoid. See "Air cells, mastoid"
  maxillary, 611, 611.1, 615–616.3
    accessory ostia, 613
    duct (ostium), 517, 610, 616.2
    medial wall, 615
    roots of teeth, 615, 616, **616.3**
  paranasal, 608.1–620.1
  pericardial; oblique; 440, 441
    transverse, 436, 441
  petrosal; inferior, 512, **543.3, 643**
    superior, 512, **643**
    phrenico-costal. See "Recess, pleural"

Sinus (*cont.*)

Sinus (*cont.*)
    pleural. See "Recess, pleural"
    prostatic, 208
    renal, 181.1, 183
    sagittal, 502–504
    sigmoid, **504,** 508, 512, **643**
    sphenoidal, **609–612,** 614.1, 619–620.1
    straight, 503
    tarsal, 336, 345 (see text)
    transverse, 504, **508**
    venous, in dura mater, 502–**504, 643**
    vertebral venous, 390, 493
Skull—
    from above, 498
    anterior view, 459, 460
    at birth, 602
    exterior of base, 569, 570
        lines, transverse, 571, 571.2
    interior of base, 507–512
    lateral view, 461, 462
    pole, posterior, 485
    posterior view, 485
    surface anatomy, 499
Slit, nasal, 508
"Snuff-box" 73–76, 79
Sole, 325–331
Space—
    cone of muscles, within, 471.2
    intercostal, 405–410
    lateral pharyngeal, **579, 639**
    palmar, **65,** 70 (see text)
    perineal; deep, 192 (see text)
        superficial, **201, 205, 228** (see text)
    popliteal. See "Fossa, popliteal"
    Prussak's, 641
    quadrangular of arm, 32, 33
    recto-vaginal, 241
    retropharyngeal, **458, 535, 584**
    retropubic, **203,** 205, 236, **241**
    subaponeurotic of scalp (dangerous
        area), 458, 498.1, 591
    subarachnoid, 203, 484, 522.1
    suprasternal, 458, **527**
    triangular of arm, 32
Sphenoid bone—
    of child, 619
    from above, 507–512
    from behind, 619.2
    from below, 569, 570
    from front, **463, 619.1**
    lateral side, 557, **558**
Sphincter. See "Muscle, sphincter"
Spine—
    angular. See "S., of sphenoid"
    iliac; anterior, 242
        posterior, 243, 480
    ischial, 222, **243,** 273
    mental (genial), 553.1
    "kissing," 379
    nasal—
        anterior, 460, 461
        of frontal bone, **464,** 605, **608**
        posterior, 569, **570,** 580
    of pterygoid, 608
    of scapula, 2, 25
    of sphenoid, 508, **558, 570**
        key position, 571.1
    suprameatal, 462, 499, **557**
    trochlear, 518
    of vertebra. See "Vertebra"
Spleen, **149–153,** 179

Spleen (*cont.*)
    accessory, 152
    arterial supply, 132, **135,** 153, **158**
Spondylolisthesis, 382, 383
Squama—
    of occipital bone, 486, 570
    of temporal bone, **462,** 557, 558, 645
Stapes, 633 (see text), 636, **638**
Sternebra, 393
Sternum, **11,** 391, **393–395**
    anomalies of, 396, 397
    relation to pericardium, 432
    relation to pleura, 413.2
Stomach, 125–129
    arteries of, 132
    bed of, 134, 135, **149**
    nerves of, 133
Substance, perforated, anterior, 506
Sulcus—See also "**Groove**"
    intertubercular (bicipital), 1
    chiasmatic (optic), 508, **512**
    coronary (Groove, atrio-ventricular),
        434, 435
    interventricular, 434, 435
    pre-auricular of ilium, 222
    sigmoid, **497,** 512
    terminalis; of heart, **433**
        of tongue, 578 594 (see text)
Sustentaculum tali, **311, 314,** 315, 344
Sutural (Wormian) bones, 485, **487,** 488
Suture—
    coronal (frontal), 462
    intermaxillary, 460
    internasal, 460
    lambdoid, 462, **485**
    metopic, 460, 602A
    occipito-mastoid, 485
    parieto-mastoid, 485
    petro-squamous, 510, 645.1
    sagittal, 485
Sympathetic. See "Trunk, & Ganglion"
Symphysis—
    menti, 460
    pubis, 109, 203, 209
    sterno-manubrial, 404
Synchondrosis—
    of first costal cartilage, 393 (see text)
    neurocentral, 359, 360
    spheno-occipital, 511
Synergist (muscle), 86.3
Synostosis, sacro-iliac, 223.1
    of vertebrae, 377
Synovial fold. See "Pad of fat"
    sheath, 69.1
System; digestive, diagram of, 124

Taenia [Tenia] coli, **162,** 164, 169
Talus, **311–315,** 333–337, **344,** 345
Tarsus, of eyelid, 470
Teeth, 580, 601–604
    maxillary sinus, 615, 616, 616.3
    nerve supply, 654, 655
    permanent, 601–601.5
        erupting, 603, 604
    primary, 602.1, 602.2
Tegmen tympani, 558, 569, **633.1,** 640
Tela choroidea, 506
Temporal bone—
    in child, 645–647
    from below, 570
    lateral view, 461, 462

Temporal bone (*cont.*)
    from within, 510, 512
Tendo calcaneus (Achillis), **304,** 308, 316–
        320
Tendon, central of perineum (perineal
        body), 229
    conjoint [Falix inguinalis], 110–112
        female, 123
Tenia coli (Taenia), **162,** 164, 169
Tentorium cerebelli, **503,** 504, **514,** 572
Testis, 116–119, 203
    cross-section, 114
Thigh, cross-section;
    hip joint level, 281
    above middle, 264
Thorax, bony, 391, 392
Thymus, **448,** 458, 528
Thyroid. See "Cartilage" and "Gland"
Tibia, 294, 310, **315**
    muscle attachments, **265,** 288, 295–298,
        303, 316
Tissue, adipose. See "Fat"
    extraperitoneal [subperitoneal], 190, 205
Tongue—
    dorsum, 594
    muscles; extrinsic, 596.1
        intrinsic, 592
    nerve distribution, 593
    posterior third of, 578, 587
    side of, 548
    sections, 591, 595
Tonsil—
    lingual, 587 (see text)
    pharyngeal (nasopharyngeal), 579, 587
    palatine, 576, **585,** 587
        bed, 588–590
        blood supply, 586
        cross-section, 584
        sensory nerves, 659
Torus of auditory tube, 587
Trabeculae; carneae, 444, 445
    septomarginal, 444, 445.1
Trachea—
    arterial supply, 454
    in neck; 621, 623, 624
        interior of, 632
        relations of, 529–532, 534, 536
    in superior mediastinum;
        cross-section, 430
        front view, 448–452
        right side, 428
Tract—
    iliotibial, **258–260,** 264, **267–269**
        insertion, 295, 296
        at knee, 294, 299, 301
    olfactory, 506
    optic, 506
Tragus, 469
Trapezium bone. See "Carpus"
Trapezoid bone. See "Carpus"
Triangle and **Trigone**—
    anal, 192.1
    of auscultation, 24
    of bladder, 208, 234
    carotid, 540, 541, 542
    deltopectoral, 13
    digastric. See "Tr. submandibular"
    femoral (of Scarpa), 258, 259
    lumbar, 24, 173 (see text), 478
    of neck; anterior, 541, 542
        posterior, 472–476

Triangle and **Trigone** (*cont.*)
  submandibular (digastric), 540, 541, 542
  submental, 527, **540**
  suboccipital, 491, 492 (see text)
  urogenital; female, 224–230
    male, 192.1
  vertebro-costal (lumbocostal), 190, 191
Triquetrum. See "Carpus"
Trochanter; greater, **242, 243,** 270–276
  lesser, **242, 243,** 272–276
Trochlea—
  of humerus, 1, 51, **55**
  of orbit, 519, 521
  peroneal, 312
  of talus, 311–313
    definition, 312
Truncus arteriosus, 446.3
Trunk—
  of brachial plexus, 476
  brachio-cephalic (innominate art.), 432–435, 448–450, **452,** 531, **536**
  broncho-mediastinal (Lymph), 453
  celiac (artery), 132.1, 133.1, 179, 188
  costo-cervical, 452, 536A, **561**
  jugular (Lymph), **453,** 533 (see text)
  lumbo-sacral, 190, 213 (see text)
  pulmonary (artery), 433, 434, 436
  subclavian (Lymph), **453,** 533 (see text)
  sympathetic—
    in abdomen, 178–179, **190, 191**.3
    in neck, 531, **534,** 537, **561,** 573
    in pelvis, 213
    in thorax, 410, **428,** 429
  thyro-cervical, 536A, 561
  vagal, 133, (149), 179, **180**
Tube—
  auditory; medial view, **639**
    lateral view, 576, **577**
    orifice (mouth), tympanic, **639,** 641
      pharyngeal, **587,** 588, 609, **639**
    isthmus, **639,** 641
    bony part, **569,** 571.1
    cross-section, 554
    schemes, 633–633.2
  pharyngo-tympanic. See "Tube auditory"
  uterine (Fallopian), 232, 233, 236
Tuber, Tubercle, Tuberosity—
  accessory, of 12th thoracic, 369
  adductor, 242, 243
  articular, of sacrum, 374
    of temporal bone, 558, 569
  of atlas; anterior, 367, **561**–563
    posterior, 563
  of auricle (Darwin's), 469
  bicipital, of radius, 1, **51,** 52
  of calcaneum; anterior, 314, **342**
    lateral and medial, 315
    tuber, 313
  carotid, 367, 561
  corniculate, 627, 632
  of cricoid, 622, 623
  cuneiform, 627, 632
  deltoid, 1, 2
  of epiglottis, 631
  frontal, 459, 462
  genial. See "Spine, mental"
  gluteal, 243
  of humerus, 1, 2, 26
  of iliac crest, 242, 243
  intercondylar, of tibia, 294
  of ischium, 222, **243,** 273

Tuber, Tubercle, Tuberosity (*cont.*)
  jugular, 508, **512, 564**
  lateral, of 12th thoracic, 369
  of Lister, 94
  mammillary. See "Process"
  of maxilla, 558, 619.2
  mental, 460, 553
  of metacarpal V, 62
  of metatarsal V, 312, 313
  of navicular bone, **311,** 313, 314
  omentale of liver, 136, 147
  of palatine bone. See "Process, pyramidal"
  parietal, 462, 602
  peroneal. See "Trochlea, peroneal"
  pharyngeal, 569
  postglenoid, 462, 557
  pterygoid, **569,** 580, 608
  pubic, 109, 219, 242, 274
  radial (bicipital), 1, **51,** 52
    dorsal (of Lister), 2, **94**
  of rib, **398,** 411
  of sacrum, 222
  scalene (Lisfranc), 399
  of scaphoid, 62, 66, 72, **95**
  sellae, 508, 512
  for serratus anterior, 399
  spinous, of sacrum, 374
  of talus, 313, 315
  of thyroid cartilage, 621, 623
  tibial, 242
    intercondylar, 294
  for transverse lig. of atlas, 367, **563**
  on transverse process, 366
  transverse, of sacrum, 374
  of trapezium (crest), 62, **95**
  of ulna, 51, 52
  of vertebra; anterior, 367, 368
    posterior, 367, 368
  of zygoma, 462, **557**
Tubules, seminiferous, 114
Tunica vaginalis testis, 114, 116, 119
Tunnel—
  for lumbricals (gutter), 70
  osseo-fibrous; of foot, 322
    of hand, 69, 72 (see text)
  tarsal (sinus), 336, 345 (see text)
Turbinate bone. See "Concha"
Tympanic bone, 461, 557, 558
  in child, **645,** 646, 647
Tympanum, 633–637, 640–641

Ulna, **1, 2, 52**
  cross-sections, 104.1
  lower end, 90–94
  muscle attachments, 58, 77
  upper end, 49–51
Umbilicus, 107
Uncus, 506
Urachus, 205, **233**
Ureter—
  parts of, 182, 104.2
  in abdomen, **148** (text), **165, 179,** 191.3
  anomalies of, 186, 187
  arteries, 189
  in female pelvis, 233–**235, 238**
  in male pelvis, **202,** 207–208.1, **210**
Urethra—
  female, 232.1, 236
    external orifice of, 227, 228
  male;

Urethra; male (*cont.*)
  parts, 182, 197
  interior, 199.1, 208
  section; cross, 200, 201
    median, 203
  nerve supply, 214
Uterus, 232–236
  retroverted, 238
  suspensory mechanism, 241
  masculinus. See "Utricle, prostatic"
Utricle; of ear, 650
  prostatic, 203, 208 (unlabelled)
Uvula of palate, 578, 581

Vagina, 232.1, **234, 236,** 241
  orifice of, 227, 230
  section; cross, **196.1,** 231, 241
    median, 236
  vestibule of, 225
Vaginae synoviales. See "Sheath, synovial"
Vallecula, epiglottic, 599
Valve—
  anal, 196.1, 203
  of heart:
    aortic, **436, 445, 446**–446.3
    atrio-ventricular, 444–446
    of coronary sinus, 443
    mitral [l. atrioventricular], 445
    of pulmonary trunk, 436, 444, 446.3
    semilunar. See "V., aortic and of pulmonary trunk"
    tricuspid [r. atrioventricular], 444, 446
    of vena cava inferior, 443
  spiral (fold) in cystic duct, 156
  of veins—
    axillary, 21
    femoral, 255, 281
    great (long) saphenous, 225
    internal jugular, 543.3
    subclavian, 21, 543.3
Variations. See "Anomalies"
Vas deferens [Ductus], 115, **210**
  near bladder, 205–**207**
  at pelvic brim, **202,** 216
  near testis, 114, 118
Vasa recta, intestinal, **162,** 166, 167

VEINS AND VENAE—
  for veins synonymous with arteries, see "Arteries"
  auricular, posterior, **467,** 471.3
  of axilla, 21
  axillary, 21
  azygos, **428,** 453, **455**
    arch of, **428,** 450–452
    anomaly, 457
  basilic, **4–6, 21,** 44, 80
  basi-vertebral, 386, **390**
  brachiocephalic (innominate), **449, 453,** 455, 536
    on side view, 428, 429
  cardiac, **433, 438, 440**
  cava inferior—
    anomalies, 185–186
    in abdomen, 148, 179, 191.3
    on cross-section, 178, 431
    at liver, **136,** 139
    within pericardial sac, 440–443
    peritoneal relations, 177
    pleural aspect, 428
    tributaries, **188.2**

Veins and Venae (*cont.*)

VEINS AND VENAE (*cont.*)
   cava superior, **433,** 441, **449,** 455
      right side, 428
         on section, 436, 440
         surface anatomy, 432
   cephalic, **4–6,** 13–16, 44
   cerebral, great, 504
   cervical; deep, 491–493
      transverse, **471.3** (472), **542**
   circumflex femoral, 257
      iliac, superficial, 245, **252,** 257
   of clitoris, 228
   colic, 135
   comitans of nerve XII, 545
   condylar emissary, 493
   cubital, 4, **44**
   cystic, 146, 146.1
   digital, 5, 6
   diploic, 501
   epigastric, inferior, 106, 112
      superficial, 105, 252
   facial—
      (anterior) facial, **466,** 467, **541,** 543
      common facial, 541, 543
      retromandibular (post. facial), **471.3,**
         541
   femoral, 254–257
      valves, 255, 281
   foot, dorsum of, 245–247
   of gall-bladder, 146, 146.1
   gastrocolic, 135
   hand, superficial, 5, **6,** 73
   hemi-azygos, **455**
   hepatic, 137.1, **139, 179, 188.2**
   inguinal, superficial, **105,** 245, 252, 257
   innominate. See "V. brachiocephalic"
      front view, **449, 453,** 455, 536
      side view, 428, 429
   intercostal; posterior, 455
      superior, 428, **429,** 430, **455,** 456
   jugular—
      anterior, **21,** 543, 566
      external, 467, **472,** 543
      internal, 529–531, 533, 534
         and accessory nerve, 566
         in carotid triangle, 541, 542
         and inf. root of ansa, 566.2
         diagram of, 543.3
         deep to parotid region, **552, 577**
         seen from post. triangle, 473, **475**
         below tympanum, 640
   of limb, superficial—
      lower, 105, 245–247
      upper, 4, 5, 6, 44
   lingual, 543.3
   lumbar, ascending, **188.3,** 390
   mastoid emissary, 491–493
   maxillary (internal), 543
   median cubital, 4, **44**

VEINS AND VENAE (*cont.*)
   mesenteric, inferior, 132.2, **135,** 165
      superior, **135,** 153 (see text)
   of neck;
      connecting, **527,** 543, **566**
      deep, 543.3
      superficial, 543
   oblique, of left atrium, 440, 456
   obturator, abnormal, 210, 212
   occipital, **471.3,** 491–**493,** 543.3
   ophthalmic, 504
   palatine, 582
   paratonsillar, 588, 589 (see text)
   of pelvis, female, 234, **238**
      male, 210
   of penis, 199–201
   pharyngeal, 543.3, 589 (not labelled)
   portal, **135,** 142, 146, **148,** 153
      diagram, 132.2
      intrahepatic course, 138
   porta-caval, 160.1
   profunda cervicis. See "V., cervical, deep"
      femoris, **257,** 259
   prostatic, 208
   pudendal, external, 245, **252**
   pulmonary, 428, 429, **434, 435**
      in lung, 415, 416, 418, 421
      in pericardium, 440, 441
   renal, 135, 151, **179, 188.2,** 455
   retromandibular, 471.3, 541
   saphenous—
      great (long), 245
         near ankle, 321
         at knee, 263
         upper end, 251–258
      small (short), **246,** 247, **285**
   scapular, transverse. See "V., suprascapu-
      lar"
   splenic, 132.2, **135, 149,** 151
   superficial—
      hand, 5, 6
      lower limb, 245–247
      upper limb, 4–6, 44
   supra-orbital, **466,** 543
   suprascapular, **21,** 474, **475,** 543
   supratrochlear, 543
   temporal, superficial, 543
   testicular, **114,** 165, **179,** 188.2
   thyroid—
      inferior, 528, **529,** 534
      middle, **529,** 543.3
      superior, 529, 530, **534, 541**
   transverse scapular. See "V., suprascapu-
      lar"
   uterine, 234
   vertebral, plexus, 390, 493, **600**
   vesical, 208, 234
Venae comitantes—
   of brachial artery, 21

Venae comitantes (*cont.*)
   of femoral artery, 257
   of hypoglossal nerve, 545
Ventricle—
   of brain, 495, 609
   of heart; exterior, of, 433–435, 440
      interior of left ventricle, 445
      interior of right ventricle, 444
   of larynx (sinus), 629, 631, **632**
Vertebra, 357–383, 392
   anomalies, 375–383, 489
   articulated, 363, 384–389, 538
   cervical, 367, 368, 563
   homologies, 365
   lumbar, 371, 372
   as a measuring rod, 104.2
   movements, 366
   sacrum and coccyx, 373, 374
   thoracic, 369, 370
   typical, 357, 358
Vertex, 460
Vesicle, seminal, 197, 205–207
Vessels. See "Artery, Vein, Lymphatic"
Vestibule—
   bulb of (in female), 228
   of bony labyrinth, 633, **649,** 650.1
   of larynx, 631.1
   of mouth, 591
   of nose, 609
   of vagina, 225, 229
Vincula tendinum, 88
Vomer, 460, 570, 580, **605**

W_{all—}
abdominal, anterior, 105–**112**
      female, 120–123
      posterior, 24, 173–175, **190**
         structures on, 165, 177, **179**
   pelvic, 210, 213, 216, 217
   thoracic, 405–411
Wing of sphenoid. See also "Sphenoid
   bone"
   greater, 462, 507, 518
   lesser, 507, 512, 518
Wormian bones. See "Sutural bones"
Wrist—
   dorsal aspect, 77–79, 86–87
   palmar aspect, 59–62.1, **66–72**
   radial aspect, 73–76
   ulnar border, 80–82

X_{iphoid.} See "Process xiphoid"

Z_{one,} orbicular, **275,** 282
Zygoma, 462, 466, **557**
Zygomatic bone, 461, **557**
   bipartite, 557.1

Bruce R. Webber

Bruce R. Webber